Atlas of Hip Surgery

Edited by
R. Bauer, F. Kerschbaumer, and S. Poisel

with contributions by

R. Bauer
F. Kerschbaumer
E. Nieder
S. Poisel
H. Wagner
M. Wagner

494 illustrations by G. Spitzer, S. Cull, R. Henkel, and S. Spitzer

1996
Georg Thieme Verlag Stuttgart · New York
Thieme Medical Publishers Inc., New York

Library of Congress Cataloguing-in-Publication Data

Atlas of Hip Surgery / ed. by R. Bauer . . . With contributions by R. Bauer . . . Ill. by G. Spitzer . . . – Stuttgart ; New York : Thieme ; New York : Thieme Med. Publ., 1996
Einheitssacht.: Orthopädische Operationslehre <engl.>
NE: Bauer, Rudolf [Hrsg.]; Spitzer, Gerhard [Ill.]; EST

Translated by John Grossman, M.A.

This book is an authorized and revised translation of the German edition published and copyrighted 1994 by Georg Thieme Verlag, Stuttgart, Germany.
Title of the German edition:
Orthopädische Operationslehre, Band II/1: Becken und untere Extremität

Typesetting by Druckhaus Götz GmbH,
D-71636 Ludwigsburg
Printed in Germany by K. Grammlich GmbH
D-72124 Pliezhausen

ISBN 3-13-102461-5 (GTV, Stuttgart)
ISBN 0-86577-601-6 (TMP, New York) 1 2 3 4 5 6

Addresses

Bauer, R., Prof. Dr.
Head, Orthopädische Universitätsklinik,
Anichstr. 35, 6020 Innsbruck, Austria

Kerschbaumer, F., Prof. Dr.
Head, Abteilung für Rheumaorthopädie,
Orthopädische Universitätsklinik,
Marienburgstr. 2, 60528 Frankfurt, Germany

Nieder, E., Dr.
Endoklinik,
Holstenstr. 2, 22767 Hamburg, Germany

Poisel, S., Prof. Dr.
Institut für Anatomie der Universität,
Müllerstr. 59, 6010 Innsbruck, Austria

Wagner, H., Prof. Dr.
Head, Orthopädische Klinik Wichernhaus,
90592 Schwarzenbruck/Nürnberg, Germany

Wagner, M., Dr.
Orthopädische Klinik Wichernhaus,
90592 Schwarzenbruck/Nürnberg, Germany

Preface

Our first atlas, *Operative Approaches in Orthopedic Surgery and Traumatology,* was rewarded with high sales in its many editions (German, English, French, Italian, Japanese, and Spanish) for its novel presentation of surgical procedures. Following the same concept—namely, color illustrations with concise accompanying text—we then published the three German volumes on orthopedic operations: *Spine; Pelvis and Lower Extremities;* and *Shoulder and Upper Extremities.*

The basis for this atlas is, in addition to the operative experience of the authors, the anatomic substrate. We have also taken all the major approaches for the discussed operations from the *Atlas of Operative Approaches in Orthopedic Surgery and Traumatology* and compiled them in the introductory chapter. In the following chapters, the most tried-and-true techniques and standard operative procedures are presented step by step, including the indications, pitfalls, and complications.

Taking the international market into consideration, we have divided the contents of the entire work in accord with nosological and topographical specialization into individual volumes covering the spine, hip, knee, tumor surgery and amputations, pediatric orthopedics, and upper extremities, the first two of which are now published. In this way, the specialist has the possibility of purchasing individual volumes dealing with his or her particular field of interest.

We would like to thank the authors, without whose contributions this atlas would not have been possible. Then we would like to extend our thanks to Dr. G. Hauff, Mr. A. Menge, and the staff at Thieme for their cooperation and the high quality of their work. We are grateful to the graphic artists, Ms. S. Cull, Mr. R. Henkel, Prof. G. Spitzer, and S. Spitzer who transformed their sketches from the operating theater and dissection table into excellent illustrations. The dissection of cadavers was done at the Institute for Anatomy of the University of Innsbruck, Austria, for which our thanks go to Prof. W. Platzer.

Autumn 1995

R. Bauer, Innsbruck
F. Kerschbaumer, Frankfurt
S. Poisel, Innsbruck

Contents

1 Approaches

R. Bauer
F. Kerschbaumer
S. Poisel

Pelvis

Posterior Approach to the Hip Joint

Primary Indications

- Arthroplasty
- Acetabular fractures and fractures of the posterior column of the pelvis
- Tumors

Positioning and Incision

The patient is usually placed in a lateral position for arthroplasty.

The patient may also be positioned prone for internal fixation of a fracture of the posterior column of the pelvis.

In the lateral position, anterior and posterior supports are required to stabilize the trunk and pelvis. The leg is draped to permit free movement. The curved incision begins approximately two finger widths below the posterior superior iliac spine, coursing distally across the greater trochanter (Fig. 1.**1**).

After dividing the subcutaneous tissues, the surgeon splits the fascia lata. This incision is then extended proximally, parallel to the fibers of the gluteus maximus. The surgeon must now maximally internally rotate the leg to avoid damaging the sciatic nerve when the short external rotators are cut. The short rotators should be cut one finger width medially of their insertion (see Fig. 1.**2**), to permit them to be reattached later.

The detached external rotators are retracted posteriorly and protected with a blunt retractor.

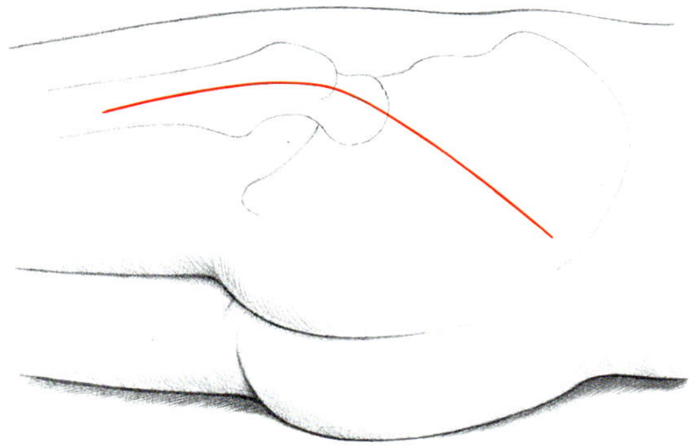

Fig. 1.**1** The posterior approach to the hip joint. Positioning and incision.

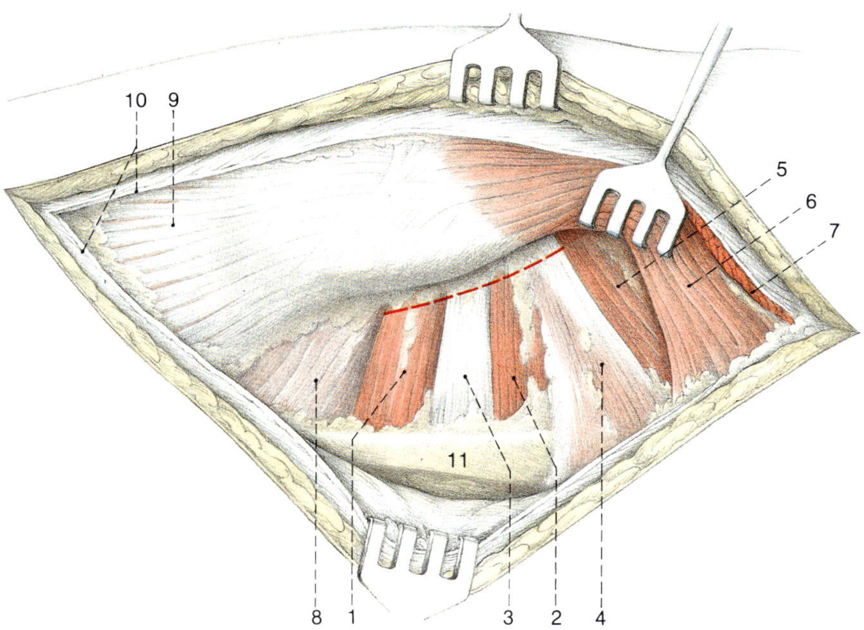

Fig. 1.**2** With the leg in internal rotation, the short external rotators and the piriformis are tenotomized.

1 Gemellus inferior
2 Gemellus superior
3 Obturator internus
4 Piriformis
5 Gluteus minimus
6 Gluteus medius
7 Gluteus maximus
8 Quadratus femoris
9 Vastus lateralis
10 Fascia lata
11 Sciatic nerve

Exposure of the Hip Joint

The gluteus medius and gluteus minimus muscles are retracted anteriorly. A "T" incision is made to open the joint capsule (Fig. 1.**3**). Two curved Hohmann retractors can be inserted around the femoral neck to expose it more completely. If broad exposure of the acetabulum is required, as in total hip arthroplasty, the greater trochanter can be osteotomized (Fig. 1.**4**). Before performing the osteotomy, the surgeon should insert a sound beneath the gluteal musculature to gauge thr proper plane of osteotomy. To avoid damaging the blood supply to the femoral head, the osteotomy should not be made too low on the femur. Alternatively, the surgeon may employ a gable-shaped osteotomy using two osteotomes.

After the osteotomy of the greater trochanter is completed, the greater trochanter with the attached gluteal musculature is retracted proximally, and a sharp Hohmann retractor is impacted into the ilium (Fig. 1.**5**). This permits increased exposure of the acetabulum and the femoral head. If the hip must be dislocated, this is done with the leg flexed and adducted in internal rotation.

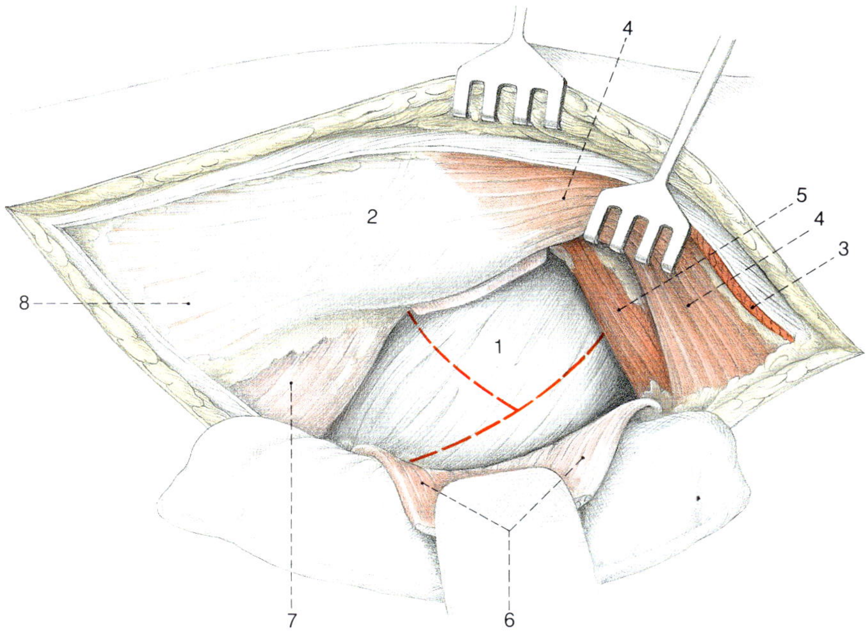

Fig. 1.**3** With the short external rotators retracted, the capsule of the hip joint is opened with a "T" incision.

1 Hip joint capsule
2 Greater trochanter
3 Gluteus maximus
4 Gluteus medius
5 Gluteus minimus
6 Piriformis, gemelli, obturator internus, and obturator externus.
7 Quadratus femoris
8 Vastus lateralis

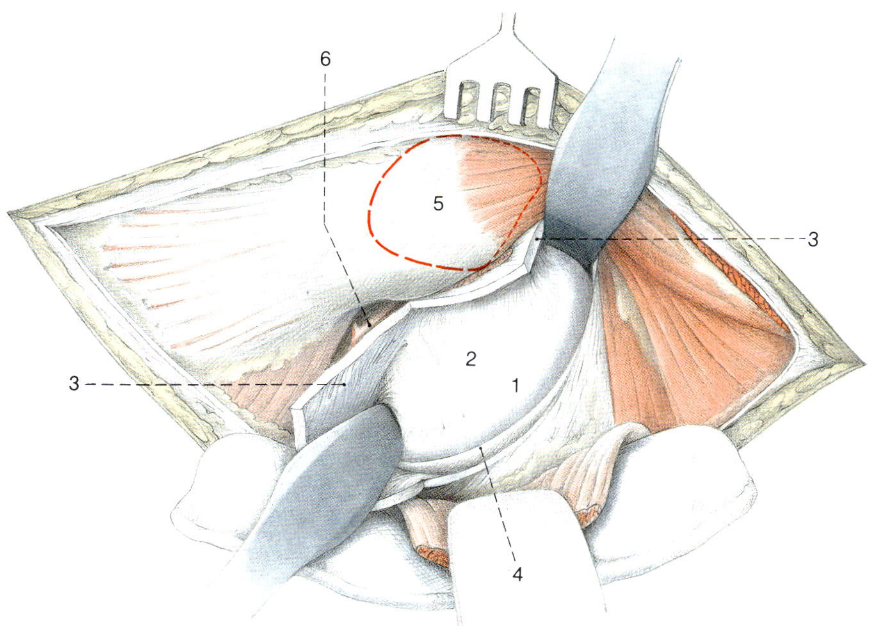

Fig. 1.**4** With the hip joint open, the femoral neck can be more completely exposed by inserting two curved Hohmann retractors around it. If necessary, the greater trochanter can be osteotomized (dotted line).

1 Femoral head
2 Femoral neck
3 Joint capsule
4 Acetabular labrum
5 Greater trochanter
6 Deep branch of the medial femoral circumflex artery

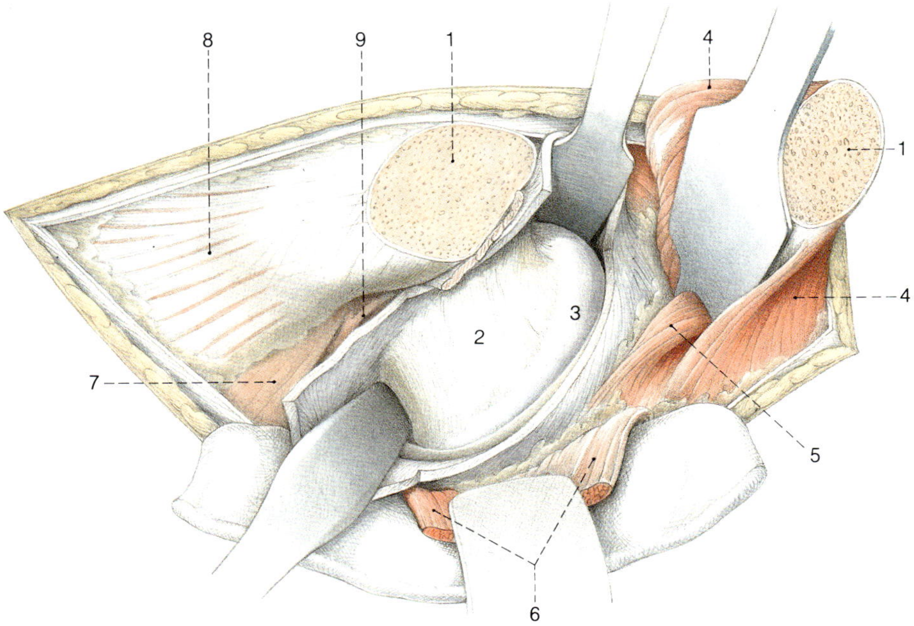

Fig. 1.**5** Hip joint following osteotomy of the greater trochanter. The gluteal musculature with the attached trochanter is retracted proximally and a sharp Hohmann retractor is impacted into the ilium.

1 Cut surface of the greater trochanter
2 Femoral neck
3 Femoral head
4 Gluteus medius
5 Gluteus minimus
6 Piriform muscle, gemellus muscles, and interal obdurator
7 Quadratus femoris
8 Vastus lateralis
9 Deep branch of the medial femoral circumflex artery

Exposure of the Posterior Column of the Pelvis

If the posterior column of the pelvis is to be exposed, the incision in the gluteus maximus may have to be extended proximally (Fig. 1.**6**). If this is the case, osteotomy of the greater trochanter is unnecessary. A Cobb elevator is used to retract the short external rotators posteriorly. A curved periosteal elevator is used to expose the greater sciatic notch; here, a curved Hohmann retractor may be carefully used. Care should be taken to avoid placing too much tension on the retractor, as this may damage the sciatic nerve.

If further exposure of the posterior column of the pelvis to the ischium is required, the skin incision may be extended distally, and the tendinous attachment of the gluteus maximus to the femur may be incised. This allows the surgeon to retract the short external rotators posteriorly, permitting exposure of the ischium as far as the ischial tuberosity. If increased exposure of the proximal ilium is required (as with acetabular or pelvic fractures), the surgeon can subperiosteally dissect the gluteal musculature after osteotomy of the greater trochanter, exposing the ilium as far as the anterior inferior iliac spine.

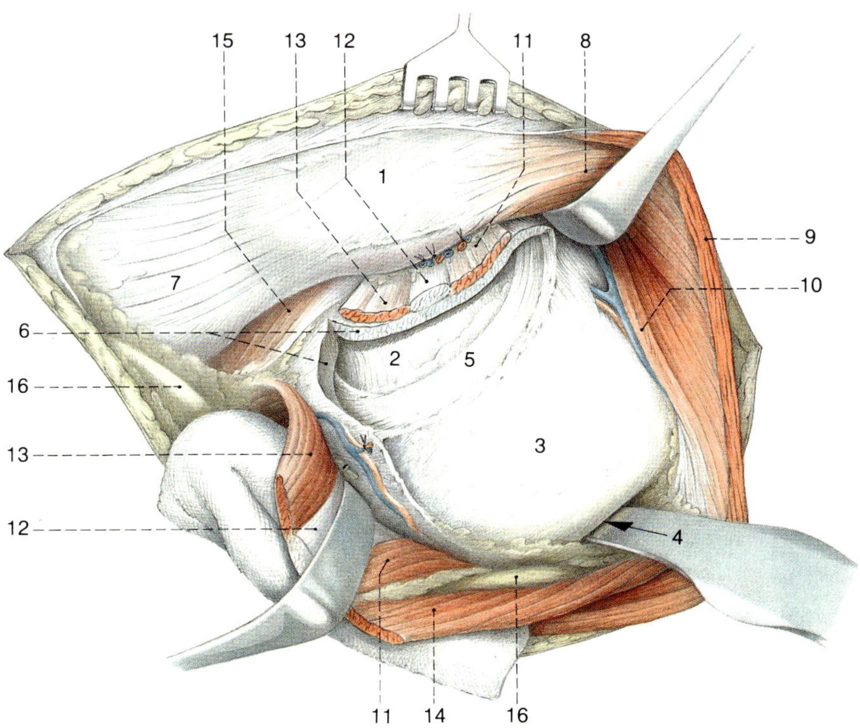

Fig. 1.**6** Exposure of the posterior column of the pelvis and the greater sciatic notch after extending the incision proximally and distally.

1 Greater trochanter
2 Femoral neck
3 Body of the ischium
4 Greater sciatic notch
5 Acetabular labrum
6 Hip joint capsule
7 Vastus lateralis
8 Gluteus medius
9 Gluteus maximus
10 Gluteus minimus
11 Gemellus superior
12 Obturator internus
13 Gemellus inferior
14 Piriformis
15 Quadratus femoris
16 Sciatic nerve

Anatomical Site

In Figure 1.**7**, the gluteus maximus has been divided perpendicular to the direction of the fibers, exposing the blood vessels and nerves that supply it. The fatty tissue surrounding the sciatic nerve has been removed. The sciatic nerve generally extends distally between the piriformis and the gemellus superior, but it can also penetrate the piriformis. Note the course of the medial femoral circumflex artery and its position with respect to the short external rotators.

Closure

The wound is closed by suturing the fascia lata and the fibers of the gluteus maximus. When a trochanteric osteotomy has been performed, the greater trochanter must first be reattached and secured by wire in two planes. Normally it is not necessary to reattach the short rotators.

Hazards

In revision surgery, the sciatic nerve may be obscured by scar tissue. Exposure of the nerve is recommended in such cases. The superior gluteal vessels can be damaged when the greater sciatic notch is exposed. If the anatomic joint is to be preserved, the surgeon should take care to avoid damaging the branch of the medial femoral circumflex artery that supplies the femoral head (Figs. 1.**4** and 1.**5**).

Note

Posterior approaches to the hip joint have been described as "posterolateral approaches" by Gibson, Marcy, and Fletcher, and by Moore and others.

Posterior approaches with the patient prone have been described by Kocher, by Langenbeck, and by Henry, and others.

There are no major differences in the approaches, although details such as the exposure of the acetabulum and direction of dislocation of the hip vary.

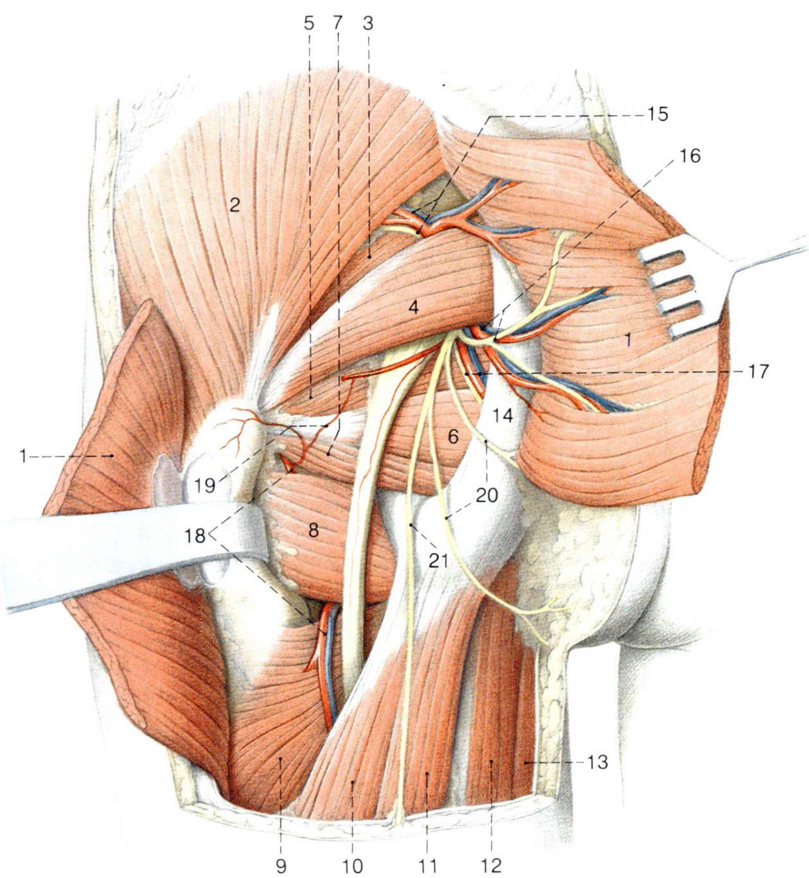

Fig. 1.**7** Anatomical site. The gluteus maximus has been split transversely (left).

1 Gluteus maximus
2 Gluteus medius
3 Gluteus minimus
4 Piriformis
5 Gemellus superior
6 Obturator internus
7 Gemellus inferior
8 Quadratus femoris
9 Adductor minimus
10 Long head of the biceps femoris
11 Semitendinosus
12 Adductor magnus
13 Gracilis
14 Sacrotuberous ligament
15 Superior gluteal artery and vein, superior gluteal nerve
16 Inferior gluteal artery and vein, inferior gluteal nerve
17 Internal pudendal vessels and pudendal nerve
18 Medial femoral circumflex artery
19 Anastomosis to the inferior gluteal artery
20 Inferior clunial nerves
21 Posterior femoral cutaneous nerve

Bauer Transgluteal Approach

Primary Indications

- Total hip arthroplasty
- Fractures of the femoral neck
- Osteotomy of the femoral neck
- Treatment of slipped capital femoral epiphysis
- Synovectomy of the hip joint

Positioning and Incision

The patient is positioned supine with a cushion beneath the buttocks. The skin incision extends about 15 cm in a slight curve, and is centered over the greater trochanter. The incision begins approximately one hand width posterior to the anterior superior iliac spine, coursing distally across the greater trochanter (Fig. 1.**8**). After dividing the subcutaneous tissue and the fascia lata parallel to the skin incision, the surgeon splits the anterior third of the gluteus medius, the gluteus minimus, and the vastus lateralis parallel to the direction of their fibers (Fig. 1.**9**). Electrocautery is used to subperiosteally dissect the tendinous and periosteal tissues between the gluteus medius and the vastus lateralis of the bone in a single layer.

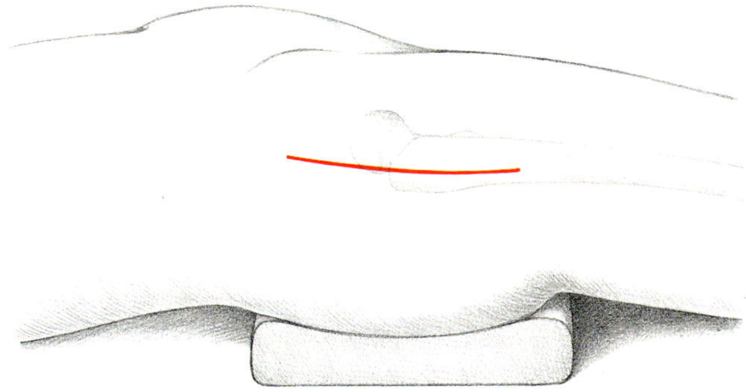

Fig. 1.**8** The transgluteal approach to the hip joint. Positioning and incision.

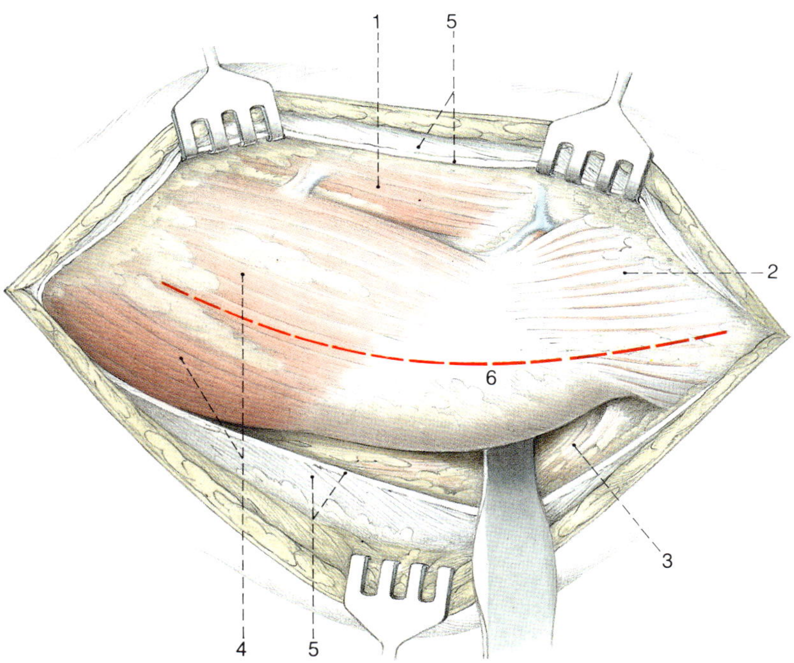

Fig. 1.**9** The transgluteal approach to the hip joint. The gluteaus medius and the vastus lateralis are incised at the boundary between the lateral and anterior thirds of the muscle (right leg is shown).

1 Tensor fasciae latae
2 Vastus lateralis
3 Gluteus maximus
4 Gluteus medius
5 Fascia lata
6 Greater trochanter

Exposure of the Hip Joint Capsule

Using a Cobb elevator, the surgeon exposes the anterior capsule. A curved Hohmann retractor is inserted between the origin of the rectus and the anterior wall of the acetabulum. On the cranial side, a Hohmann retractor is placed between the joint capsule and the gluteus medius, and an additional one is placed further distally between the iliopsoas and the joint capsule. If necessary, a second anterior Hohmann retractor may be inserted distal to the large curved retractor. The capsule is opened with a broad "T" incision made close to the acetabulum (Fig. 1.**10**). After the capsule has been opened, two Hohmann retractors may be inserted between the capsule and the femoral neck. This procedure does not endanger the blood supply to the femoral neck (Fig. 1.**11**).

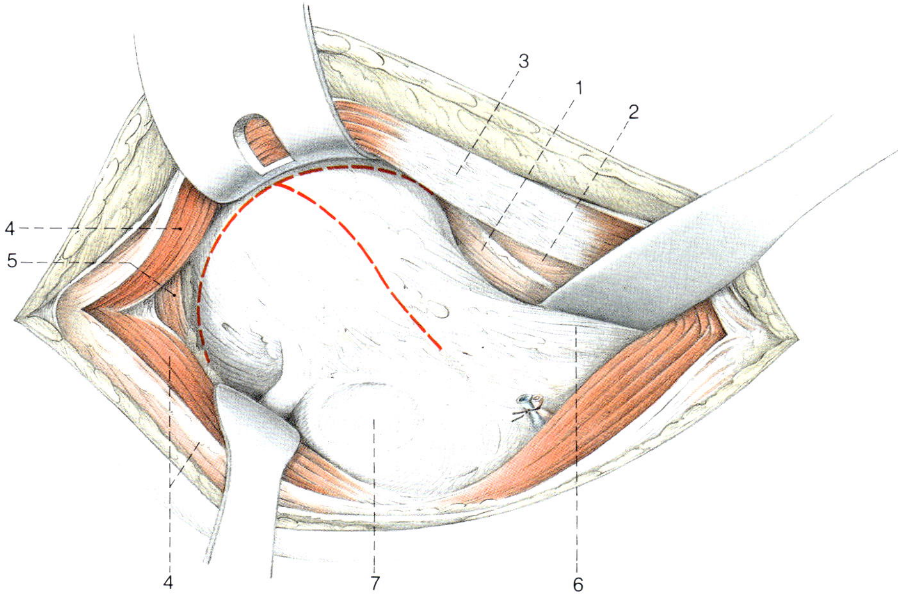

Fig. 1.**10** The muscle layer consisting of the gluteus medius and minimus, the tendinous and periosteal tissues at the greater trochanter, and the vastus lateralis is retracted toward the anterior. After the capsule of the hip joint is exposed, Hohmann retractors are inserted. The capsule is opened with a "T" incision.

1 Iliopsoas
2 Vastus intermedius
3 Vastus lateralis
4 Gluteus medius
5 Gluteus minimus
6 Iliofemoral ligament
7 Gluteus minimus bursa

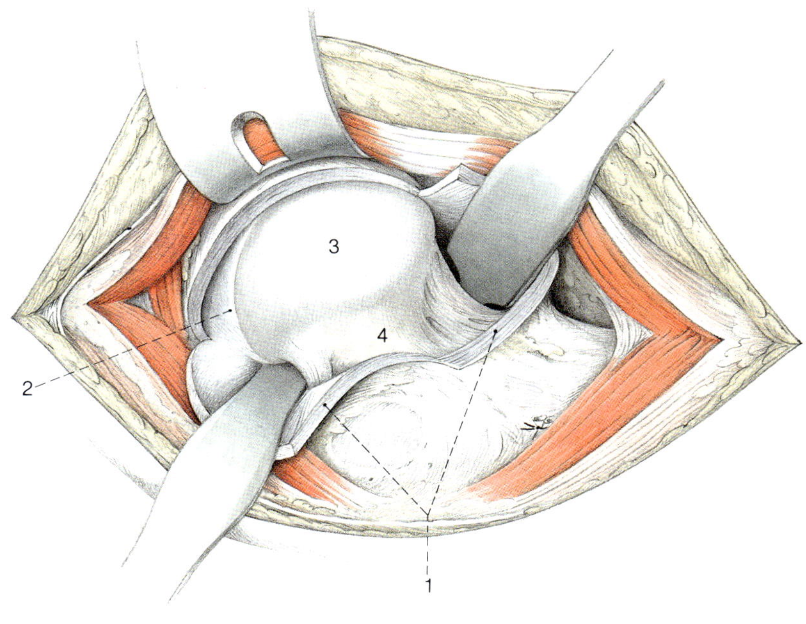

Fig. 1.**11** Hip joint after opening the capsule. Hohmann retractors have been placed behind the femoral neck with the leg adducted in maximum external rotation.

1 Joint capsule
2 Acetabular labrum
3 Femoral head
4 Femoral neck

Anatomical Site

As can be seen in Figure 1.**12**, the advantage of the transgluteal approach is that the gluteus minimus with its broad layer of muscle tissue protects the superior gluteal nerve from being pinched by the retractors. The separation of the gluteus medius from the iliac crest and the greater trochanter improves the exposure of the superior gluteal nerve. Further advantages of this approach are the broader exposure of the femoral neck, the proximal part of the hip joint capsule, and the femoral neck osteotomy plane when implanting a total hip.

Closure

The wound is closed by suturing the muscles that have been split parallel to the direction of their fibers (gluteus medius, gluteus minimus, and vastus lateralis; Fig. 1.**13**). The fascial and periosteal layers above the greater trochanter are securely sutured.

Note

The authors routinely use the transgluteal approach in total hip arthroplasty. Osteotomy of the greater trochanter is rarely necessary when using this approach.

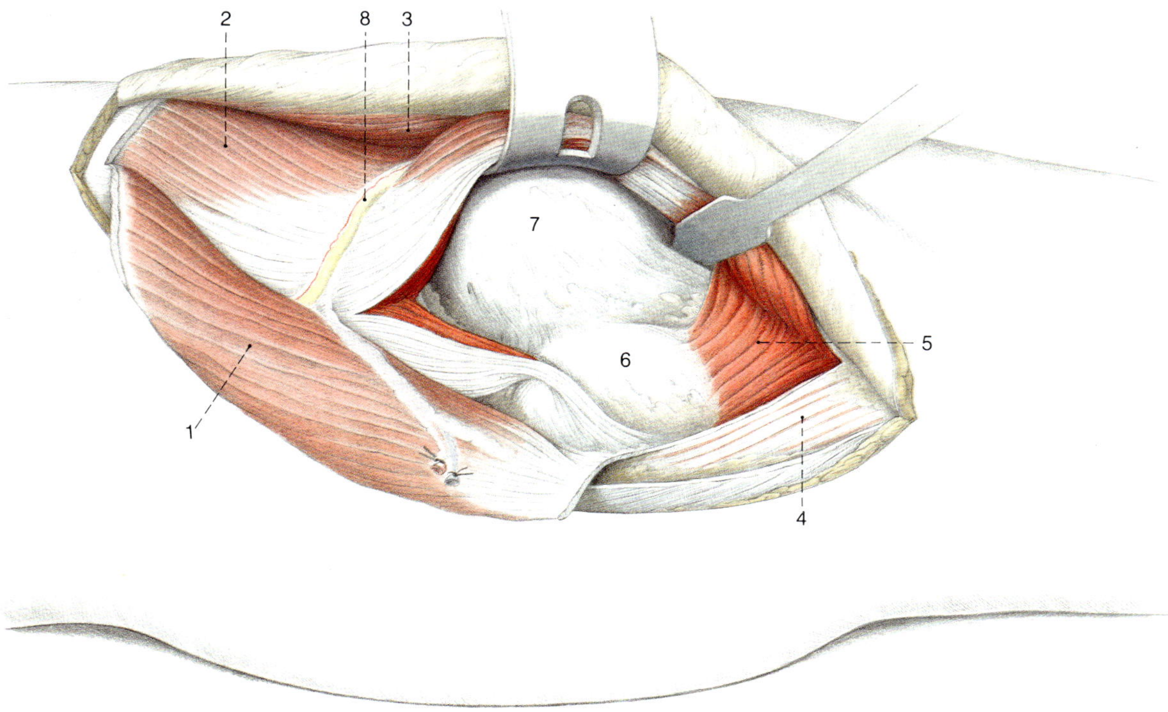

Fig. 1.**12** Anatomical site. Exposure of the superior gluteal nerve in the transgluteal approach. The gluteus medius has been partially separated from the iliac crest and the greater trochanter, creating a posterior flap.

1 Gluteus medius
2 Gluteus minimus
3 Tensor fasciae latae
4 Vastus lateralis
5 Vastus intermedius
6 Greater trochanter
7 Femoral head
8 Superior gluteal nerve

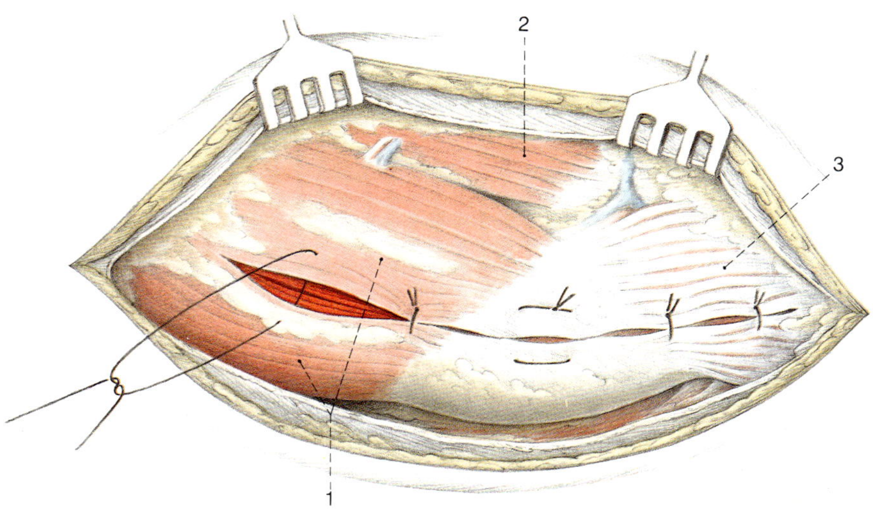

Fig. 1.**13** The musculature is closed with interrupted sutures.

1 Gluteus medius
2 Tensor fasciae latae
3 Vastus lateralis

References

Anson BJ, McVay CB. Surgical Anatomy; vol 1. Philadelphia: Saunders; 1971.

Banks SW, Laufmann H. An Atlas of Surgical Exposures of the Extremities. Philadelphia: Saunders; 1968.

Bauer RF, Kerschbaumer F Poisel S, Oberthaler W. The transgluteal approach to the hip joint. Arch Orthop Traumat. 1979; 95:47.

Cosentino R. Atlas of Anatomy and Surgical Approaches in Orthopaedic Surgery; vol 11. Springfield, Ill.: Thomas; 1973.

Fahey JJ. Surgical approaches to bones and joints. Surg Clin N Amer. 1949; 29:65.

Gibson A. Posterior exposure of the hip joint. J Bone Jt Surg. 1950; 32B:183.

Henry A. Extensile Exposure. Edinburgh: Churchill-Livingstone; 1973.

Honnart F. Voies d'abord en chirurgie orthopedique et traumatologique. Paris: Masson; 1978.

Hoppenfeld S, de Boer P. Surgical Exposures in Orthopaedics. Philadelphia: Lippincott; 1984.

Lanz T von, Wachsmuth W. Praktische Anatomie, Bd. I/4. Berlin: Springer; 1972.

McFarland B, Osborne G. Approach to the hip. J Bone Jt Surg. 1954; 36B:364.

Marcy GH, Flechter RS. Modification of the posterolateral approach to the hip for insertion of femoral head prosthesis. J Bone Jt Surg. 1954; 36A:142.

Moore AT. The self-locking metal hip prosthesis. J Bone Jt Surg. 1957; 39A:811.

Nicola T. Atlas operativer Zugangswege in der Orthopädie. Munich: Urban & Schwarzenberg; 1971.

Platzer W. Volume 1: Bewegungsapparat. In: Taschenatlas der Anatomie. 4th ed. Kahle E, Leonhardt H, Platzer W. eds, 1979. Stuttgart: Thieme; 1984.

Ruedi T, Hochstetter AHC, Schlumpf R. Operative Zugänge zur Osteosynthese. Berlin: Springer; 1984.

Schauwecker F. Osteosynthesepraxis. Stuttgart: Thieme; 1981.

Smith-Petersen MN. Approach to and exposure of the hip joint for mold arthroplasty. J Bone Jt Surg. 1949; 31A:40.

2 Reconstructive Hip Surgery

H. Wagner
M. Wagner

Using Fluoroscopy in the Operating Room

With the Patient Supine

Visualization of the Hip Joint

Indications

Verifying the position of the femoral neck or head, verifying the position of implants, locating the roof of the acetabulum for corrective osteotomies, verifying coverage of the femoral head, and using Kirschner wire to determine the horizontal plane.

Technique

If the hip joint is to be visualized in an anteroposterior projection, the patient is placed supine on a radiolucent operating table (Figs. 2.**1** and 2.**2**). The sterilely draped, C-shaped arm of the fluoroscope is brought into position above the hip from the contralateral side. A long Kirschner wire can be placed over the hip parallel to the iliac spina to mark the horizontal plane of the pelvis in the fluoroscopic image.

When the femoral neck is visualized in the lateral plane (Lauenstein view), the patient is placed supine with the leg externally rotated 90° and the knee flexed at a right angle (Figs. 2.**3** and 2.**4**). To visualize the femoral neck in the lateral plane as it would appear with the patient standing erect, the calf must be positioned over the contralateral leg parallel to the surface of the table with the knee flexed at a right angle. If the hip is limited and this degree of external rotation is not feasible, then the pelvis should be rotated to place the calf in this position.

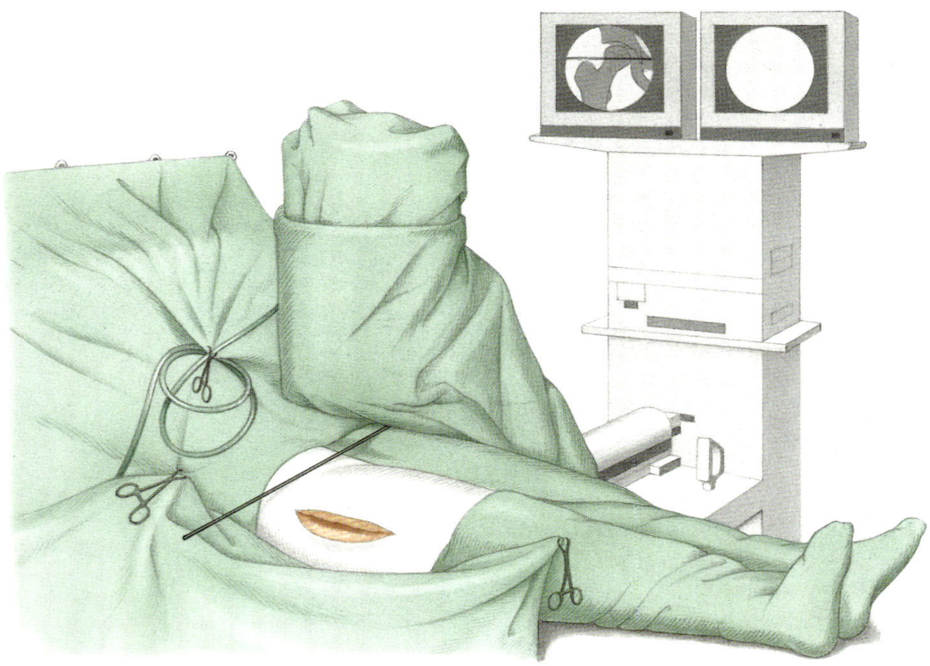

Fig. 2.**1** Anteroposterior fluoroscopy of the hip joint. The patient is supine on a radiolucent operating table. The two monitors of the image intensifier can be seen in the background.

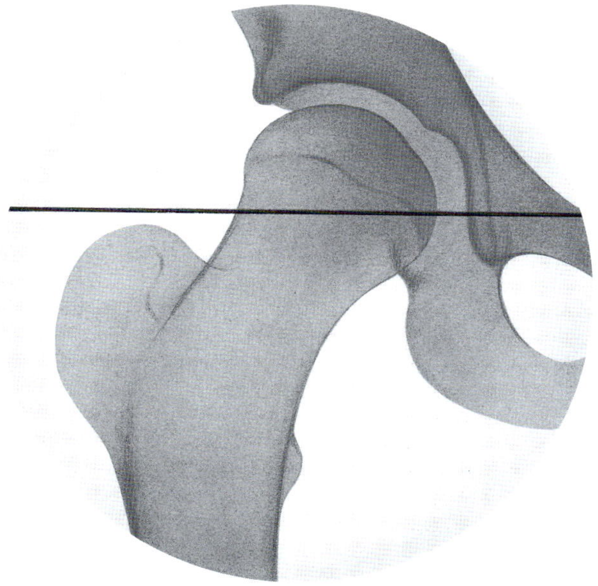

Fig. 2.**2** The image shows the anteroposterior view of the hip joint with the Kirschner wire marking the horizontal plane.

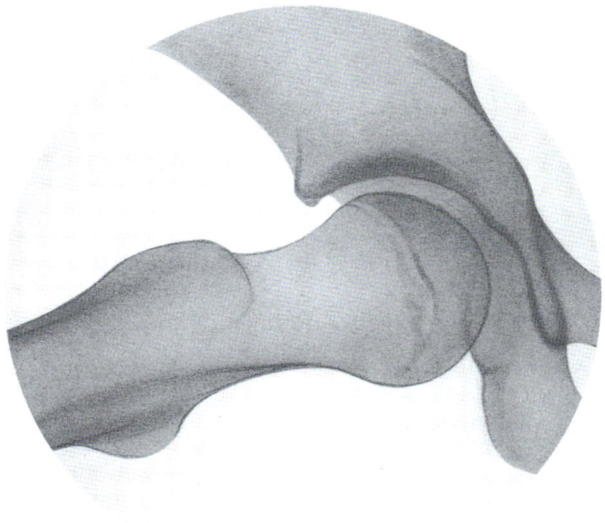

Fig. 2.**4** The image shows the lateral view of the femoral neck.

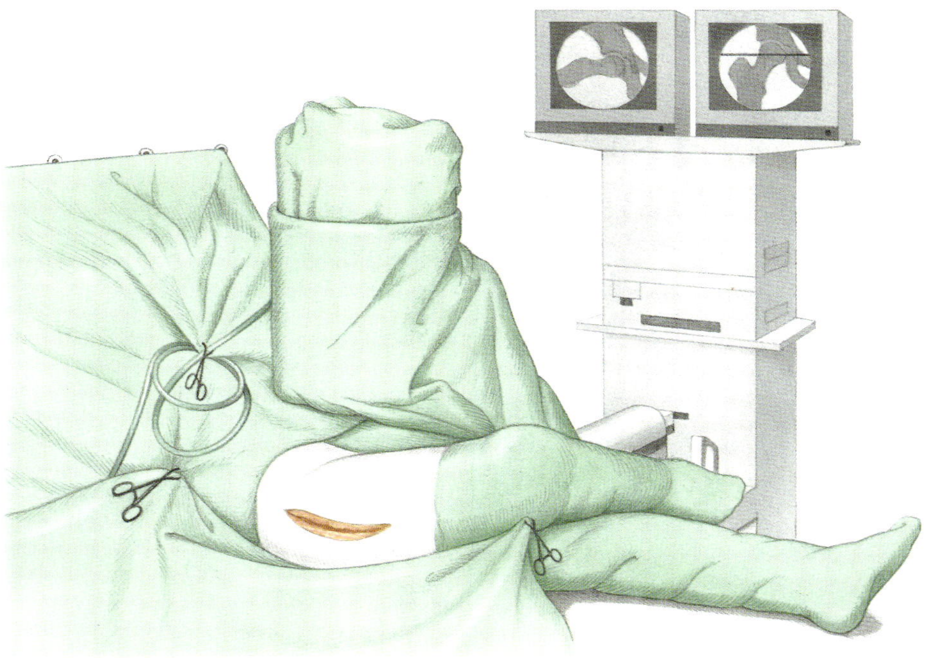

Fig. 2.**3** Lateral fluoroscopy of the femoral nack. The patient is supine on a radiolucent operating table. The leg is externally rotated 90°, and the knee is flexed at a right angle.

Measuring the Length of the Femur

Indications

Preoperative planning, including shortening osteotomies, valgus intertrochanteric osteotomies to prevent an increase in leg length, and in all other osteotomies performed on the femur to adjust leg length.

Technique

Measurements are made with the patient supine on a radiolucent table. The joint is visualized in the center of the monitor image (Fig. 2.**5**). The position of the tip of the pointer is marked on the skin (Figs. 2.**6** and 2.**7**). The pointer should be at least 1 meter long to protect personnel from excessive radiation exposure. When leg length is measured in the operating room under sterile conditions, the position may be marked with a fine clamp attached to the skin or incision sheeting instead of marking the skin with a marking pen.

The same procedure is repeated at the knee. (Figs. 2.**8** and 2.**9**). The distance between the two marks is then measured. This yields a very accurate measurement of the length of the femur. A long tape measure or cerclage wire may be used for measuring the distance.

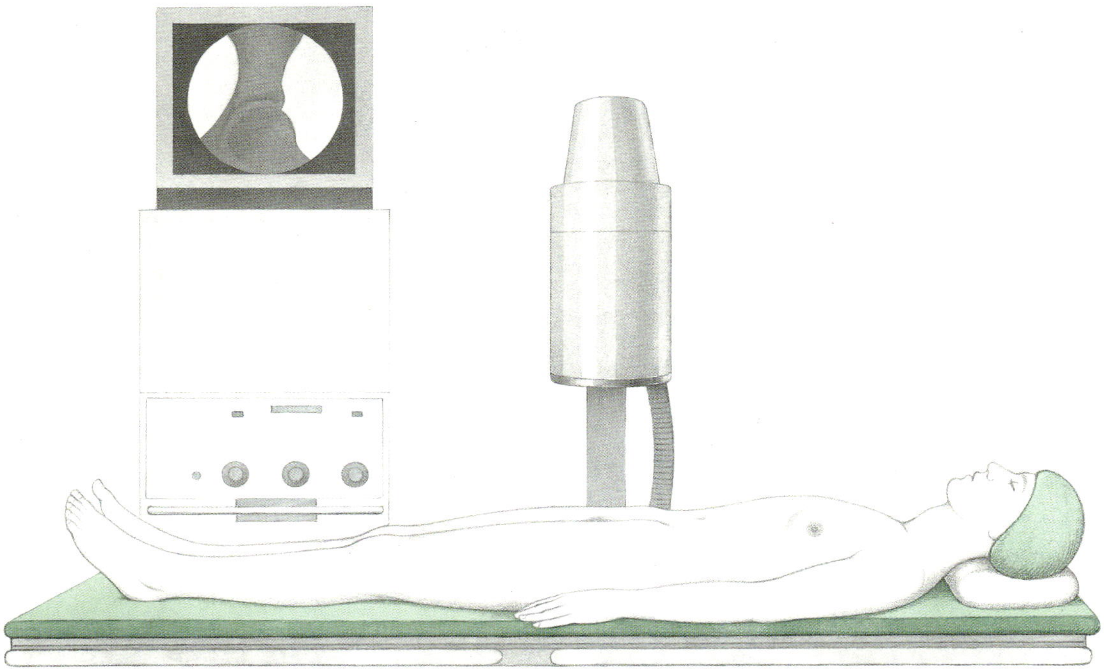

Fig. 2.**5** Measuring the length of the femur is done with the patient lying supine on a radiolucent table. The C arm of the image intensifier is brought into position above the hip, and the joint appears in the center of the monitor.

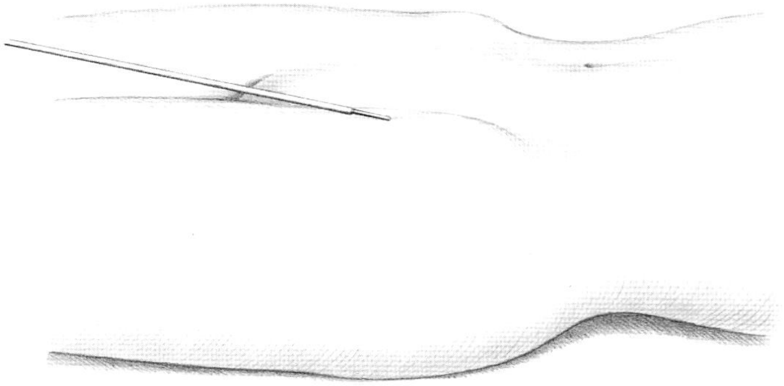

Fig. 2.**6** The tip of a long pointer is placed on the skin, resting over the joint. Joint and pointer appear in the center of the monitor.

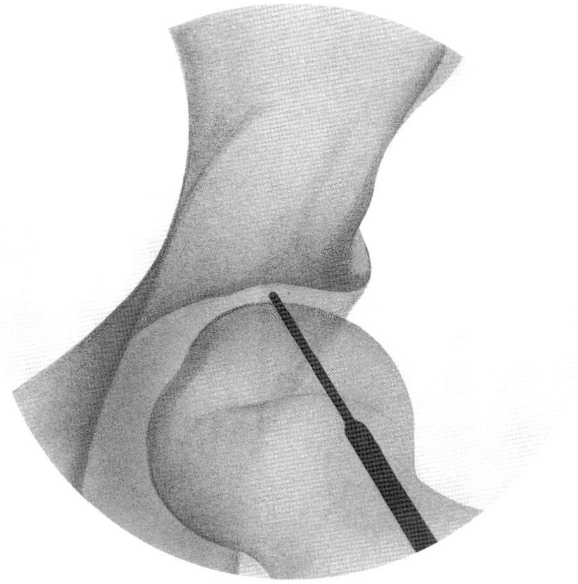

Fig. 2.**7** The image shows the tip of the pointer superimposed on the joint.

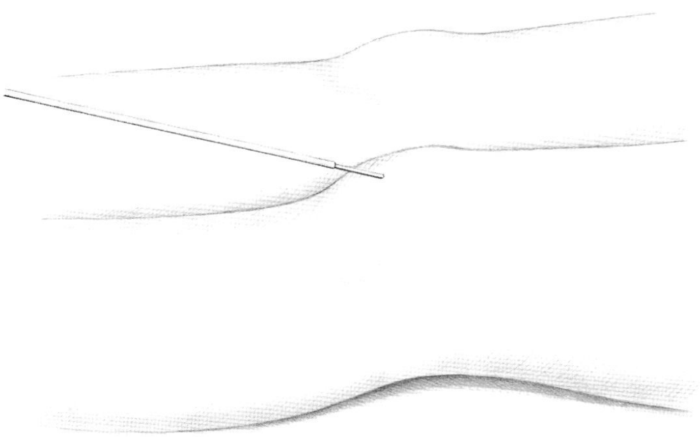

Fig. 2.**8** The tip of a long pointer is placed on the skin, resting over the knee joint.

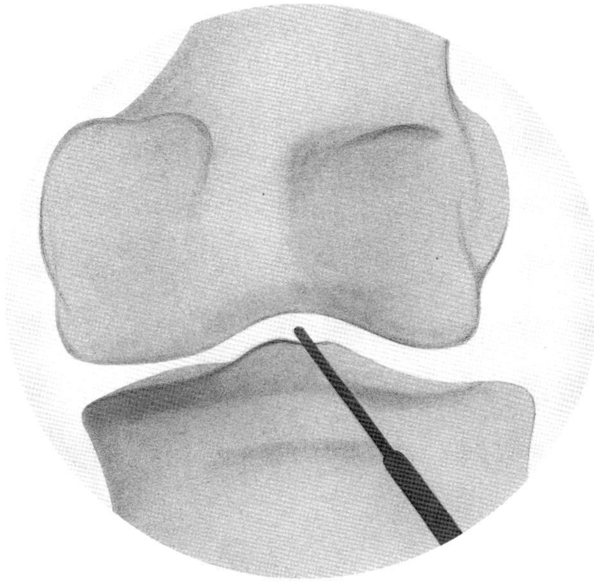

Fig. 2.**9** The image shows the tip of the pointer superimposed on the knee joint.

With the Patient Positioned Laterally

Indications

Verifying the position of implants when using the posterior approach to the hip joint.

Technique

The C arm of the image intensifier is not draped, but additional sterile draping is applied to the patient. The arm is positioned over the patient, and the hip is visualized in an anteroposterior projection (Fig. 2.**10**).

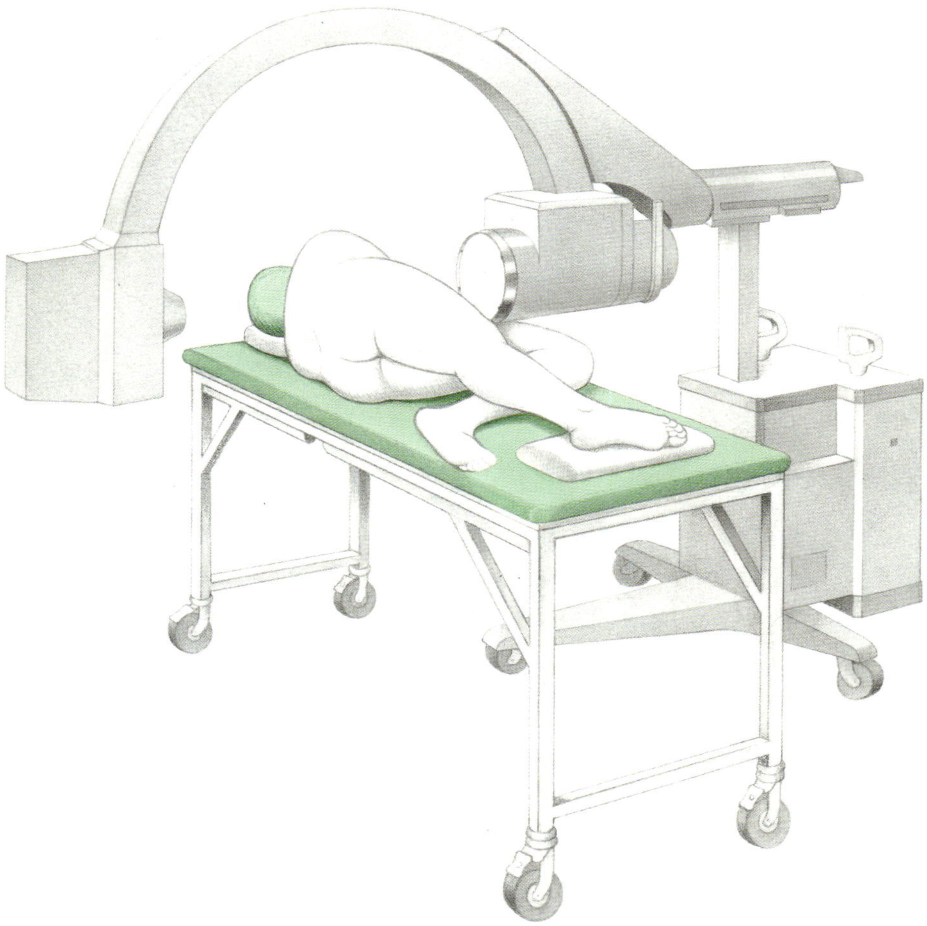

Fig. 2.**10** Position of the C arm when imaging the hip joint with the patient in the lateral position.

General Hip Surgery

Arthrocentesis of the Hip Joint

Indications

Aspiration of septic, aseptic, or bloody fluid; injection of medications; arthrography.

Positioning

The patient is positioned appropriately for the planned procedure. A radiolucent table permits fluoroscopy.

Technique

Arthrocentesis of the hip joint may be performed from any direction if the surgeon carefully avoids neurovascular structures. The patient is usually supine, and an anterior approach is used. This has definite advantages for orientation: With the patient supine, the anterior superior iliac spine, the symphysis, and the femoral artery distal to the inguinal ligament are readily palpable; in slender patients, even the anterior inferior iliac spine and the joint capsule are palpable. When aspirating the joint anteriorly, the surgeon feels the characteristic firm resistance of the iliofemoral ligament (which is fused with the anterior joint capsule) as the cannula is inserted into the joint. When this resistance is overcome, the tip of the cannula has entered the joint capsule. The image intensifier can be used for orientation with the patient supine.

When warranted by particular findings, lateral or posterior approaches may also be performed with the patient positioned appropriately.

The best approach direction of the cannula depends on the respective findings. Care should be taken to avoid injury to the articular cartilage. If a large amount of fluid has collected in the hip joint, aspiration is easy to perform because the joint capsule is expanded, and the cannula punctures it well before reaching the articular cartilage. When aspirating a joint capsule that lies close to the head of the femur, insert the cannula into the inferior section of the joint, where the joint capsule is generally relaxed. This applies in particular to subluxed hips, in which there is a wide cavity between the femoral head and the acetabular fossa. However, arthrocentesis is often not feasible in a hip with degenerative joint disease where scar tissue is present.

The surgeon first locates the anterior superior iliac spine and the pubic symphysis. The midpoint on the line defined by these two points is where the femoral artery crosses the medial segment of the femoral head; the pulse of the artery can be readily felt at this point. In adults, the best insertion point for the cannula lies 3 cm lateral and 6 cm distal to this point because the cannula is lateral of the femoral nerve (Fig. 2.**11**). In children, the distances are proportionally smaller. At the point of entry, a skin incision about 2 mm long is made with a narrow scalpel to prevent the cannula from carrying skin particles into the subcutaneous tissues.

The cannula is advanced at a superior angle of approximately 25° and a posterior angle of approximately 45°, meeting the firm resistance of the joint capsule with the iliofemoral ligament. The capsule can be palpated and penetrated with the cannula. The fluid in the capsule then drains through the cannula. If the capsule does not contain any fluid, Ringer's solution may be injected. If the cannula is positioned correctly, this can be done easily. If the Ringer's solution can only be injected under high pressure, this is an indication that

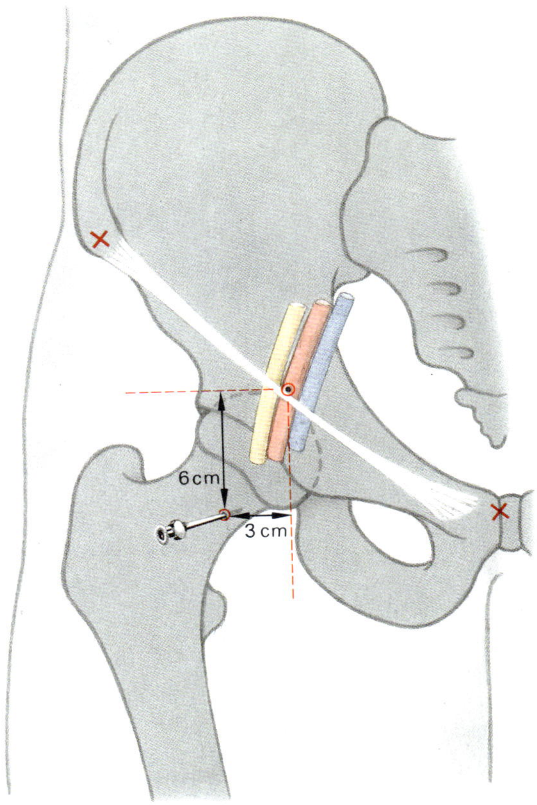

Fig. 2.**11** Landmarks for anterior arthrocentesis of the hip with the patient supine.

the tip of the cannula is not in the joint. It should be advanced or inserted from a different direction as required. The position of the cannula can be easily verified using fluoroscopy. A return flow (or rapid sequence of drips) of Ringer's solution from the capsule is another reliable sign that the tip of the cannula is positioned correctly. If viscous fluid flows out of the cannula, the surgeon may be certain of having punctured the joint capsule.

On rare occasions, aspiration of the hip joint is performed with the patient positioned laterally with the leg adducted. Here, the cannula is inserted above the apex of the greater trochanter, and the surgeon may target the anterior superior, superior, and posterior superior portion of the capsule of the hip joint. The remainder of the procedure is performed as described previously (Fig. 2.**12**).

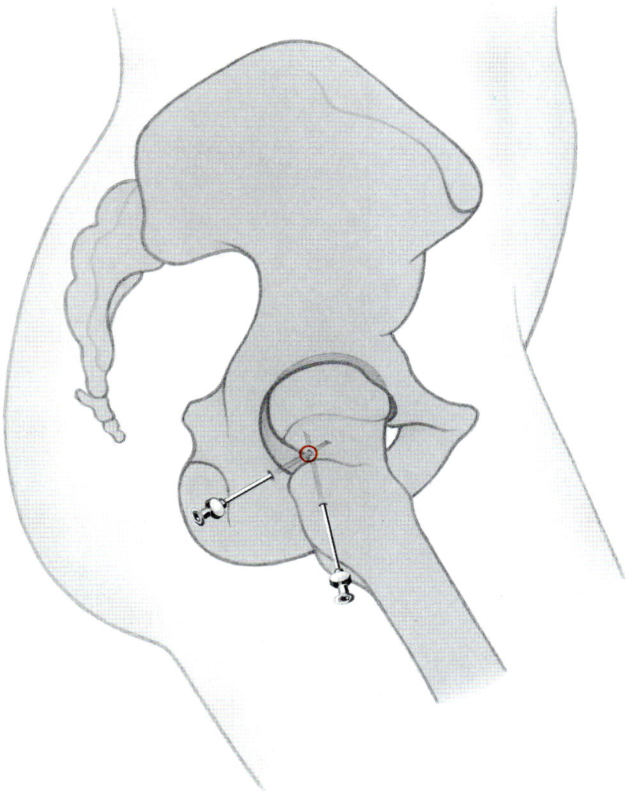

Fig. 2.**12** Arthrocentesis of the hip with the patient positioned laterally with the leg adducted. The cannula is inserted superior to the greater trochanter and advanced into the capsule.

Arthrography of the Hip

Indications

Visualizing intra-articular structures that do not appear in plain radiographs, such as the joint capsule, articular cartilage, intra-articular connective tissue structures, and chondral fragments.

The contrast medium used in arthrography expands the joint capsule, making it possible to visualize how the capsule unfolds or adheres. Any interposed soft-tissue structures are also revealed.

Positioning

The patient is generally positioned supine on a radiolucent table, facilitating the use of fluoroscopy for orientation.

Technique

In arthrography, radiopaque liquid or radiolucent gaseous contrast media are injected into the hip by means of arthrocentesis. These contrast media show up in the radiograph and help visualize the surrounding structures. In double-contrast arthrography, radiopaque and radiolucent contrast media are used simultaneously. This procedure is more complicated, but it can provide more detailed radiographic findings.

Arthrography of the hip must be performed under sterile conditions. This is best done in the operating room with the patient sterilely prepped and draped. After aspirating the hip, the surgeons verifies the correct position of the cannula within the capsule by injecting Ringer's solution into the capsule. The surgeon should feel no resistance initially, but increasing resistance as the solution is injected. When the syringe is removed, there should be a return flow or a rapid sequence of drips of Ringer's solution from the cannula. Viscous fluid flowing out of the cannula is a reliable indication that the tip of the cannula is positioned correctly within the joint capsule.

Now the contrast medium is injected into the joint. A great advantage of using a syringe is that the surgeon can feel and maintain the pressure under which the contrast medium is injected. While injecting the contrast medium, the surgeon should monitor the gradual expansion of the capsule with fluoroscopy to ensure optimum filling. To protect surgical staff from excessive radiation exposure, the cannula and syringe should be connected by extension tubing that permit the surgeon's hands to remain outside of the radiation beam (Fig. 2.**13**).

Gas arthrography produces radiographs that permit the surgeon to assess the intra-articular soft-tissue structures (Fig. 2.**14**). Carbon dioxide gas is commonly used as a contrast medium. It has the advantage of being quickly absorbed if it inadvertently enters the venous bloodstream, greatly reducing the risk of a gas embolism. Atmospheric air is flushed from the system by filling the syringe and connecting hose with Ringer's solution. Then the gas is drawn into the syringe through a sterile hose connection to the cylinder and the Ringer's solution is gradually flushed out.

Fig. 2.**13** Arthography of the hip joint of a child (with carbon dioxide) under sterile conditions in an operating room. The cannula lies in the left hip and is connected to the contrast-medium syringe via an extension tube. The system is first filled with carbon dioxide gas from a pressurized cylinder.

1 Sterilely draped image intensifier
2 Carbon dioxide cylinder
3 Sterile extension tube for filling the syringe.

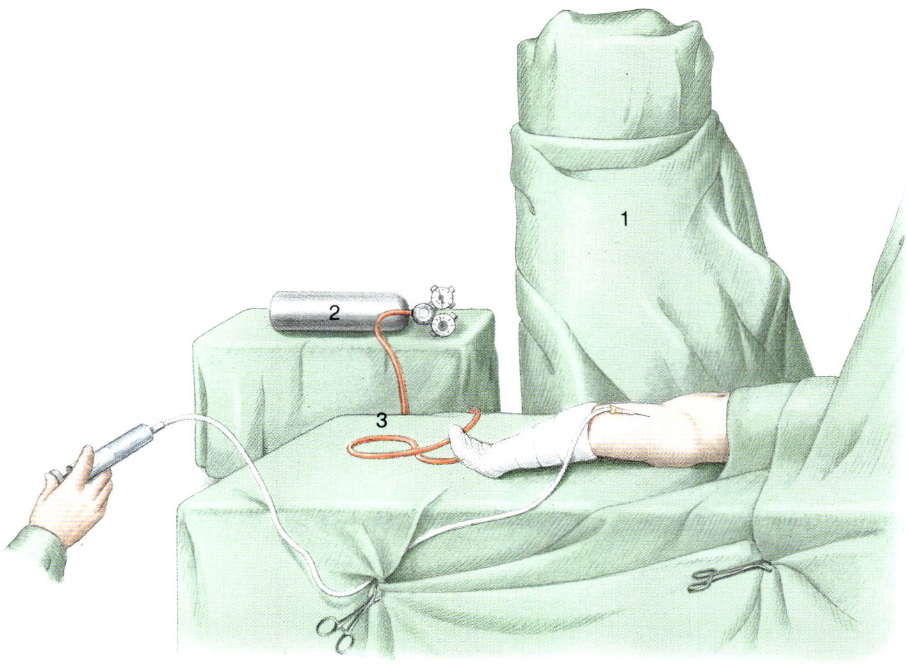

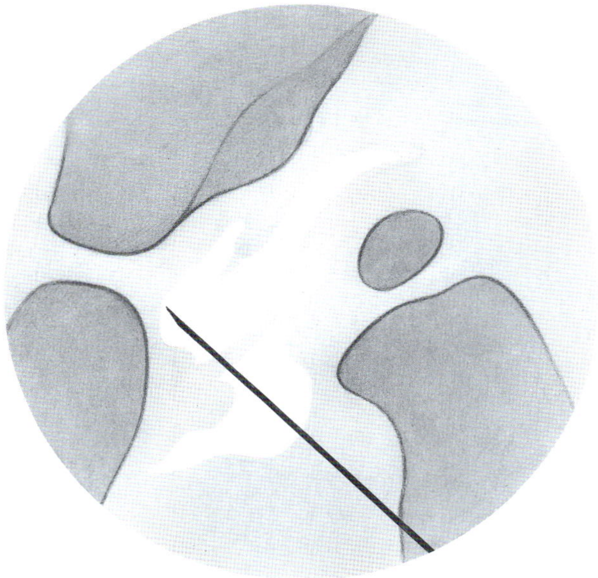

Fig. 2.**14** Gas arthrography of a dislocated hip in a child. The femoral head is displaced, and the joint capsule is only partially unfolded, indicating intra-articular adhesion. The articular cartilage, the acetabular labrum, the elongated ligament of the femoral head, and the distended pulvinar are readily discernible.

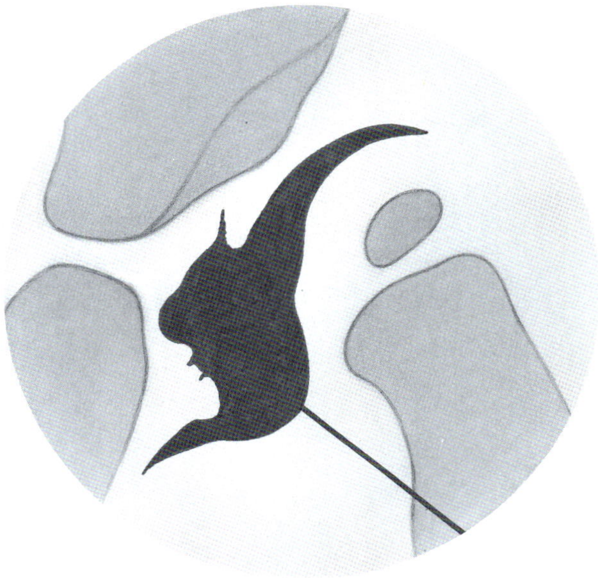

Fig. 2.**15** Radiopaque arthrography of the same hip shown in Fig. 2.**14**. The peripheral structures are well defined, whereas the central soft-tissue structures are obscured by the contrast medium.

When a radiopaque contrast medium is used in arthrography, the syringe and connecting hose are filled with liquid contrast medium, which is injected into the hip through the cannula. Radiopaque arthrography provides high-contrast images of the intra-articular structures (Fig. 2.**15**). However, only the peripheral soft-tissue structures are revealed by the contrast medium; central structures are wholly or partially obscured.

In double-constrast arthrography, the radiopaque liquid is injected into the hip first. After the joint is put through its range of motion, the contrast medium is drained. Next, the joint is filled with carbon dioxide. Radiopaque liquid contrast medium adheres to the capsule walls (synovial membrane, interposed soft-tissue structures, and articular cartilage), while the radiolucent gas lightens the capsule interior (2.**16**). This produces impressive radiographs in which the light interior of the capsule is framed by thick dark lines.

The surgeon should remember that redundancy in the capsule may form folds or potential spaces, which neither liquid nor gas contrast medium can penetrate. Arthrography cannot detect these structures, regardless of the contrast media used. As the contrast medium dilates the capsule, these folds are distended. The potential spaces become actual spaces and may be visualized. With capsular distension, however, the lateral displacement of the femoral head increases. The surgeon should take this into consideration when assessing the arthrogram.

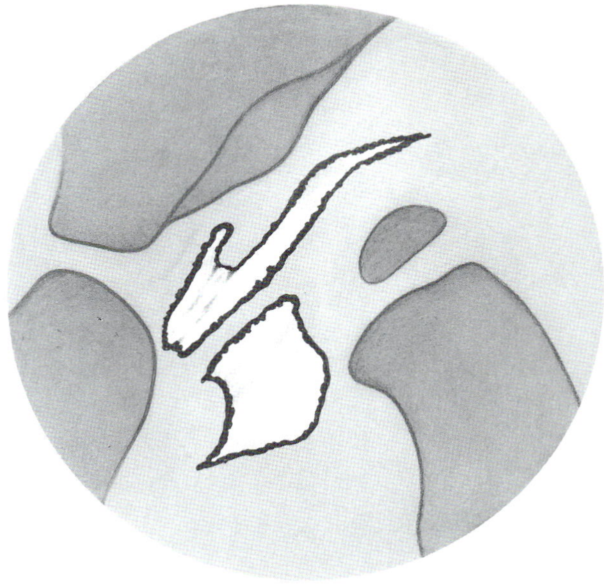

Fig. 2.**16** Double-contrast arthrography of the same hip shown in Fig. 2.**14**. Radiopaque liquid contrast medium adheres to the surface of the soft-tissue structures, while the carbon dioxide gas makes the capsule interior appear lighter.

Hip Surgery

Hip Surgery Using an Anterior Approach

Indications

Broad exposure of the hip in treating degenerative joint disease (inflammation, formation of scar tissue, ossification), deformities in the immediate proximity of the joint, and traumatic injuries. The approach is used for hip surgery, synovectomy, and corrective surgery involving the acetabulum.

Positioning and Incision

With the patient positioned supine, a curved skin incision is made parallel to the iliac crest, beginning lateral of the anterior superior iliac spine and coursing distally to the middle of the lateral thigh.

Technique

The anterior approach is the most challenging and versatile approach to the hip. It permits broad exposure of the hip and the lateral and medial surface of the iliac wing, and can be easily extended as far as necessary. A further advantage of the incision is that it courses along the dividing line between the femoral and gluteal neurovascular structures. A disadvantage is that it may require separating muscles from their origins over a broad area, which requires particular caution.

The skin incision courses 2–3 cm lateral of the iliac crest (Fig. 2.**17**). After splitting the muscle fascia parallel to its fibers, the surgeon transects the tensor fasciae latae and retracts it laterally. The medial fascia is kept in place to protect the lateral femoral cutaneous nerve (Fig. 2.**18**), which lies medial to the incision. After the deep layer of the fascia has been split, the rectus femoris and ascending branch of the lateral femoral circumflex artery (Fig. 2.**19**) are visible. Limited exposure of the hip capsule may now be obtained by retracting the pericapsular fat, and a partial capsulectomy can be performed without significant risk to the surrounding musculature.

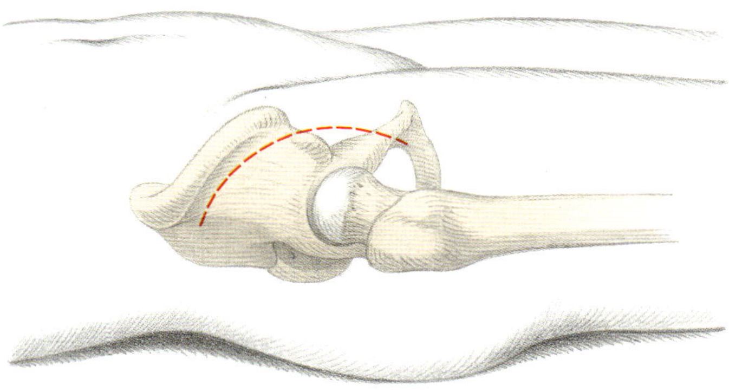

Fig. 2.**17** In the anterior approach to the hip, the skin incision courses 2–3 cm lateral of the iliac crest.

Fig. 2.**18** After the muscle fascia is split parallel to the direction of its fibers, the tensor fasciae latae is dissected from the medial fascia and retracted laterally.

1 Iliac crest
2 Anterior superior iliac spine
3 Sartorius
4 Superficial layer of the fascia lata
5 Deep layer of the fascia lata
6 Tensor fasciae latae
7 Iliotibial tract

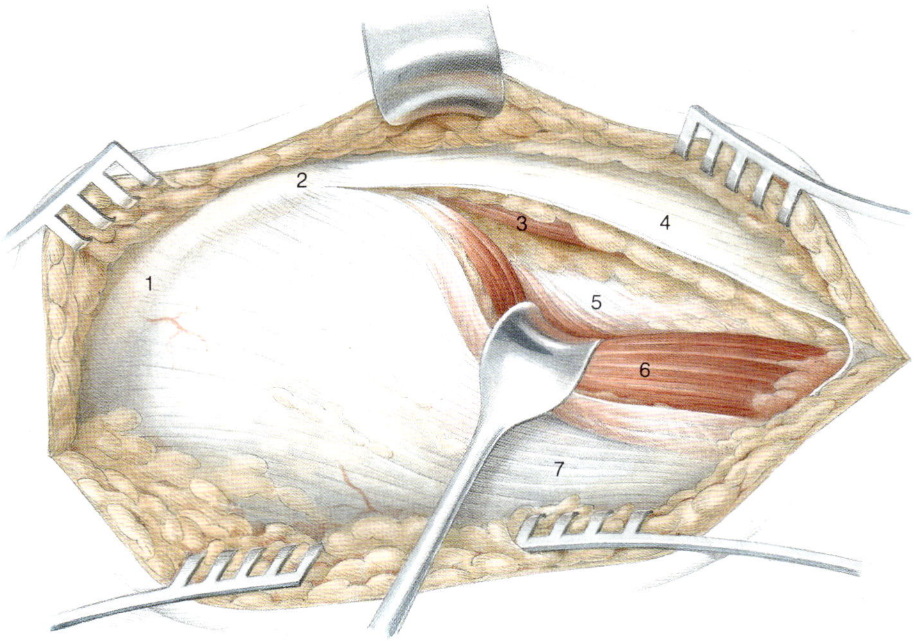

Fig. 2.**19** After the deep layer of the fascia has been split, the sartorius is retracted medially, and the tensor fasciae latae laterally. The rectus femoris with its two heads of origin and the ascending branch of the lateral femoral circumflex artery are visible is the deepest layer.

1 Iliac crest
2 Anterior superior iliac spine
3 Sartorius
4 Rectus femoris
5 Direct origin of the rectus femoris
6 Reflected origin of the rectus femoris
7 Ascending branch of the lateral femoral circumflex artery
8 Tensor fasciae latae
9 Iliotibial tract

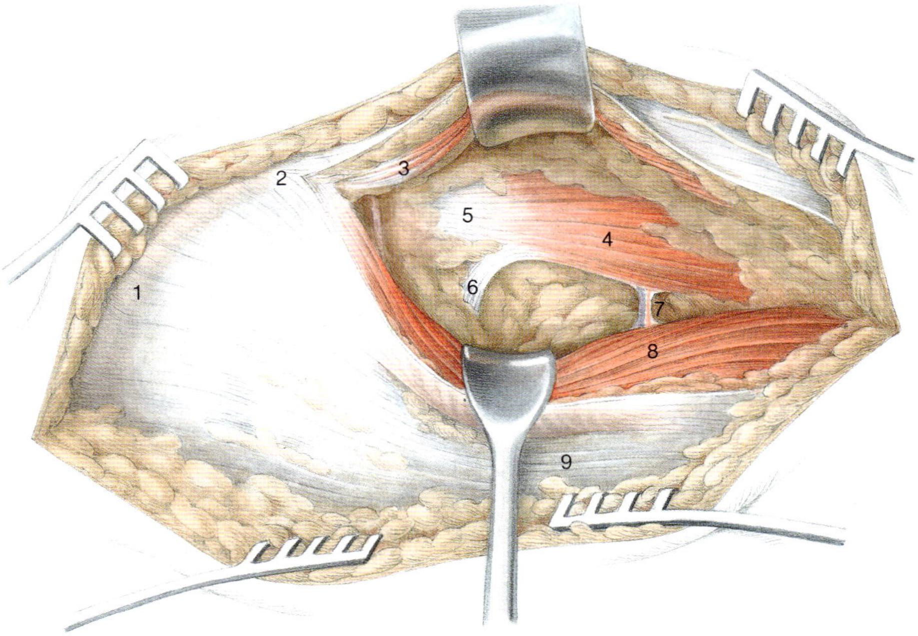

Broader exposure of the hip requires more extensive soft-tissue dissection. The tensor fasciae latae and the gluteus medius are successively dissected from the lateral surface of the iliac wing. After the pericapsular fat is retracted, the capsule of the hip is clearly visible beneath the origin of the rectus femoris (Fig. 2.**20**). This degree of exposure is often sufficient for limited surgical procedures about the hip.

If more extensive exposure of the hip is required, the direct and reflect origins of rectus femoris are resected (Fig. 2.**21**). When severe soft-tissue contracture is present or the anterior margin of the ilium and anterior capsule or the inner surface of the ilium must be visualized, the the soft-tissue structures are dissected from the anterior superior iliac spine and the inner surface of the iliac wing. A broad blunt elevator is in-

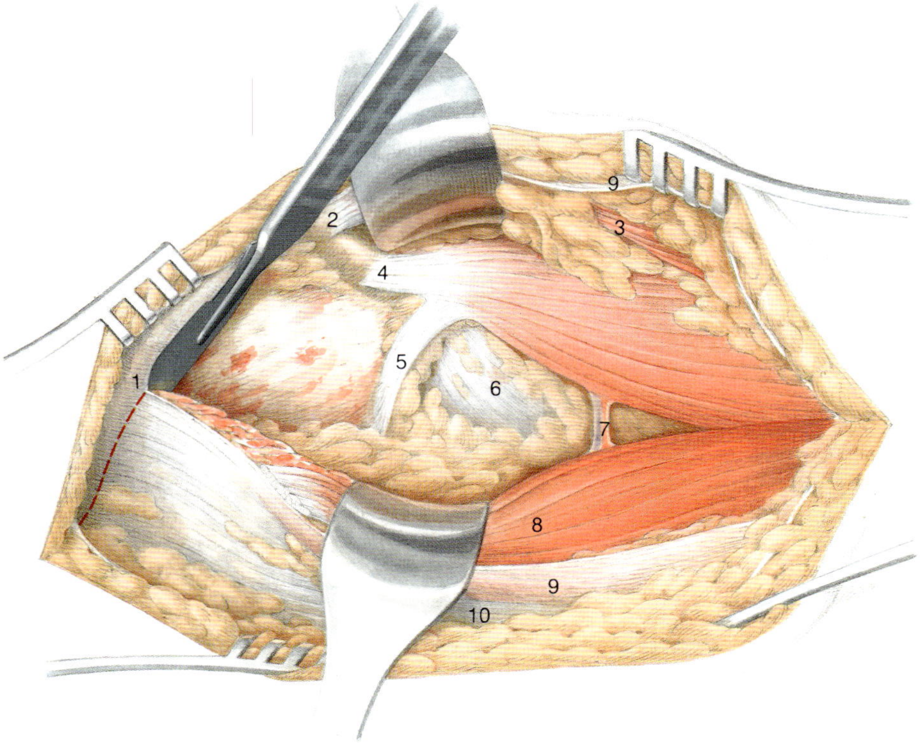

Fig. 2.**20** The musculature covering the hip is dissected along the outer surface of the iliac wing, exposing the joint capsule.

1 Iliac crest
2 Anterior superior iliac spine
3 Sartorius
4 Direct origin of the rectus femoris
5 Reflected origin of the rectus femoris
6 Hip joint capsule
7 Ascending branch of the lateral femoral circumflex artery
8 Tensor fasciae latae
9 Fascia lata
10 Iliotibial tract

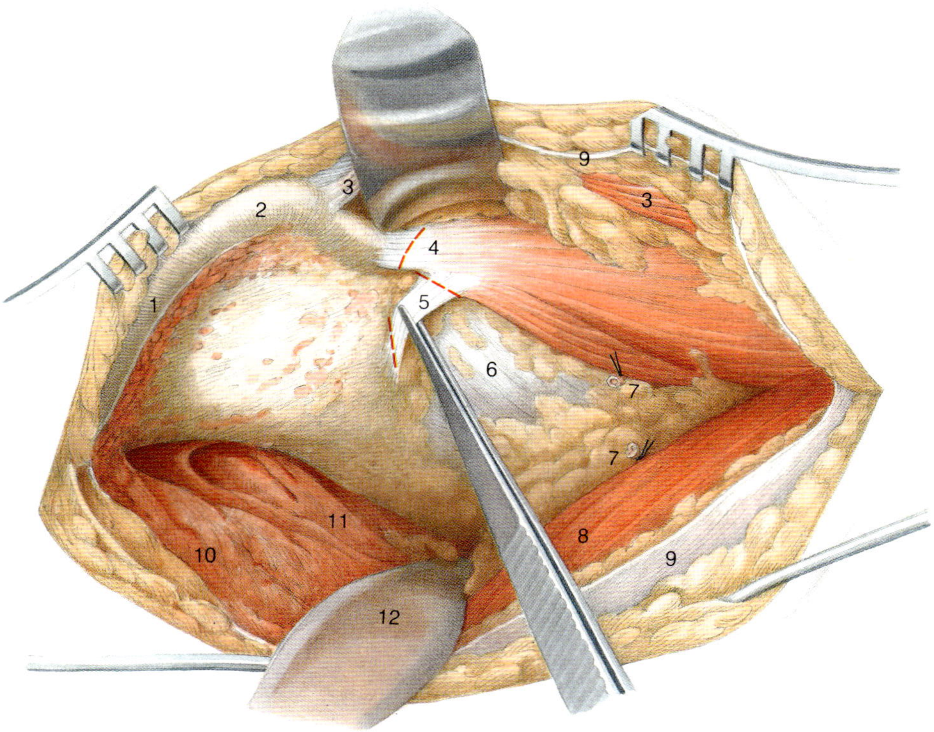

Fig. 2.**21** Dissecting the rectus lfemoris by resecting the reflected origin and transecting the direct origin.

1 Iliac crest
2 Anterior superior iliac spine
3 Sartorius
4 Direct origin of the rectus femoris
5 Reflected origin of the rectus femoris
6 Hip joint capsule
7 Ascending branch of the lateral femoral circumflex artery
8 Tensor fasciae latae
9 Fascia lata
10 Gluteus medius
11 Gluteus minimus
12 Elevator in the greater sciatic notch

serted under the soft tissue on the medial surface of the ilium and lifted. The surgeon first severs the sartorius and the inguinal ligament at the iliac spine with a scalpel (Fig. 2.**22**). Then the iliacus can be bluntly retracted from the medial surface of the ilium; if necessary, it can be retracted posteriorly as far as the sacroiliac joint.

The surgeon lifts the anterior soft tissue using a short, sharp-tipped elevator impacted in the pubis and retracts the pelvic and trochanteric musculature posteriorly with a blunt elevator in the greater sciatic notch (Fig. 2.**23**). This exposes two-thirds of the circumference of the hip capsule. The surgeon opens the capsule with a "T" incision, taking care not to dam-

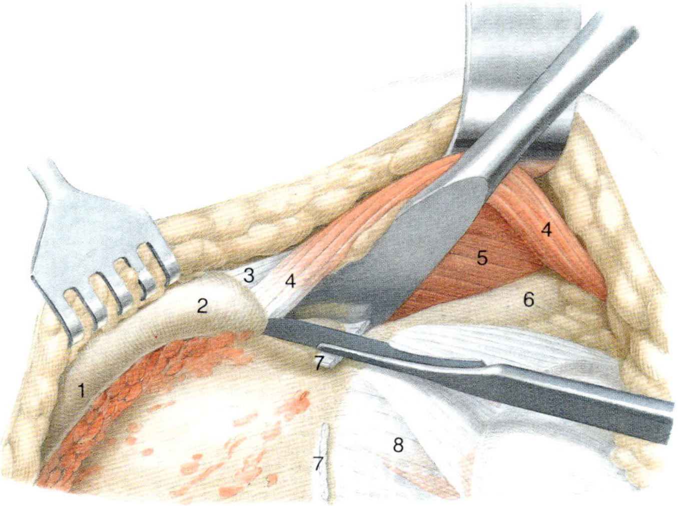

Fig. 2.**22** Dissecting the soft-tissue structures from the medial side of the anterior superior iliac spine and the inner surface of the ilium.

1 Iliac crest
2 Anterior superior iliac spine
3 Inguinal ligament
4 Sartorius
5 Iliopsoas
6 Pubic ramus
7 Transected rectus femoris
8 Hip joint capsule

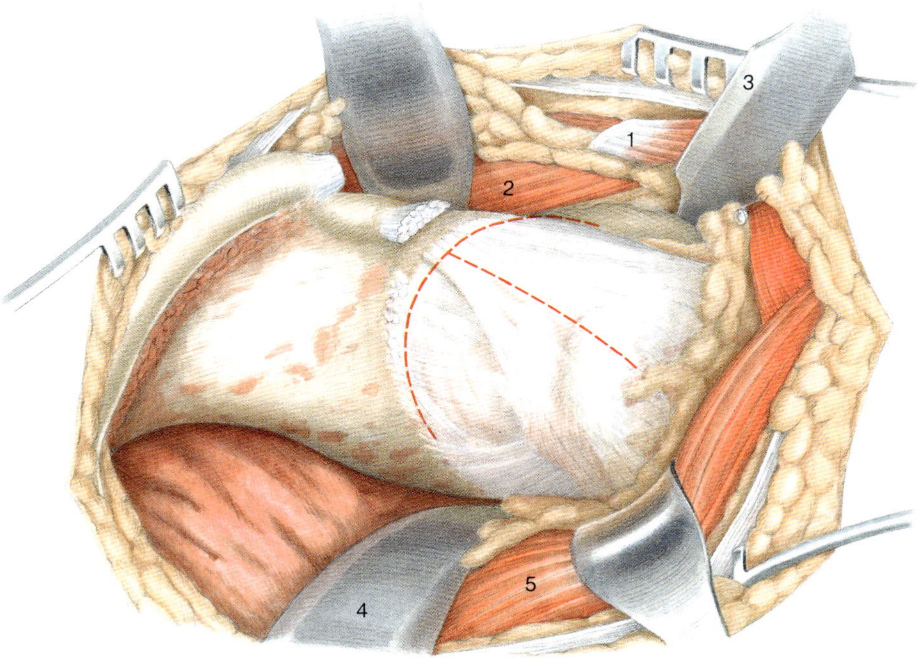

Fig. 2.**23** The anterior soft tissue is lifted using a short, sharp-tipped elevator impacted in the pubis, and the pelvic and trochanteric musculature is retracted posteriorly with a blunt elevator in the greater sciatic notch. The capsule is opened with a "T" incision.

1 Sartorius
2 Iliopsoas
3 Short, sharp-tipped elevator impacted in the pubis
4 Blunt elevator in the greater sciatic notch
5 Tensor fasciae latae

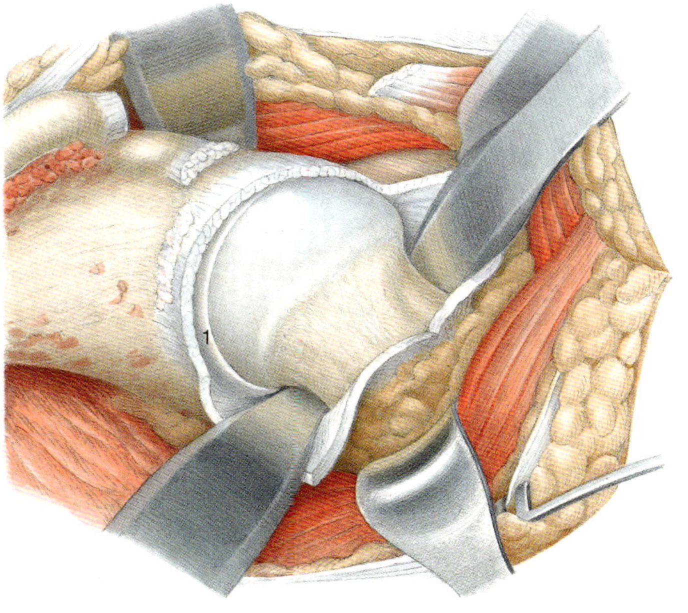

Fig. 2.**24** Broad exposure of the hip joint after opening the incised capsule.

1 Acetabular labrum

age the acetabular labrum or the cartilage of the femoral head. Opening the two capsule flaps exposes the joint completely (Fig. 2.**24**). The surgeon can now perform a synovectomy or capsulectomy, or dislocate the hip with the leg flexed and adducted in external rotation.

It is not always necessary to suture the capsule when closing the wound; reattaching the musculature is more important. The direct origin of the rectus femoris is reattached to the anterior inferior iliac spine, the inguinal ligament and the sartorius to the anterior superior iliac spine, and the gluteus medius and tensor fasciae latae to the iliac crest (Fig. 2.**25**). Secure fixation of the muscular origins may require suture to the bone via drill holes or suture anchors. Excessive tension on the pelvic and trochanteric musculature can be effectively relieved by alternately incising the superficial muscle fascia perpendicular to the direction of its fibers.

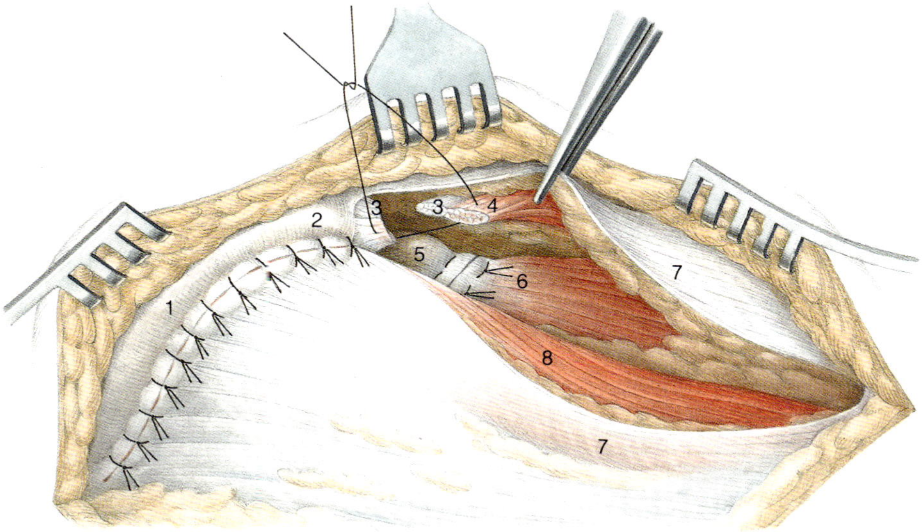

Fig. 2.**25** Reattaching the musculature.

1 Iliac crest
2 Anterior superior iliac spine
3 Inguinal ligament
4 Sartorius
5 Anterior inferior iliac spine
6 Rectus femoris
7 Fascia lata
8 Tensor fasciae latae

Hip Surgery Using an Anterolateral Approach

Indications

The anterolateral approach provides limited exposure of the anterior hip, yet it does so with minimal soft-tissue detachments. In hip surgery, this option should be weighed against the extensive exposure of the anterior approach before beginning. The anterolateral approach offers the additional advantage of permitting simultaneous exposure of the proximal femur.

Positioning and Incision

With the patient positioned supine, a longitudinal skin incision is made that begins at the apex of the greater trochanter and courses distally (Fig. 2.**26**).

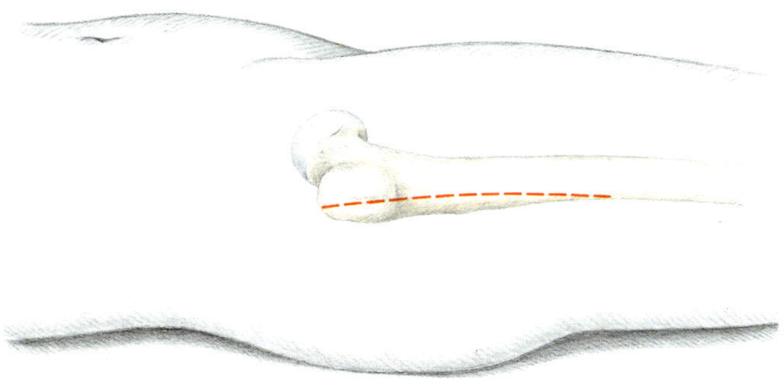

Fig. 2.**26** In the anterolateral approach, the longitudinal skin incision begins at the apex of the greater trochanter and courses distally.

Technique

After the fascia is split, the hip joint is exposed between the tensor fasciae latae and the vastus lateralis without significant damage to the musculature of the hip. Broad exposure of the proximal femur is also possible.

The anterior margin of the gluteus medius is conservatively detached from its insertion on the greater trochanter to provide access to the anterior surface of the hip joint capsule (Fig. 2.**27**). The pericapsular fat is retracted from the anterior surface of the joint capsule with a sharp periosteal elevator, exposing the entire anterior capsule (Fig. 2.**28**). The reflected origin of the rectus femoris is now visible in the deep layer. Elevators are inserted on the superior, medial, and inferior sides of the femoral neck, providing broad exposure of the joint capsule (Fig. 2.**29**). The surgeon opens the capsule with a "T" incision, taking care not to damage the acetabular labrum or the cartilage of the femoral head.

The capsule flaps are opened like doors, providing access sufficient for performing a partial synovectomy or partial capsulectomy (Fig. 2.**30**). Further soft-tissue dissection is necessary if the hip is to be dislocated or a prosthesis implanted.

Closure is begun by suturing the anterior margin of the gluteus medius back to its insertion on the greater trochanter (Fig. 2.**31**). After placing a subfascial drain, the surgeon closes the fascia lata with a secure vertical mattress suture, overlapping the lips of the wound (Fig. 2.**32**). The wound is then closed in layers.

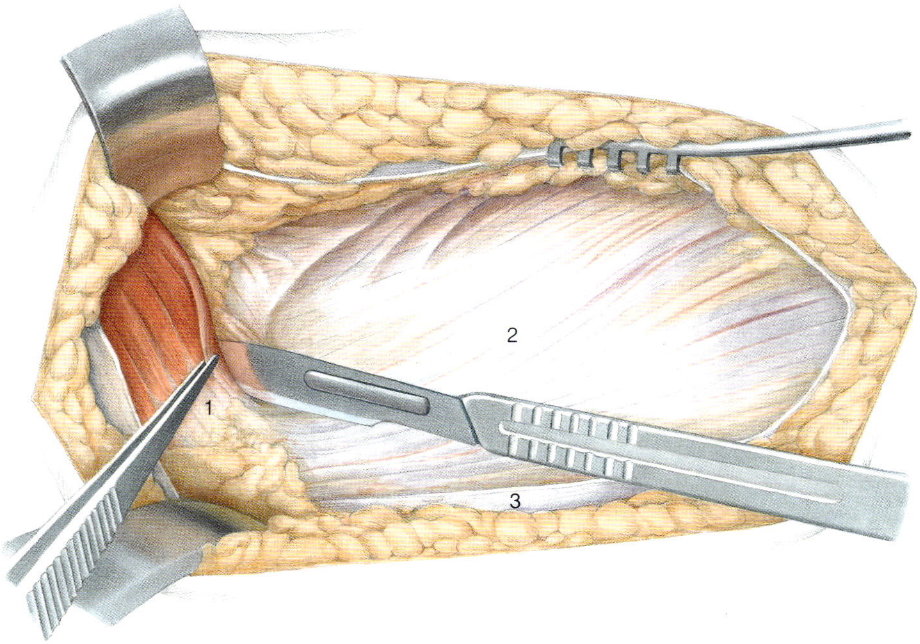

Fig. 2.**27** After the fascia lata is split, the anterior margin of the gluteus medius is conservatively detached from its insertion on the greater trochanter.

1 Gluteus medius
2 Vastus lateralis
3 Fascia lata, divided longitudinally

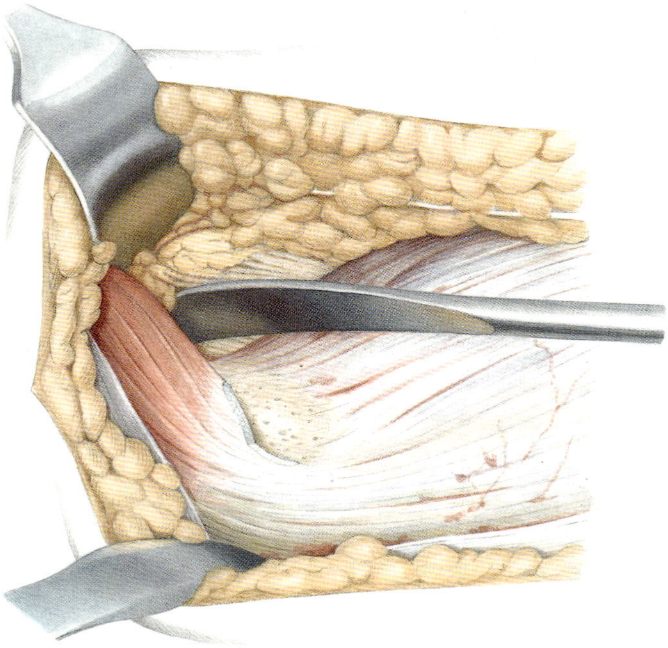

Fig. 2.**28** The pericapsular fat is retracted from the anterior surface of the joint capsule with a sharp periosteal elevator.

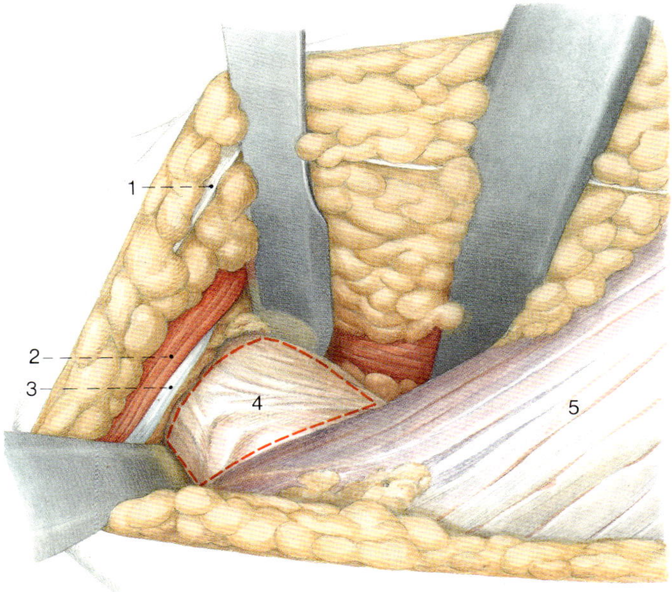

Fig. 2.**29** The reflected origin of the rectus femoris is visible in the deep layer. Elevators are inserted on the superior, medial, and inferior sides of the femoral neck, providing broad exposure of the joint capsule, which is then incised.

1 Fascia lata
2 Gluteus medius
3 Reflected origin of the rectus femoris
4 Hip joint capsule
5 Vastus lateralis

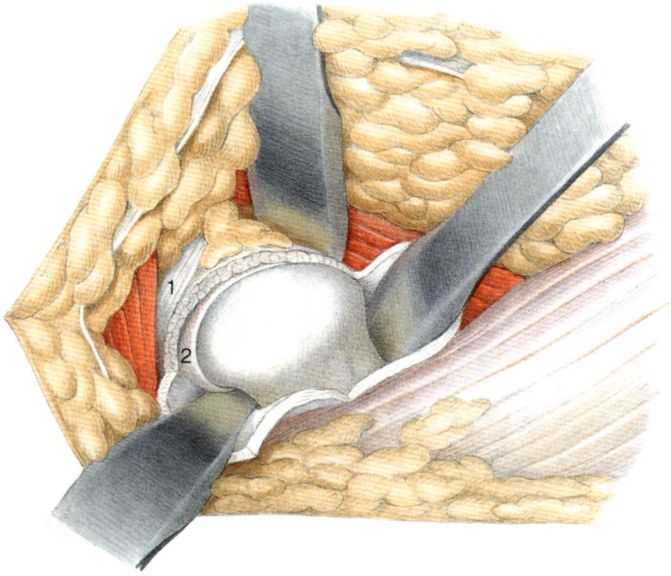

Fig. 2.**30** Opening the door-like capsule flaps provides broad exposure of the hip joint.

1 Reflected origin of the rectus femoris
2 Acetabular labrum

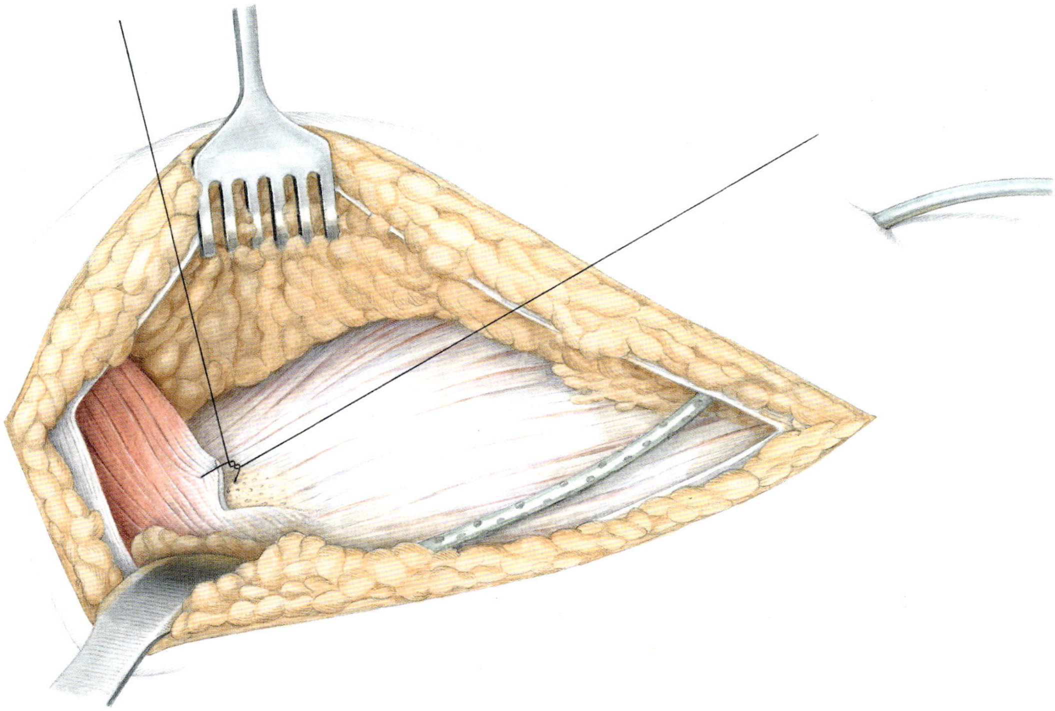

Fig. 2.**31** Closure is begun by reattaching the anterior margin of the gluteus medius to its insertion on the greater trochanter.

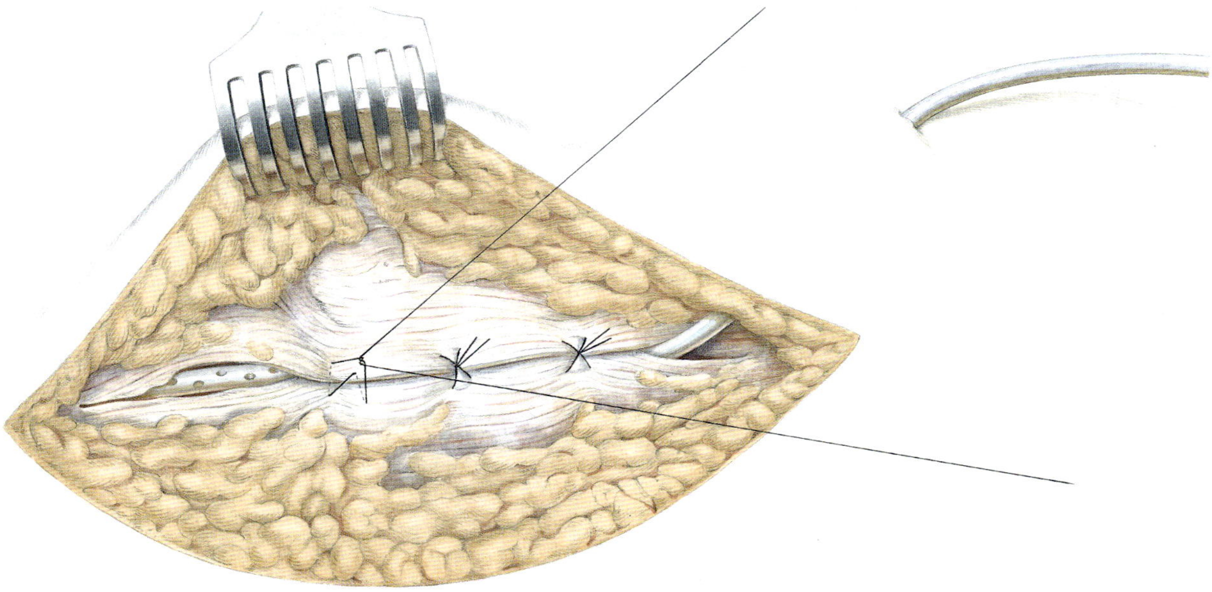

Fig. 2.**32** The fasica lata is closed with a vertical mattress suture, overlapping the lips of the wound.

Hip Surgery Using the Bauer Transgluteal Approach

Indications

The transgluteal approach permits broad lateral exposure of the hip joint and the proximal femur. Its range of indications is the same as with the anterolateral approach; synovectomy of the hip, open reduction and internal fixation of femoral neck fractures, femoral neck osteotomies, slipped capital femoral epiphysis, and total hip arthroplasty. Compared with the anterolateral approach, the transgluteal approach has the advantage of greater simplicity with broader exposure of the hip. However, the procedure requires extensive dissection of the gluteus medius and vastus lateralis.

Positioning and Incision

With the patient positioned supine, a longitudinal skin incision is made which courses across the greater trochanter (see Fig. 1.**8**).

Technique

After dividing the fascia lata parallel to the skin incision, the surgeon splits the gluteus medius, the gluteus minimus, and the vastus lateralis parallel to the direction of their fibers. The anterior half of the tendinous insertion of these muscles is dissected off the greater trochanter in a single layer to preserve the soft-tissue envelope laterally and posteriorly (see Fig. 1.**9**).

With the anterior joint capsule exposed, elevators are placed between the rectus femoris and the anterior acetabular labrum, superiorly between the capsule and the gluteus minimus, inferiorly between the capsule and the iliopsoas tendon. The surgeon opens the capsule with a "T" incision, taking care not to damage the acetabular labrum or the cartilage of the femoral head (see Fig. 1.**10**).

After opening the capsule widely, the surgeon places blunt Hohmann retractors between it and the lateral and medial femoral neck (see Fig. 1.**11**). The surgical options permitted by this exposure range from synovectomy to dislocation of the hip for total joint arthroplasty.

When the wound is closed, the divided musculature is approximated and sutured. Retention sutures are used to close the incision in the tendinous insertions of the two muscles over the greater trochanter (see Fig. 1.**13**). After placing a suction drain, the surgeon closes the fascia lata with an overlapping retention suture.

Hip Surgery Using the Posterior Approach

Indications

The posterior approach primarily exposes the posterior hip with minimal soft-tissue detachment through a small incision. This approach is indicated primarily in treating acetabular fractures, in arthroplasty, and in excising localized tumors.

Positioning and Incision

The patient is generally positioned laterally with the leg draped to permit free movement; the prone position is used only if the procedure so requires. The skin incision begins at the intertrochanteric crest and extends 3 cm distally, parallel to the direction of the fibers of the gluteus maximus and the fascia lata (see Fig. 1.**1**). The incision may be extended distally as far as necessary if exposure of the femur is required. In adipose patients, the lateral position has the advantage that gravity causes the excess soft tissue to fall away from the incision, and the distance between the skin and the hip joint is shorter. This reduces venous stasis and bleeding.

Technique

When the fascia lata and gluteus maximus are divided parallel to the direction of their fibers and retracted, the cushion of fatty tissue covering the short external rotators and the sciatic nerve is exposed. Always expose the sciatic nerve when using the posterior approach; often there will be perineural adhesions that can now be removed, and the nerve is most easily protected when exposed. The subfascial cushion of fatty tissue is retracted laterally when exposing the sciatic nerve and then returned to its original position. It should not be resected because it has an important protective function.

With the leg in internal rotation, the surgeon severs the short external rotators and the piriformis at the intertrochanteric crest (see Fig. 1.**10**). The surgeon should preserve a strip of tissue 1 cm wide at the insertion to facilitate subsequent reattachment. If this is not possible due to scarring, then the short external rotators may later be reattached to the bone.

The musculature is dissected from the joint capsule and retracted posteriorly, the gluteus medius and gluteus minimus are lifted with an elevator, and another elevator is inserted at the lower margin of the femoral neck. The surgeon now makes a "T" incision in the broadly exposed capsule (see Fig. 1.**3**), and opens the flaps like doors (see Fig. 1.**4**). Two elevators can be inserted on either side of the femoral neck to increase exposure of the hip joint.

If the capsule remains limited, as is often the case when there is severe periarticular scarring, a trochanteric osteotomy can be performed to improve exposure (see Fig. 1.**5**). Before performing the osteotomy, the surgeon should insert a narrow curved elevator anteriorly to gauge the proper plane of osteotomy and to prevent damage to the blood supply to the femoral neck.

If the hip is to be dislocated, this is done posteriorly with the leg flexed and in internal rotation. When closing the wound, the surgeon must securely reduce the osteotomized greater trochanter and verify that the sciatic nerve is not damaged by the sutures when the external rotators are reattached. When closing the fascia lata, make sure that the hip musculature is under sufficient tension to ensure stability.

Surgical Correction of a Snapping Hip

Indication

In a snapping hip, the iliotibial tract moves anteriorly and posteriorly over the greater trochanter when the hip is flexed, extended, and rotated in flexion. This generally occurs when the patient stands or walks. This phenomenon is palpable at the greater trochanter, but can be so severe that it is visible or audible. The large bursa located between the greater trochanter and the iliotibial tract can become inflamed by mechanical irritation, causing severe pain.

The snapping hip phenomenon is not necessarily pathologic; often the patient has the "ability" to induce and control the phenomenon voluntarily, so that surgical treatment is not necessarily indicated. However, surgical intervention is often indicated when the condition is accompanied by severe pain, loss of function, weakness, and rapid onset of fatigue.

Pronounced thickening of the iliotibial tract can be observed in a snapping hip; the gluteus maximus can be seen to fan out into posterior margin of the iliotibial tract, and its superior fibers are closer to horizontal than normal (Fig. 2.**33**). The tension of the iliotibial tract exerts an anterior pull on the tract, while the gluteus maximus exerts a posterior pull. With the hip flexed, or if the femur is in external rotation, the iliotibial tract is anterior to the greater trochanter. With the hip extended, or if the femur is in internal rotation, the gluteus maximus pulls the iliotibial tract posteriorly across the greater trochanter. The result is a forceful snapping motion. The common treatment of suturing the iliotibial tract leaves these tensile mechanisms intact, which explains the frequency of recurrence.

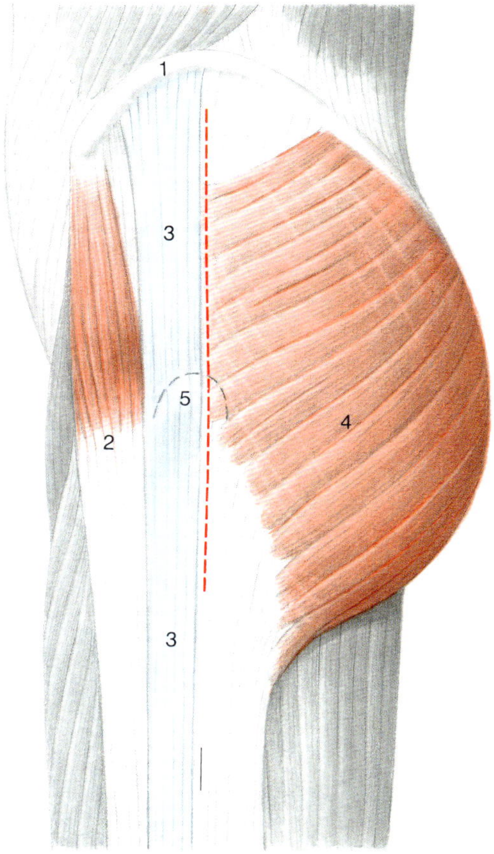

Fig. 2.**33** Snapping hip with pronounced thickening of the iliotibial tract. The superior fibers of the gluteus maximus are closer to horizontal than normal.

1 Iliac crest
2 Tensor fasciae latae
3 Iliotibial tract
4 Gluteus maximus
5 Position of the greater trochanter (dotted line)

Positioning and Incision

The patient is positioned laterally. The skin incision is made across the posterior margin of the greater trochanter (Fig. 2.**35**). Positioning the patient laterally with the leg draped to permit free movement permits the surgeon to intraoperatively verify elimination of the snapping mechanism.

Technique

The snapping phenomenon is reliably eliminated by improving the way tensile forces act on the anatomic structures. The gluteus maximus is dissected from the posterior margin of the iliotibial tract with a longitudinal incision extending distally 5 cm from the apex of the greater trochanter. This causes the iliotibial tract to retract anteriorly. The posterior edge of the incision is sutured to the greater trochanter and the tendon of the gluteus medius and the gaping split in the fascia lata is left open (Fig. 2.**34**). The iliotibial tract now remains anterior to the greater trochanter in every movement and the snapping action is eliminated. The longitudinal incision in the fascia lata does significantly affect the tension acting on the lateral hip, nor does it significantly impair hip stability.

When the subcutaneous fatty tissue is retracted, the fascia lata appears as a broad band. After this, the thickened iliotibial tract can be seen anteriorly, and the gluteus maximus posteriorly. The dividing line between the two is sharply demarcated (Fig. 2.**36**). The fascia lata is incised with a scalpel along the dividing line between the iliotibial tract and the gluteus maximus (Fig. 2.**37**). Using a sharp periosteal elevaotor, the surgeon carefully separates all the muscle fibers from the iliotibial tract.

After the incised fascia is retracted, a large thick-walled trochanteric bursa (often inflamed) generally appears on the outer surface of the greater trochanter. This bursa is resected completely (Fig. 2.**38**).

The posterior edge of the incised fascia is retracted to the posterior margin of the greater trochanter and fixed in this position. The anterior edge of the incised fascia with the iliotibial tract automatically retracts to behind the anterior margin of the greater trochanter. The posterior edge of the incised fascia with the gluteus maximus is securely fixed with several sutures to the posterior margin of the greater trochanter, the posterior margin of the gluteus medius tendon, and the vastus lateralis (Fig. 2.**39**). The broad gap in the fascia, extending 5 cm distally from the apex of the greater trochanter, is left open when the wound is closed. Fine fascial tissue will soon form to bridge the gap. The surgeon closes the wound over a suction drain.

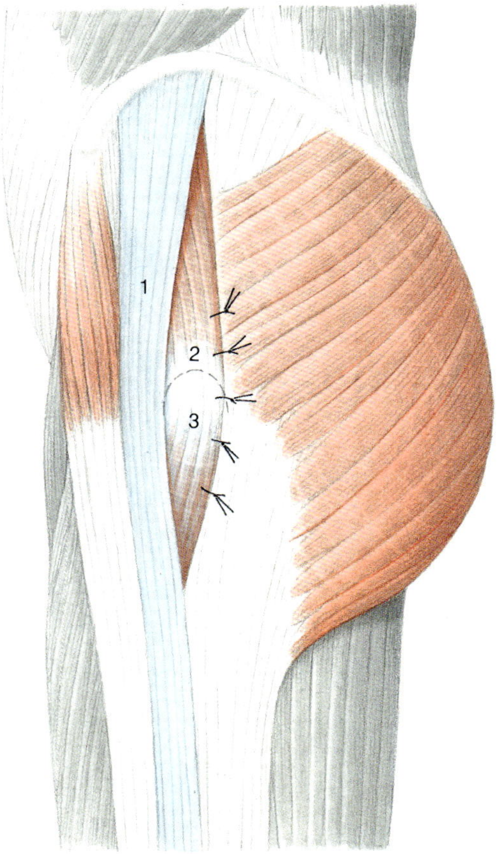

Fig. 2.**34** The posterior incised edge of the fascia lata is sutured to the tendon of the gluteus medius, the posterior margin of the greater trochanter, and the tendon of the vastus lateralis. The gaping incision in the fascia lata posterior to the iliotibial tract is left open.

1 Iliotibial tract
2 Tendon of the gluteus medius
3 Vastus lateralis

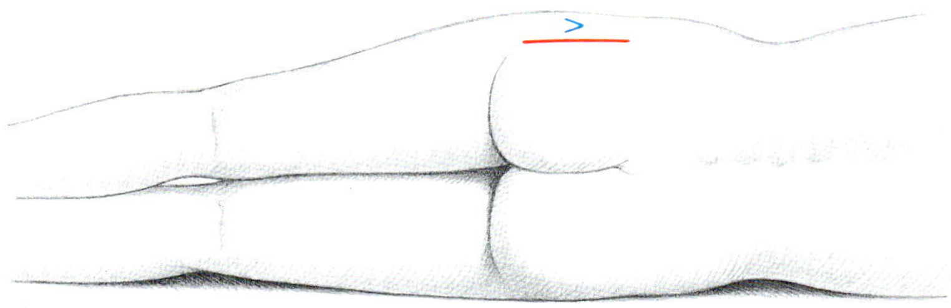

Fig. 2.**35** Lateral positioning and incision for surgical treatment of a snapping left hip. The skin incision is made across the posterior margin of the greater trochanter.

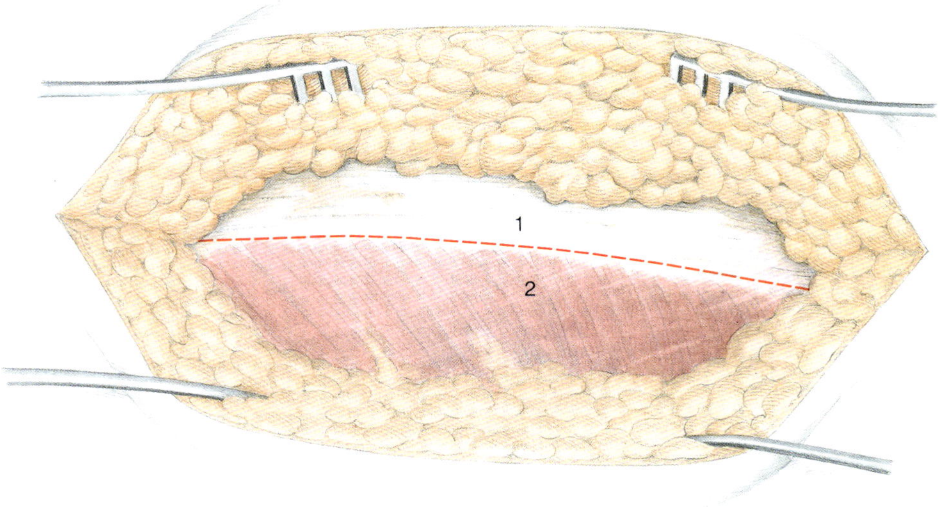

Fig. 2.**36** When the subcutaneous fat is retracted, the sharply demarcated dividing line between the thickened iliotibial tract and the gluteus maximus is exposed.

1 Iliotibial tract
2 Gluteus maximus

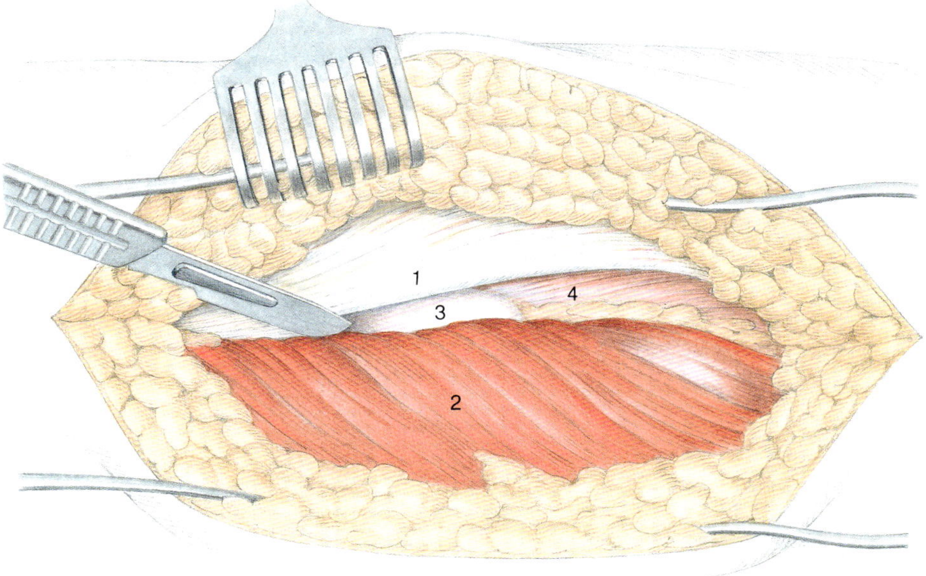

Fig. 2.**37** The fascia lata is incised along the anterior margin of the gluteus maximus. The distended trochanteric bursa and the gluteus medius are now visible in the deep layer.

1 Iliotibial tract
2 Gluteus maximus
3 Trochanteric bursa
4 Gluteus medius

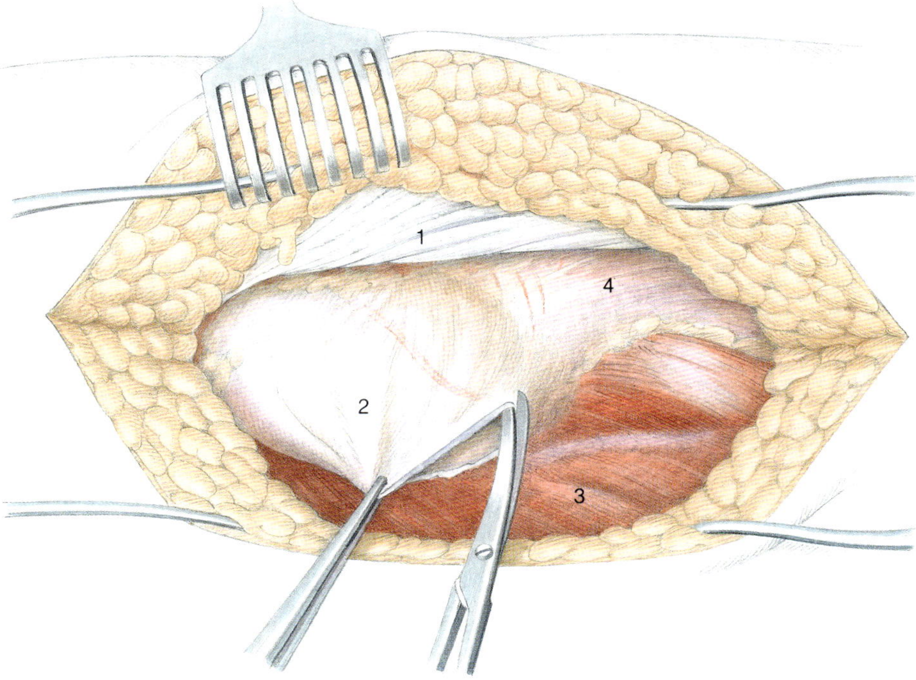

Fig. 2.**38** The thick-walled trochanteric bursa is resected.

1 Iliotibial tract
2 Trochanteric bursa
3 Gluteus maximus
4 Gluteus medius

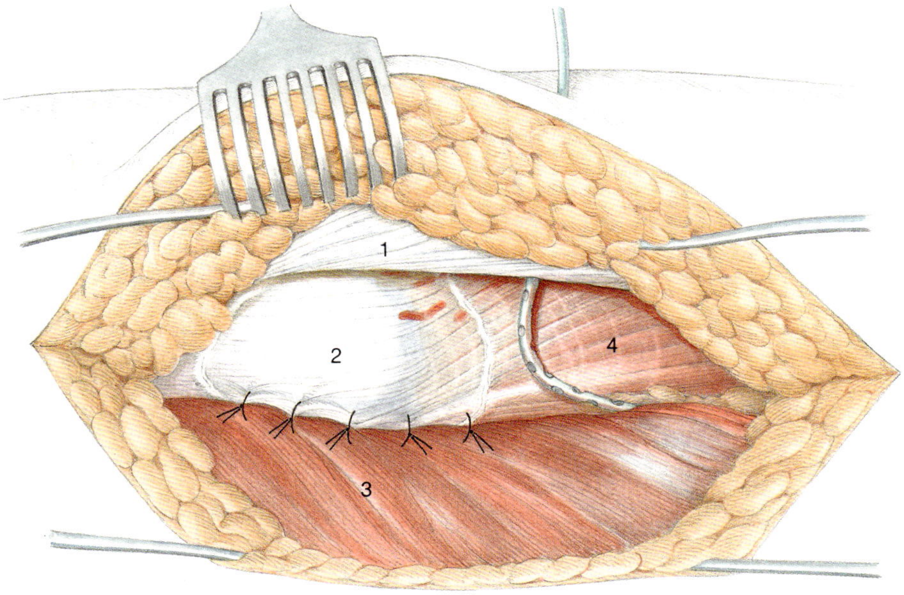

Fig. 2.**39** The posterior edge of the incised fascia with the gluteus maximus is securely fixed with several sutures to the posterior margin of the greater trochanter, the posterior margin of the gluteus medius tendon, and the vastus lateralis. The anterior edge of the incised fascia with the iliotibial tract automatically retracts to behind the anterior margin of the greater trochanter and does not require fixation.

1 Iliotibial tract
2 Greater trochanter
3 Gluteus maximus
4 Gluteus medius

Acetabular Surgery

Open Reduction of a Developmentally Dislocated Hip Using an Anterior Approach

Indications

Congenital subluxation or dislocation of the hip or teratologic dislocation if radiological and arthrographic findings or previous conservative treatment have shown that closed reduction will not be successful. The surgical treatment is most effective on children between 6 and 18 months old.

Positioning and Incision

The patient is positioned supine for the anterior approach. Since soft tissue is easily displaced in infants, a short skin incision is sufficient, keeping in mind that the scar will become larger as the child grows.

Technique

The soft-tissue structures that inhibit reduction are resected to permit the femoral head to enter the acetabulum so that it is in direct contact with the articular surface of the acetabulum. Even slight remaining lateral displacement will inevitably result in dislocation.

The dislocation of the joint has expanded the joint capsule and elongated the ligament of the head of the femur. The acetabular labrum no longer fits snugly against the femoral head and has drawn together in the form of a ring, shortening the transverse acetabular ligament. In addition to these deformities, the lack of compression from the femoral head results in hyperplasia of the pulvinar.

When closed reduction is attempted, all of these soft-tissue structures can help inhibit reduction:

The shrunken acetabular labrum, drawn together distally by the transverse acetabular ligament, reduces the size of the acetabular opening, preventing the femoral head from deeply engaging the acetabulum. The elongated ligament of the head of the femur and enlarged pulvinar cover the floor of the acetabulum and do not leave sufficient space to deeply engage the femoral head. In addition to his, the expanded joint capsule impinges between the greater trochanter and the roof of the acetabulum and prevents the proximal femur from reaching a sufficiently medial position.

Correct open reduction requires the removal of all these soft-tissue impediments: The superior and anterior sections of the joint capsule, the ligament of the head of the femur and the transverse acetabular ligament are resected, and the size of the pulvinar is reduced accordingly. Lastly, radial posterosuperior and anterosuperior incisions are made in the shrunken acetabular labrum so that it can unfold and remain in intimate contact with the femoral head after reduction. Such a thorough removal of the impediments to reduction is only possible through a surgical approach that exposes the entire circumference and roof of the acetabulum. Partial removal of the impediments will limit the reliability of the reduction.

The curved skin incision extends approximately 4 cm and courses 1 cm lateral of and parallel to the iliac crest, equally proximal and distal to the anterior superior iliac spine (Fig. 2.**40**). When the subcutaneous fatty tissue is retracted, the anterior margin of the fascia of the tensor fasciae latae is split parallel to the direction of its fibers. The medial fascia is retracted medially to protect the lateral femoral cutaneous nerve embedded in the fatty tissue. The surgeon then dissects the tensor fasciae latae and the anterior section of the gluteus medius from the outer surface of the ilium (Fig. 2.**41**). After elevating the sartorius to expose the rectus femoris with its two heads of origin, the surgeon exposes the joint capsule and the lateral surface of the ilium (Fig. 2.**42**). The reflected origin is resected. Now, the soft-tissue attachments of the joint capsule, visible as a snow white body, must be carefully dissected. This significantly reduces bleeding and improves exposure. The iliopsoas tendon and the distal surface of the anterior inferior iliac spine now come into view in the deep layer of the wound. Finally, the surgeon incises the joint capsule along the acetabular labrum, taking care not to damage the labrum or the cartilage of the femoral head (Fig. 2.**43**).

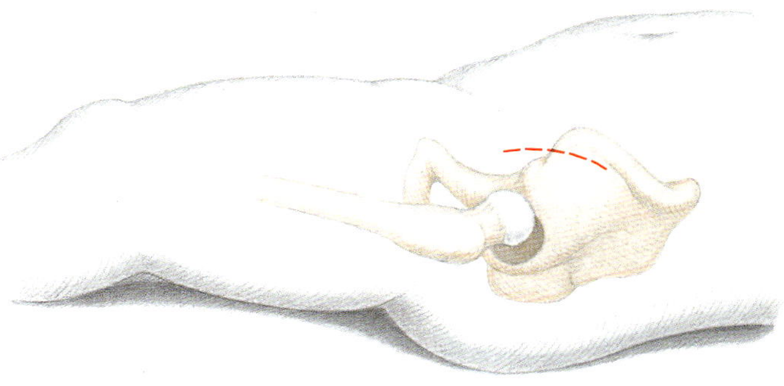

Fig. 2.**40** Positioning and incision for open reduction of a dislocated left hip. The skin incision 1 cm lateral of and parallel to the iliac crest.

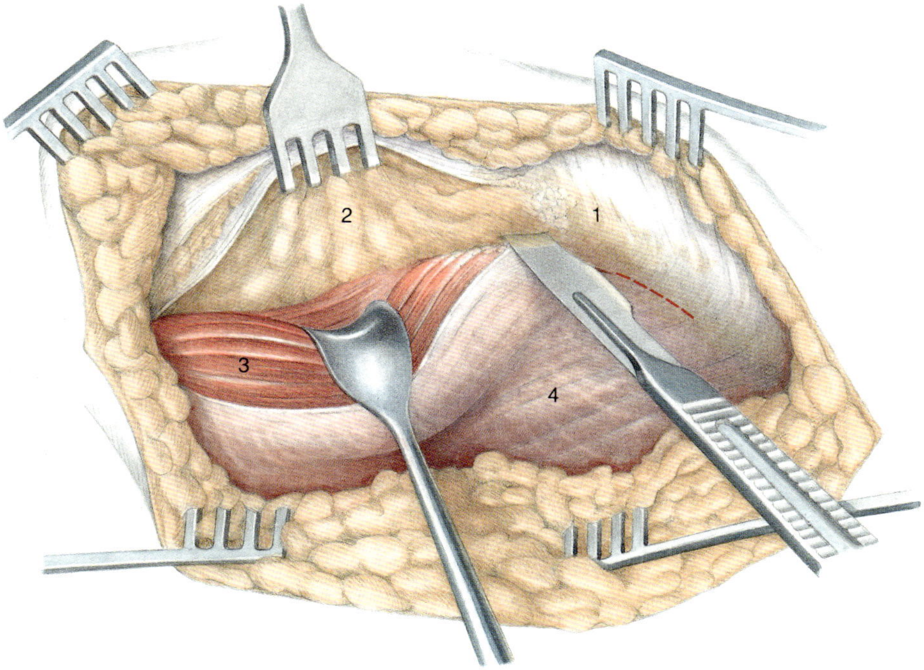

Fig. 2.**41** After the fascia above the tensor fasciae latae is split parallel to the direction of its fibers, the tensor fasciae latae and the anterior section of the gluteus medius are dissected from the outer surface of the ilium.

1 Anterior superior iliac spine
2 Medial fascia covering the lateral femoral cutaneous nerve
3 Tensor fasciae latae
4 Gluteus medius

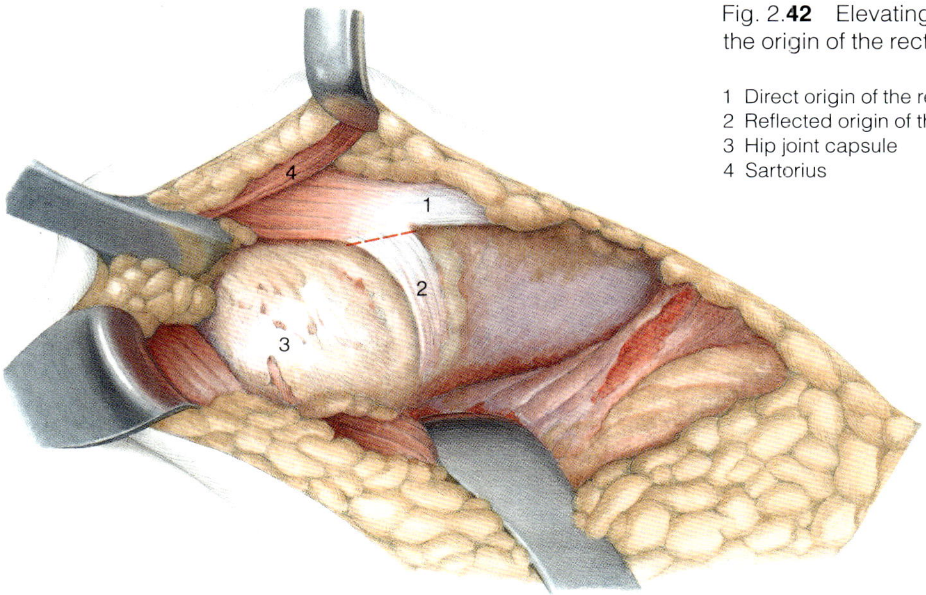

Fig. 2.**42** Elevating the sartorius exposes the joint capsule and the origin of the rectus femoris. The reflected origin is resected.

1 Direct origin of the rectus femoris
2 Reflected origin of the rectus femoris
3 Hip joint capsule
4 Sartorius

The iliopsoas is lifted and narrow elevators are inserted medially at the pubis and distally at the hip joint capsule. The surgeon then resects the anterior section of the joint capsule, taking care not to damage the acetabular labrum (Fig. 2.**44**). With the leg in external rotation, the femoral head is even more prominent beneath the acetabular labrum. The surgeon lifts the widened and elongated ligament of the head of the femur with a fine bone hook and severs it at the fovea capitis, taking care not to damage the articular cartilage (Fig. 2.**45**).

Fig. 2.**43** Elevating the direct origin of the rectus femoris exposes the iliopsoas tendon in the deep layer of the wound.

1 Iliopsoas tendon
2 Direct origin of the rectus femoris
3 Anterior inferior iliac spine
4 Hip joint capsule

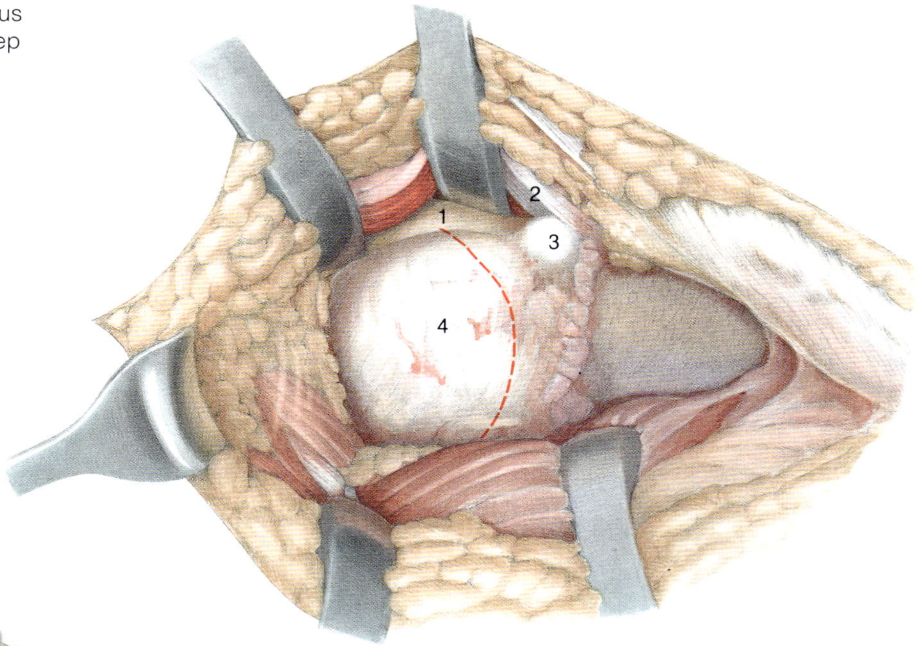

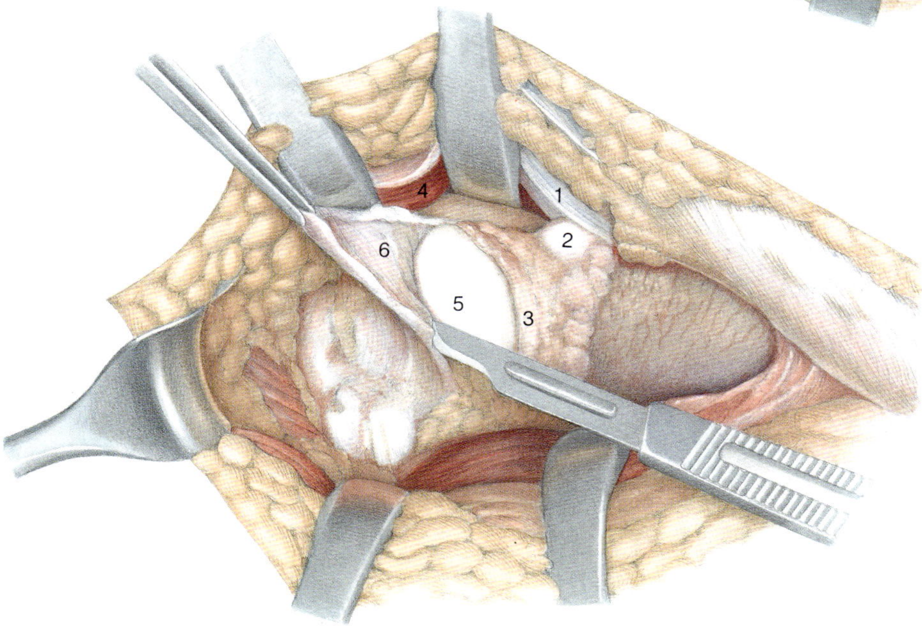

Fig. 2.**44** A narrow elevator inserted into the pubis is now used to lift the iliopsoas and the direct origin. A second elevator is inserted distally outside the capsule at the femoral neck. This broadly exposes the joint capsule. The surgeon then resects the anterior section of the joint capsule, taking care not to damage the acetabular labrum.

1 Direct origin of the rectus femoris
2 Anterior inferior iliac spine
3 Acetabular labrum
4 Iliopsoas
5 Femoral head
6 Hip joint capsule

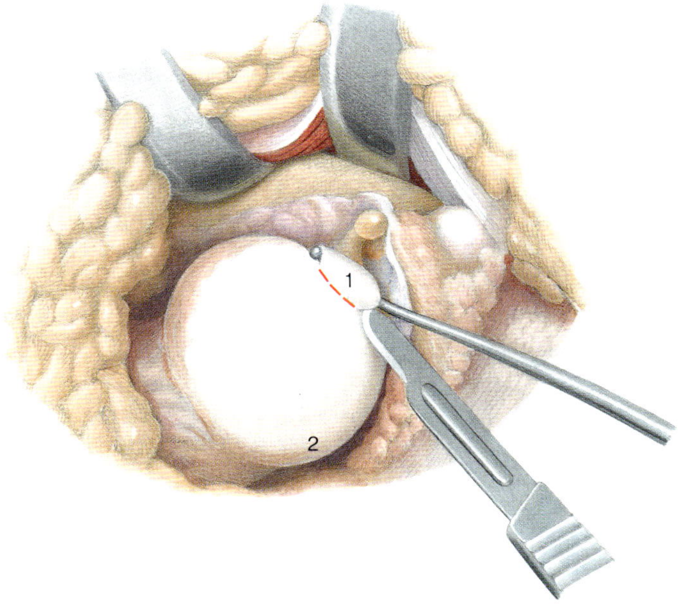

Fig. 2.**45** With the leg in external rotation, the surgeon lifts the ▶ widened and elongated ligament of the head of the femur with a narrow bone hook and transects it at the fovea capitis, taking care not to damage the articular cartilage.

1 Ligament of the head of the femur
2 Head of the femur

After the ligament of the head of the femur has been severed, the femoral head can be completely removed from beneath the acetabular labrum. With the leg flexed, the femoral head can be posteriorly dislocated, exposing the entire circumference of the acetabulum. The ligament of the head of the femur and part of the pulvinar are resected in the acetabular fossa. Part of the fatty tissue of the pulvinar is left in place (Fig. 2.**46**). The transverse acetabular ligament is resected at the respective union with the posterior and anterior sides of the acetabular labrum and removed (Fig. 2.**47**). The acetabular fossa now contains only the remainder of the pulvinar, and resecting the transverse acetabular ligament eliminates the distal narrowing of the acetabulum. The acetabular labrum is now rolled in against the articular surface. Radial postero-

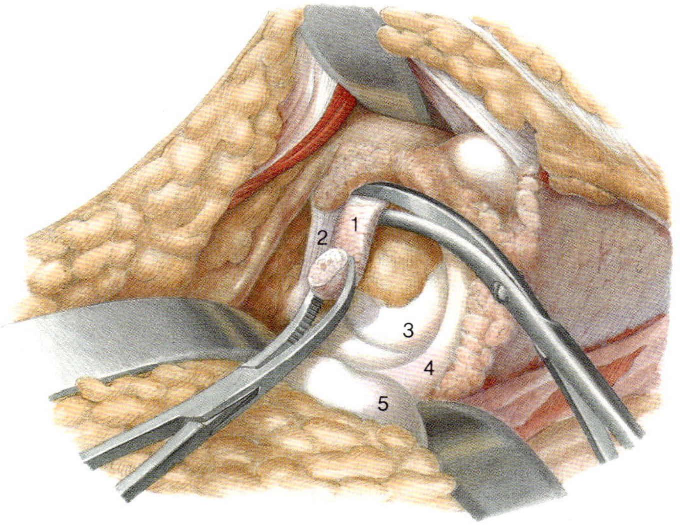

Fig. 2.**46** With the leg flexed in external rotation, the femoral head can be posteriorly dislocated as far as the posterior margin of the acetabulum, exposing the entire circumference of the acetabulum. The ligament of the head of the femur is resected in the acetabular fossa along with part of the pulvinar.

1 Ligament of the head of the femur
2 Transverse acetabular ligament
3 Lunate surface
4 Acetabular labrum
5 Femoral head

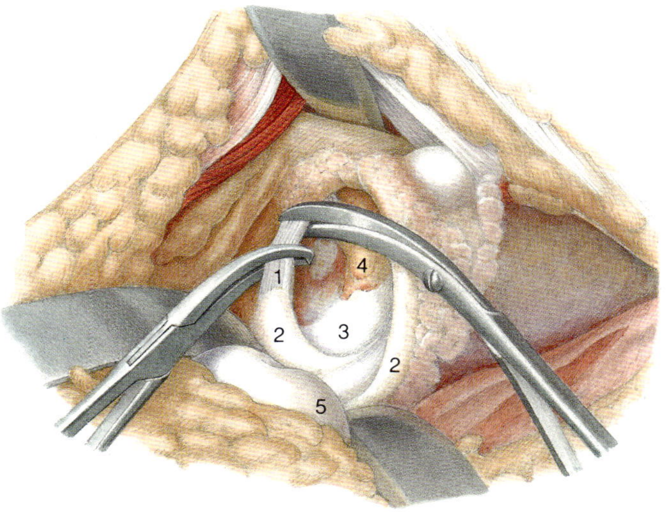

Fig. 2.**47** The transverse acetabular ligament is resected at the respective union with the posterior and anterior sides of the acetabular labrum and removed. This relieves the shrunken acetabular labrum and the acetabular fossa can be distally opened.

1 Transverse acetabular ligament
2 Acetabular labrum
3 Lunate surface
4 Acetabular fossa with pulvinar
5 Femoral head

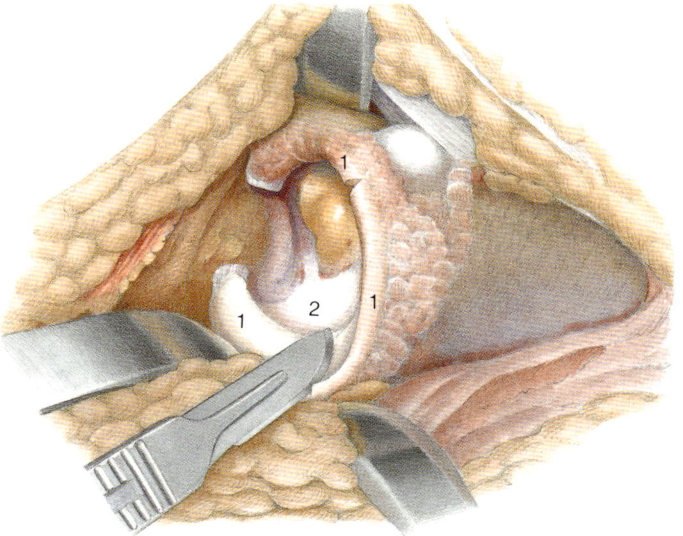

Fig. 2.**48** Radial posterosuperior and anterosuperior incisions are made in the acetabular labrum so that it can unfold and fit snugly against the articular surface of the femoral head.

1 Acetabular labrum
2 Lunate surface

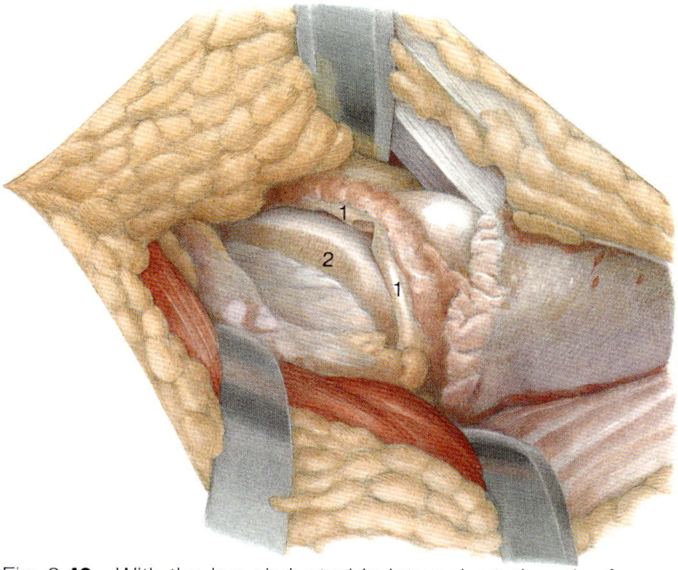

Fig. 2.**49** With the leg abducted in internal rotation, the femoral head is inserted beneath the acetabular labrum deep into the acetabulum. The incised, relieved labrum fits snugly against the femoral head.

1 Acetabular labrum
2 Femoral Head

superior and anterosuperior incisions are made in the acetabular labrum so that it can unfold and fit snugly against the articular surface of the femoral head after the dislocation is reduced. Avoid resecting the labrum because this could produce ossification on the acetabular margin (Fig. 2.**48**). With the leg abducted in internal rotation, the femoral head is inserted beneath the acetabular labrum deep into the acetabulum. The mobilized labrum fits snugly against the articular surface of the femoral head. After the dislocation has been reduced and the femoral head deeply engages the acetabulum, the distance between the greater trochanter and the acetabular margin is very short, and the remaining sections of the capsule might impede medial positioning (Fig. 2.**49**).

With the leg abducted in internal rotation, the surgeon reattaches the musculature to the ilium. After placing a fine suction drain, he or she closes the wound (Fig. 2.**50**). The skin incision is closed with a continuous fine-subcutaneous suture (Fig. 2.**51**). The surgeon should make every effort to avoid superficial scarring.

A plaster hip spica to keep the leg slightly abducted and internally rotated is applied for 3 weeks postoperatively. The belly portion of the cast is removed 1 week postoperatively to permit practicing hinge motion by sitting up. Three weeks postoperatively, the surgeon should assess whether a derotation osteotomy of the proximal femoral is required. In rare cases, an intertrochanteric osteotomy will be required during surgical reduction.

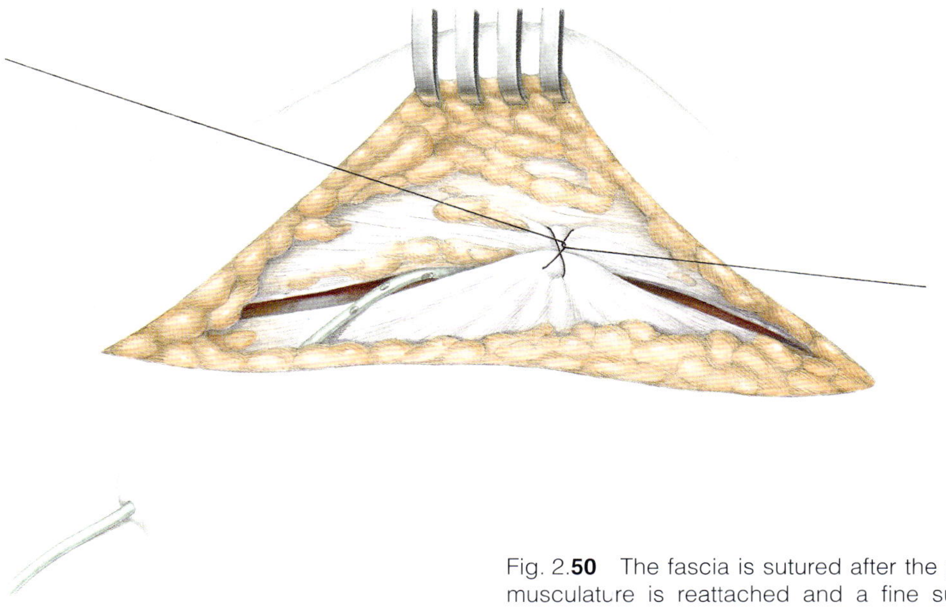

Fig. 2.**50** The fascia is sutured after the pelvic and trochanteric musculature is reattached and a fine suction drain has been placed.

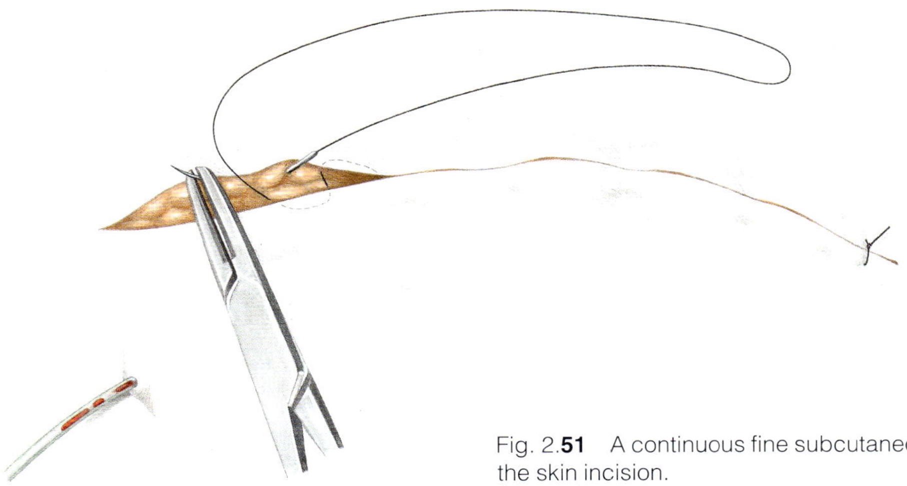

Fig. 2.**51** A continuous fine subcutaneous suture is used to close the skin incision.

Shelf Procedures

Indications

For surgical treatment of congenital dislocation of the hip in children where there is insufficient coverage of the femoral head and flattening of the acetabulum.

Typically, there is a dysplastic acetabulum with increasing subluxation; the radius of curvature of the acetabulum is greater than that of the femoral head, and the femoral head moves superiorly and inferiorly in the flattened acetabulum when the leg is abducted or adducted (Fig. 2.**52**). Radiographic follow-up generally reveals gradually increasing superior migration in these hips. A single radiographic examination revealing incomplete coverage of the femoral head in the skeletally immature patient does not provide sufficient information for prognosis and is not an indication for surgery. A cetabular surgery is only indicated when radiographic follow-up reveals increasing subluxation, or fluoroscopy demonstrates joint instability and the possibility of spontaneous healing can be excluded. Shelf procedures are indicated not only to widen the roof of the acetabulum, but also to stabilize the joint.

Positioning and Incision

An anterior approach is used with the patient positioned supine.

The skin incision courses 1.5 cm lateral of and parallel to the iliac crest. After the fascia lata is split, the lateral surface of the ilium and the joint capsule are exposed between the tensor fasciae latae and the sartorius.

Technique

The classic shelf procedures (Fig. 2.**53a** and **b**) have attempted to improve the superior support of the femoral head and reduce the tendency to sublux by widening the roof of the acetabulum over the joint capsule. The disadvantage of this procedure is that this support is not provided with articular cartilage; joint capsule interposed between the bone graft and the femoral head acts as the missing articular surface. The durability of the interposed capsule is limited. In addition to this, these shelf procedures do not alter the curvature of the acetabulum. In the authors' modified procedure described in the following section, an osteotomy is performed similarly to a crescentic acetabular osteotomy. Crescent-shaped gouges are used between the two superior arms of the triradiate cartilage to facilitate shaping the roof of the acetabulum. The corrected position of the superior acetabulum is secured by autologous or allograft bone chips implanted in the gap created by the osteotomy (Fig. 2.**54**).

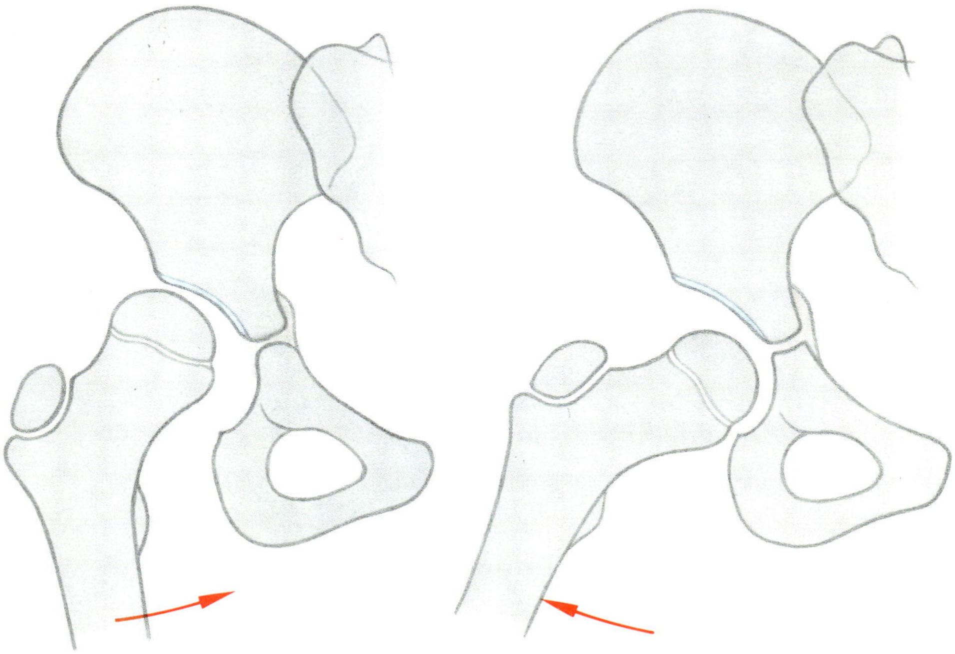

Fig. 2.**52** The typical indication for a shelf procedure is a flattened acetabulum whose radius of curvature is greater than that of the femoral head so that the femoral head migrates superiorly and inferiorly n the acetabulum when the leg is abducted or adducted. This phenomenon is accompanied by joint instability and a tendency toward lateral displacement or subluxation.

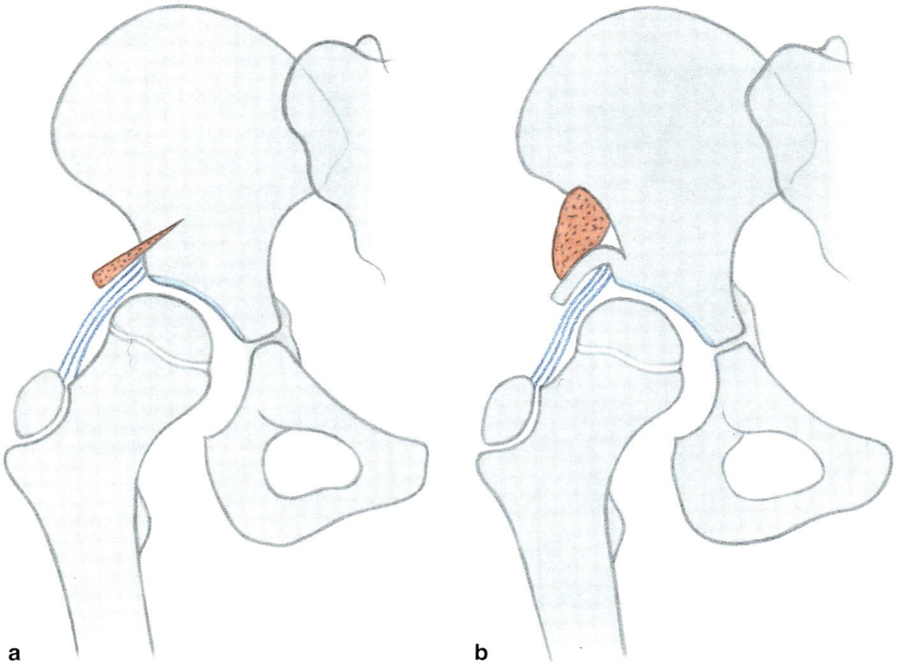

Fig. 2.**53a** and **b** Examples of classic shelf procedures:
a In the Spitzy shelf procedure, a bone wedge is inserted into the ilium superior to the margin of the acetabulum outside of the joint capsule. The graft widens the roof of the acetabulum and supports the femoral head superiorly. The anatomic articular surface is not widened, rather the interposed joint capsule acts as the missing articular surface.
b In the Wilson shelf procedure, a corticocancellos flap is excised from the lateral surface of the ilium and bent distally. This bone flap is held in position by a bone wedge inserted superior to it. In this procedure also, the interposed joint capsule acts as an extension of the articular surface and the curvature of the acetabulum is not altered.

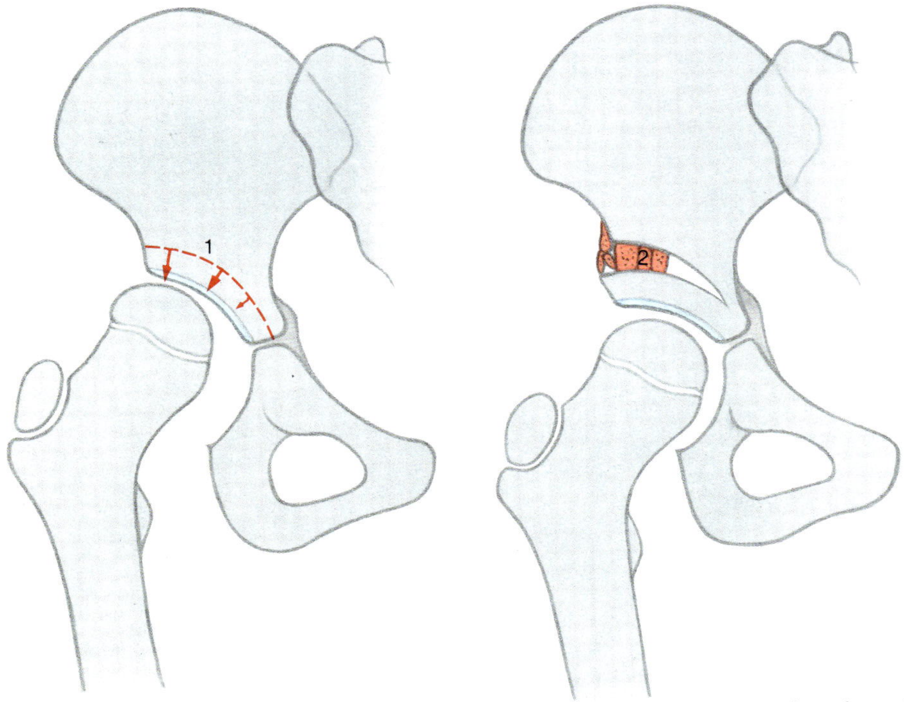

Fig. 2.**54** Shelf procedure with corrective shaping of the roof of the acetabulum. A crescent-shaped incision is made around the superior section of the dysplastic acetabulum. This section is then mobilized and its cartilaginous articular surface molded to fit the femoral head. The gap created by the osteotomy is filled with bone chips.

1 A crescent-shaped osteotomy is performed arount the superior portion of the acetabulum, parallel to the articular surface.
2 After the superior part of the acetabulum is molded to fit the femoral head, the resulting deep gap created by the osteotomy is filled with bone chips.

The skin incision courses 1.5 cm lateral of and parallel to the iliac crest, extending laterally and distally from the anterior superior iliac spine in a gentle curve (see Fig. 2.**17**). The edges of the wound are retracted, broadly exposing the fascia lata and iliac crest. The tensor fasciae latae and sartorius are clearly visible beneath the fascia lata. The thin fascia is split above the anterior margin of the tensor fasciae latae parallel to the direction of its fibers. The tensor fasciae latae is bluntly dissected from the medial fascial septum. The muscular septum covering the lateral surface of the sartorius and the fatty tissue beneath it that covers the lateral femoral cutaneous nerve is retracted medially. This procedure protects the cutaneous nerve (see Fig. 2.**18**).

The origin of the rectus femoris, the joint capsule, and the anterior margin of the ilium are now exposed in the deep layer of the wound (see Fig. 2.**19**). The tensor fasciae latae, gluteus medius, and gluteus minimus are dissected one after the other from the iliac wing until the joint capsule margin is sufficiently exposed (see Fig. 2.**20**). The reflected origin of the rectus femoris is resected and the direct origin dissected so that the anterior section of the capsule margin is also accessible (see Fig. 2.**21**). A marker wire is inserted into the ilium at the planned osteotomy site superior to the margin of the capsule to indicate the correct osteotomy level (Fig. 2.**55**). The position of the marker wire is verified with fluoroscopy (Fig. 2.**56**).

The surgeon makes a crescent-shaped cut around the acetabulum superior to the triradiate cartilage with a wide osteotome whose radius of curvature matches that of the acetabulum. When making the cut, he must maintain a distance of 5–7 mm from the articular surface (distance varies according to the patient's age) so that the layer of bone mobilized will be thick enough to prevent a fracture of the articular surface (Fig. 2.**57**). Penetration of the osteotome toward the triradiate cartilage is monitored with fluoroscopy (Fig. 2.**58**).

The crescentic osteotomy around the acetabulum is performed gradually with extreme care and verified with fluoroscopy to prevent unintentional injury, particularly to the triradiate cartilage. As soon as the osteotomy has been completed and the osteotome has attained a sufficient depth, it is levered distally, widening the gap created by the osteotomy (Fig. 2.**59**). In children, the bone is pliable and can be readily molded to the required contour. A narrow bone spreader can be used to widen the osteotomy gap.

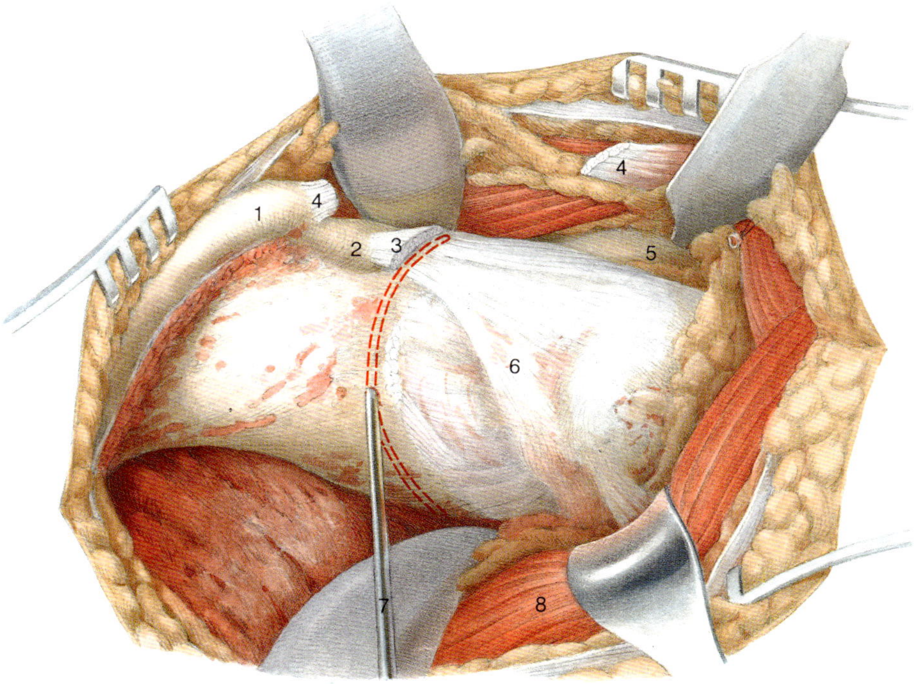

Fig. 2.**55** After the direct origin has been dissected and the capsule broadly exposed, a marker wire is inserted into the ilium superior to the roof of the acetabulum to mark the osteotomy level.

1 Anterior superior iliac spine
2 Anterior inferior iliac spine
3 Direct origin of the rectus femoris (dissected)
4 Sartorius
5 Pubis
6 Hip joint capsule
7 Marker wire indicating osteotomy site
8 Tensor fasciae latae

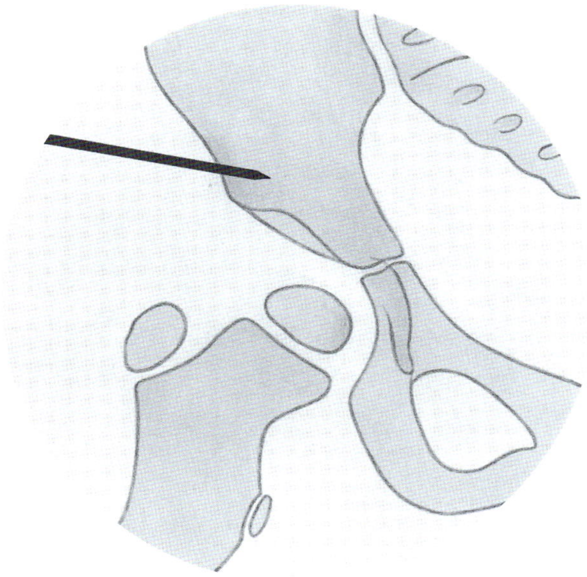

Fig. 2.**56** The position of the marker wire is verified with fluoroscopy.

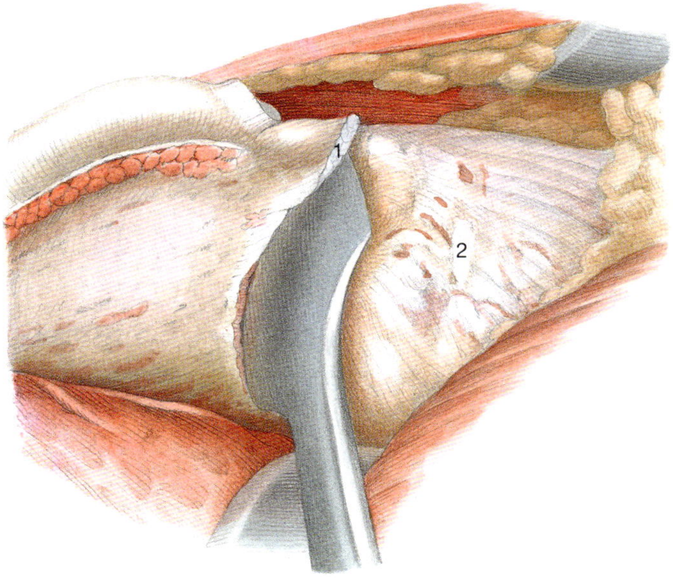

Fig. 2.**57** With a wide gouge, the curvature radius of which matches that of the acetabulum, a crescent-shaped cut is made around the acetabulum superior to the triradiate cartilage at the marked position.

1 Direct origin of the rectus femoris (transected)
2 Hip joint capsule

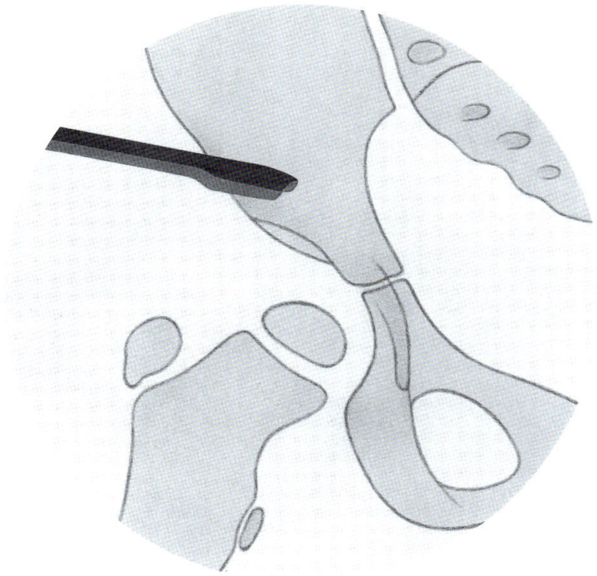

Fig. 2.**58** Penetration of the gouge toward the triradiate cartilage is monitored with fluoroscopy.

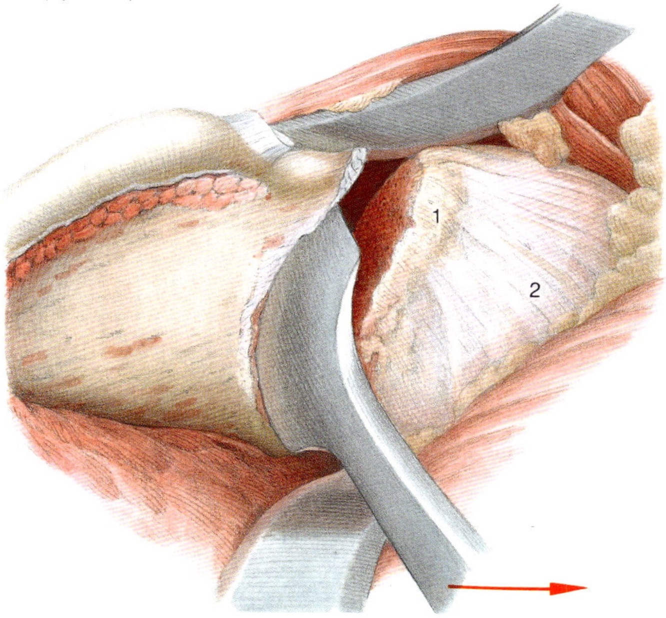

Fig. 2.**59** After the osteotomy has been completed, the gouge is levered distally, widening the gap created by the osteotomy and pressing the roof of the acetabulum down onto the femoral head.

1 Osteotomized roof of the acetabulum
2 Hip joint capsule

The corrected position of the roof of the acetabulum is secured by a wedge-shaped corticocancellous bone allograft implanted in the gap created by the osteotomy perpendicular to the osteotomy plane (Fig. 2.**60**). In most cases, three grafts placed at equal intervals along the osteotomy plane will be sufficient to prevent deformation of the articular surface. Cancellous bone chips are taken with a narrow gouge from the lateral surface of the iliac crest, distal to the cartilaginous apophysis and are inserted between the bone wedges to accelerate integration (Fig. 2.**61**). The results of the shelf procedure and the stability of the joint with the leg in abduction and adduction are verified with fluoroscopy (Fig. 2.**62**).

The rectus femoris is reattached to the anterior inferior iliac spine (Fig. 2.**63**). The pelvic and trochanteric musculature is securely sutured to the iliac crest (Fig. 2.**25**). After a suction drain has been inserted, the thin fascia above the tensor fasciae latae is sutured with fine suture material, and the wound is closed in layers.

The acetabular bone graft is strong enough that it does not require any additional external fixation. However, small children are more easily cared for when placed in a generously padded cast that permits limited motion.

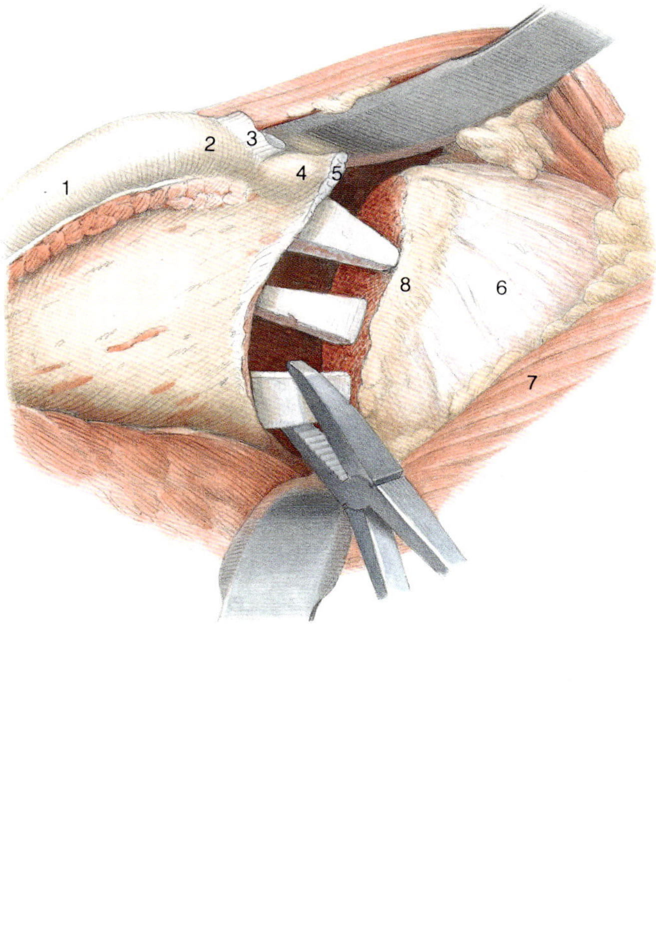

Fig. 2.**60** To secure the corrected position of the roof of the acetabulum, corticocancellous bone chips (from the bone bank) are implanted in the gap created by the osteotomy perpendicular to the osteotomy plane.

1 Iliac crest
2 Anterior superior iliac spine
3 Sartorius
4 Anterior inferior iliac spine
5 Dissected direct origin of the rectus femoris
6 Hip joint capsule
7 Tensor fasciae latae
8 Roof of acetabulum in corrected position

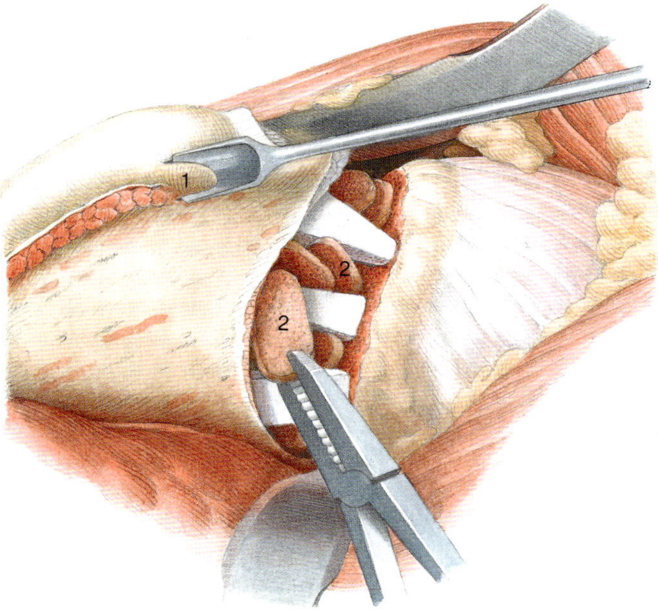

Fig. 2.**61** Cancellous bone chips are taken with a narrow gouge from the lateral surface of the iliac crest, distal to the cartilaginous apophysis and inserted between the bone wedges in the gap created by the osteotomy.

1 Removing chips from the lateral surface of the iliac crest
2 Cancellous chips in the osteotomy gap

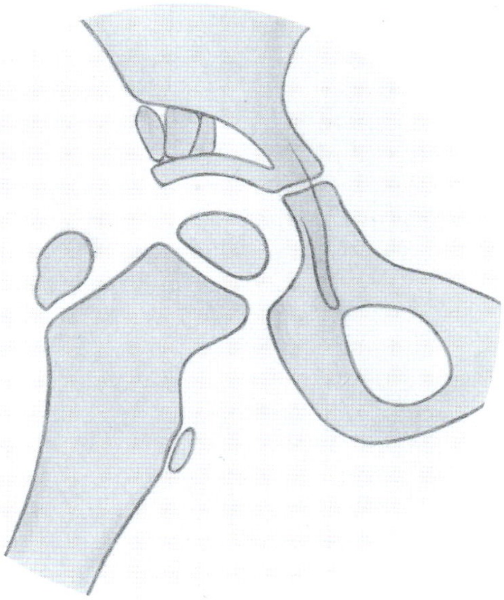

Fig. 2.**62** The results of the shelf procedure with the leg in abduction and adduction are verified with fluoroscopy.

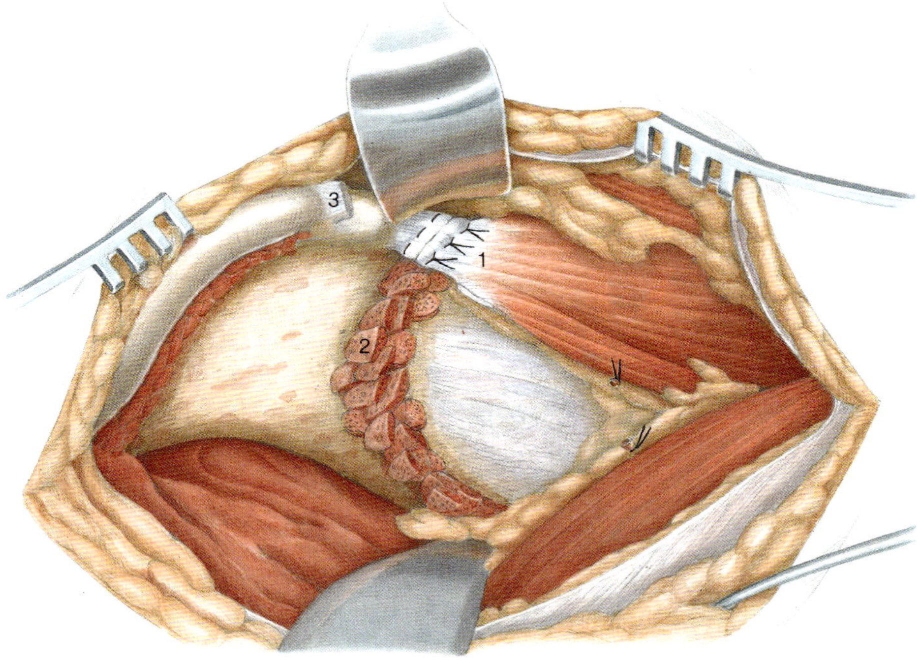

Fig. 2.**63** The rectus femoris is securely sutured to the anterior inferior iliac spine.

1 Rectus femoris
2 Cancellous chips in the osteotomy gap
3 Sartorius (dissected)

Acetabular Osteotomy

Indication

For surgical treatment of congenital dislocation of the hip with acetabular insufficiency after the triradiate cartilage has closed.

Positioning and Incision

The patient is positioned supine for the anterior approach. The skin incision courses 2 cm lateral of the iliac crest (see Fig. 2.**17**).

Technique

An extra-articular crescentic osteotomy mobilizes the dysplastic acetabulum, leaving the capsule intact. Using crescent-shaped gouges, the surgeon separates the acetabulum from the underlying bone with a hemispherical cut around the acetabulum that is concentric with the articular surface. The acetabulum is then shifted laterally and anteriorly with respect to the underlying bone to achieve the best possible coverage of the femoral head. The acetabular osteotomy can be performed in three versions:

Type I: Simple periacetabular osteotomy to correct the position of the acetabulum (Fig. 2.**64**).

Type II: If the center of the dysplastic acetabulum is too far superior and Shenton's line is interrupted, the position of the mobilized acetabulum is corrected and the acetabulum is inclined distally a maximum of 15 mm. Further distal inclination risks increased intra-articular compression (Fig. 2.**65**).

Type III: If the center of the dysplastic acetabulum is too far lateral, the periacetabular osteotomy is combined with a transverse osteotomy of the ilium superior to the acetabulum (similar to a pelvic osteotomy), and the joint is shifted medially. Both the periacetabular osteotomy and the transverse osteotomy of the ilium have the same radius of curvature, so that all the osteotomy surfaces will fit together after the positions of the fragments have been corrected (Fig. 2.**66**).

In all three versions of the acetabular osteotomy, the fragments are stabilized with internal fixation. This eliminates the need for a cast and permits mobilization of the hip immediately postoperatively.

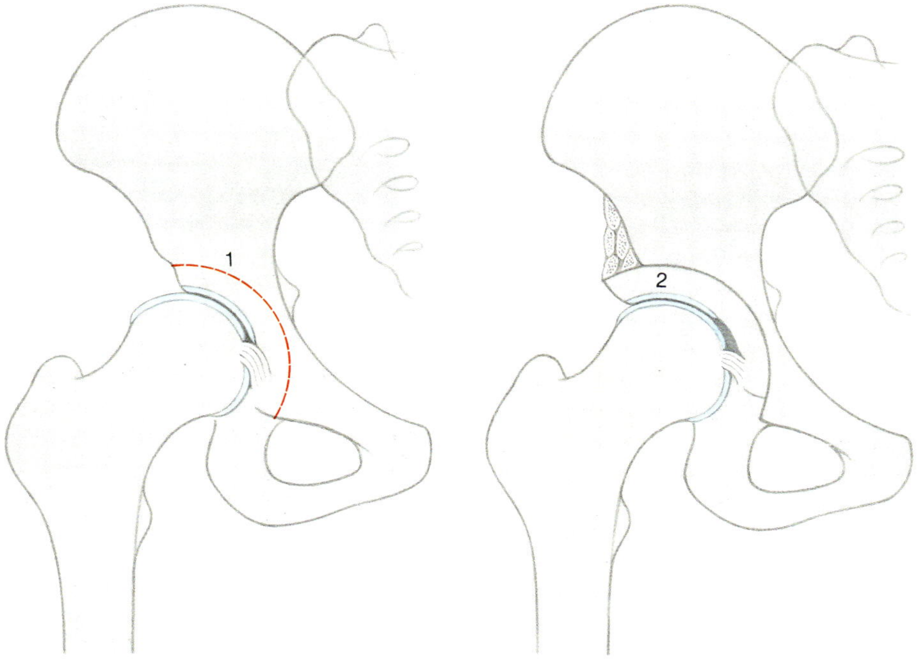

Fig. 2.**64** Type I crescentic acetabular osteotomy. The dysplastic acetabulum is shifted laterally and anteriorly within the hemispheric periacetabular osteotomy.

1 Hemispheric periacetabular osteotomy surface
2 Mobilized acetabulum shifted to correct position

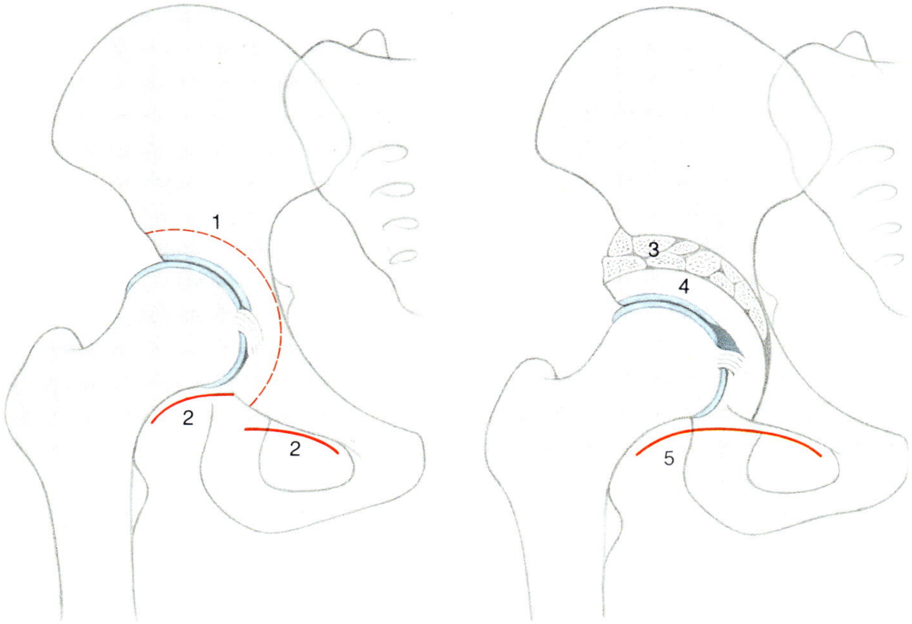

Fig. 2.**65** Type II crescentic acetabular osteotomy. The osteotomized dysplastic acetabulum is shifted to the correct position and inclined distally. The gap created by the osteotomy is filled with cancellous bone chips.

1 Hemispheric periacetabular osteotomy surface
2 Interrupted Shenton's line
3 Cancellous bone chips in the gap created by the osteotomy
4 Mobilized acetabulum shifted to correct position
5 Restored Shenton's line

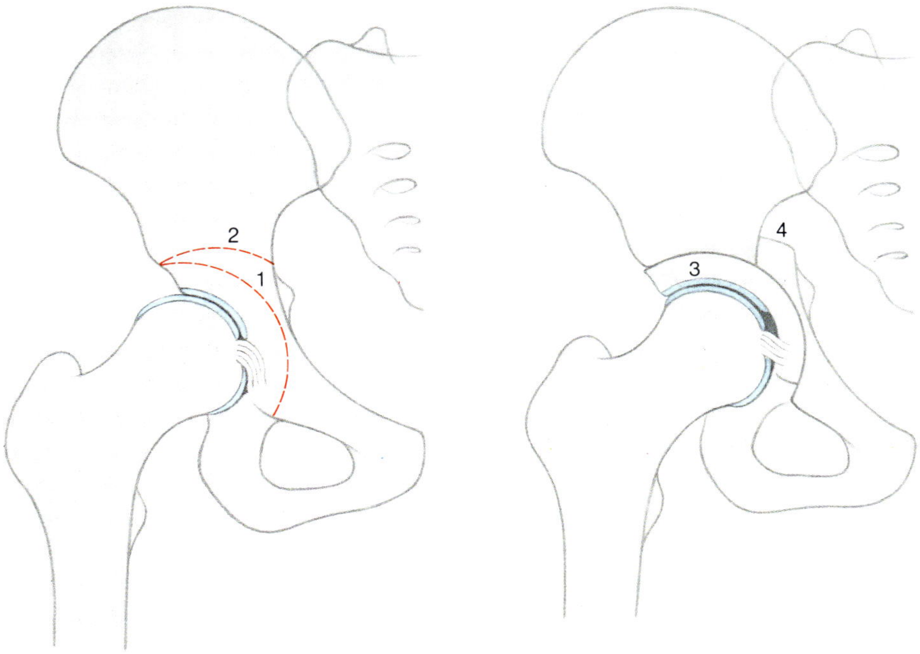

Fig. 2.**66** Type III crescentic acetabular osteotomy. The osteotomy around the dysplastic acetabulum is combined with a matching crescentic transverse osteotomy of the ilium. This permits the entire joint to be shifted medially after the position of the dysplastic acetabulum is corrected.

1 Hemispheric periacetabular osteotomy surface
2 Transverse osteotomy of the ilium with matching radius of curvature
3 Mobilized acetabulum shifted to correct position
4 Protrusion in terminal line after hip joint is shifted medially

After the skin incision has been made and the subcutaneous fatty tissue retracted, the muscular fascia above the anterior margin of the tensor fasciae latae is split parallel to the direction of its fibers. The medial fascia is kept in place to protect the lateral femoral cutaneous nerve, which lies medial of the incision. The tensor fasciae latae is dissected from the medial fascia and retracted laterally (see Fig. 2.**18**). After the deep layer of the fascia has been split, the rectus femoris and ascending branch of the lateral femoral circumflex artery with its adjacent veins are visible. The sartorius is retracted medially (see Fig. 2.**19**). The surgeon now gradually dissects the tensor fasciae latae and the gluteus medius from the lateral surface of the iliac wing. This must be done with great care to avoid splitting the resected origins of the muscles (see Fig. 2.**20**). Now the surgeon resects the reflected origin of the rectus femoris and dissects the direct origin from the anterior inferior iliac spine. He then ligates and severs the ascending branch of the lateral femoral circumflex artery and its adjacent veins (see Fig. 2.**21**).

To gain unrestricted access to the anterior margin of the hip joint capsule, the medial surface of the ilium must also be exposed. This is done by dissecting the sartorius and, if necessary, the inguinal ligament from the anterior superior iliac spine. Together with the iliopsoas, they are lifted and medially retracted (see Fig. 2.**22**). Safely performing the osteotomy requires exposing as much of the acetabular circumference as possible because most of the osteotomy is performed with the unaided eye. This means that the joint capsule is exposed from the obturator foramen anteriorly to the greater sciatic notch posteriorly (Fig. 2.**67**). A marker wire is inserted superior to the proximal capsule margin at the site of the acetabular osteotomy (approximately 12 mm proximal to the articular surface). The distance between the marker wire and the articular surface is verified with fluoroscopy (Fig. 2.**68**). The distance between the osteotomy and the articular surface is very important. If it is too short, the mobilized acetabulum will be too thin and fragile; if it is too long, the osteotomy will be too far from the hip joint, which can significantly complicate the correction.

The crescentic acetabular osteotomy is performed using wide crescent-shaped gouges, which make a hemispherical cut (Fig. 2.**69**). Gouge sets with a radius of curvature of 40–50 mm that can be matched to the diameter of hip joint are used. Each set consists of three gouges with the same radius of curvature. The first or A gouge corresponds to a standard gouge with a defined radius of curvature and is used to cut out a broad 3-mm wide groove in the iliac cortex (which is often quite dense at this site) starting at the marked site and coursing around the margin of the capsule in an arc. The second or B gouge looks somewhat like an ice-cream scoop. It is inserted into the groove cut in the cortex and deepens the osteotomy around the acetabulum, cutting through most of the cancellous bone. The third or C gouge has the same scoop-shaped appearance, but is longer. It is inserted into the osteotomy gap and used to sever the remaining cancellous bridge between the superior ischium and the osteotomized acetabulum. All three gouges are sharp at their tips and dull on their sides to prevent damage to soft tissue.

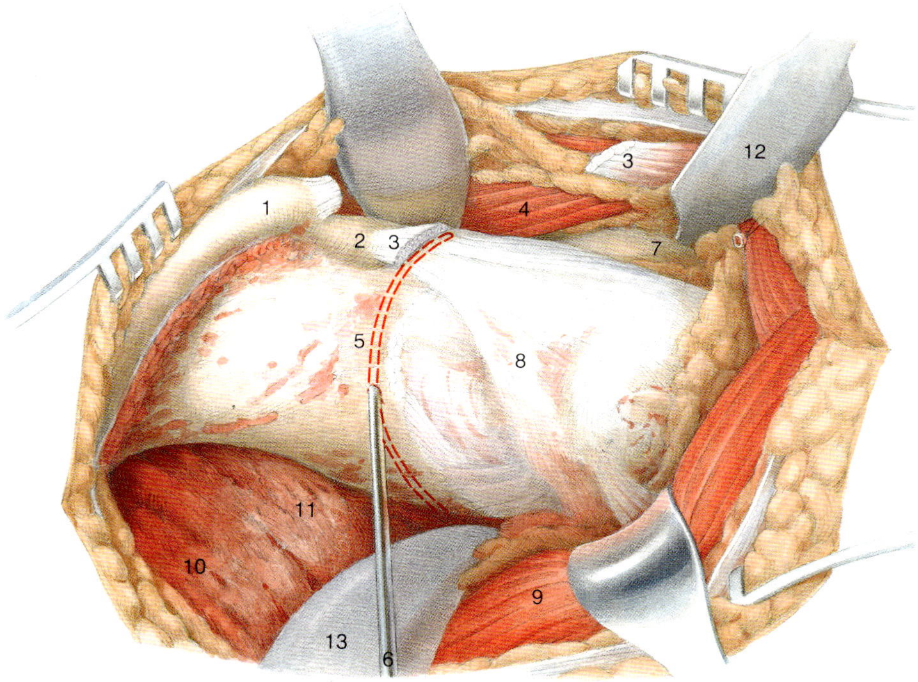

Fig. 2.**67** After the pelvic margin of the joint capsule has been broadly exposed, a marker wire is inserted at the site of the acetabular osteotomy. The double dotted lines mark the curve of the osteotomy.

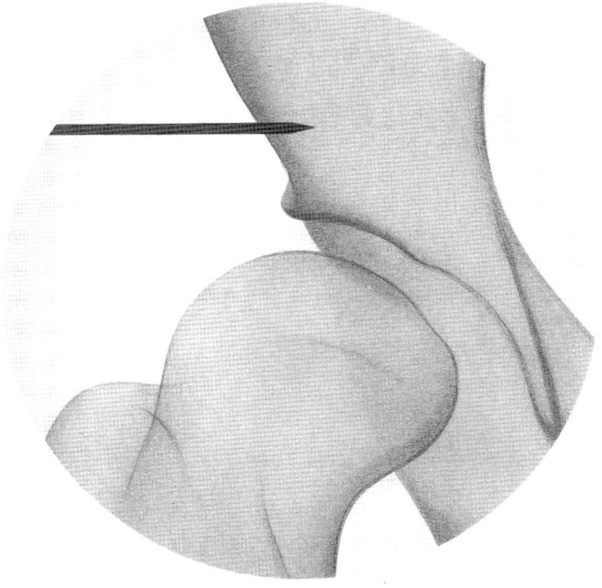

Fig. 2.**68** The distance between the marker wire and the articular surface is verified with fluoroscopy.

The crescentic acetabular osteotomy is performed in two stages. After the A gouge (whose radius of curvature is chosen in preoperative planning) has cut a cortical groove at the marked osteotomy level, the surgeon inserts the B gouge into the groove and drives it about 15 mm into the cancellous bone (Fig. 2.**70**). The gouge cuts around the acetabulum, splitting the teardrop figure. The orientation of the gouge is verified with fluoroscopy (Fig. 2.**71**) as often as necessary. The floor of the acetabulum is generally thickened in a dysplastic hip, so that acetabular circumference is shorter than in a normal hip. This simplifies the periacetabular osteotomy and makes it easier to separate the acetabulum from the bone behind it.

As soon as the correct position of the gouge has been verified, the surgeon begins the osteotomy anteriorly, making the cut with the unaided eye, yet verifying the position of the gouge with fluoroscopy (Fig. 2.**72**). Because of the hypoplasia of the anterior margin of the acetabulum, the gouge passes beyond the medial cortex of the ilium, its path curving farther distally to medially enter the pubic rami, which it then severs. The path of the gouge through the teardrop figure is verified with fluoroscopy (Fig. 2.**73**).

The posterior section of the osteotomy is also performed with the unaided eye. Between the posterior margin of the capsule and the greater sciatic notch, the surgeon can follow the edge of the acetabular gouge as far as the spine of the ischium (Fig. 2.**74**). This is the most difficult part of the osteotomy. The surgeon must allow for the configuration of the dysplastic acetabulum. When it reaches the distal end of the posterior acetabular margin, the gouge must come back out of the bone laterally right next to the margin of the joint capsule. Sometimes it will be necessary to use a gouge with a lesser radius of curvature for this distal posterior section of the osteotomy. In a grossly flattened acetabulum with a large radius of cur-

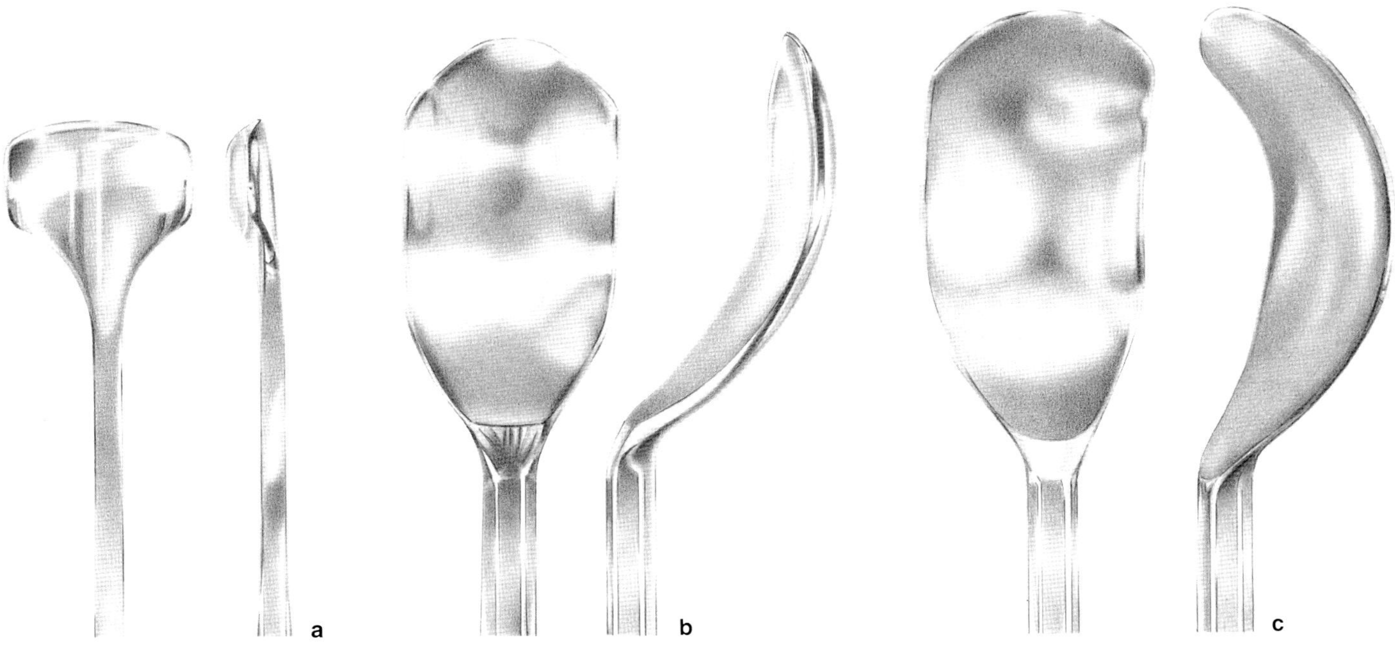

Fig. 2.**69** Gouges with identical radii of curvature for the crescentic acetabular osteotomy.

a A gouge for cutting curved groove in the cortex
b B gouge for acetabular osteotomy in cancellous bone
c C gouge for removing the remaining cancellous bridge between the superior ischium and the osteotomized acetabulum

Fig. 2.**70** The B gouge is inserted into the cortical groove and driven about 15 mm into the cancellos bone.

1 Anterior superior iliac spine
2 Anterior inferior iliac spine
3 Pubic ramus
4 Obturator foramen
5 Hip joint capsule
6 B gouge

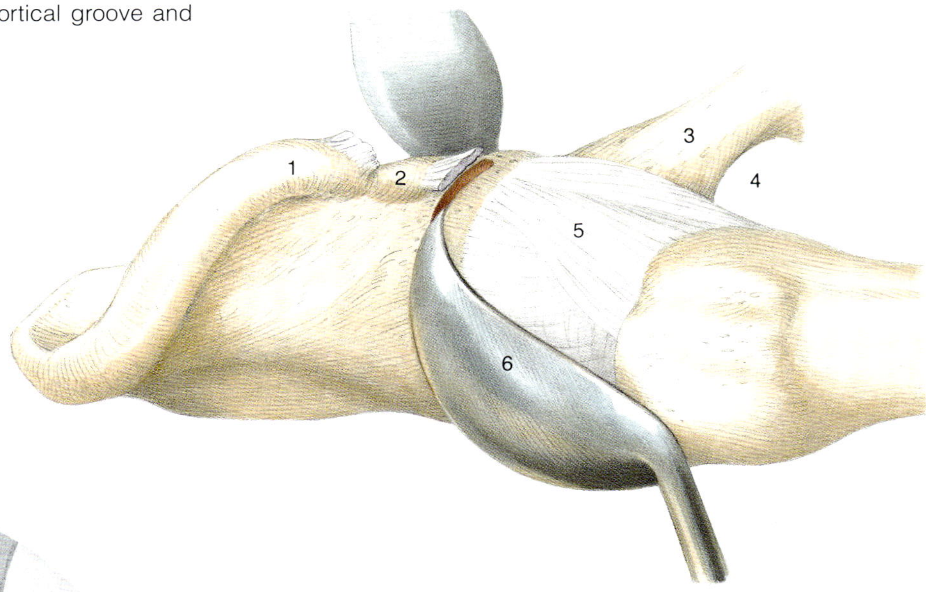

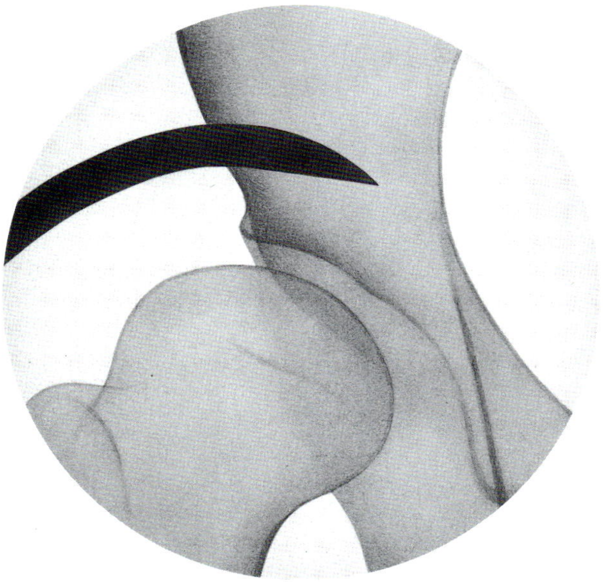

Fig. 2.**71** The orientation of the gouge is verified with fluoroscopy, repeatedly if necessary. The tip of the gouge should point toward the middle of the underlying bone medial of the acetabulum.

Fig. 2.**72** The osteotomy begins anteriorly. The osteotomy itself is performed with the unaided eye, yet the position of the gouge is verified with fluoroscopy. Near the dysplastic anterior acetabular margin, the gouge passes beyond the medial cortex of the ilium, curving farther distally and medially entering the superior aspect pubis, which it severs.

1 Anterior superior iliac spine
2 Anterior inferior iliac spine
3 Pubic ramus
4 Obturator foramen
5 Hip joint capsule
6 B gouge

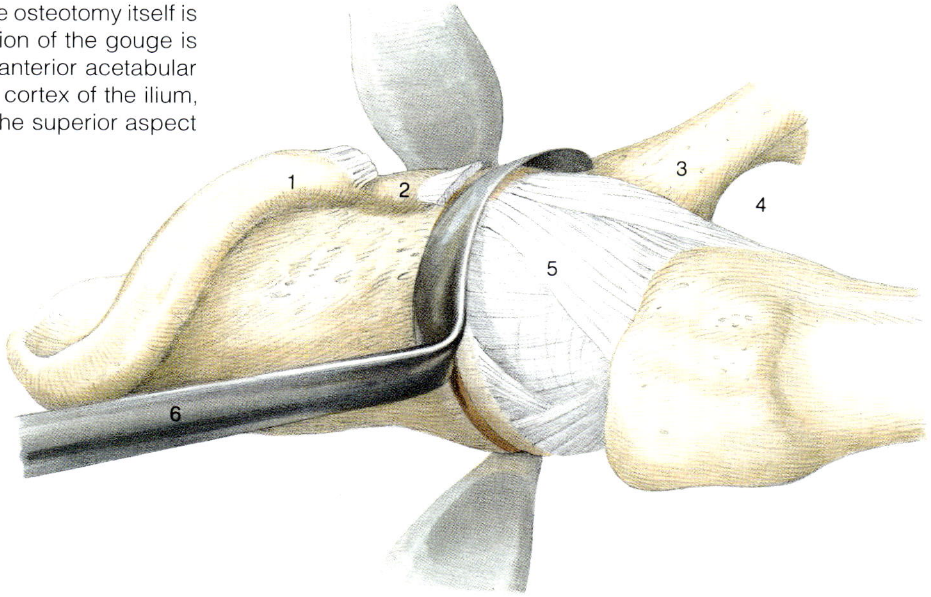

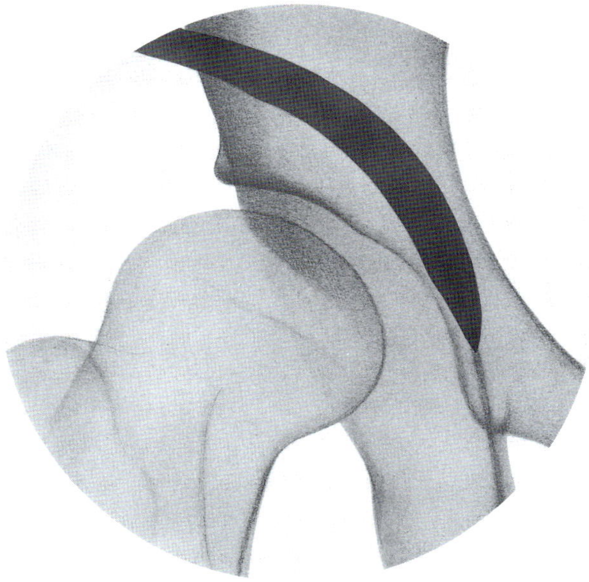

Fig. 2.**73** The path of the gouge through the underlying bone medial of the acetabulum is verified with fluoroscopy.

vature, there is the danger that the osteotomy might extend too far into the pubic rami, making a correction difficult or even impossible. Given proper consideration, this problem can be avoided.

When the anterior and posterior sections of the osteotomy have been completed, the acetabulum is mobilized to the extent that bone spreaders can be used to widen the gap created by the osteotomy (Fig. 2.**75**). The acetabulum is now connected to the superior aspect of the ischium only by a narrow bridge of cancellous bone or by a few fibers of the posterior margin of the capsule. The surgeon can palpate these connections and sever them with the C gouge through the osteotomy gap.

The acetabulum can now be shifted laterally and anteriorly with respect to the underlying bone to achieve the best possible coverage of the femoral head. The dislocation of the acetabulum is often impeded by the remaining parts of the ischiocapsular ligament. These structures can be palpated through the gap created by the osteotomy and severed. They can often be separated by simple manipulation; with the femur abducted, the anterior margin of the acetabulum is pulled laterally with a sharp retractor, while using an elevator inserted in the osteotomy gap as a lever to push the posterior margin of the acetabulum anteriorly.

The corrected position of the acetabulum is verified with fluoroscopy. A long Kirschner wire laid on the patient parallel to the connecting line of the iliac spine represents the horizontal reference plane for the acetabular correction (Fig. 2.**76**).

The position of the acetabulum is stabilized with internal fixation. This keeps the acetabulum in the corrected position. Stability of the osteotomy itself is maintained by the broad area of contact between the rough cancellous bone surfaces in the hemispherical osteotomy. Internal fixation permits early mobilization.

Internal fixation is achieved using two semitubular plates, each with one sharp fork-shaped end. First, the plates are driven into the cancellous bone between the inner and outer tables of the osteotomized acetabular fragment. Then they are fastened to the ilium with screws. This provides sufficient stability. The bone graft is placed on the shelf created by the osteotomy (Fig. 2.**77**).

In the type II acetabular osteotomy, the osteotomy gap is widened to a maximum of 15 mm. Internal fixation is achieved by the same method. The widened osteotomy is filled with bone chips (Fig. 2.**78**).

Fig. 2.**74** The posterior section of the osteotomy is performed without visual aids. Between the posterior margin of the capsule and the greater sciatic notch, the surgeon can follow the edge of the acetabular gouge as far as the spine of the ischium.

1 Point at which pubis is osteotomized.
2 Tip of the acetabular gouge level with the spine of the ischium.

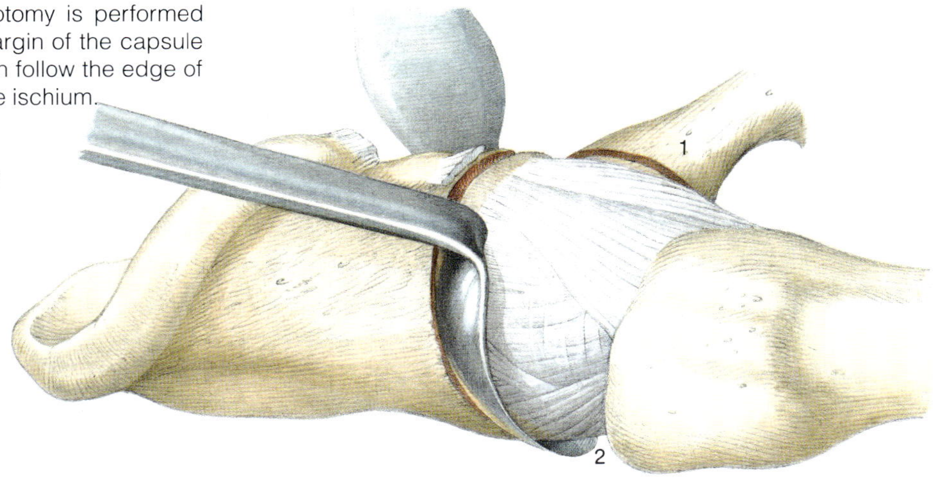

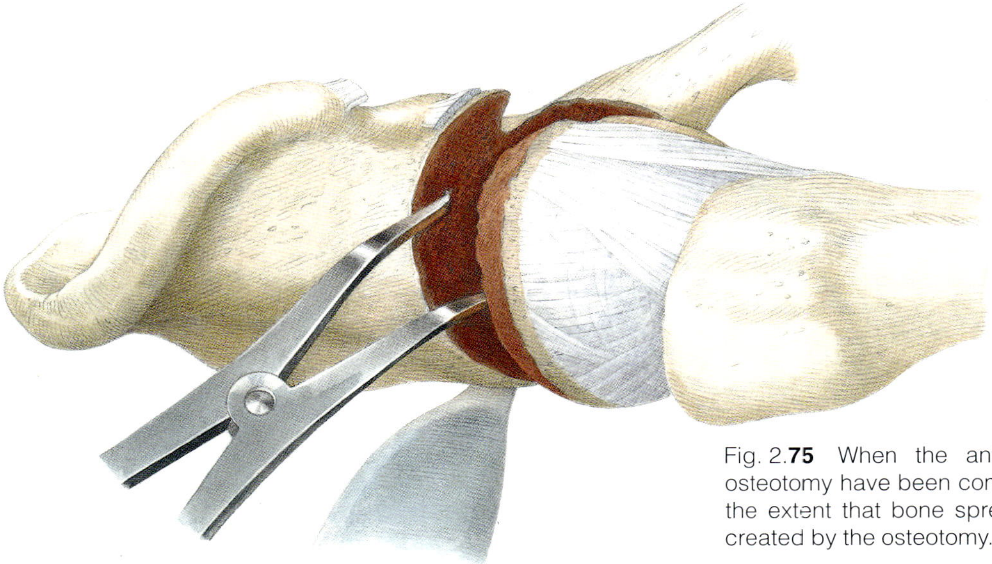

Fig. 2.**75** When the anterior and posterior sections of the osteotomy have been completed, the acetabulum is mobilized to the extent that bone spreaders can be used to widen the gap created by the osteotomy.

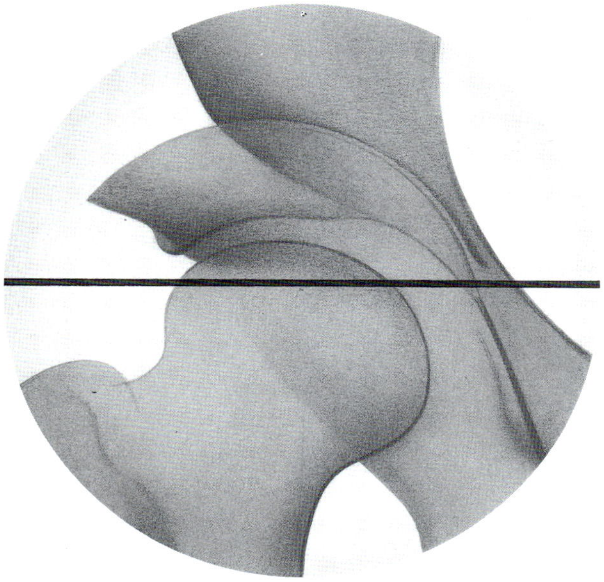

Fig. 2.**76** The corrected position of the acetabulum is verified with fluoroscopy. A long Kirschner wire laid on the patient parallel to the connecting line of the iliac spine represents the horizontal reference plane for the acetabular correction.

In the type III acetabular osteotomy, a transverse osteotomy of the ilium is performed after a periacetabular osteotomy to mobilize the acetabulum. This permits shifting the hip medially to correct its lateral displacement. First, the medial surface of the ilium must be exposed for the transverse osteotomy. A sharp curved periosteal elevator is advanced subperiosteally along the medial surface of the ilium toward the greater sciatic notch (Fig. 2.**79**). Then, a blunt elevator with the same curvature is inserted into the greater sciatic notch. The tip of the elevator is visible laterally deep in the greater sciatic notch. A Gigli saw should be used at least for the posterior part of the transverse osteotomy of the ilium because the bone is extremely brittle and an osteotome might cause the bone to splinter. This would endanger adjacent soft tissue and complicate the realignment of the pelvic fragments.

The Gigli saw can be pulled through the greater sciatic notch with a long thin clamp, but it is best to use a guide instrument. The guide instrument consists of a thin-walled flattened tube with the same radius of curvature as the elevator already in place. The guide instrument is inserted into the greater sciatic notch between the elevator and the medial surface of the pelvis. A metal strip with an eyelet at its tip is fed through the tube. The Gigli saw is tied to the eyelet with a strong thread and pulled through the greater sciatic notch (Fig. 2.**80**). The ilium is then osteotomized along the edge of the previous periacetabular osteotomy (Fig. 2.**81**). As the surgeon makes the transverse cut from posterior to anterior, he moves the Gigli saw distally so that the path of the saw describes an arc that follows the periacetabular osteotomy. The gap created by the osteotomy is opened with a bone spreader inserted laterally. The surgeon then smooths and rounds the superior osteotomy surface with the A gouge for a snug fit with the mobilized acetabulum (Fig. 2.**82**).

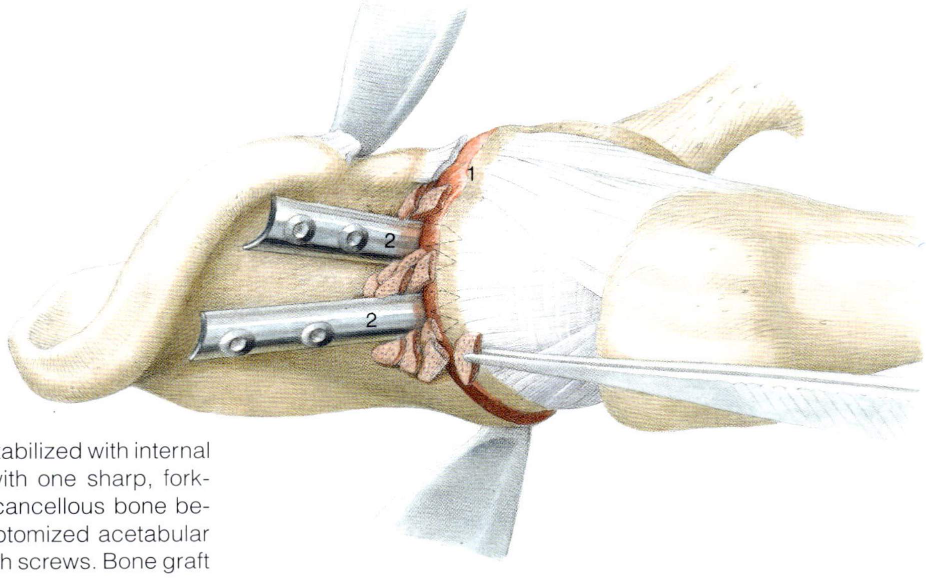

Fig. 2.**77** The position of the acetabulum is stabilized with internal fixation with two semitubular plates, each with one sharp, fork-shaped end. The plates are driven into the cancellous bone between the inner and outer tables of the osteotomized acetabular fragment and then fastened to the the ilium with screws. Bone graft is placed on the shelf created by the osteotomy.

1 Shelf created by shifting tables to corrected position
2 Semitubular plates with their fork-shaped ends impacted in the acetabulum and their shafts fastened to the ilium with bone screws

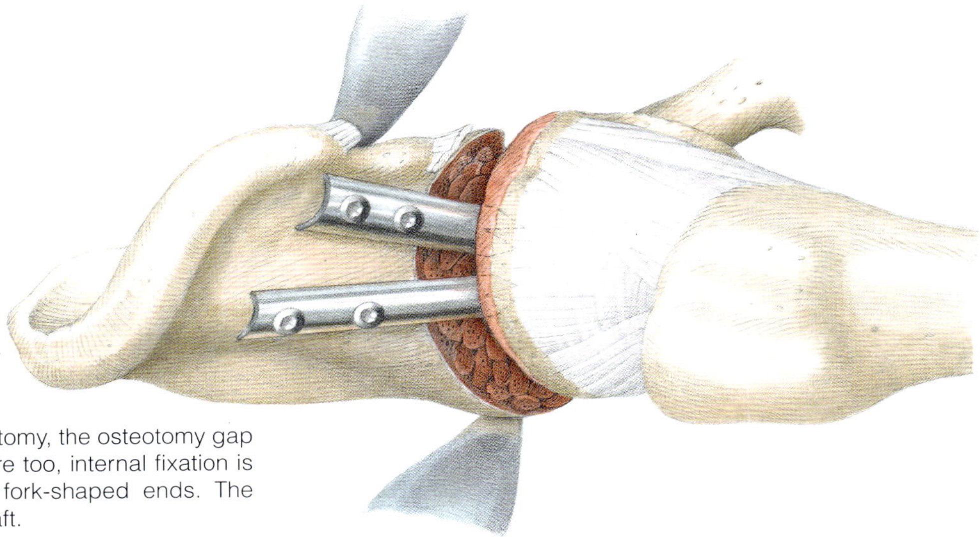

Fig. 2.**78** In the type II acetabular osteotomy, the osteotomy gap is widened to a maximum of 15 mm. Here too, internal fixation is achieved with semitubular plates with fork-shaped ends. The widened osteotomy is filled with bone graft.

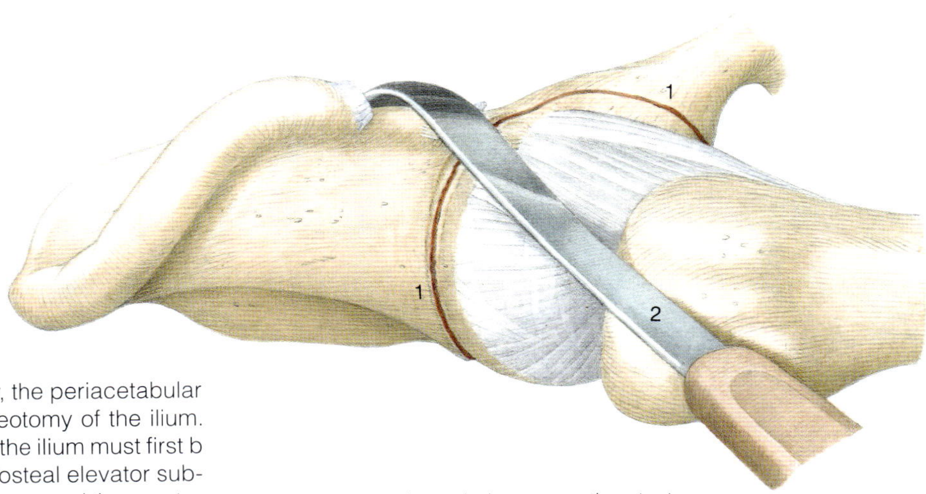

Fig. 2.**79** In the type III acetabular osteotomy, the periacetabular osteotomy is combined with a transverse osteotomy of the ilium. Before this can be done, the medial surface of the ilium must first b e exposed by advancing a sharp, curved periosteal elevator subperiosteally along the medial surface of the ilium toward the greater sciatic notch.

1 Completed periacetabular crescentic osteotomy
2 Sharp curved periosteal elevator

Kirschner wires are used to shift and stabilize the fragments in the type III acetabular osteotomy. First, two or three 2.5-mm Kirschner wires are inserted superiorly into the mobilized acetabulum between the margin of the capsule and the edge of the osteotomy. The wires are inserted deep enough that their tips just barely protrude from the medial cancellous osteotomy surface (Fig. 2.**83**). The surgeon can use the Kirschner wires as a handle for maneuvering the acetabulum into position. The wires are bent superiorly so that they will be parallel to the iliac wing when the acetabulum is in a slightly overcorrected position. Then they are cut flush with the iliac crest and bent toward the ilium to form right angles, so that they can later be inserted into holes drilled in the iliac wing (Fig. 2.**84**).

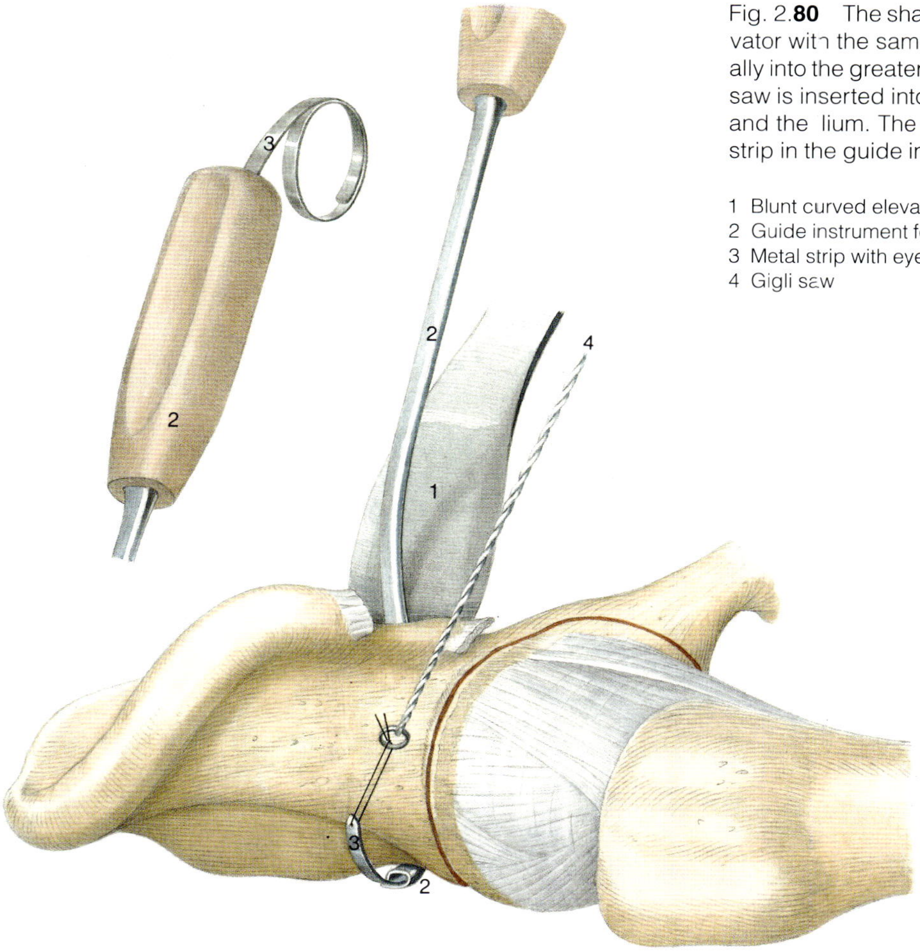

Fig. 2.**80** The sharp periosteal elevator is replaced by a blunt elevator with the same radius of curvature, which is advanced medially into the greater sciatic notch. The guide instrument for the Gigli saw is inserted into the greater sciatic notch between the elevator and the lium. The Gigli saw is attached to the eyelet of the metal strip in the guide instrument and fed around the ilium.

1 Blunt curved elevator at the medial surface of the ilium
2 Guide instrument for the Gigli saw
3 Metal strip with eyelet fed through the tube of the guide instrument
4 Gigli saw

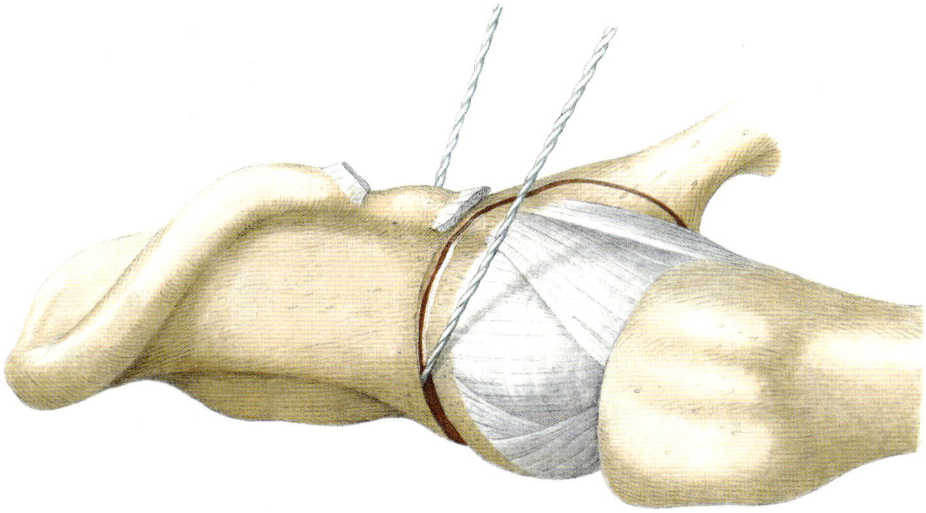

Fig. 2.**81** The ilium is osteotomized with the Gigli saw along the edge of the previous periacetabular crescentic osteotomy.

With the acetabulum in its corrected position, a clamp is applied to the Kirschner wires and fastened to the ilium with a bone screw. As the surgeon tightens the screw, the acetabulum and distal pelvic fragment are drawn medially into their final position (Fig. 2.**85**). The clamp can be fashioned from a semitubular plate.

Fig. 2.**82** The gap created by the osteotomy is opened wide with a bone spreader. The superior osteotomy surface is smoothed and rounded with the A gouge for a snug fit with the mobilized acetabulum.

1 Bone spreader
2 A gouge

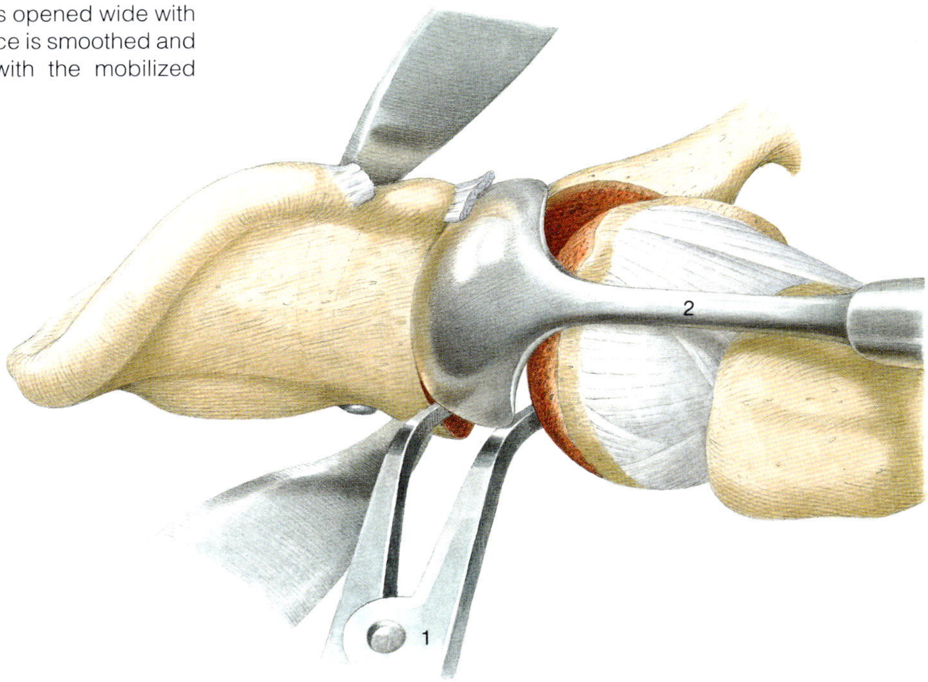

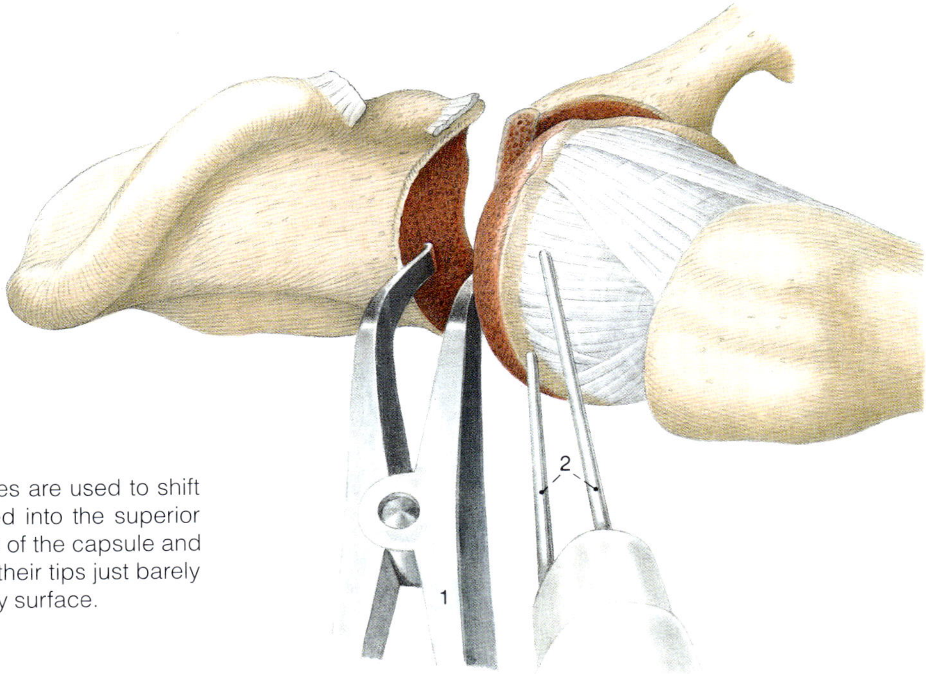

Fig. 2.**83** Two or three 2.5-mm Kirschner wires are used to shift and stabilize the fragments. They are inserted into the superior margin of the acetabulum between the margin of the capsule and the edge of the osteotomy, deep enough that their tips just barely protrude from the medial cancellous osteotomy surface.

1 Bone spreader
2 2.5-mm Kirschner wires

When closing the wound, the surgeon first securely sutures the rectus femoris to the anterior inferior iliac spine (Fig. 2.**86**), then reattaches the sartorius, the inguinal ligament, and the pelvic and trochanteric musculature to the iliac crest (see Fig. 2.**25**).

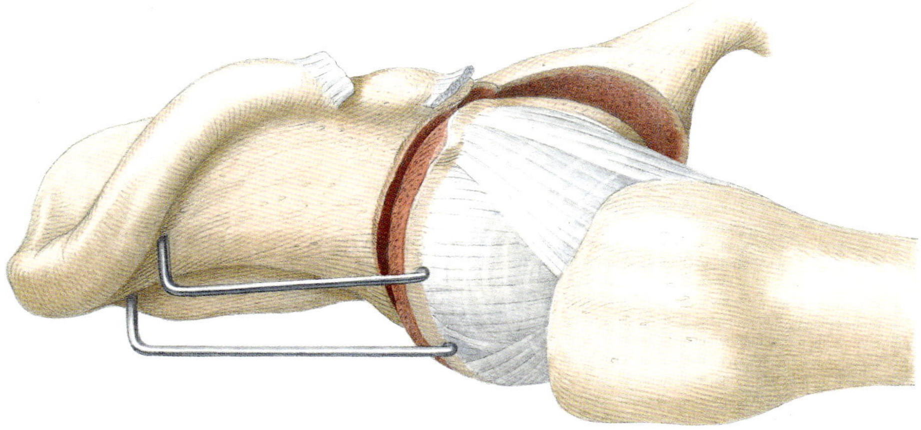

Fig. 2.**84** The Kirschner wires are bent superiorly so that they will be parallel to the iliac wing when the acetabulum is in a slightly overcorrected position. They are cut flush with the iliac crest and bent toward the ilium to form right angles, so that they can later be inserted into holes drilled in the iliac wing.

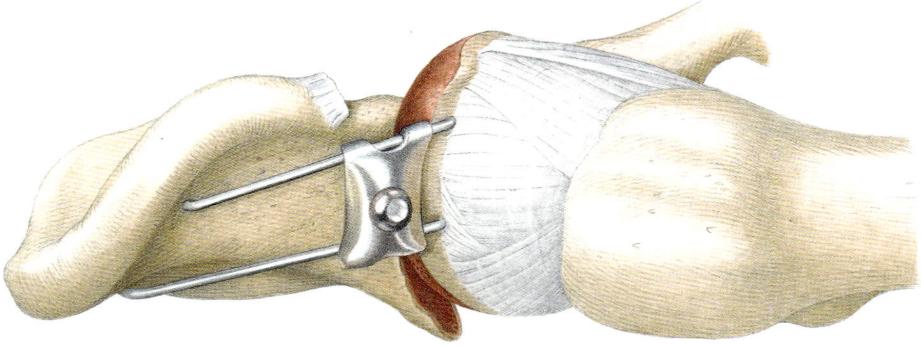

Fig. 2.**85** With the acetabulum in its corrected position, a clamp is applied to the Kirschner wires and fastened to the ilium with a bone screw. Tightening the screw draws the acetabulum and distal pelvic fragment medially into their final position.

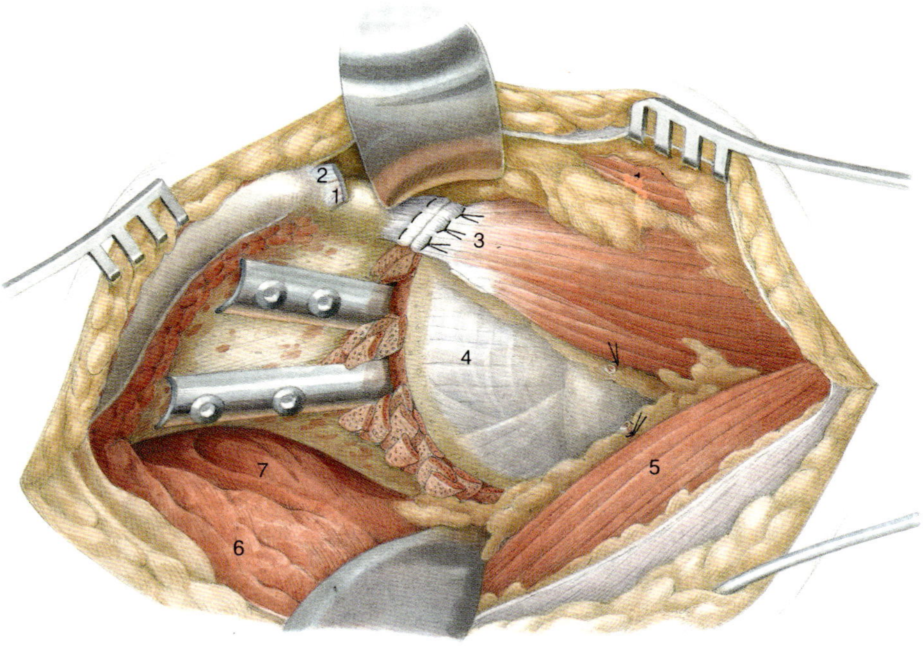

Fig. 2.**86** When closing the wound, the rectus femoris is securely sutured to the anterior inferior iliac spine.

1 Sartorius
2 Inguinal ligament
3 Rectus femoris
4 Hip joint capsule
5 Tensor fasciae latae
6 Gluteus medius
7 Gluteus minimus

Salter Pelvic Osteotomy (Innominate Osteotomy)

Indication

Congenital dislocation of the hip with flattening of the acetabulum and insufficient coverage of the femoral head, provided that the articular surfaces are not severely deformed and the femoral head can be deeply inserted into the acetabulum with the leg abducted in internal rotation. Surgery is contraindicated where there is persistent lateral displacement of the femoral head. The osteotomy is best performed in children when the symphysis is still mobile and future growth will compensate for the pelvic deformation induced by the procedure.

Positioning and Incision

The patient is positioned supine for the ilioinguinal approach.

Technique

After a transverse osteotomy of the ilium is performed superior to the roof of the acetabulum between the greater sciatic notch and the anterior inferior iliac spine (Fig. 2.**87**), the distal pelvic fragment is rotated laterally and distally around the symphysis so that the dysplastic acetabulum covers the femoral head. The corrected position is secured by a solid wedge-shaped bone graft taken from the anterior iliac wing and inserted into the gap created by the osteotomy and by two threaded wires that bridge the osteotomy (Fig. 2.**88**).

The Salter pelvic osteotomy has the advantage of being a relatively simple operation in wich the acetabulum is rotated to bring articular cartilage into position above the femoral head.

The disadvantage of the procedure is that it creates a pelvic deformity that shifts the hip joint distally and laterally, wich can increase soft-tissue tension. However, in a growing child, this deformity can at least partially correct itself over time without reducing the coverage of the femoral head.

Resecting a relatively large wedge of bone from the anterior iliac wing for a graft is not without risk. It distorts the shape of the pelvis and reduces the size of the origin of the tensor fasciae latae. An initial abductor tenotomy is indicated when hip abduction is limited. With the leg draped to permit free movement, a skin incision is made beginning at the middle of the iliac crest and coursing parallel to the inguinal ligament toward the symphysis (Fig. 2.**89**).

After the subcutaneous fatty tissue has been retracted and the fascia split, the muscular site between the tensor fasciae latae and the sartorius is exposed. The apophysis of the iliac crest is split longitudinally. The two halves of the apophysis are spread apart and the lateral and medial surfaces of the ilium are exposed by subperiosteally dissecting the soft tissue as far as the greater sciatic notch (Fig. 2.**90**). The rectus femoris is dissected from its origins and retracted distally, and the iliopsoas is released by cutting several transverse notches in the tendinous part of the muscle. The pelvic aspect of the cap-

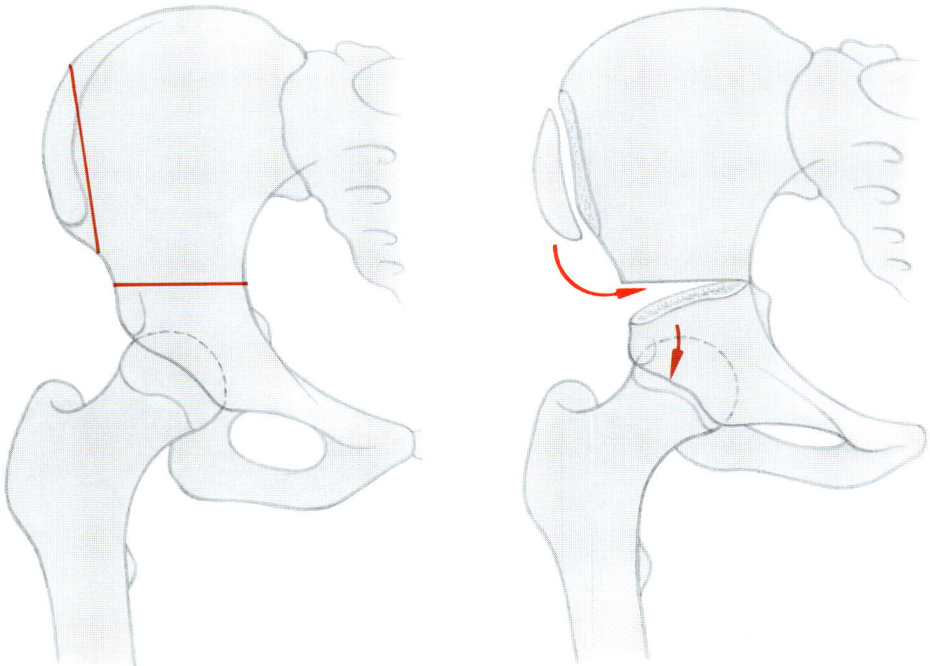

Fig. 2.**87** Principle of the Salter pelvic osteotomy. After a transverse osteotomy of the ilium beginning immediately superior to the ischiadic spine and extending to the superior margin of the anterior inferior iliac spine, the distal pelvic fragment is rotated laterally and distally around the symphysis so that the dysplastic acetabulum covers the femoral head.

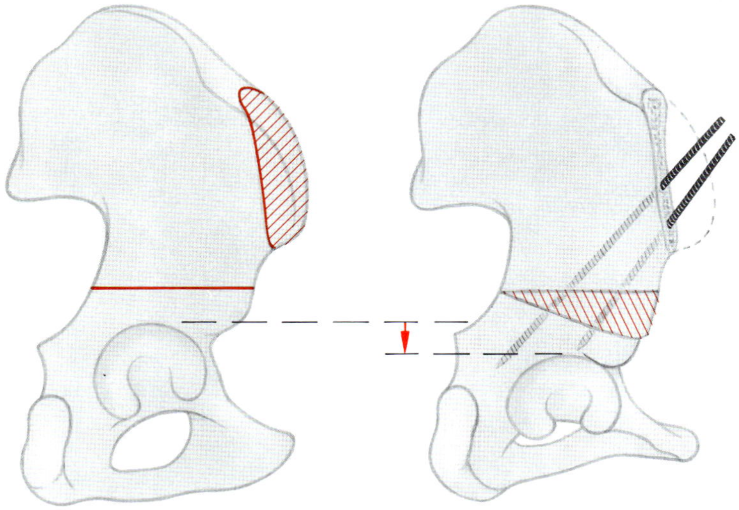

Fig. 2.**88** The corrected position is secured by a solid wedge-shaped bone graft taken from the anterior aspect of the ilium and inserted into the gap created by the osteotomy and by two threaded wires that bridge the osteotomy.

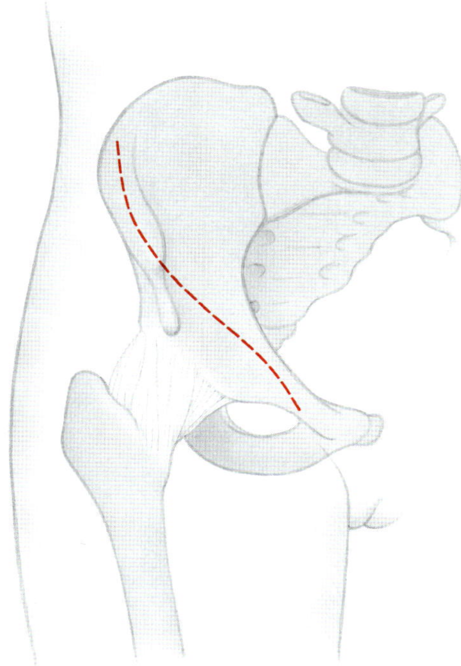

Fig. 2.**89** A ilioinguinal approach is used to expose the pelvis. A skin incision is made that begins at the middle of the iliac crest and courses parallel to the inguinal ligament toward the symphysis.

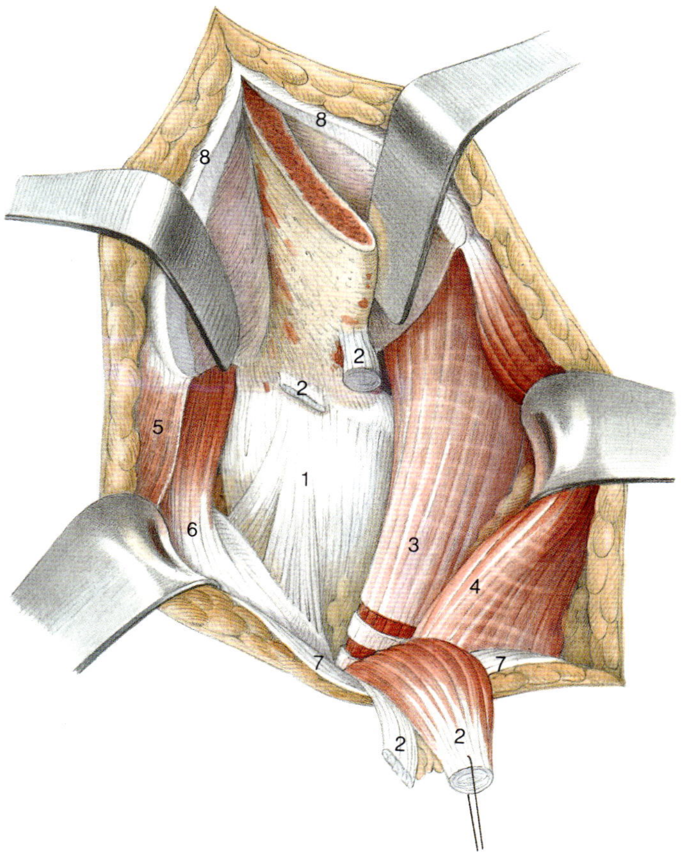

Fig. 2.**90** The muscular site between the tensor fasciae latae and the sartorius is exposed. The apophysis of the iliac crest is split longitudinally. The two halves of the apophysis are spread apart and the lateral and medial surfaces of the ilium are exposed by subperiosteally dissecting the soft tissue as far as the greater sciatic notch. The rectus femoris is dissected from its origins and retracted distally, and the iliopsoas is released by making several transverse incisions in the tendinous part of the muscle.

1 Hip joint capsule
2 Rectus femoris
3 Iliopsoas with distal transverse notches
4 Sartcrius
5 Tensor fasciae latae
6 Gluteus medius
7 Fascia lata
8 Apophysis of the iliac crest.

sule is broadly exposed. Thorough, meticulous exposure of the ilium is necessary if the operation is to be performed safely. Protecting the adjacent soft tissue with blunt elevators, the surgeon then passes a Gigli saw through the greater sciatic notch (Fig. 2.**91**).

The osteotomy of the ilium begins at the distal part of the greater sciatic notch, courses perpendicular to the iliac wing, and ends anteriorly immediately superior to the anterior inferior iliac spine. The surgeon removes a bone wedge that includes the lateral and medial cortex. This is later grafted into the gap created by the osteotomy. To dislocate the distal fragment, the leg is maximally abducted, flexed 90°, and externally rotated 90° while holding the proximal pelvic fragment with a forceps. With strong distal and lateral traction applied to the thigh, the distal fragment is rotated distally, laterally,

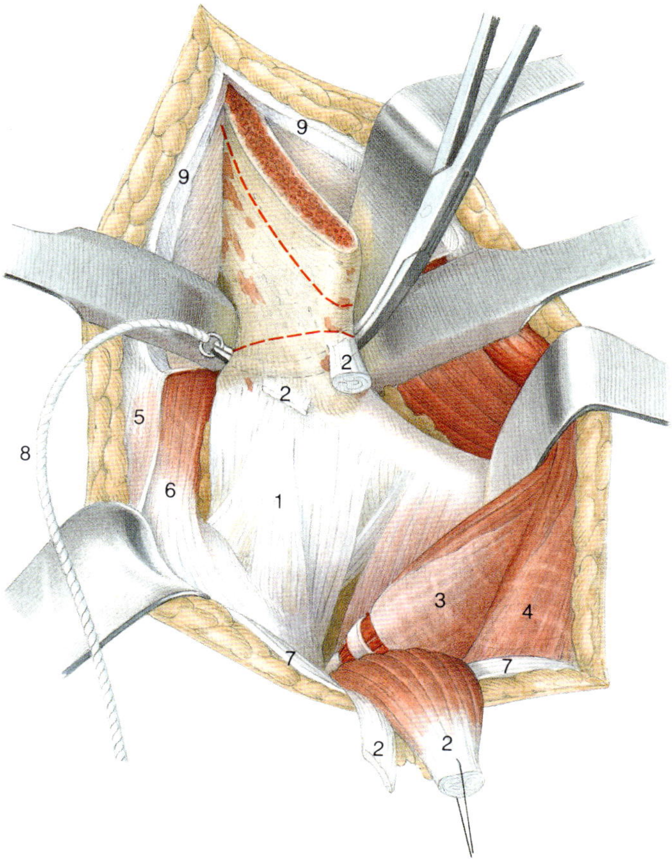

Fig. 2.**91** Blunt elevators are insected medially and laterally into the greater sciatic notch to protect adjacent soft tissue, and a Gigli saw is passed through the greater sciatic notch to osteotomize the ilium.

1 Hip joint capsule
2 Rectus femoris
3 Iliopsoas
4 Sartorius
5 Tensor fasciae latae
6 Gluteus medius
7 Fascia lata
8 Gigli saw
9 Apophysis of the iliac crest

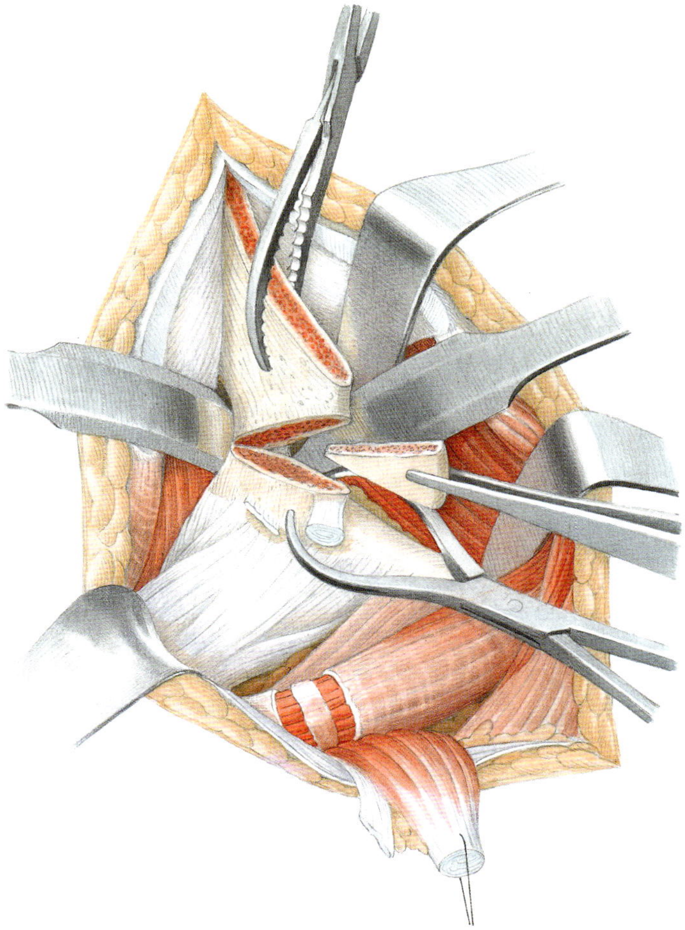

Fig. 2.**92** The leg is flexed, abducted, and externally rotated while the proximal pelvic fragment is held with a forceps and the distal fragment is rotated distally, laterally, and anteriorly with a second forceps. During this procedure, strong distal and lateral traction is applied to the thigh. The wedge-shaped bone graft from the iliac crest is then securely inserted into the gap of the osteotomy as it opens anteriorly.

and anteriorly with a second forceps, opening the gap created by the osteotomy anteriorly. The two pelvic fragments should remain in contact posteriorly because the rotation of the distal fragment would otherwise not be sufficient, and the hip would be shifted too far distally, with corresponding increase in leg length. The wedge-shaped bone graft from the iliac crest is now inserted anteriorly into the gap created by the osteotomy (Fig. 2.**92**). When the traction on the thigh is released, soft-tissue tension holds the bone wedge into place between the pelvic fragments. The surgeon then stabilizes the osteotomy and graft with two threaded wires. The wires extend from anterior margin of the graft removal site on the proximal fragment to the posterior part of the distal fragment, passing diagonally through the osteotomy without affecting the hip joint (Fig. 2.**93**). The dissected musculature is then reattached and the wound closed.

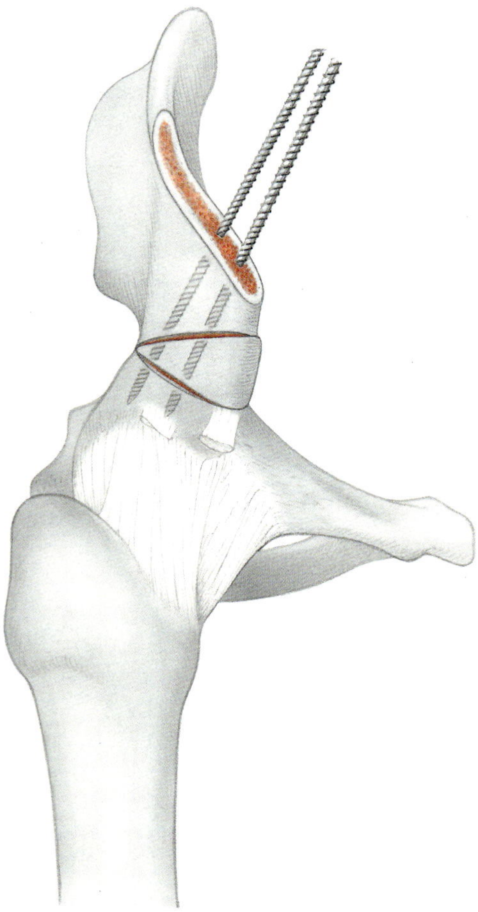

Fig. 2.**93** Two threaded wires that diagonally bridge the osteotomy are inserted to stabilize the osteotomy and graft.

Sutherland Pelvic Osteotomy (Double Innominate Osteotomy)

Indication

Congenital dislocation of the hip where there is flattening of the acetabulum and insufficient coverage of the femoral head. The objective of the operation is to rotate the dysplastic acetabulum anteriorly and bring articular cartilage into position above the femoral head. A major requirement for the procedure is that the articular surfaces are not severely deformed and the femoral head can be deeply inserted into the acetabulum with the leg abducted in internal rotation; the articular surfaces must be congruent. Surgery is contraindicated where there is persistent lateral displacement of the femoral head. The osteotomy is best performed in children when the symphysis is still mobile and future growth will be able to compensate for the pelvic deformation induced by the procedure.

Positioning and Incision

The patient is positioned supine on a radiolucent table to permit the use of intraoperative fluoroscopy. The procedure requires two approaches: the ilioinguinal approach for the pelvic osteotomy and a suprapubic transverse incision for osteotomy of the pubic ramus. An indwelling catheter is inserted for a few days to empty the urinary bladder (Fig. 2.**94**).

Technique

The operation is an extension of the Salter pelvic osteotomy. In addition to the typical Salter osteotomy, the pubic ramus is osteotomized between the symphysis and obturator foramen. This is done to facilitate mobilizing the distal pelvic fragment with the acetabulum and to permit making a larger correction with less soft-tissue tension and lateral displacement. This surgical procedure is significantly more complicated than the Salter pelvic osteotomy.

First, a Salter pelvic osteotomy is performed as described previously. The wound is temporarily closed with a subcutaneous suture. Next, a transverse suprapubic incision is made. After retracting the edges of the wound, the surgeon locates and retracts the spermatic cords or Hunter's ligaments laterally. The rectus abdominis and the pyramidalis are dissected from the superior aspect of the pubic ramus, and the periosteum is split above the anterior margin of the pubic ramus (Fig. 2.**95**). The origins of the adductor longus and gracilis are subperiosteally dissected from the anterior sur-

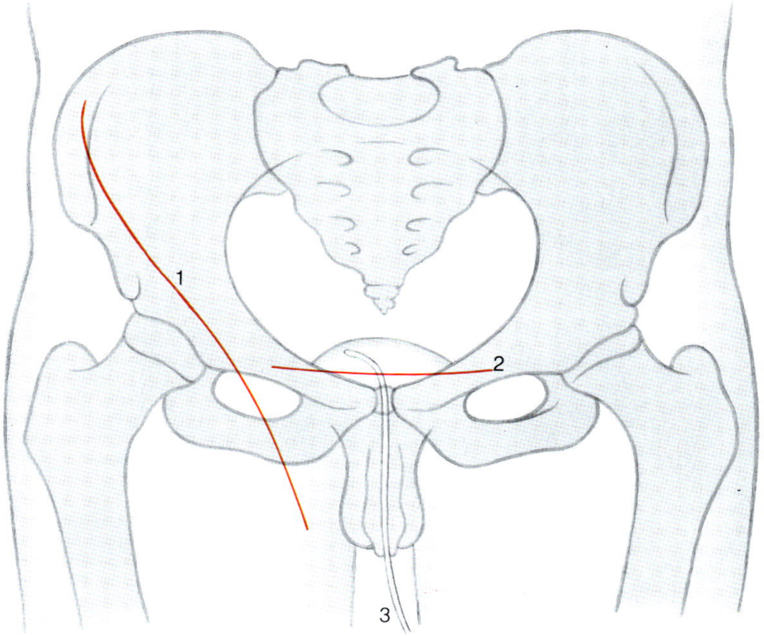

Fig. 2.**94** Approaches for the Sutherland double pelvic osteotomy.

1 Ilioinguinal approach
2 Suprapubic approach
3 Indwelling catheter

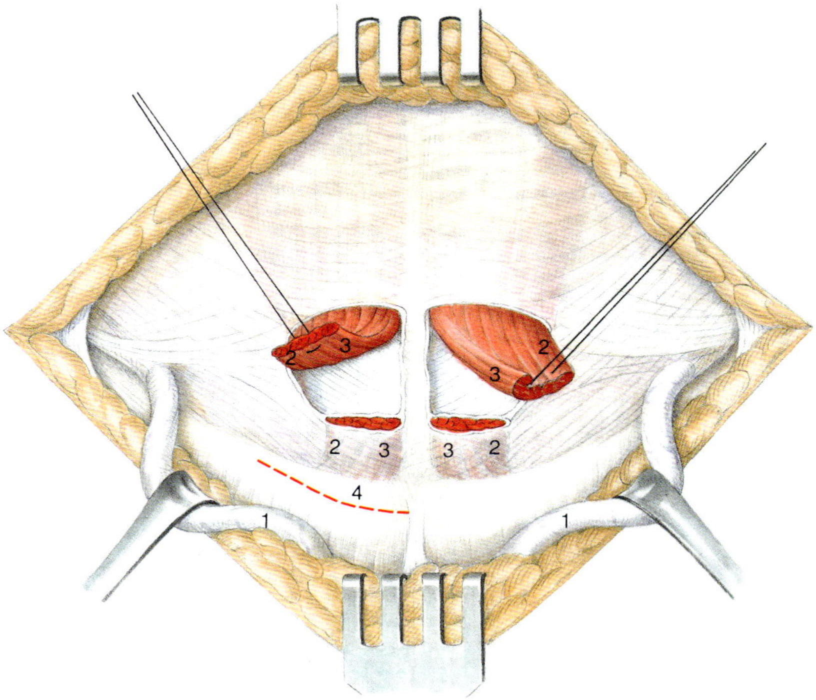

Fig. 2.**95** Exposure of the pubic ramus and symphysis. The rectus abdominis and the pyramidalis are dissected from the superior aspect of the pubic ramus, and the spermatic cords or Hunter's ligaments are retracted laterally. The periosteum is split above the anterior margin of the pubic ramus.

1 Spermatic cord
2 Rectus abdominis
3 Pyramidalis
4 Periosteal incision above the pubic ramus

face of the pubis (Fig. 2.**96**). The surgeon next locates the exact position of the symphysis by inserting a marker wire into the symphysis and verifying its position with fluoroscopy. A marker wire is inserted at the site of the osteotomy. Its position is also verified with fluoroscopy (Fig. 2.**97**). The surgeon then uses a sharp curved periosteal elevator to subperiosteally dissect the soft tissue from the entire circumference of the pubis at the marked location. To avoid any injury to the adjacent soft tissue, one should remain strictly subperosteal in the dissection (Fig. 2.**98**). A segment about 1 cm wide is resected from the pubic ramus at the marked osteotomy site (Fig. 2.**99**). The pubic ramus is then lifted anteriorly, while its soft-tissue attachments are subperiosteally retracted laterally until the pubic ramus is sufficiently mobilized (Fig. 2.**100**).

The surgeon now reopens the initial incision, and corrects the position of the pelvic fragments through both incisions.

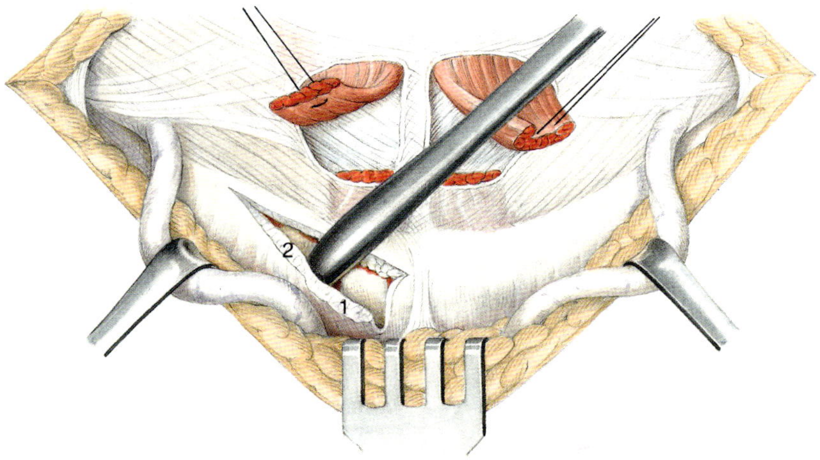

Fig. 2.**96** The origins of the gracilis and adductor longus are subperiostelly dissected from the anterior surface of the pubic ramus.

1 Gracilis
2 Adductor longus

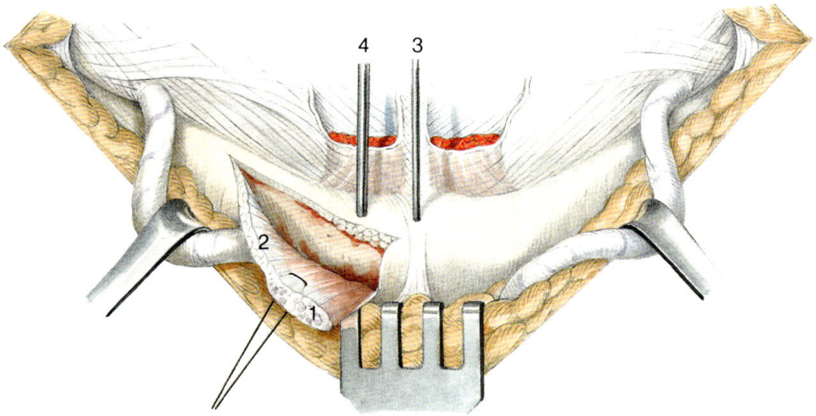

Fig. 2.**97** Locating the symphysis and the osteotomy site. Both positions are verified with fluoroscopy.

1 Gracilis
2 Adductor longus
3 Index needle marking the symphysis
4 Marker wire marking the osteotomy site on the pubis

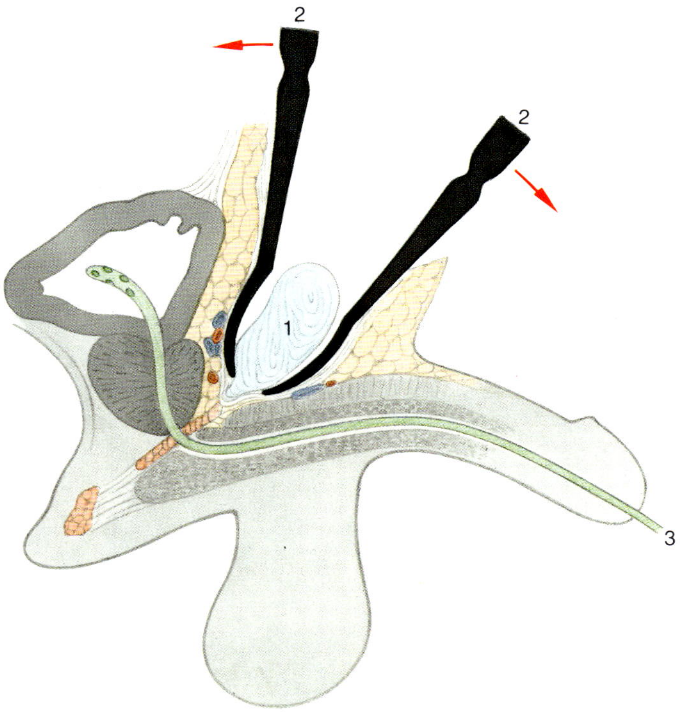

Fig. 2.**98** Subperiosteal dissection of the pubis at the marked location with sarp-curved periosteal elevators.

1 Pubis
2 Sharp curved periosteal elevator
3 Indwelling catheter

Using a holding forceps applied to the anterior inferior iliac spine, he or she moves the distal fragment distally and anteriorly; the pubic ramus is gripped with a bone clamp and dislocated superiorly and medially (Fig. 2.**101**). The surgeon then reduces the dislocation of the symphysis, using one or two threaded wires that bridge the symphysis to transfix the pubic ramus and stabilize it in its corrected position. At this stage of the procedure, the surgeon performs a Salter osteotomy as described previously, using threaded wires to stabilize the wedge-shaped graft (Fig. 2.**102**).

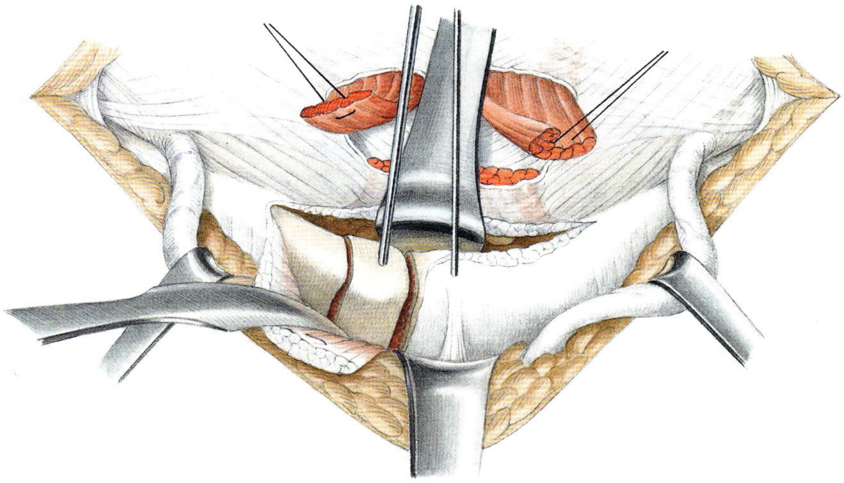

Fig. 2.**99** Osteotomy of the pubis. A segment about 1 cm wide is resected.

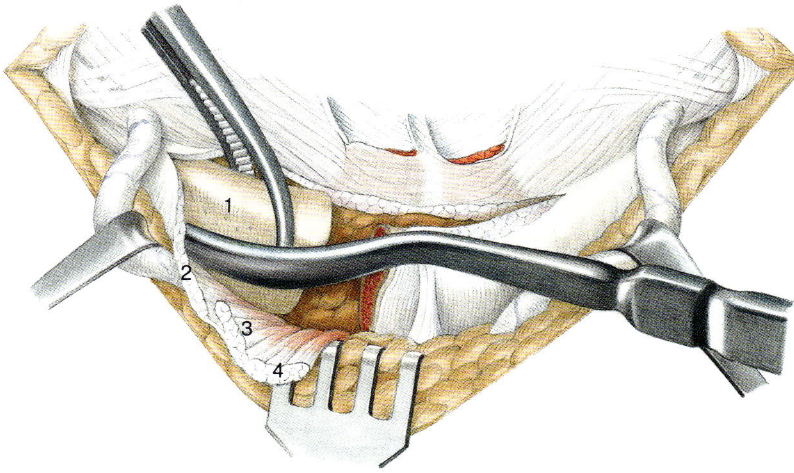

Fig. 2.**100** After the osteotomy, the pubis is lifted anteriorly while its soft-tissue attachments are retracted laterally.

1 Pubis
2 Pectineus
3 Adductor longus
4 Gracilis

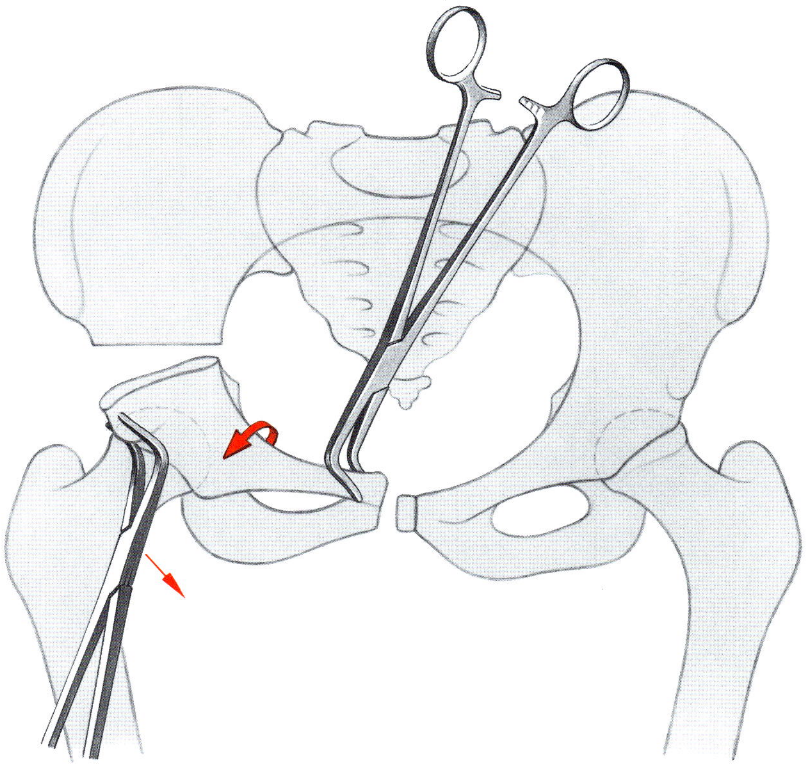

Fig. 2.**101** The distal pelvic fragment is rotated into the corrected position with two forceps.

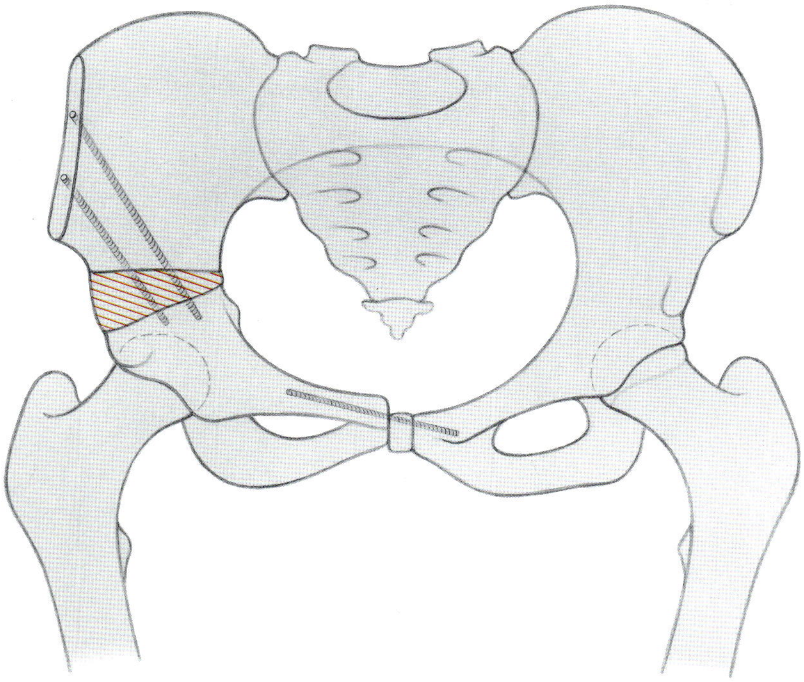

Fig. 2.**102** The osteotomy of the pubis is stabilized with one or two threaded wires that bridge the symphysis and transfix the pubis. Then a Salter pelvic osteotomy is performed, in which a wedge-shaped graft from the wing is inserted into an osteotomy superior to the acetabulum and fixed with threaded wires.

Steel Pelvic Osteotomy (Triple Innominate Osteotomy)

Indication

Congenital dislocation of the hip with flattening of the acetabulum and insufficient coverage of the femoral head. The requirements of articular congruity, lack of degenerative changes, and seating of the femoral head are the same as for the Salter and the Sutherland osteotomies.

Principle

The Steel triple pelvic osteotomy has the same objectives and essentially proceeds in the same manner as the Salter and Sutherland methods. However, the operation is considerably more complicated because the patient's position must be changed intraoperatively and two incisions are made through wich three separate osteotomies are performed (1) on the inferior aspect of the ischium, (2) on the ilium superior to the acetabulum, and (3) on the pubic ramus (Fig. 2.**103**).

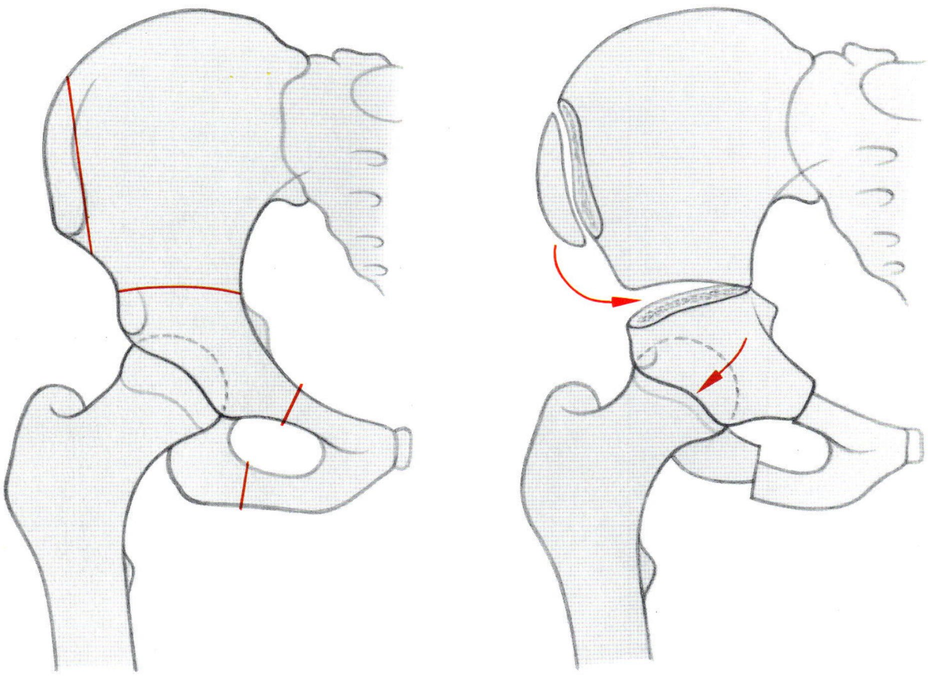

Fig. 2.**103** Principle of the Steel triple pelvic osteotomy. A Salter osteotomy of the ilium superior to the acetabulum and osteotomies of the inferior aspect of the ischium and the pubic ramus are performed. The position of the acetabulum is corrected by rotating the fragment created by these osteotomies.

Positioning and Incision

The patient is placed in lithotomy position for the initial osteotomy. The approach to the ilium is made through a diagonal skin incision across the ischial tuberosity (Fig. 2.**104**). The patient is than positioned supine for the second and third osteotomies, and the approach to the pubis is made through an ilioinguinal skin incision.

Surgical Technique

With the patient in lithotomy position, a diagonal skin incision is made, wich courses across the ischial tuberosity from posteromedial to anterolateral (Fig. 2.**104**). After splitting the fascia, the surgeon retracts the distal margin of the gluteus maximus posterolaterally, exposing the ischial tuberosity with its muscular attachments and the sacrotuberous ligament (Fig. 2.**105**).

The biceps femoris, semitendinosus, and semimembranosus are dissected from the ischium and retraced superiorly. The periosteum over the inferior aspect of the ischium is split (Fig. 2.**106**). The surgeon carefully subperiosteally dissects the soft tissue anteriorly from the ischial tuberosity to expose the inferior aspect of the ischium. Two elevators are then inserted (Fig. 2.**107**). A flat osteotome is now used to anteriorly separate the inferior aspect of the ischium from the ischial tuberosity. The osteotomy courses diagonally from posteromedial to anterolateral. The previously dissected hamstrings are then reattached to the ischium (Fig. 2.**108**), and the fascia over the gluteus maximus is sutured (Fig. 2.**109**). The wound is then closed in layers and the patient positioned supine.

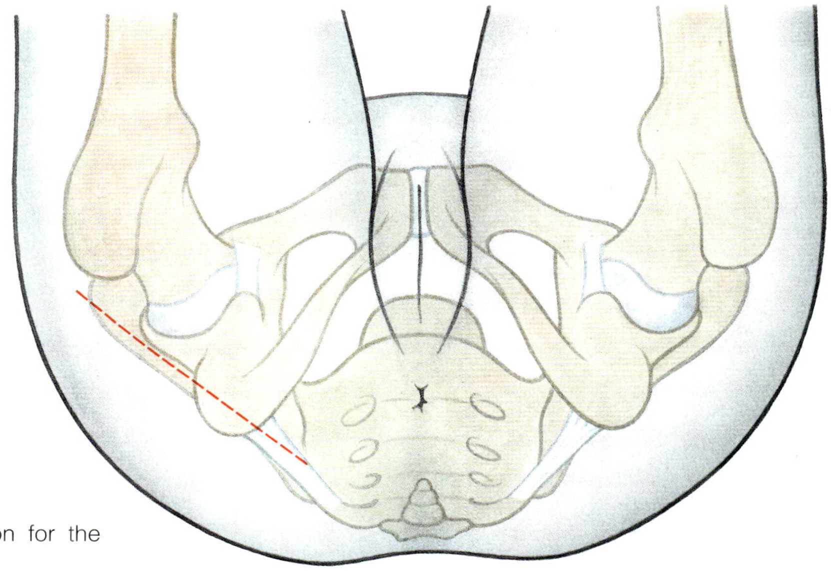

Fig. 2.**104** The patient is placed in lithotomy position for the osteotomy of the inferior aspect of the ischium.

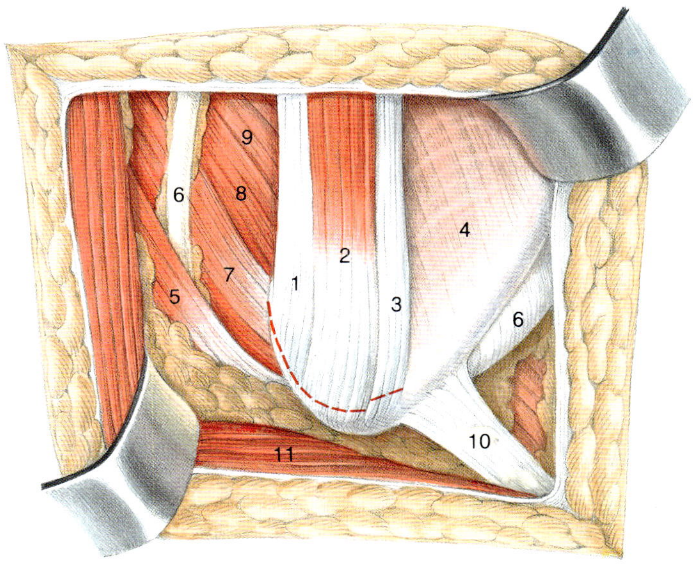

Fig. 2.**105** A diagonal skin incision is made that courses across the ischial tuberosity, and the soft-tissue attachments of the ischium are exposed.

1 Biceps femoris
2 Semitendinosus
3 Semimembranosus
4 Adductor magnus
5 Piriformis
6 Sciatic nerve
7 Obturator internus
8 Gemellus inferior
9 Quadratus femoris
10 Sacrotuberous ligament
11 Gluteus maximus

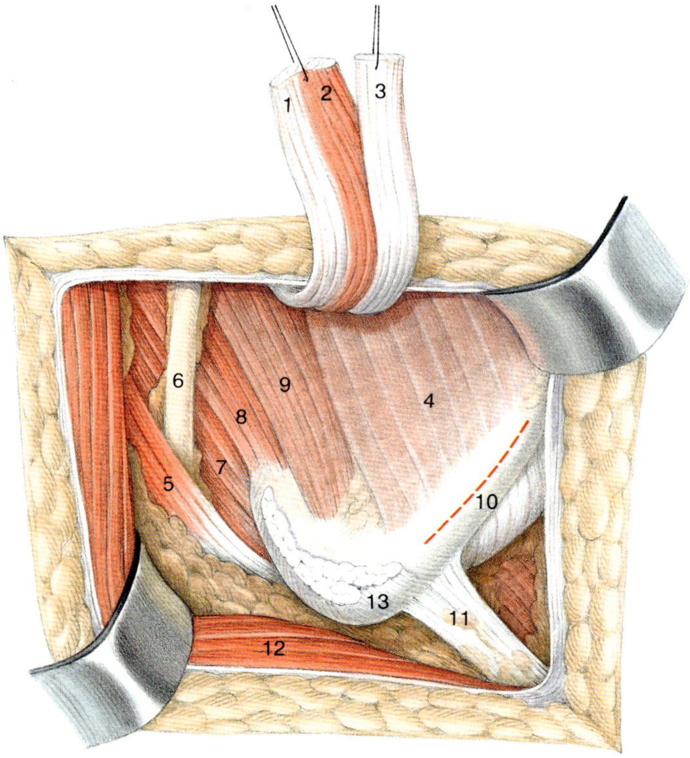

Fig. 2.**106** Exposure of the inferior aspect of the ischium. The biceps femoris, semitendinosus, and semimembranosus are dissected from the ischium and folded back superiorly. The periosteum over the inferior aspect of the ischium is incised longitudinally.

1 Biceps femoris
2 Semitendinosus
3 Semimembranosus
4 Adductor magnus
5 Piriformis
6 Sciatic nerve
7 Obturator internus
8 Gemellus inferior
9 Quadratus femoris
10 Inferior aspect of the ischium
11 Sacrotuberous ligament
12 Gluteus maximus
13 Ischial tuberosity

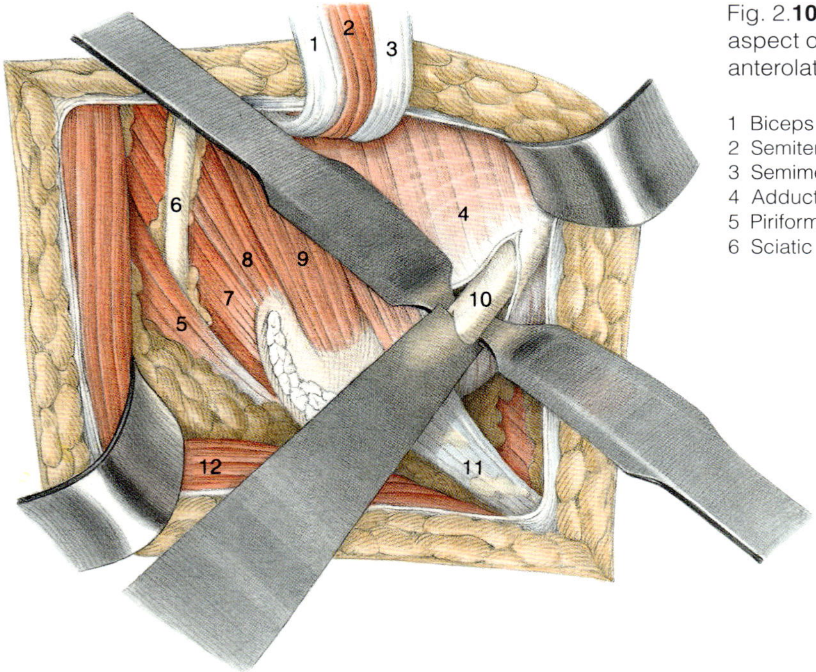

Fig. 2.**107** Subperiosteal exposure and osteotomy of the inferior aspect of the ischium coursing diagnonally from posteromedial to anterolateral.

1 Biceps femoris
2 Semitendinosus
3 Semimembranosus
4 Adductor magnus
5 Piriformis
6 Sciatic nerve
7 Obturator internus
8 Gemellus inferior
9 Quadratus femoris
10 Inferior aspect of the ischium
11 Sacrotuberous ligament
12 Gluteus maximus

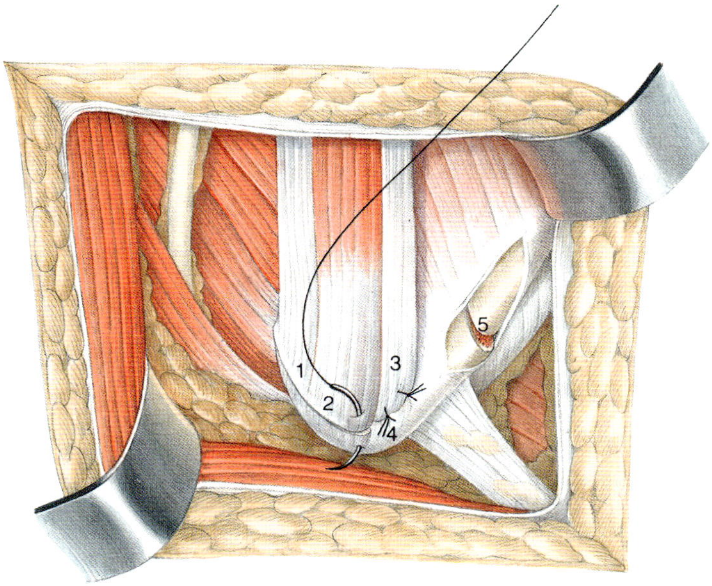

Fig. 2.**108** Reattaching the hamstrings to the ischium.

1 Biceps femoris
2 Semitendinosus
3 Semimembranosus
4 Ischial tuberosity
5 Osteotomy of the inferior aspect of the ischium

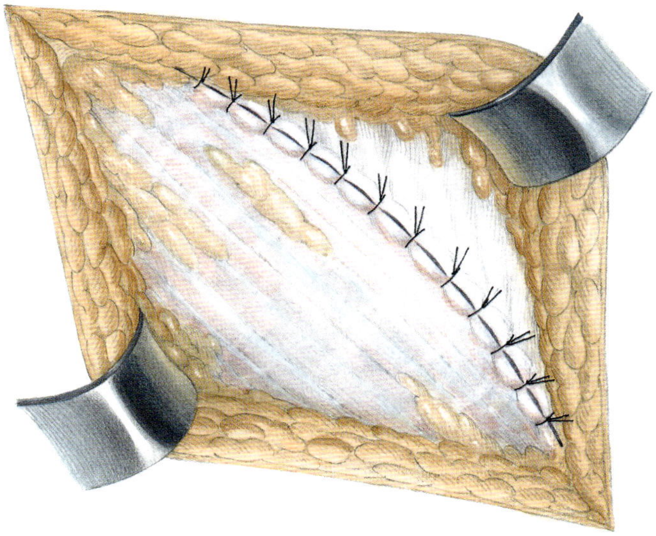

Fig. 2.**109** Sutured gluteus maximus.

The surgeon uses an ilioinguinal approach to expose the ilium superior to the acetabulum (see Fig. 2.**89**) in the same manner described with the Salter osteotomy. The apophysis of the iliac crest is split longitudinally. The surgeon subperiosteally dissects the two halves of the apophysis and the musculature from the lateral and medial surfaces of the ilium until the greater sciatic notch is accessible from both sides. The rectus femoris and pectineus are dissected from their origins, and the iliopsoas is released and extended by cutting several transverse notches in the tendinous part of the muscle (Fig. 2.**110**).

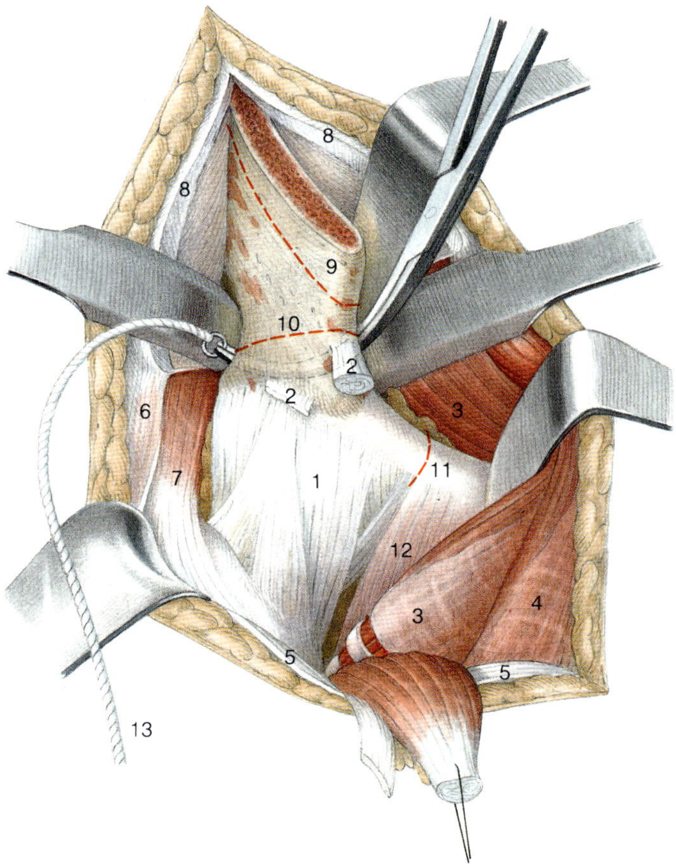

Fig. 2.**110** Subperiosteal dissection of the ilium after splitting the apophysis of the iliac crest. The rectus femoris is dissected from its two origins and retracted distally. The iliopsoas is released by making several transverse incisions in the tendinous part of the muscle distal to the hip joint.

1 Hip joint capsule
2 Rectus femoris
3 Iliopsoas with distal transverse notches
4 Sartorius
5 Fascia lata
6 Tensor fasciae latae
7 Gluteus medius
8 Apophysis of the iliac crest
9 Bone wedge to be inserted in gap created by osteotomy
10 Ilium
11 Pubis osteotomy
12 Pectineus
13 Gigli saw

Finally, the pubic ramus immediately adjacent to the acetabulum is subperiosteally exposed and the soft tissue retracted with a blunt elevator. The pubic ramus is then osteotomized between the pubic tubercle and the anterior margin of the acetabulum (Fig. 2.**111**).

Blunt elevators are inserted laterally and medially into the greater sciatic notch, overlapping each other in the deep layer of the wound. With the soft tissue protected by the elevators, the surgeon inserts a Gigli and transects the ilium superior to the acetabulum. The osteotomy extends from the distal part of the greater sciatic notch to the superior margin of the anterior inferior iliac spine (Fig. 2.**112**). As in the Salter osteotomy, the distal pelvic fragment is pulled into the corrected position with a bone clamp, while a second bone clamp grips the proximal fragment. The wedge-shaped graft taken from the anterior margin of the iliac wing is inserted into the gap created by the osteotomy (see Fig. 2.**92**).

The osteotomy is stabilized with two threaded wires or bone screws, which extend diagonally from the anterior section of the wing through the graft into the posterior section of the distal fragment (Fig. 2.**113**).

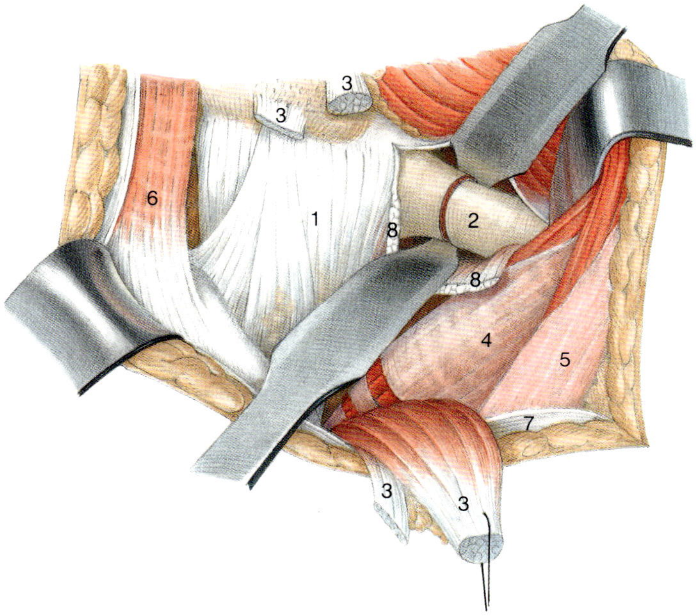

Fig. 2.**111** After the pectineus is dissected, the pubis ramus is subperiosteally exposed and osteotomized while the soft tissue is retracted with a blunt elevator.

1 Hip joint capsule
2 Transverse osteotomy of the pubic ramus
3 Rectus femoris
4 Iliopsoas
5 Sartorius
6 Gluteus medius
7 Fascia lata
8 Pectineus

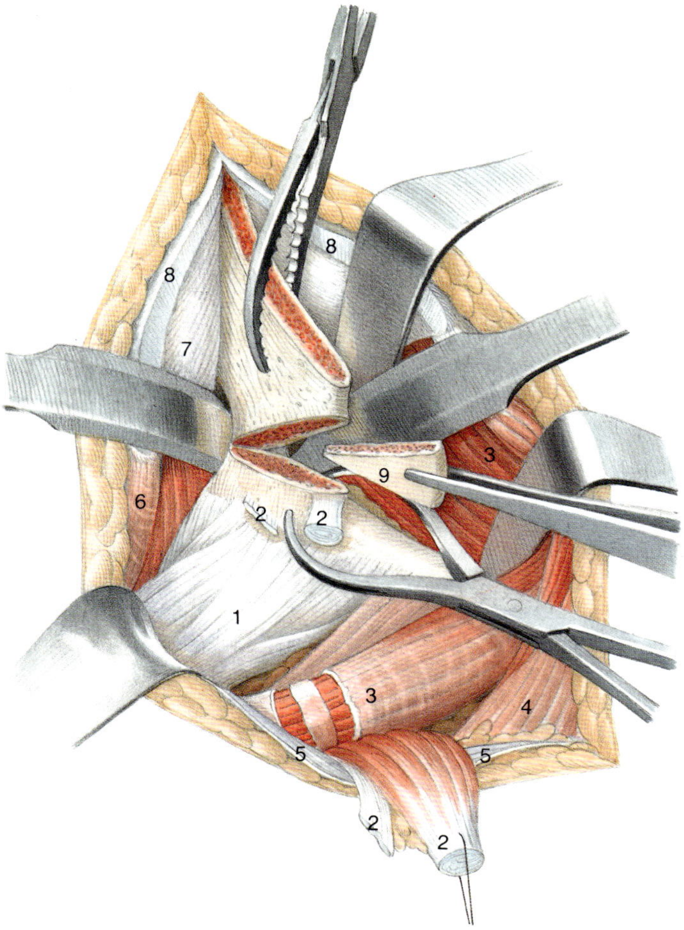

Fig. 2.**112** Blunt elevators are inserted laterally and medially into the greater sciatic notch. The ilium is transected with a Gigli fed through the greater sciatic notch.

1 Hip joint capsule
2 Rectus femoris
3 Iliopsoas
4 Sartorius
5 Fascia lata
6 Tensor fasciae latae
7 Gluteus medius
8 Apophysis of the iliac crest
9 Bone wedge to be inserted in gap created by osteotomy

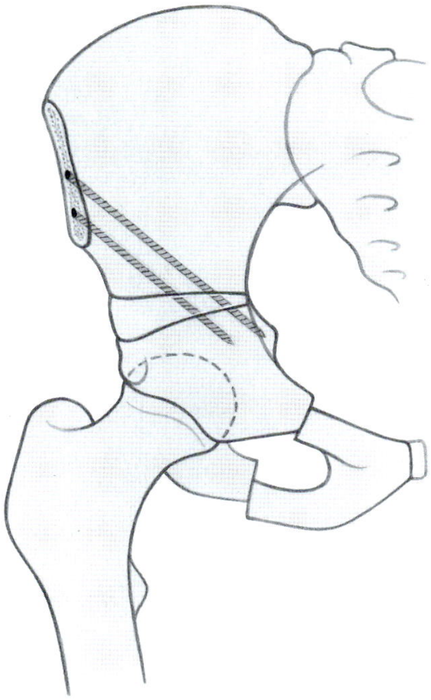

Fig. 2.**113** Osteotomy and bone wedge are fixed in the corrected position with two threaded wires or bone screws that extend diagonally to bridge the site.

Chiari Pelvic Osteotomy

Indications

1. Congenital dislocation of the hip with insufficient coverage of the femoral head, dysplastic acetabulum, and flattened articular surfaces:
   a. In growing children, to treat progressive subluxation of the femoral head or to stabilize late reduction of congenital dislocation of the hip.
   b. In adults, to increase the load-bearing articular surfaces in hip dysplasia.
2. Posttraumatic degenerative changes that are suitable for decompression.

Positioning and Incision

The patient is supine and an anterior approach is used.

Technique

The ilium is severed immediately superior to the joint capsule with a lateral osteotomy that extends medially and superiorly. The hip joint is then shifted medially with respect to the superior osteotomy surface, increasing the coverage of the femoral head. The proximal osteotomy surface thus becomes an extension of the acetabulum (Fig. 2.**114**).

Advantages:

The procedure can be performed even when the hip is severely deformed.

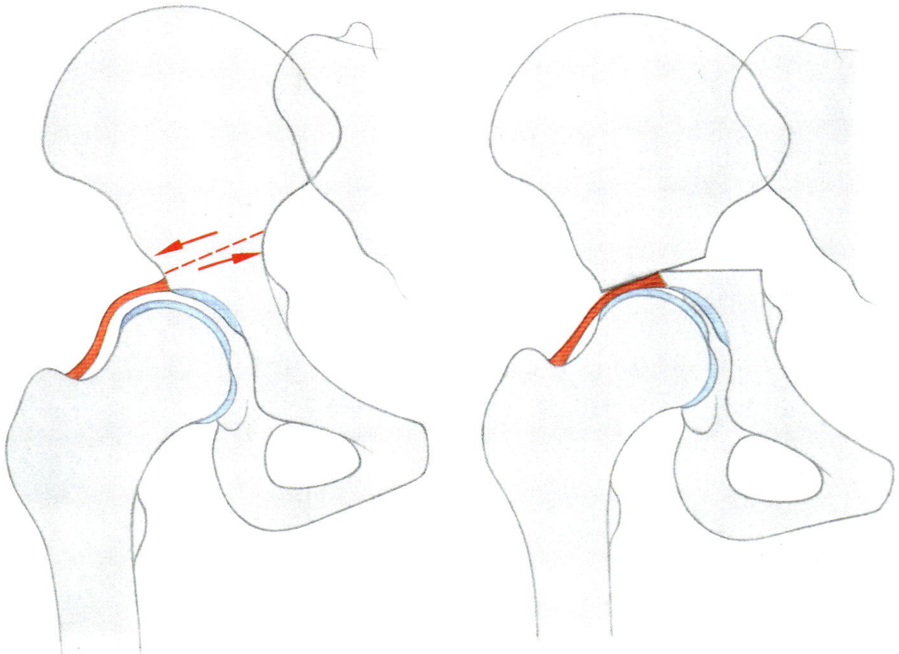

Fig. 2.**114** Principle of the Chiari pelvic osteotomy. After the ilium is severed immediately superior to the joint capsule with a lateral osteotomy that extends medially and superiorly, the hip joint is shifted medially with respect to the superior osteotomy surface. The proximal osteotomy surface thus becomes an extension of the acetabulum.

Disadvantages:

a. The interposed joint capsule substitutes for articular surface in the load-bearing area. It is less resistant to wear than hyaline cartilage.
b. Both fragments are rotated after the osteotomy; the proximal fragment around the sacroiliac joint, the distal one around the pubic symphysis. The medial shift in center of rotation of the hip is thus less than the shift in the fragments.
c. Turning the distal fragment places the cartilaginous articular surface of the dysplastic acetabulum in a steeper position, removing the stress from it.
d. Rotating both fragments creates a triangular bone gap at the anterior margin of the osteotomy in the hypoplastic anterior margin of the acetabulum. Since this can impair subsequent joint function, the gap created by the osteotomy must be filled with bone chips.

The skin incision should be made 2 cm lateral to the iliac crest (see Fig. 2.**17**). If the skin is pulled 2 cm medially, the incision can begin directly over the iliac crest. The skin will later return to its original position. It is imperative to avoid making the incision too far medially because the osteotomy itself will shift the skin medially. If the closed incision lies immediately above the iliac crest, the resulting compression could impede healing.

After the subcutaneous fatty tissue has been retracted, the fascia above the anterior margin of the tensor fasciae latae is split parallel to the direction of its fibers. The tensor fasciae latae is then retracted laterally (see Fig. 2.**18**). The outline of the rectus femoris is now visible through the deep layer of the fascia. Then the surgeon splits the deep layer of the fascia to reveal the rectus femoris with its two heads of origin and the ascending branch of the lateral femoral circumflex artery with its adjacent veins (see Fig. 2.**19**).

After the musculature is dissected from the outer surface of the iliac wing, the joint capsule is exposed (see Fig. 2.**20**). The surgeon dissects the direct origin of the rectus femoris and resects the reflected origin (see Fig. 2.**21**), exposing the joint capsule. A blunt elevator is inserted into the greater sciatic notch. The surgeon lifts the iliopsoas with a periosteal elevator and dissects the sartorius and inguinal ligament from the anterior superior iliac spine with a scalpel (see Fig. 2.**22**). After the iliopsoas is lifted to expose the margin of the acetabulum, an elevator with a short, sharp tip is impacted into the pubic ramus beneath the muscle (see Fig. 2.**65**).

The medial surface of the ilium is now exposed. A sharp curved periosteal elevator is advanced subperiosteally along the medial surface of the ilium toward the greater sciatic notch (Fig. 2.**115**). Then the periosteal elevator is removed, and a blunt elevator with the same curvature is inserted medially into the greater sciatic notch. The tip of the elevator is visible laterally in the deep layer of the wound in the greater sciatic notch. The osteotomy level at the margin of the capsule is marked with a Steinmann pin and verified with fluoroscopy (see Fig. 2.**117**). If the dysplastic acetabulum is flattened and the joint capsule extremely thick, the surgeon may have to displace the bony margin of the capsule a few millimeters with an osteotome and insert the Steinmann pin further distally.

A Gigli saw should be used at least for the posterior part of the osteotomy. The posterior margin of the ilium is extremely brittle, and an osteotome might cause the bone to splinter, endangering adjacent soft tissue in the deep pelvis. The Gigli saw can be pulled through the greater sciatic notch with a long, thin clamp, but it is safer to use a guide instrument. The guide instrument consists of a thin-walled flattened tube with the same radius of curvature at its tip as the elevator already in place. The guide instrument is inserted into the greater sciatic notch between the elevator and the medial wall of the pelvis. A metal strip with an eyelet at its tip is fed through the tube. The Gigli saw is tied to the eyelet with a strong thread and pulled through the greater sciatic notch (Fig. 2.**116**).

The lateral side of the Gigli saw is fed between the Steinmann pin and the margin of the capsule to prevent the saw from deviating from the planned osteotomy level. The medial side of the saw is inclined anteriorly so that the

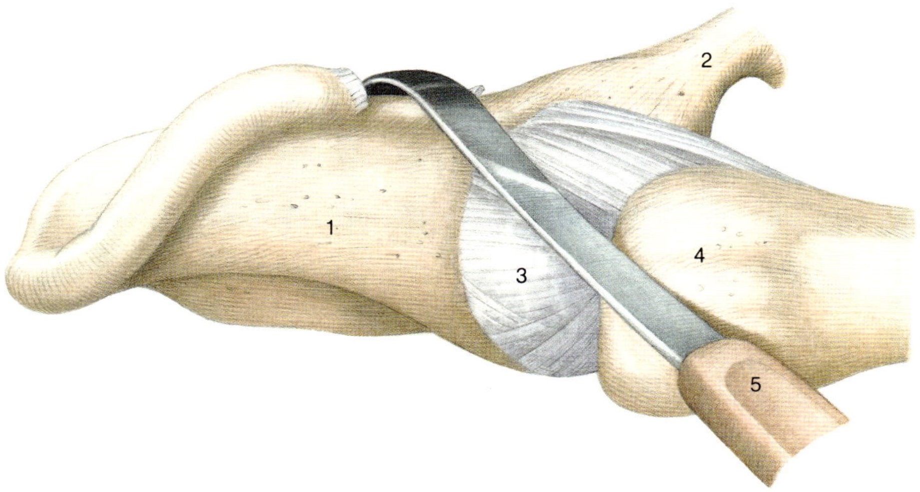

Fig. 2.**115** A sharp curved periosteal elevator is advanced subperiostelly along the medial surface of the ilium toward the greater sciatic notch.

1 Ilium
2 Pubis
3 Hip joint capsule
4 Greater trochanter
5 Sharp curved periosteal elevater

osteotomy surface rises in the coronal plane (Fig. 2.**117**). As the surgeon makes the cut, he moves the Gigli saw distally so that the path of the saw describes an arc that parallels the margin of the acetabulum (Fig. 2.**118**).

A bone spreader is laterally inserted into the osteotomy and opened to spread the osteotomy and mobilize the fragments. This makes it far easier to move them into the corrected position. Next, a second bone spreader is inserted medially into

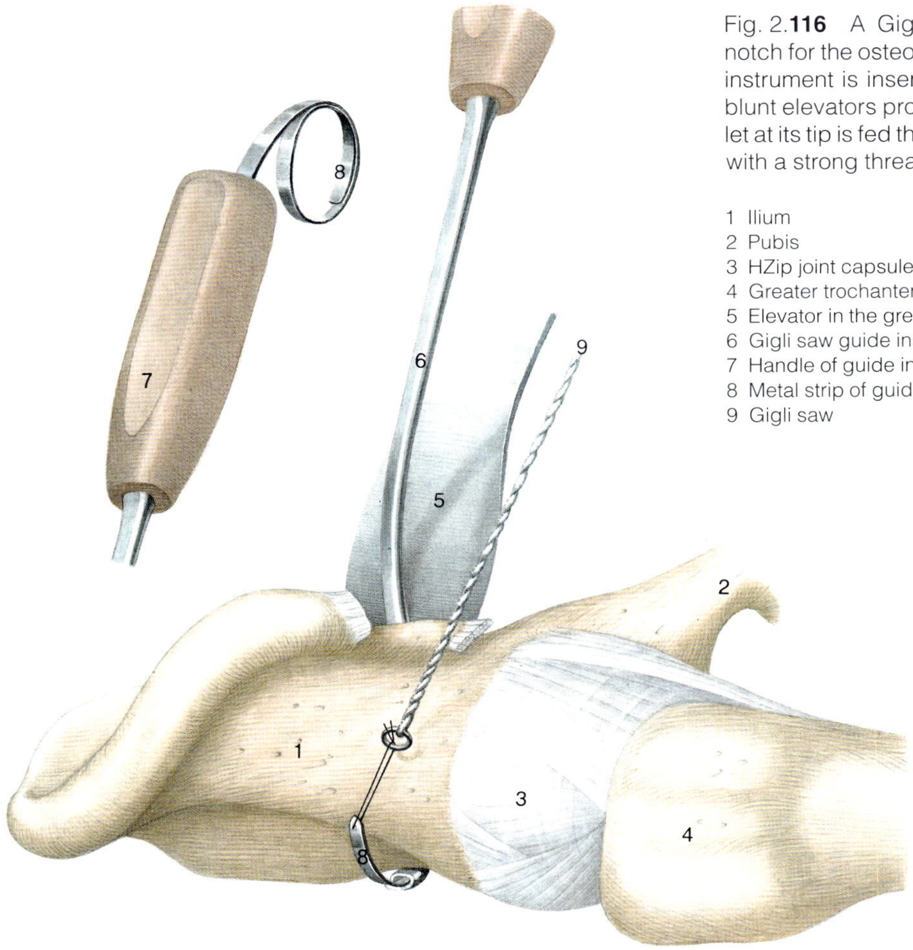

Fig. 2.**116** A Gigli saw is inserted through the greater sciatic notch for the osteotomy of the ilium. The flattened tube of the guide instrument is inserted medially into the greater sciatic notch with blunt elevators protecting the soft tissue. A metal strip with an eyelet at its tip is fed through the tube. The Gigli saw is tied to the eyelet with a strong thread and pulled through the greater sciatic notch.

1 Ilium
2 Pubis
3 HZip joint capsule
4 Greater trochanter
5 Elevator in the greater sciatic notch
6 Gigli saw guide instrument
7 Handle of guide instrument
8 Metal strip of guide instrument
9 Gigli saw

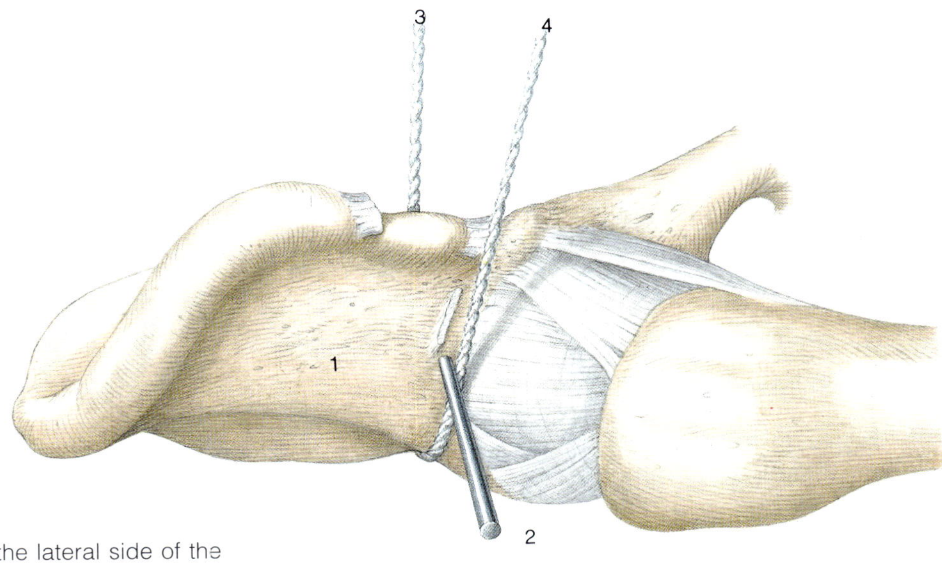

Fig. 2.**117** For the osteotomy of the ilium, the lateral side of the Gigli saw is fed between the Steinmann pin and the margin of the capsule to prevent the saw from deviating from the planned osteotomy level. The medial side of the saw is inclined anteriorly so that the osteotomy surface rises in the coronal plane.

1 Ilium
2 Steinmann pin marking the osteotomy level
3 Medial side of the Gigli saw
4 Lateral side of the Gigli saw

the osteotomy, and the first spreader is removed. By turning the bone spreader, the surgeon gradually shifts the fragments until the proximal fragment sufficiently covers the femoral head (Figs. 2.**119**–2.**121**). Shifting the pelvic fragments creates a triangular gap in the anterior margin of the osteotomy that must be filled with bone chips (Fig. 2.**122**).

The fragments are fixed in the corrected position with a screw. This eliminates the need for a cast, permits early mobilization, and accelerates healing. A cancellous screw is inserted 15 mm posterior to the anterior superior iliac spine. The screw diagonally bridges the osteotomy and engages the superior aspect of the pubic bone. A washer is used to prevent tensile forces from pulling the head of the screw into the cancellous bone of the iliac crest. Screw fixation creates sufficient compression of the fragments and permits use of the joint. The screw should be removed 8 weeks postoperatively, as it is at risk for fatigue failure. The head of the screw is readily palpable on the iliac crest beneath the skin and can later be removed under local anesthesia.

Finally, the dissected muscles are reattached to their origins with strong sutures. After placing a deep drain and suturing the fascia lata, the surgeon closes the wound in layers (see Fig. 2.**25**).

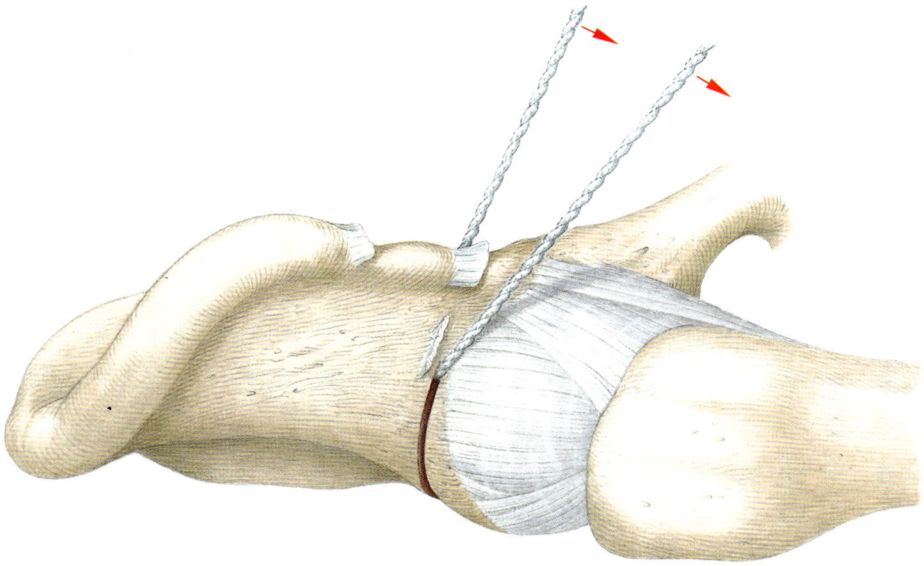

Fig. 2.**118** As the cut is made, the Gigli saw is moved distally so that the path of the saw describes an arc that parallels the articular surface.

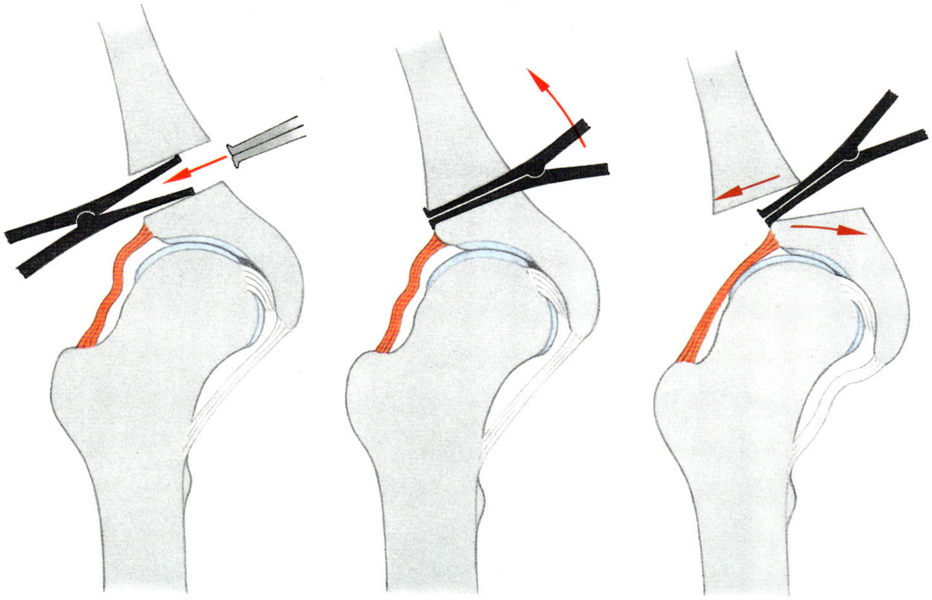

Fig. 2.**119** Principle of the Chiary osteotomy. A bone spreader of laterally inserted into the osteotomy and opened to spread the osteotomy and mobilize the two fragments. Then a second bone spreader is medially inserted into the osteotomy and slowly raised, gradually advancing the fragments.

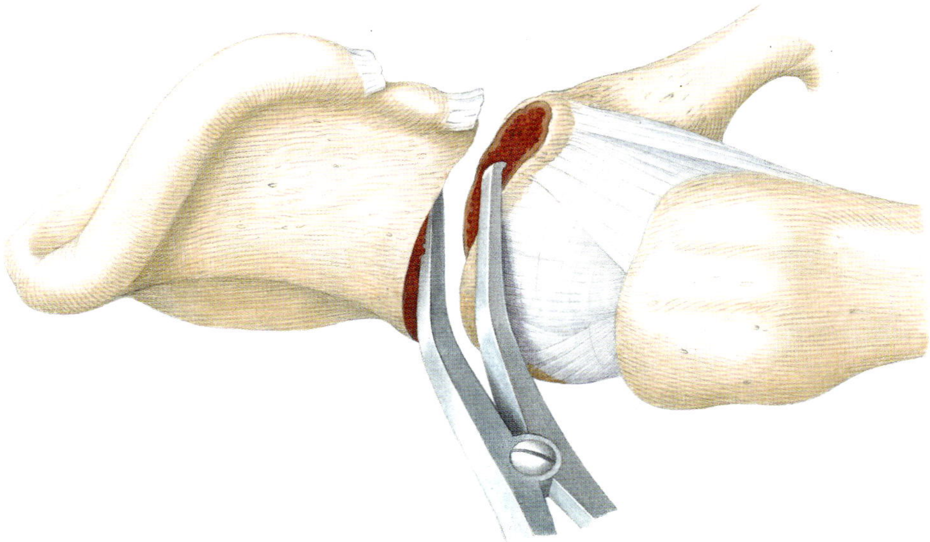

Fig. 2.**120** Laterally inserting a bone spreader into the osteotomy and opening it effectively mobilizes the two fragments.

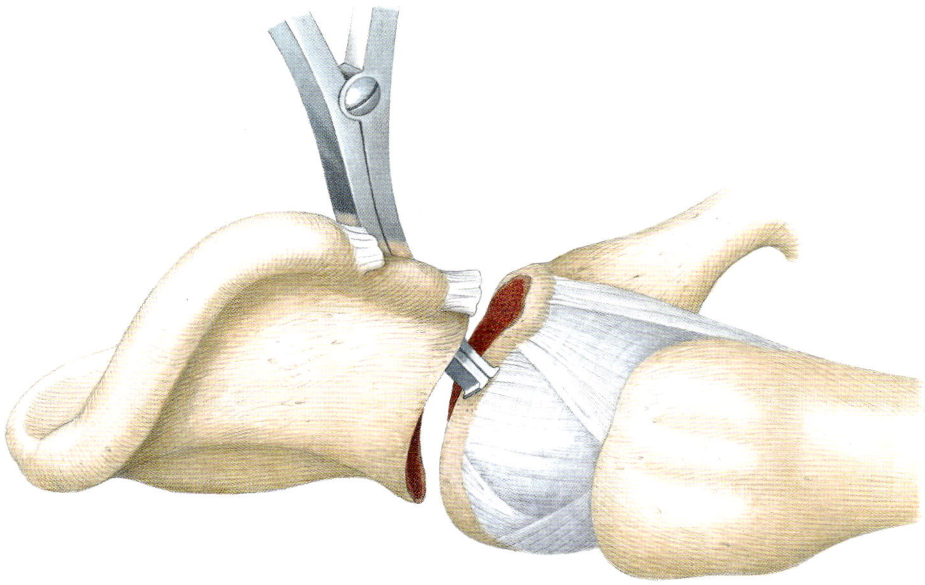

Fig. 2.**121** A second bone spreader, inserted into the osteotomy medially, engages the lateral edge of the distal frlagment and is pressed against the proximal fragment, shifting the fragments with respect to each other. Opening the bone spreader will increase the dislocation.

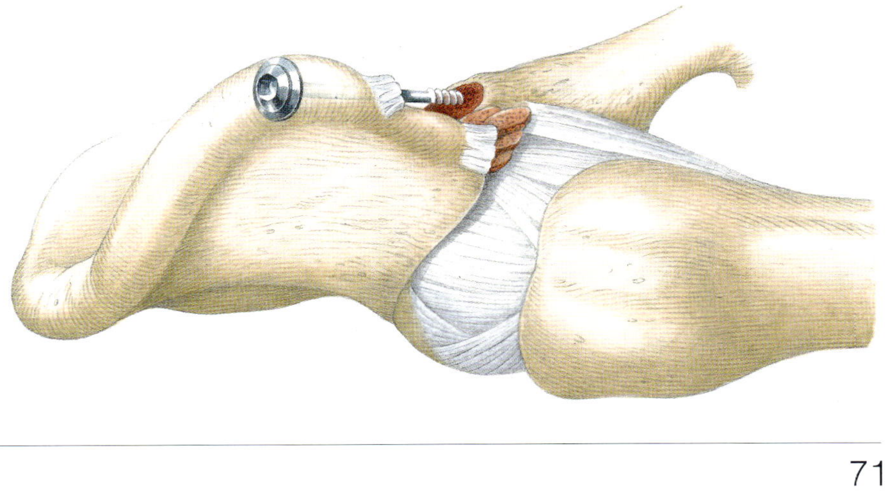

Fig. 2.**122** Internal fixation is used to maintain the corrected position and permit use of the joint. A cancellous screw is inserted 15 mm posterior to the anterior superior iliac spine. The screw diagonally bridges the osteotomy and engages the pubic ramus. The screw presses the two fragments firmly together. The bony defect created by shifting the fragments is filled with bone chips.

Proximal Femur Surgery

Preoperative Planning for Osteotomies of the Proximal Femur

Objectives

The rationale for preoperative planning is to precisely define the pathoanatomy, plan surgical objectives, plan implant usage, and evaluate alternatives. While this chapter deals with preoperative planning for osteotomies of the proximal femur, the procedures described here also apply to most leg surgery and to total arthroplasty.

In preoperative planning, the surgeon defines the problem requiring correction, prepares strategies, and develops drawings detailing the individual steps of one or more corrective procedures. If there are options, preoperative planning can be used to accurately determine the most favorable solution.

Preoperative planning dictates that the surgeon think through the procedure and draw the individual steps of the operation in the order they are to be executed prior to operating. This eliminates intraoperative planning and multiple trials, and minimizes operative delay. The procedure is shortened and surprises are minimized when the details (osteotomy sites and angles, fragment position, type and location of implants for internal fixation, and expected difference in leg length) are known and planned in advance. Preoperative planning also improves the precision of the surgery.

Radiographs

The respective bone lengths, diameters, and axes are determined extremely precisely during preoperative planning. This requires radiographs of known magnification. The use of radiographs with 15% magnification is standard. All planning templates are designed for this magnification.

To achieve this magnification, the radiologist assumes the bone lies 10 cm above the surface of the radiolucent table. The distance between the table surface and film should be 5 cm, and the distance between the focal point of the X-ray tube and film should be 115 cm (Fig. 2.**123**). In extremely obese patients, the bone may be farther from the table surface. In such cases, the radiologist should increase the distance between the X-ray tube and the film, or include a reference specimen of defined length in the same plane as the bone.

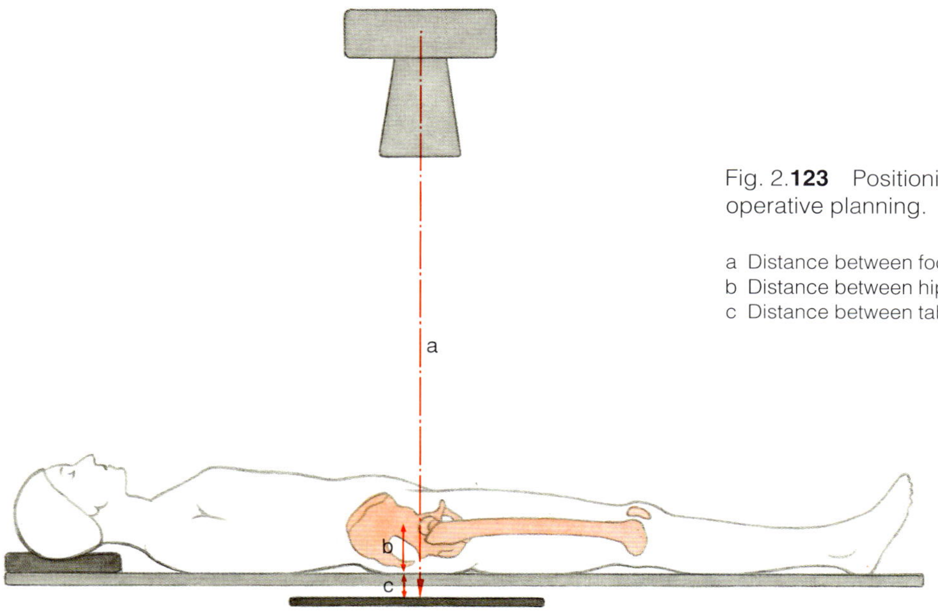

Fig. 2.**123** Positioning the patient for scale radiographs for preoperative planning.

a Distance between focal point of the X-ray tube and film = 115 cm
b Distance between hip joint and table surface = 10 cm
c Distance between table surface and film = 5 cm

Preoperative Planning Drawings

Preparing drawings requires radiographs with 15% magnification, acetate sheets, color marking pens, and planning templates for the implants to be used. The drawings are made on a horizontal translucent glass plate such as a radiograph viewer. A drawing table with a built-in illuminated translucent glass surface is more convenient because it permits placing several radiographs or drawings side by side for comparison.

Planning for an intertrochanteric varus osteotomy begins with an outline drawing of the hip joint (outline drawing A). A dotted line marks the longitudinal axis of the femur (Fig. 2.**124**). This reference line is used to determine the lateral shift of the fragments after the osteotomy and helps the surgeon avoid inadvertently placing the femur in varus or valgus when correcting the axis of the femoral neck. A solid line perpendicular to the longitudinal axis of the femur at the level of the proximal margin of the lesser trochanter marks the intertrochanteric osteotomy.

When the affected hip is severely deformed and the contralateral hip is normal, a mirror-image outline drawing of the contralateral hip can be prepared and placed beneath the drawings of the affected hip during planning.

Outline drawing B includes only the contours of the acetabulum and the dotted line representing the longitudinal axis of the femur (Fig. 2.**125**). Drawing B is laid on top of drawing A and rotated until the femoral head and femoral neck are in the desired corrected position. The resulting angle between the dotted lines representing the respective longitudinal axis of the femur on each of the drawings is the angle

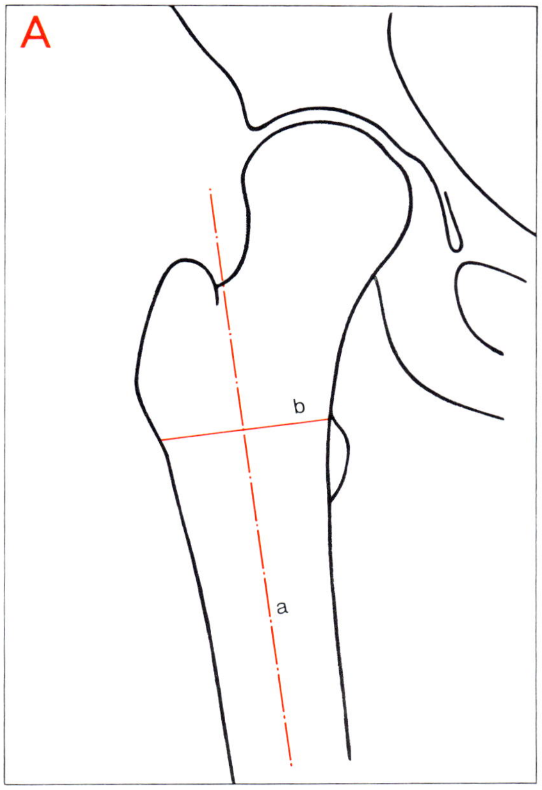

Fig. 2.**124** The longitudinal axis of the femur (a) and the intertrochanteric osteotomy (b) are marked in outline drawing A.

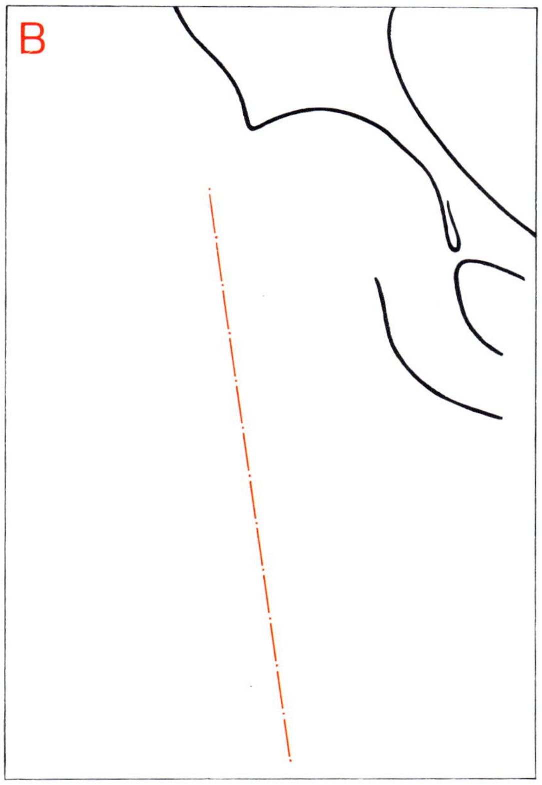

Fig. 2.**125** Outline drawing B includes only the contours of the acetabulum and the dotted line representing the longitudinal axis of the femur.

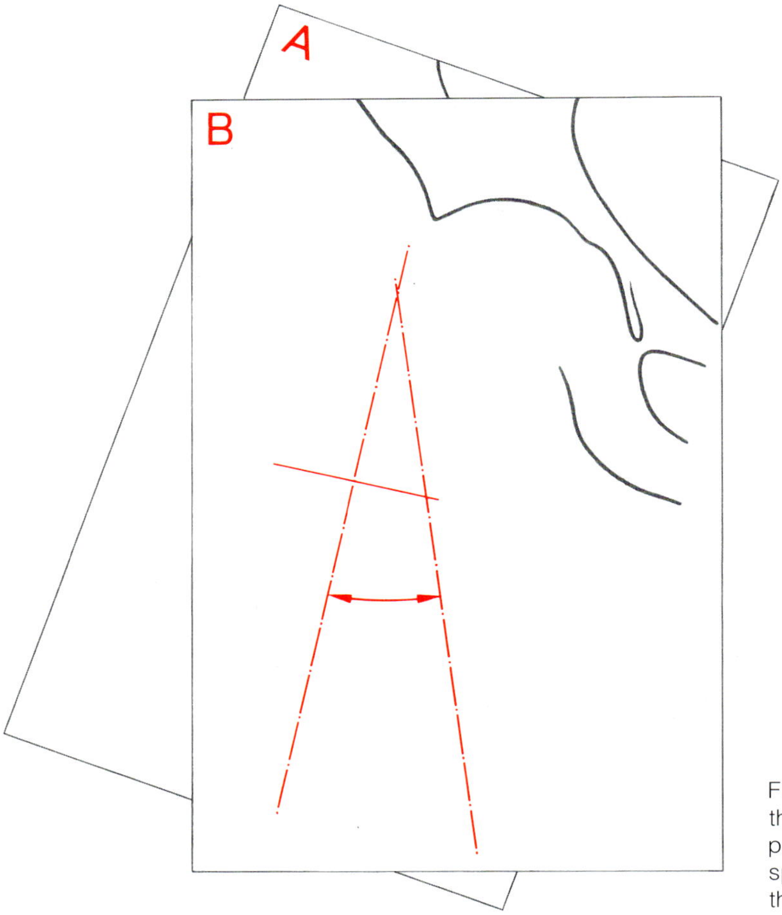

Fig. 2.**126** Drawing B is laid on top of drawing A and rotated until the femoral head and femoral neck are in the desired corrected position. The angle between the dotted lines representing the respective longitudinal axis of the femur on each of the drawings is the angle of correction.

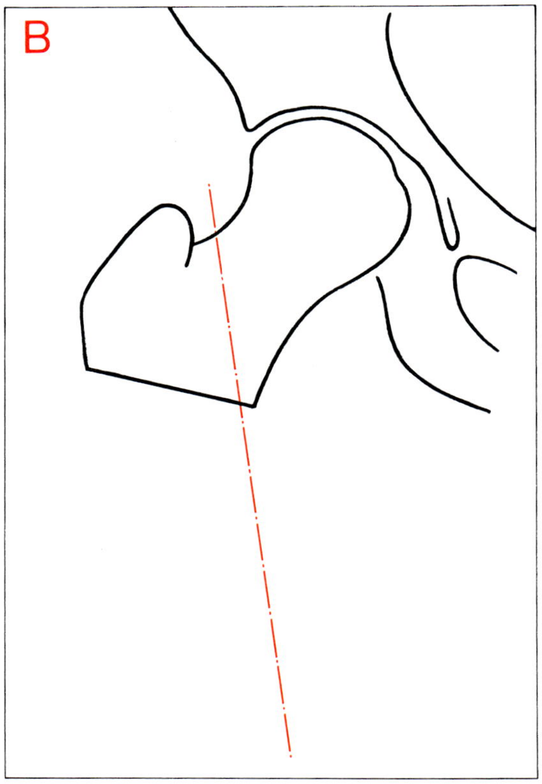

Fig. 2.**127** The proximal end of the femur proximal to the marking for the intertrochanteric osteotomy is traced on drawing B in the corrected position.

of correction (Fig. 2.**126**). The proximal end of the femur is then traced in this position on drawing B (Fig. 2.**127**).

Drawing B is then laid on top of drawing A again, and moved and rotated until the femoral shaft distal to the intertrochanteric osteotomy is below the proximal fragment of the femur and the dotted lines representing the longitudinal axis of the femur match up exactly (Fig. 2.**128**). This position reveals the required lateral displacement of the distal fragment and the inevitable change in leg length. Now the distal fragment is also traced in the corrected position (Fig. 2.**129**). Finally, the template with the osteotomy plate is laid beneath outline

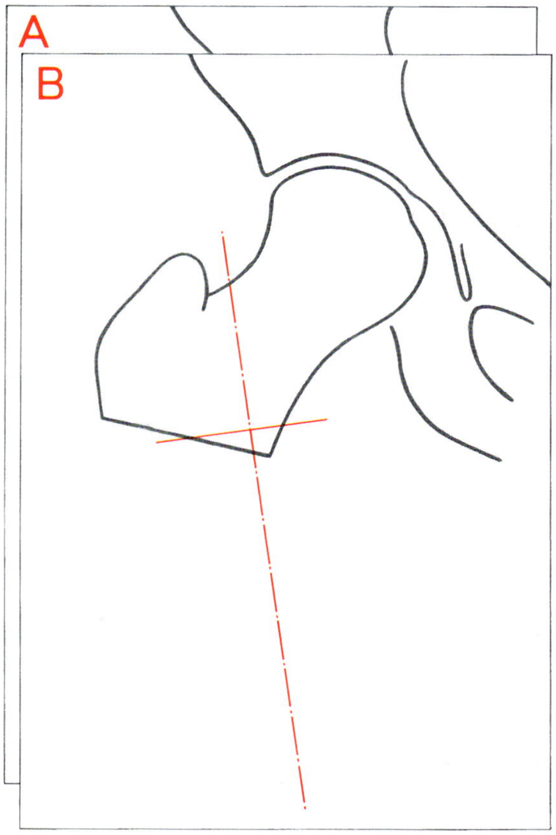

Fig. 2.**128** Drawing B is then laid on top of drawing A again and is moved and rotated until the dotted lines representing the longitudinal axis of the femur match up exactly with the fragment in the corrected position.

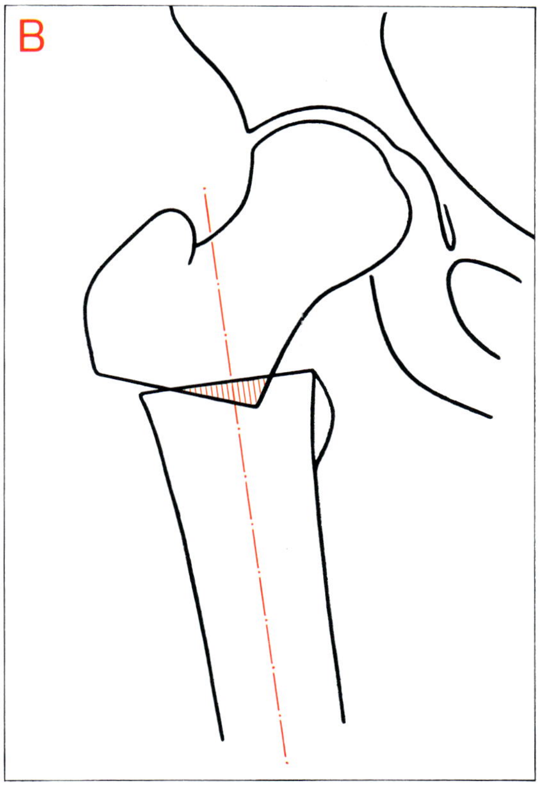

Fig. 2.**129** Then the distal fragment is also traced in the corrected position.

drawing B, and the appropriate implants are traced on the drawing (Fig. 2.**130**). Since the magnification is known, the surgeon can also record length dimensions on the planning drawing. The apex of the greater trochanter is generally used as a reference point from which the level of the osteotomy and the position of the blade of the osteotomy plate are measured. This makes the procedure more precise.

The same principles also apply to preoperative planning for more complicated surgery; each step of the procedure is planned in advance so that the surgery itself consists of implementing the preoperative planning.

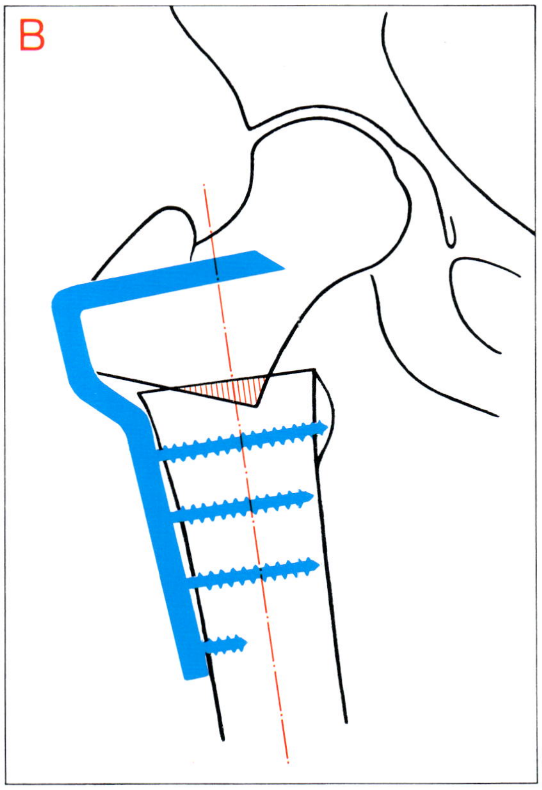

Fig. 2.**130** Finally, the template with the osteotomy plate is laid beneath outline drawing B, and the appropriate implant is selected and traced on the drawing.

Pediatric Surgery

Intertrochanteric Varus Derotation Osteotomy

Indications

- Deformity with valgus anteversion of the femoral neck where the femoral head does not sufficiently engage the acetabulum, generally in a developmentally dislocated hip.
- Legg–Calvé–Perthes disease where the margin of the acetabulum impacts a necrotic segment of the femoral head.
- Various traumatic, inflammatory, or congenital deformities of the femoral neck.

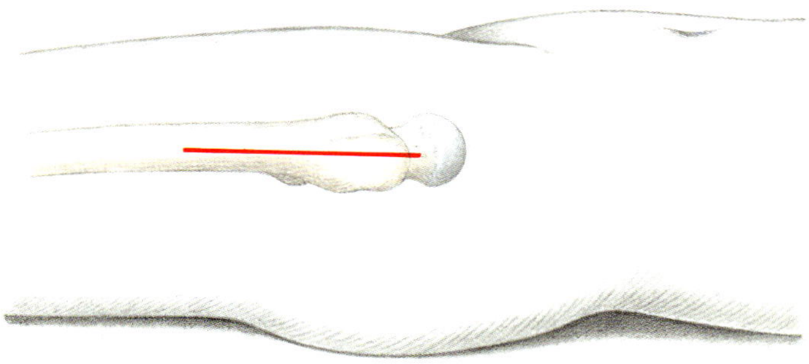

Fig. 2.**131** Positioning and incision for the intertrochanteric osteotomy. The patient is positioned supine on a radiolucent table. A longitudinal skin incision is made over the greater trochanter.

Positioning and Incision

With the patient positioned supine, a lateral approach to the proximal femur is made through a straight longitudinal skin incision (Fig. 2.**131**).

Technique

The pathologic anteversion and valgus position of the femoral neck is corrected with a varus derotation osteotomy, with the lesser trochanter maintained in its anatomic position. This normalizes the leverage of the musculature of the proximal femur. If the acetabulum is also dysplastic, the femoral head will be seated deeper into the acetabulum so that the acetabulum will engage a larger part of the articular surface.

A preoperative drawing is prepared showing the preoperative radiographic contours in the corrected position, the osteotomy, and the position of the implants (Fig. 2.**132**).

After the skin is incised on the lateral side of the hip, the fascia lata is split parallel to the direction of its fibers and retracted. The vastus lateralis is then visible in the deep layer of the wound. Its tendon is incised 5 mm distal to the most proximal aspect of the greater trochanter (Fig. 2.**133**). After splitting the vastus lateralis parallel to the direction of its fibers,

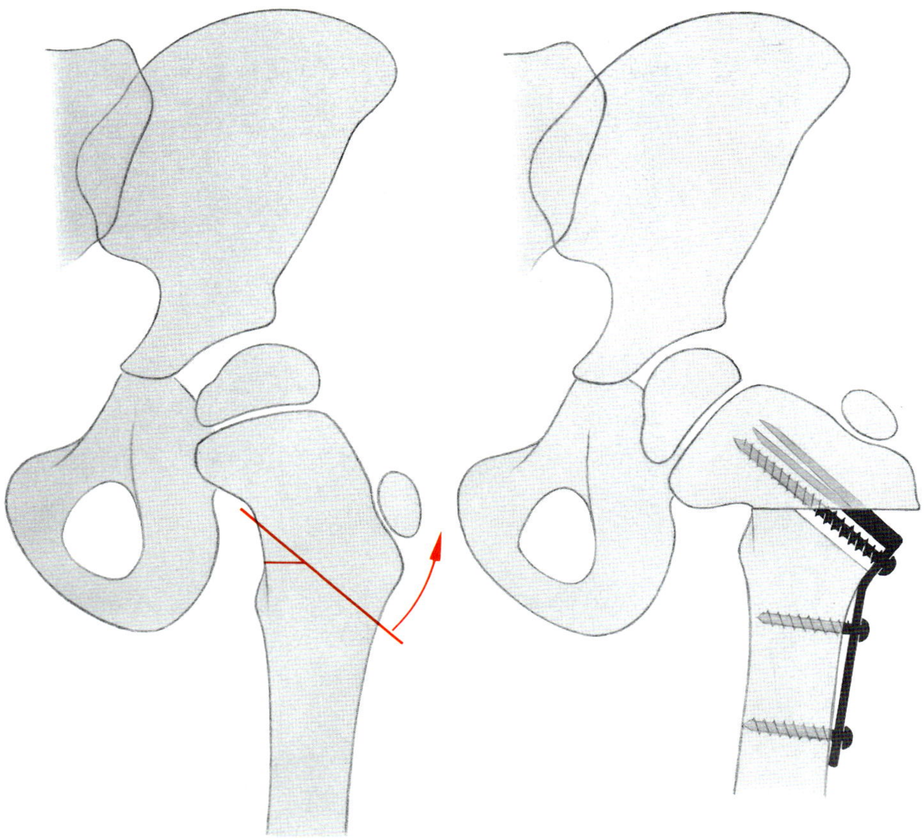

Fig. 2.**132** A preoperative planning drawing is prepared showing the corrected position of the proximal femur, the osteotomy, and the implants.

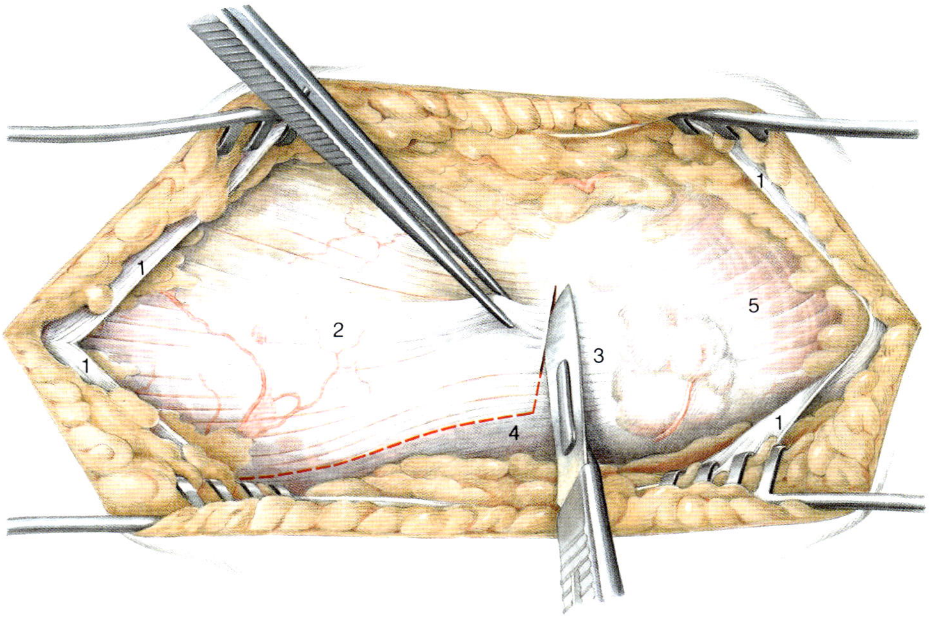

Fig. 2.**133** After the fascia lata is split parallel to the direction of its fibers and retracted, the origin of the vastus lateralis is dissected with an L-shaped incision 5 mm distal to the most proximal aspect of the greater trochanter.

1 Fascia lata
2 Vastus lateralis
3 Most proximal aspect of the greater trochanter
4 L-shaped incision in the vastus lateralis
5 Gluteus medius

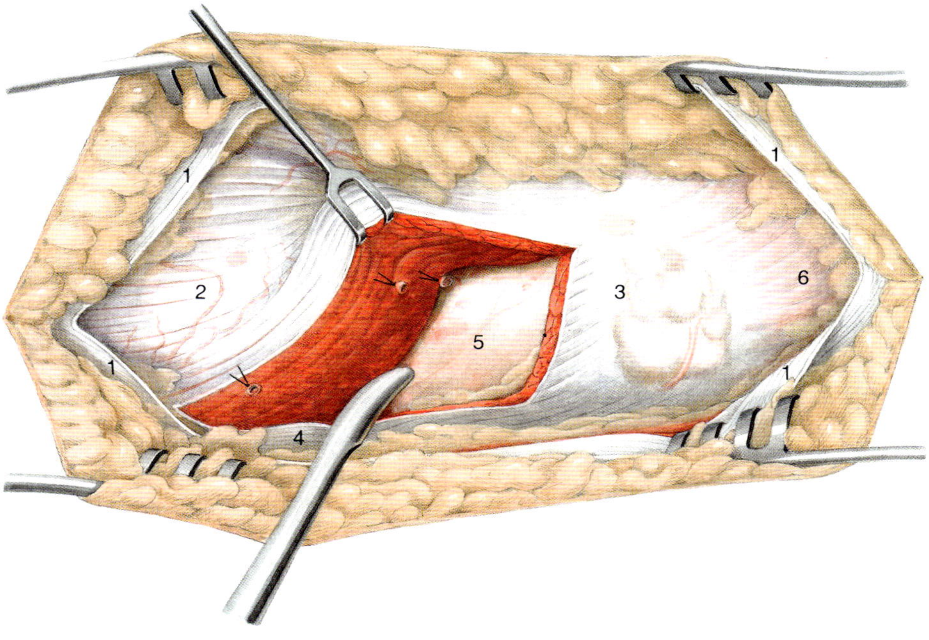

Fig. 2.**134** Dissecting the vastus lateralis from the lateral intermuscular septum and the femur with a sharp periosteal elevater.

1 Fascia lata
2 Vastus lateralis
3 Most proximal aspect of the greater trochanter
4 Lateral intermuscular septum
5 Femur
6 Gluteus medius

the surgeon carefully dissects it from the lateral intermuscular septum and the femur with a sharp periosteal elevator (Fig. 2.**134**). Narrow elevators are used to lift the musculature and expose the femur. Using a periosteal elevator and mallet, the surgeon exposes the osteotomy site on the posterior surface of the femur immediately proximal to the lesser trochanter. The cortex is exposed by dissecting the lateral intermuscular septum and the muscle origins from the linea aspera (Fig. 2.**135**). This helps to avoid injury to the adjacent veins. The surgeon now also inserts an elevator posteriorly at the osteotomy site.

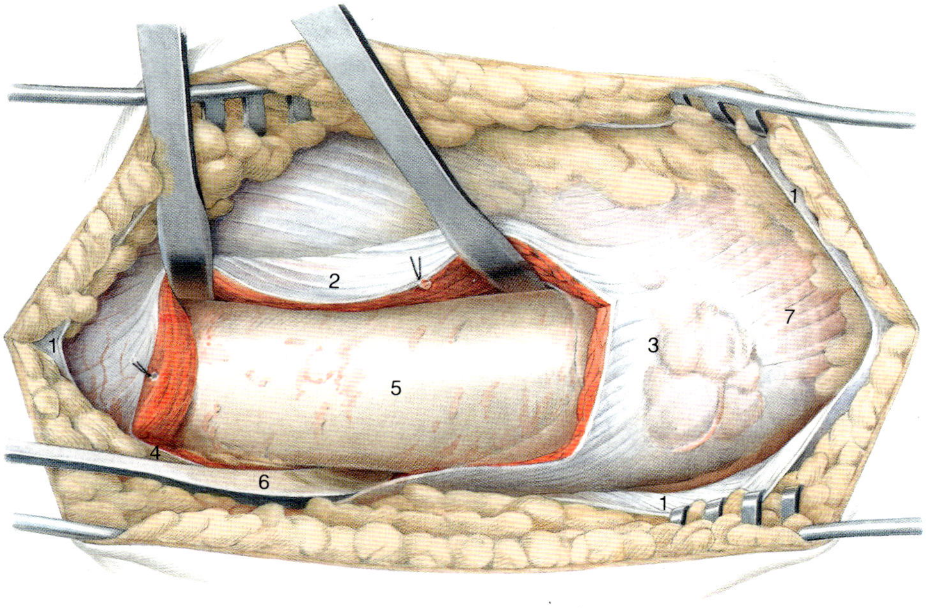

1 Fascia lata
2 Vastus lateralis
3 Most proximal aspect of the greater trochanter
4 Lateral intermuscular septum
5 Femur
6 Periosteal elevator exposing posterior femoral cortex
7 Gluteus medius

Fig. 2.**135** The osteotomy site on the posterior femoral cortex is exposed with a periosteal elevator and mallet.

The leg is then abducted and internally rotated to bring the femoral neck into the corrected position. A large marker wire is inserted into the proximal femur distal to the epiphysis of the greater trochanter. The marker wire lies in the horizontal plane (i.e., parallel to the floor of the operating room) and at a right angle to the median plane of the patient. Thus, the corrected position of the femoral neck is precisely defined and can be reliably reproduced after the intertrochanteric osteotomy. The position of the femoral neck and marker wire is verified with fluoroscopy (Fig. 2.**136**).

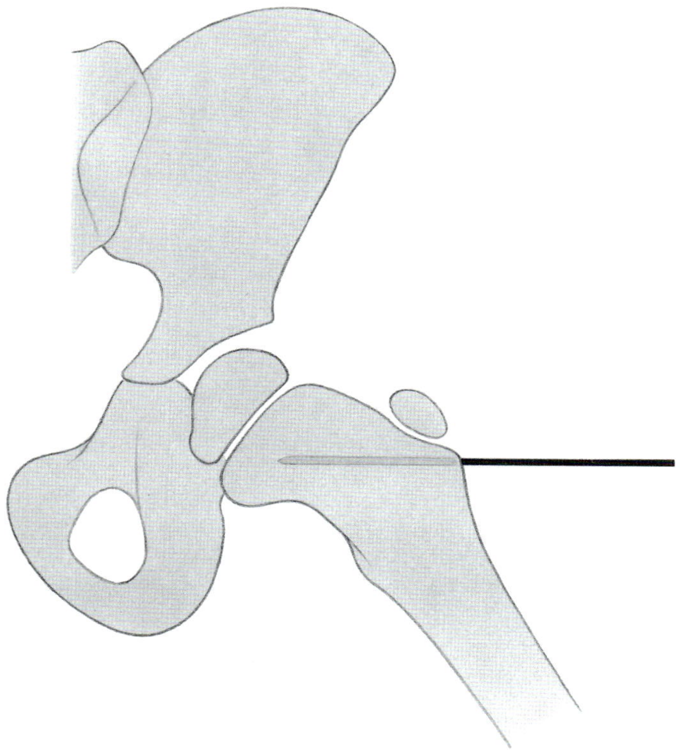

Fig. 2.**136** The leg is abducted and internally rotated to bring the femoral neck into the corrected position. A large marker wire is inserted into the proximal femur distal to the epiphyseal growth plate of the greater trochanter, parallel to the floor of the operating room, and at a right angle to the median plane of the patient.

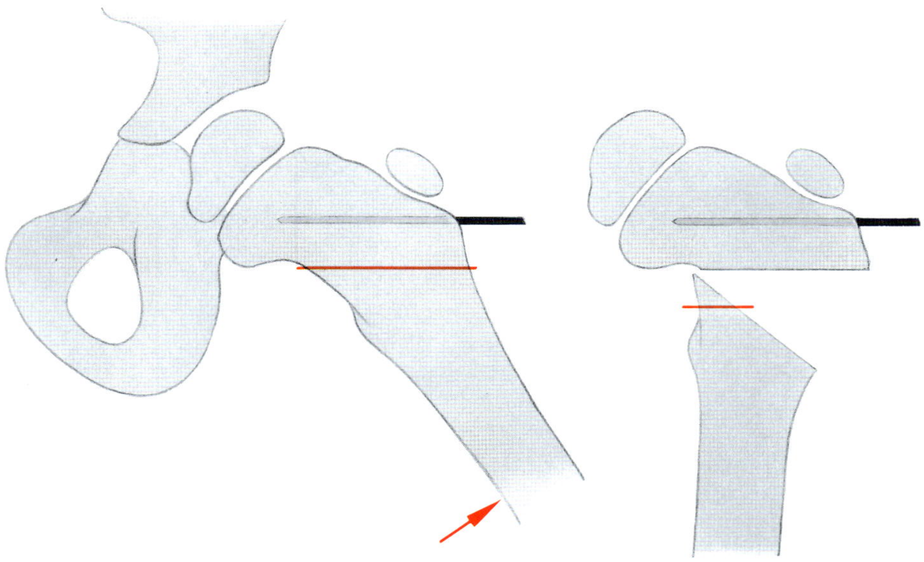

Fig. 2.**137** The osteotomy plane is vertical and parallel to the marker wire. The proximal femoral fragment with the marker wire is held in the corrected position, and the leg is adducted and externally rotated to return it to the middle position. The medial edge of the distal fragment is removed through the gap created by the osteotomy to create a contact surface between the two fragments.

The osteotomy plane is vertical and parallel to the marker wire; it lies superior to the epiphysis of the greater trochanter. Elevators are inserted to protect the surrounding soft tissue (Figs. 2.**137** and 2.**138**). The femoral neck with the marker wire is held in the corrected position, and the leg is adducted and externally rotated to return it to the middle position. This opens the gap created by the osteotomy and corrects the axial position. An osteotome inserted into the osteotomy provides a sliding surface to facilitate this correction. Preserving the lesser trochanter, the surgeon removes the medial edge of the distal fragment to create a contact surface between the two fragments. This resected wedge of bone is later inserted laterally into the gap created by the osteotomy.

The distal fragment is shifted medially with a blunt instrument (Fig. 2.**139**). The degree of medial shift depends on the length of the femoral neck. The medial shift prevents lateral displacement of the distal fragment when the varus correction of the femoral neck is made, so that the femoral shaft will remain in its original position.

A small angled plate with a bifurcate blade (a modification of Becker's plate) ist the implant of choice because it can be inserted into the proximal osteotomy surface to compress the two fragments while avoiding the epiphysis (Fig. 2.**140**). The bifurcate blade is driven into the cancellous osteotomy surface of the proximal fragment. The degree of medial shift is determined by the position of the blade in the proximal fragment; inserting the blade further medially increases the medial shift (Fig. 2.**141**). The blade is driven into the proximal osteotomy surface and fixed with a screw in the proximal fragment (Fig. 2.**142**).

To compress the two fragments, the distal screw is inserted into the shaft of the plate, slightly overcorrecting the planned medial shift. Then the proximal screw is tightened, drawing the femoral shaft toward the implant. The two fragments are

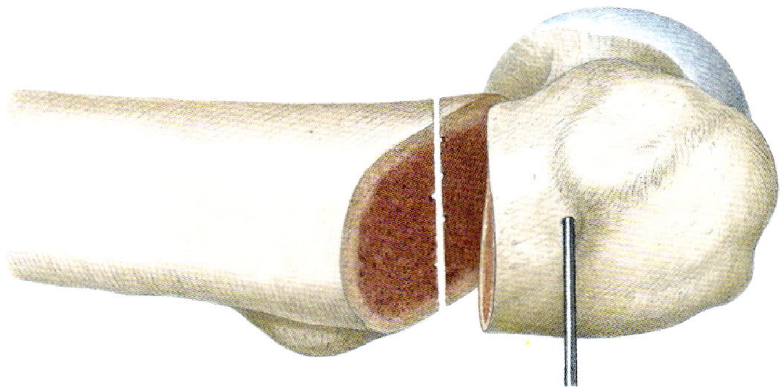

Fig. 2.**138** With the proximal femoral fragment in the corrected position, the medial edge of the distal fragment is removed through the gap created by the osteotomy.

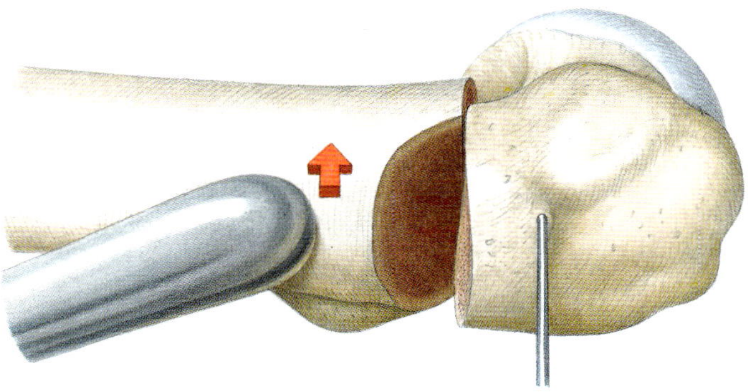

Fig. 2.**139** The distal fragment is shifted medially with a blunt instrument.

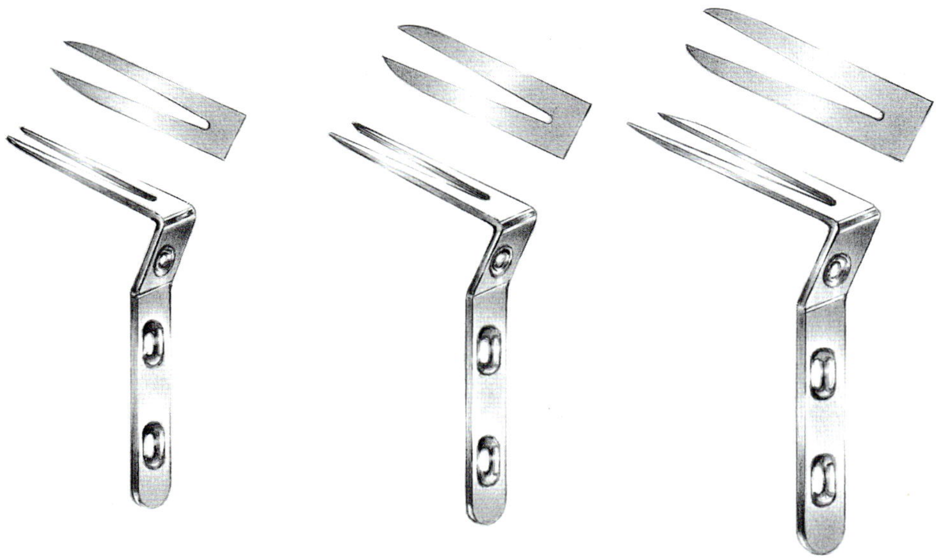

Fig. 2.**140** Small angled plate with a bifurcate blade in three sizes for internal fixation of the intertrochanteric osteotomy in children (a modification of Becker's plate).

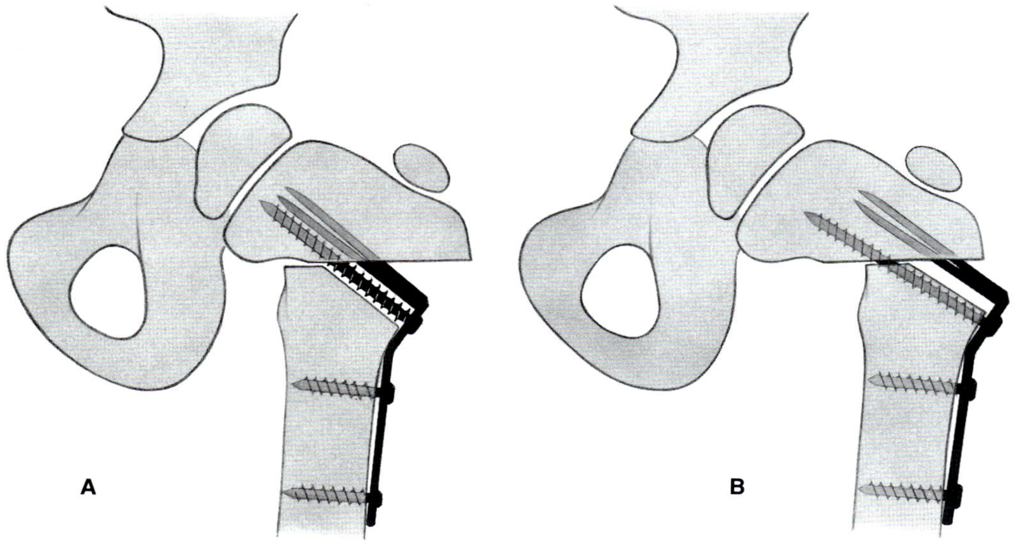

Fig. 2.**141** The degree of medial shift is determined by the position of the blade in the proximal fragment.
A: pronounced medial shaft,
B: no medial shift.

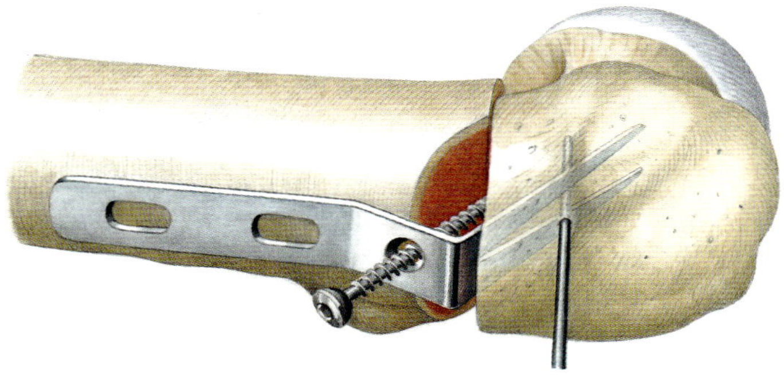

Fig. 2.**142** The blade of the angled plate is fixed with a screw in the proximal fragment.

thus rotated in opposite directions around the same center at the distal screw, compressing the medial contact point between the fragments (Fig. 2.**143**). The bone wedge removed from the medial edge of the distal fragment is inserted into the lateral gap created by the osteotomy. To strengthen fixation the plate is driven further into the bone and the most proximal screw is tightened again. This increases the compression between the two fragments (Fig. 2.**144**).

The vastus lateralis is reattached with strong sutures, preserving the important soft-tissue envelope it forms with the abductors (Fig. 2.**145**). The fascia lata is then closed over a suction drain with an overlapping suture. The wound is then closed in layers, and the skin is closed with a continuous suture before the antimicrobial film is removed (Fig. 2.**146**).

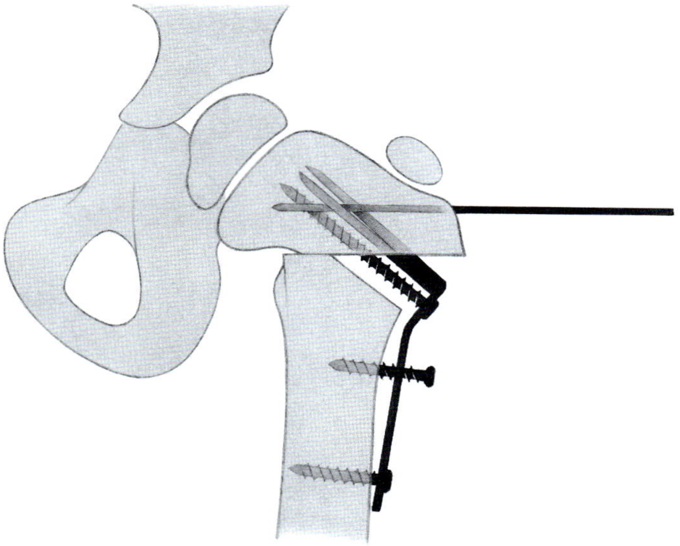

Fig. 2.**143** Compressing the two fragments. The distal screw is first inserted into the shaft of the plate, slightly overcorrecting the planned medial shift. Then the proximal screw is tightened and draws the femoral shaft toward the implant, compressing the medial contact point between the fragments.

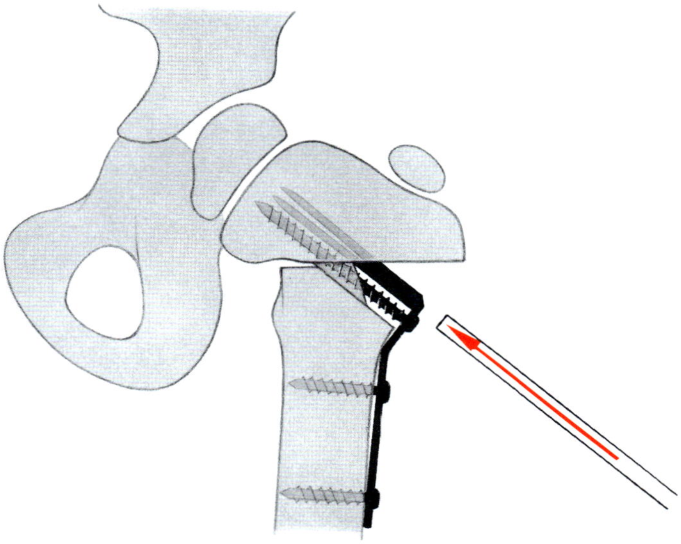

Fig. 2.**144** To strengthen fixation, the plate is driven further into the bone and the most proximal screw is tightened again.

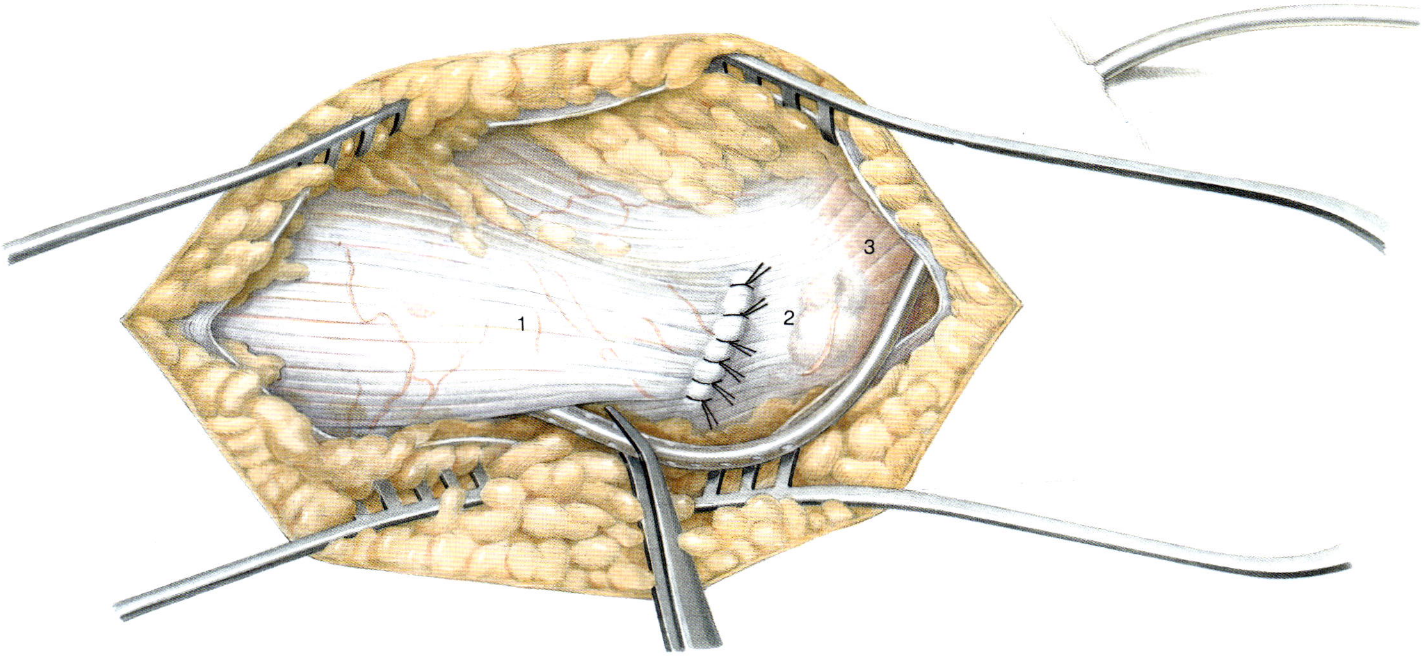

Fig. 2.**145** The vastus lateralis is reattached with strong sutures. The fascia lata is then closed over a suction drain.

1 Vastus lateralis
2 Most proximal aspect of the greater trochanter
3 Gluteus medius

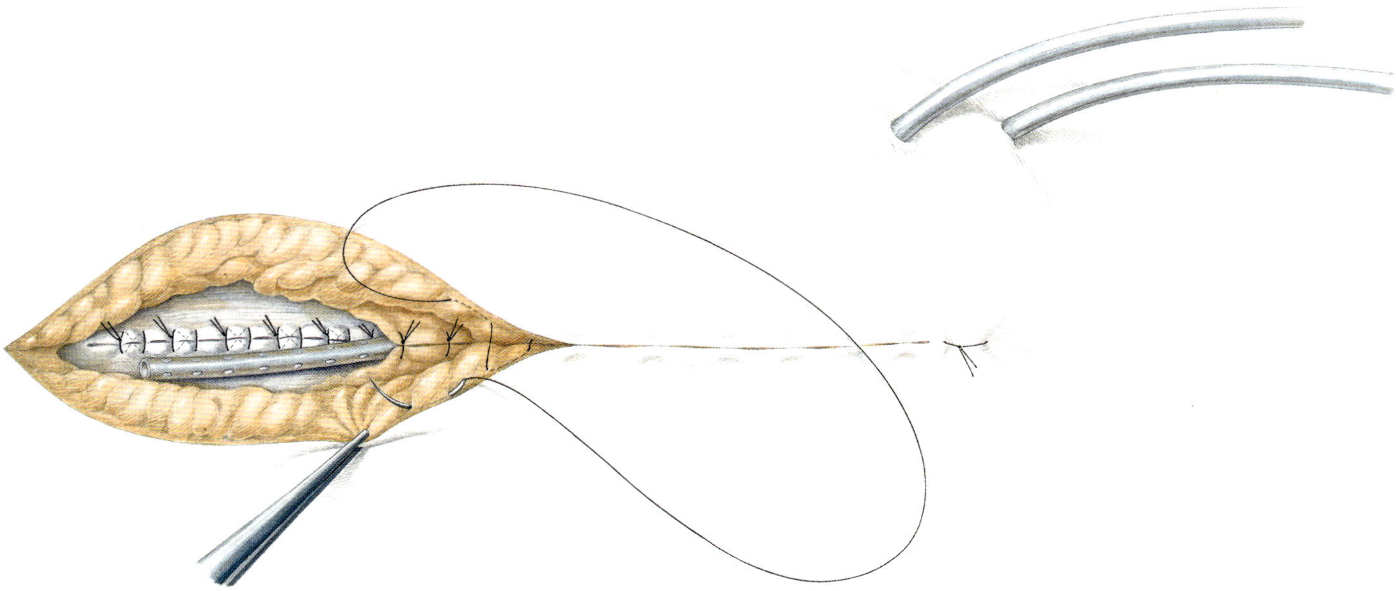

Fig. 2.**146** The wound is closed over a suction drain with a continuous suture before the antimicrobial film is removed.

Subtrochanteric Valgus Rotation Osteotomy

This procedure is used with Kirschner wire fixation for treatment of congenital coxa vara with and without subtrochanteric pseudarthrosis.

Indications

The procedure is used for surgical correction of congenital coxa vara with and without subtrochanteric pseudarthrosis, often in combination with retroversion of the femoral neck and acetabular dysplasia. This deformity is typically accompanied by shortened adductors and an adduction contracture of the hip, which prevents conventional correction of the femoral neck deformity.

Positioning and Incision

The patient is positioned supine with the leg draped free to permit movement, and a straight longitudinal skin incision is made for a lateral approach.

Technique

Since the procedure is performed on children, i.e., in skeletally immature patients, it must not interfere with epiphyseal bone growth. However, internal fixation is unavoidable due to the complicated pathologic anatomy. This requires choosing implants that ensure sufficient stability, yet avoid perforation of the epiphysis. Correcting the position of the femoral neck significantly increases leg length, and would excessively increase the existing soft-tissue tension. The tension resulting from such a correction would prevent complete adjustment of the femoral neck and produce intra-articular compression that could seriously damage the hip. The surgeon must therefore resect a segment of the distal femur to compensate for the increase in leg length produced by the valgus osteotomy of the femoral neck. This prevents an increase in soft-tissue tension (Fig. 2.**147**). After the hip joint has been stabilized, an osteotomy to compensate for the reduction in leg length can be performed at a later date. Attempting to forcefully achieve a valgus position of the femoral neck in the interest of increasing leg length will inevitably result in limited range of motion and permanent hip damage.

The skin incision courses distally from the greater trochanter on the lateral side of the hip. The fascia lata is split parallel to the direction of its fibers and retracted. This exposes the origin of the vastus lateralis. Due to the severe varus deformity of the proximal femur, the lateral margin of the femur generally protrudes from behind the origin of the vastus lateralis, displacing it anteriorly. The tendon of the gluteus maximus is scarred, thickened, and extremely hardened; there is often a wide gap in the lateral intermuscular septum distal to this tendon. The surgeon incises and dissects the origin of the vastus lateralis 5 mm distal to the most proximal aspect of the greater trochanter (Fig. 2.**148**).

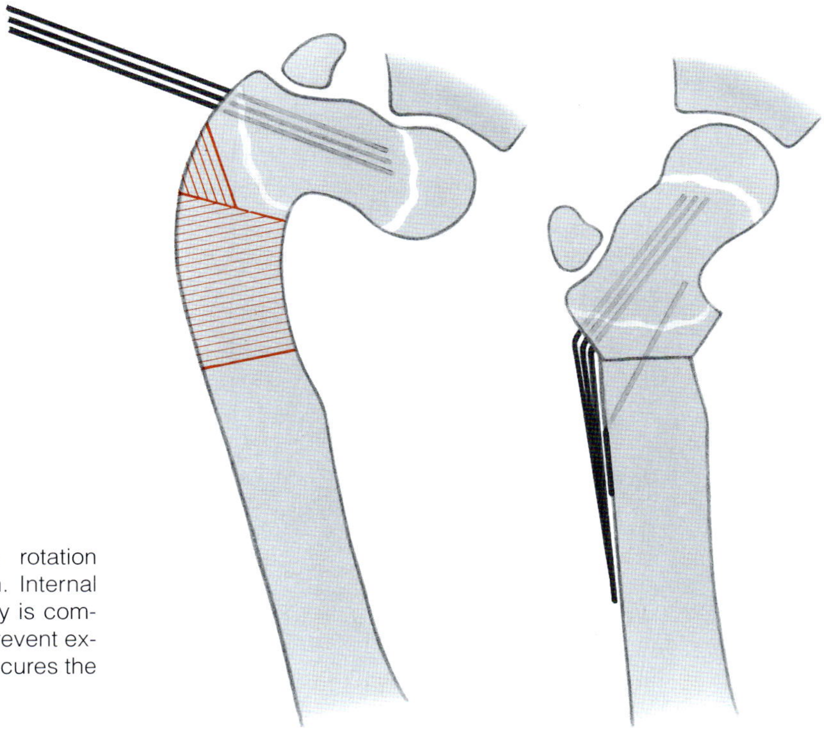

Fig. 2.**147** Principle of the subtrochanteric valgus rotation osteotomy for treatment of congenital coxa in children. Internal fixation is achieved with Kirschner wires. The osteotomy is combined with a segmental resectionof the distal femur to prevent excessive soft-tissue tension. A diagonal Kirschner wire secures the fragments against lateral displacement.

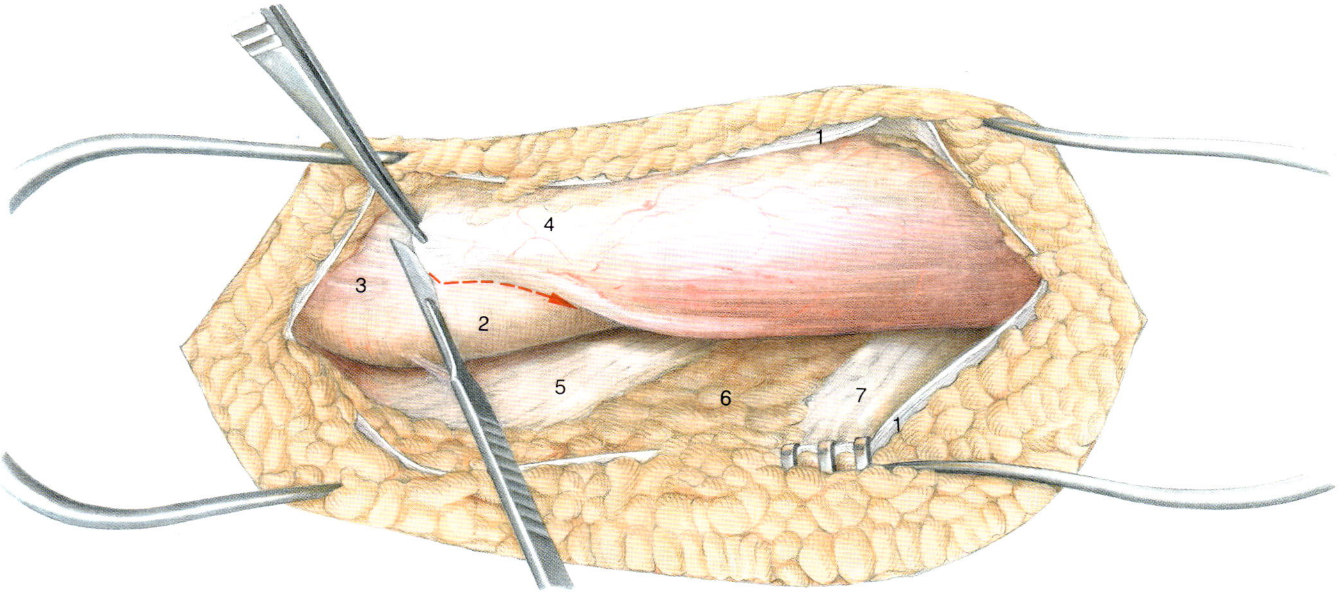

Fig. 2.**148** Lateral aspect of the hip in a patient with congenital coxa vara after the fascia lata has been incised and retracted. The origin of the vastus lateralis is dissected with an L-shaped incision immediately distal to the most proximal aspect of the greater trochanter.

1 Fascia lata
2 Femur
3 Gluteus medius
4 Vastus lateralis
5 Tendon of the gluteus maximus
6 Gap in the lateral intermuscular septum
7 Lateral intermuscular septum

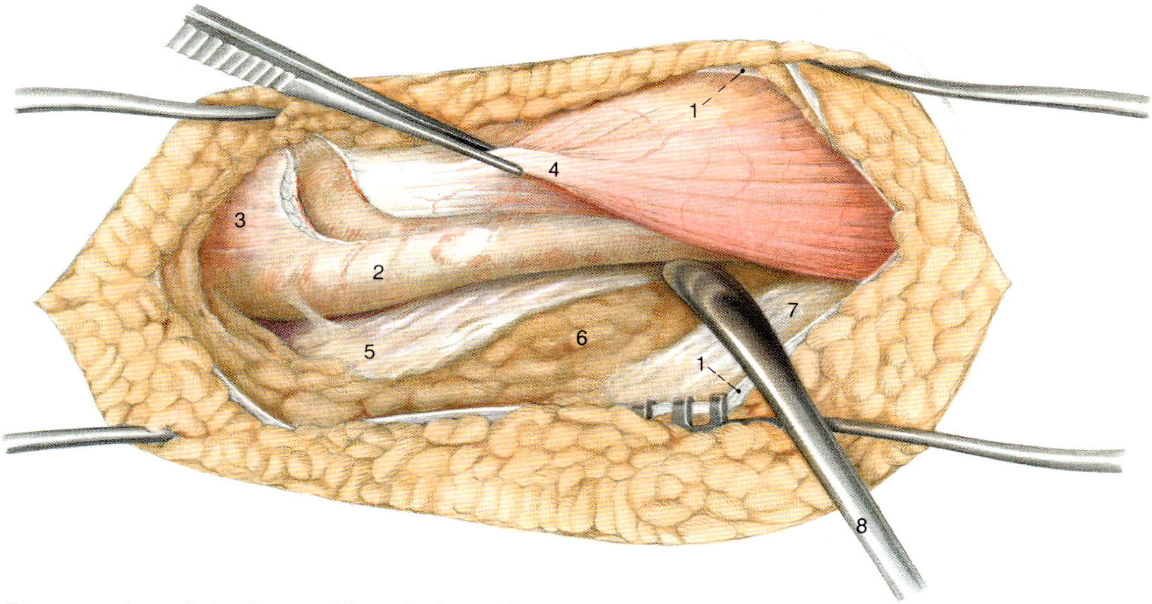

Fig. 2.**149** The vastus lateralis is dissected from the lateral intermuscular septum and the femur with a scalpel and a sharp periosteal elevator.

1 Fascia lata
2 Femur
3 Gluteus medius
4 Vastus lateralis
5 Tendon of the gluteus maximus
6 Gap in the lateral intermuscular septum
7 Lateral intermuscular septum
8 Sharp periosteal elevator

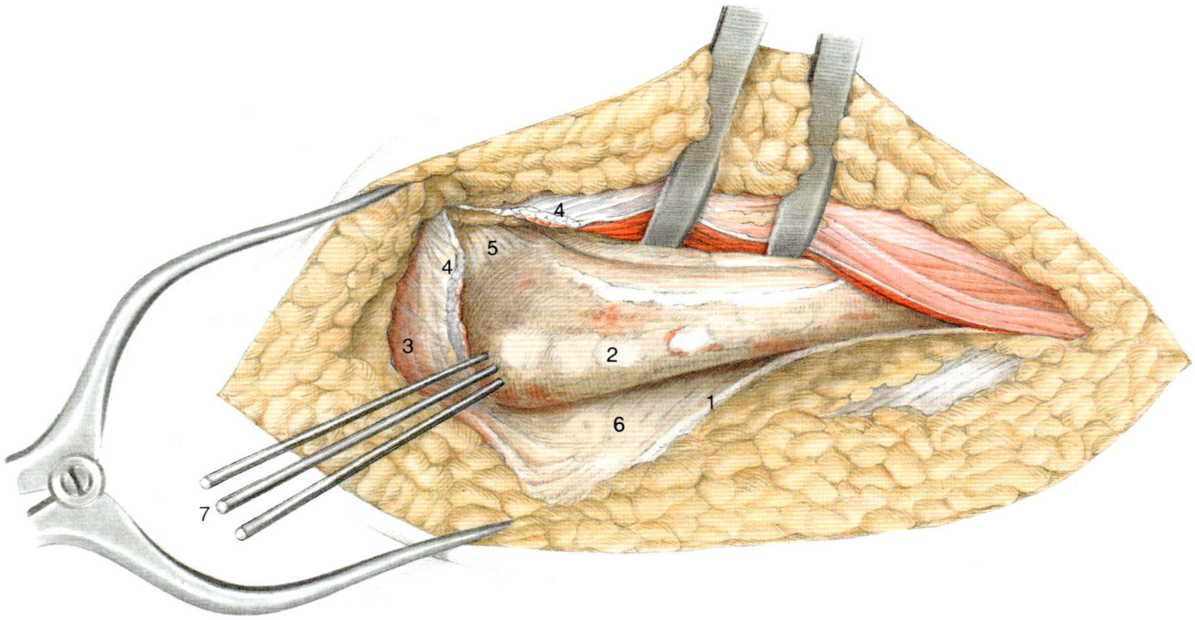

Fig. 2.**150** Elevators are inserted to lift the vastus lateralis and broadly expose the medial surface of the femur. Using fluoroscopy, the surgeon inserts three 2.5-mm Kirschner wires. They are inserted into the femoral neck along its longitudinal axis. Care must be taken not to perforate the epiphyseal growth plate.

1 Fascia lata
2 Femur
3 Gluteus medius
4 Vastus lateralis
5 Hip joint capsule
6 Tendon of the gluteus maximus
7 Three 2.5-mm Kirschner wires

The vastus lateralis is dissected from the lateral intermuscular septum and the femur with a scalpel and a sharp periosteal elevator (Fig. 2.**149**). Elevators are inserted to lift the vastus lateralis and broadly expose the medial surface of the femur. A 2.5-mm Kirschner wire is inserted into the femoral neck along its longitudinal axis, stopping immediately short of the epiphysis. After verifying the correct position of the first wire with fluoroscopy, the surgeon inserts two additional ones of the same thickness immediately beside and parallel to the first wire (Fig. 2.**150**). These three Kirschner wires are used as a handle for adjusting the position of the proximal femur and for subsequent internal fixation. The position of the wires is verified with fluoroscopy (Fig. 2.**151**).

The surgeon now exposes the site of the subtrochanteric osteotomy on the posterior surface of the femur using a periosteal elevator and mallet (Fig. 2.**152**). Elevators are inserted to protect the soft tissue, and the subtrochanteric transverse osteotomy is performed perpendicular to the surface of the bone with an oscillating saw. The distal fragment of the femur is then mobilized. A major problem encountered in congenital coxa vara is the extremely hardened scar-like thickening of the periosteum and the adjacent soft tissue on the medial surface of the femur, which initially prevents any

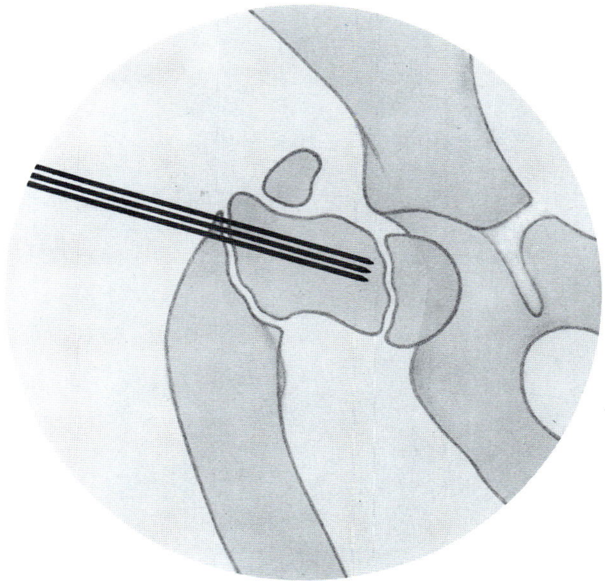

Fig. 2.**151** The position of the Kirschner wires is verified with fluoroscopy. The wires run parallel to the axis of the femoral neck, crossing the congenital pseudarthrosis and stopping short of the epiphyseal growth plate.

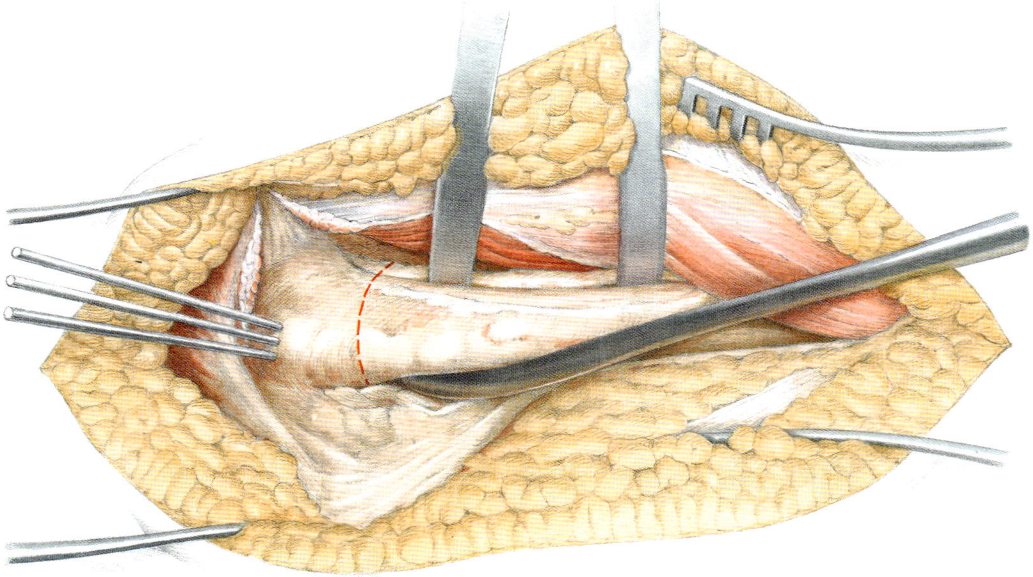

Fig. 2.**152** The osteotomy site on the femoral cortex (dotted line) is exposed with a periosteal elevator and mallet.

correction. Extensive dissection, and often resection, of these hardened soft-tissue structures is required. First, the distal fragment is retracted laterally with a forceps (Fig. 2.**153**). While holding the fragment with the forceps, the surgeon resects the hardened soft-tissue structures from the medial surface with a sharp periosteal elevator. Pulling the distal fragment anteriorly, he then resects the hardened soft-tissue structures from the posterior surface with a scalpel (Fig. 2.**154**). After this is done, extensive resection of the hardened soft-tissue structures may be necessary.

After the distal fragment has been sufficiently mobilized, the Kirschner wires are used as a handle to effect a valgus adjustment of the femoral neck until it is in an ideal position. Straightening the femoral neck in this manner increases soft-tissue tension, which pushes the distal fragment over the proximal one. When the proper soft-tissue tension has been achieved with the femoral neck in the corrected position, the surgeon marks the plane of the segmental resection on the distal fragment at the level of the proximal osteotomy surface (Fig. 2.**155**). The surgeon should refrain from resecting a shorter segment because that will increase soft-tissue tension and intra-articular compression and make it difficult to adjust the position of the femoral neck. A transverse osteotomy of the distal femoral fragment is performed at the marked site. After the segment has been removed, the two fragments can be opposed with the femoral neck in the corrected position without excessive soft-tissue tension. A Kirschner wire is inserted diagonally into the distal fragment to bridge the site of the osteotomy and stabilize the two fragments against displacement (Fig. 2.**156**). Now the retroversion of the femoral neck can be corrected by internally rotating the distal fragment.

The diagonal Kirschner wire is first bent superiorly close to the surface of the bone with a bending iron and then rotated distally with a pliers until it lies flat on the surface of the bone. If the wire does not lie completely flat, it can be rotated back and bent a bit more (Fig. 2.**157**). One after the other, the thick Kirschner wires in the femoral neck are bent distally with a bending iron until they are at an angle of 25° to the surface of the distal fragment. For the internal fixation to be stable, there must be enough distance between the wires and the surface of the distal fragment to create sufficient tension when the wires are pressed to the surface of the bone (Fig. 2.**158**). Cerclage clamps are fabricated from one-third tubu-

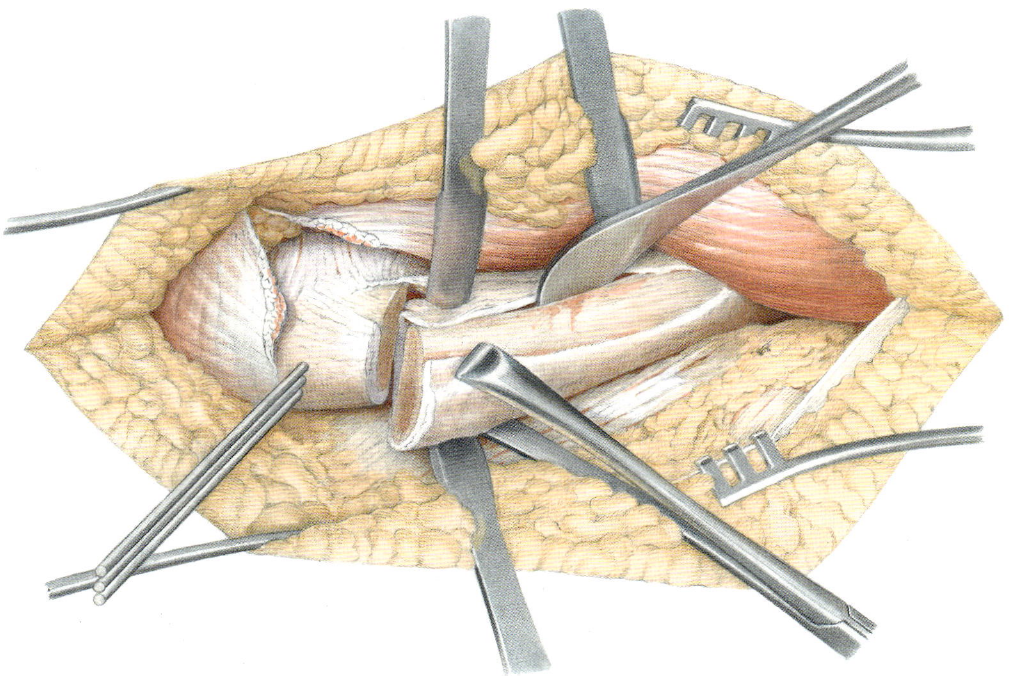

Fig. 2.**153** After the osteotomy, the distal fragment is mobilized. The fragment is retracted laterally with a forceps while the hardened soft-tissue structures on the medial surface are resected with a sharp periosteal elevator.

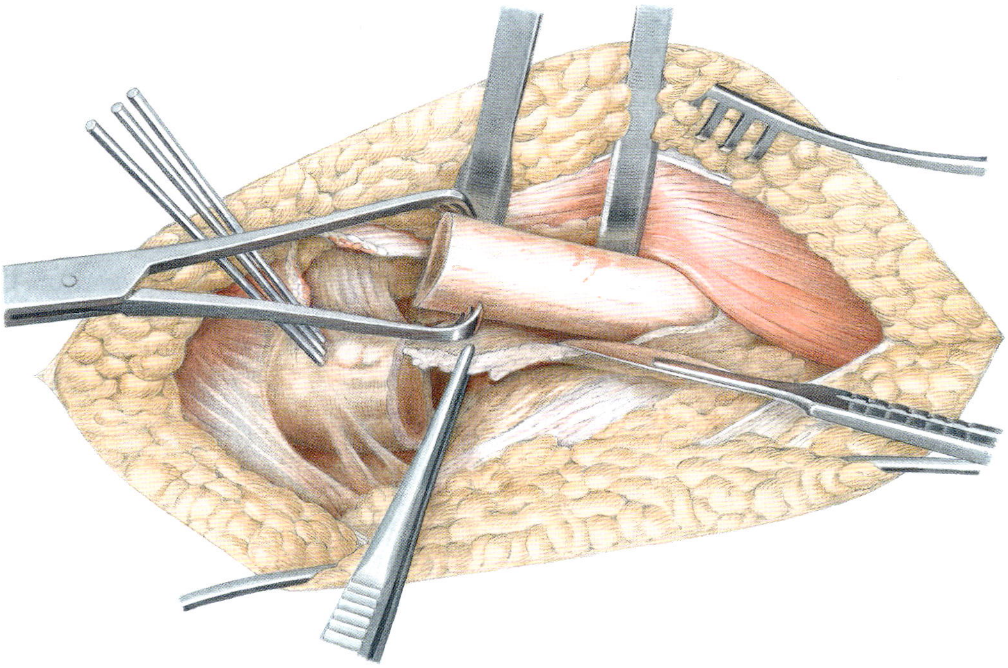

Fig. 2.**154** The distal fragment is retracted anteriorly and the hardened soft-tissue structures are resected from the posterior surface as well.

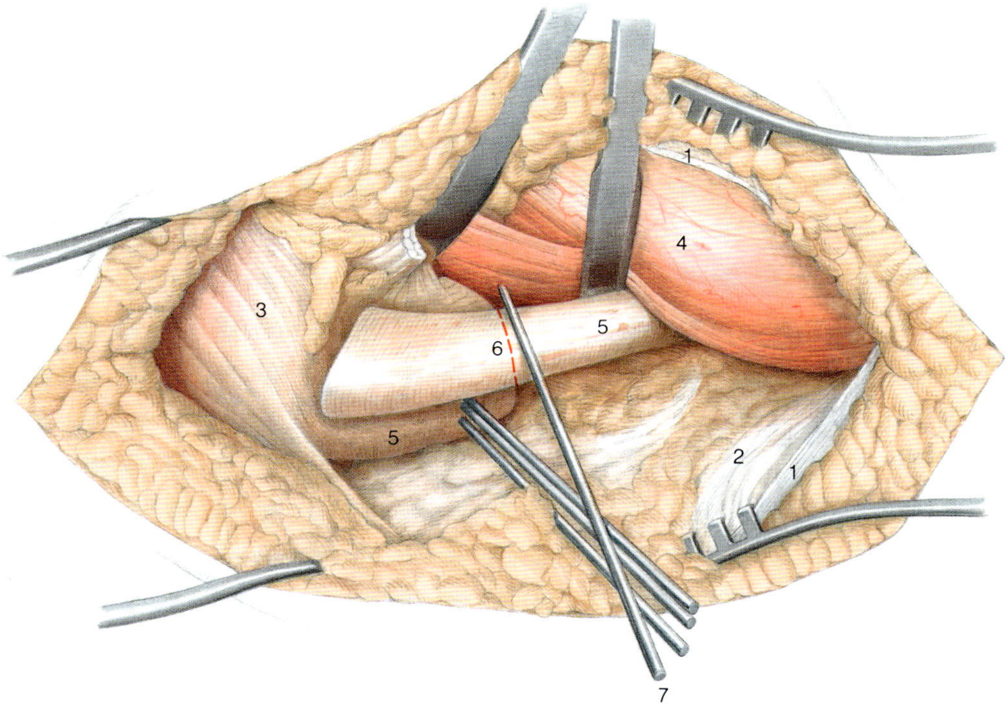

Fig. 2.**155** The femoral neck is brought into the corrected position with a valgus shift of the proximal fragment, which pushes the distal fragment past the proximal one. After the corrected position is achieved there will be slight soft-tissue tension. The level of the proximal osteotomy surface is marked on the distal fragment (dotted line). This determines the length of the segmental resection. A marker wire is inserted at the planned osteotomy site and its position is verified with fluoroscopy.

1 Fascia lata
2 Lateral intermuscular septum
3 Gluteus medius
4 Vastus lateralis
5 Femur
6 Site of segmental osteotomy
7 Marker wire for segmental osteotomy

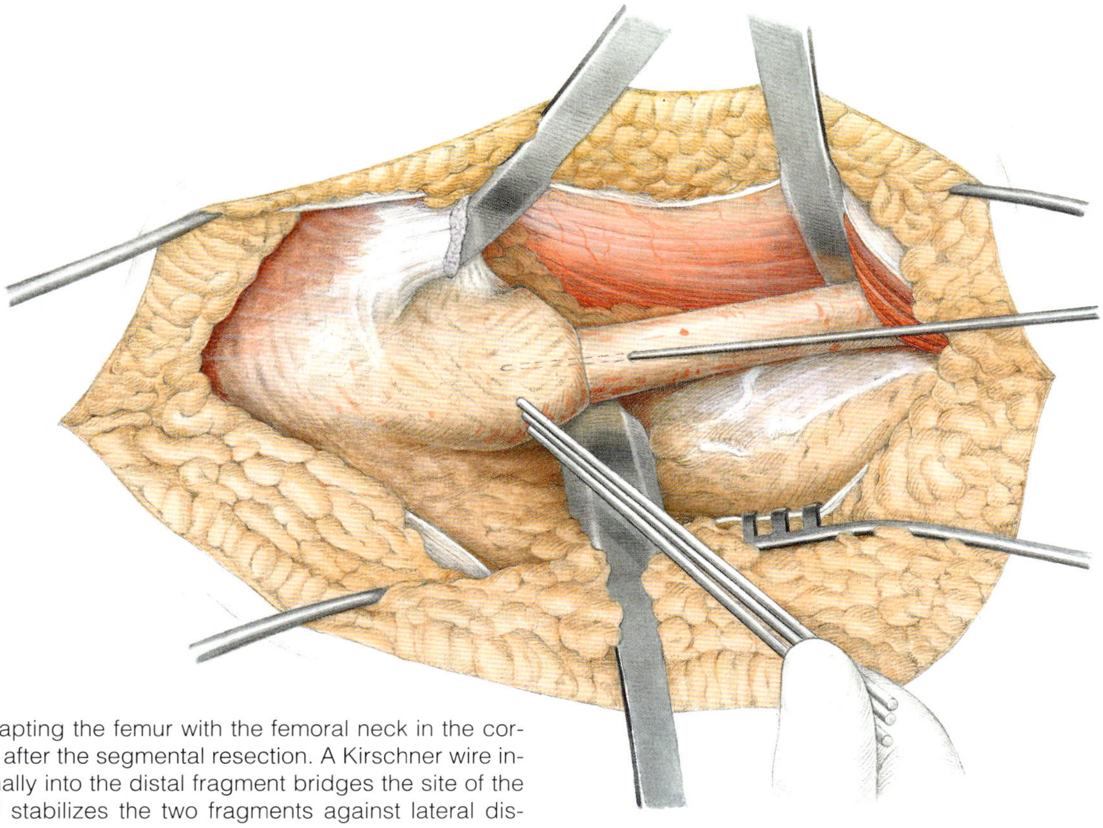

Fig. 2.**156** Adapting the femur with the femoral neck in the corrected position after the segmental resection. A Kirschner wire inserted diagonally into the distal fragment bridges the site of the osteotomy and stabilizes the two fragments against lateral displacement.

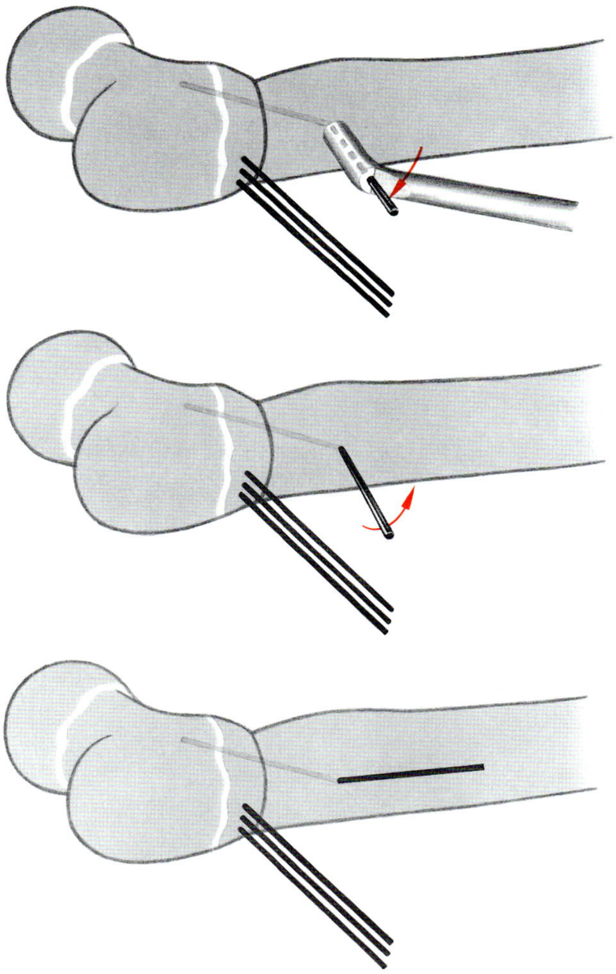

lar plate and bent in an arc to fit the surface of the bone. The Kirschner wires are then pressed against the distal fragment with a holding forceps and fastened with the fabricated clamps. First the distal clamp is applied, then the proximal one (Fig. 2.**159**). The corrected position of the fragments is verified with fluoroscopy (Fig. 2.**160**). To help accelerate bony consolidation, a narrow gouge is then used to roughen the posterior and anterior surface of the two fragments near the osteotomy. The surgeon raises "scales" in the cortex under which he inserts fine bone chips taken from the resected segment (Fig. 2.**161**).

Fig. 2.**157** The diagonal Kirschner wire is first bent superiorly at the surface of the bone and then rotated distally 180° until it lies flat on the surface of the bone.

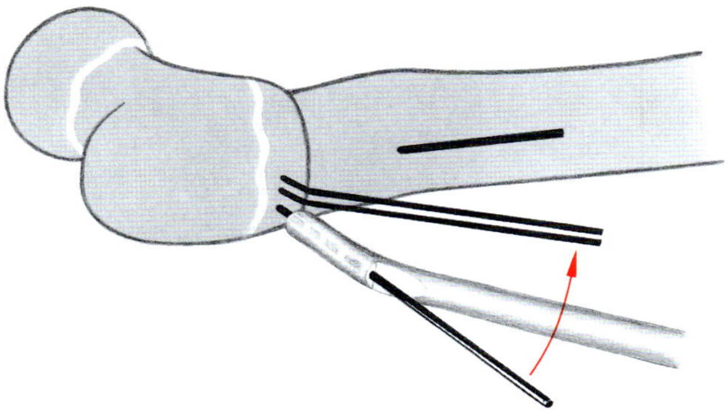

Fig. 2.**158** The thick Kirschner wires in the femoral neck are bent distally with a bending iron until they are at an angle of 25° to the surface of the distal fragment.

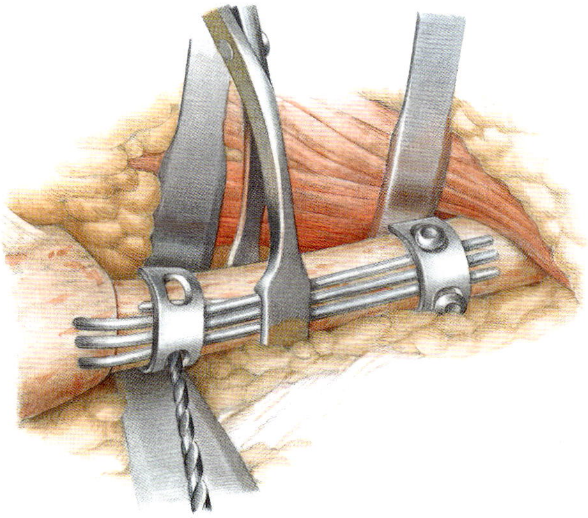

Fig. 2.**159** Cerclage clamps are fabricated from one-third tubular plate and bent in an arc to fit the surface of the bone. The Kirschner wires are then pressed against the distal fragment and held in place with a forceps while they are fastened with the clamps.

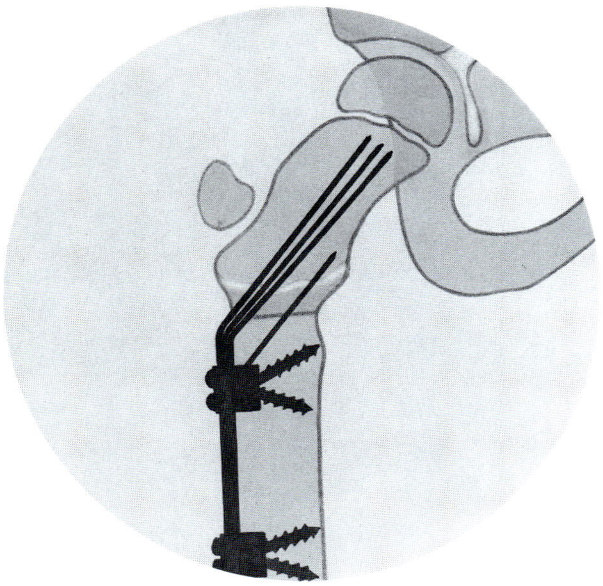

Fig. 2.**160** The corrected position of the femoral neck and the placement of the implants are verified. The illustration shows how the wires also bridge and stabilize the congenital subtrochanteric pseudarthrosis.

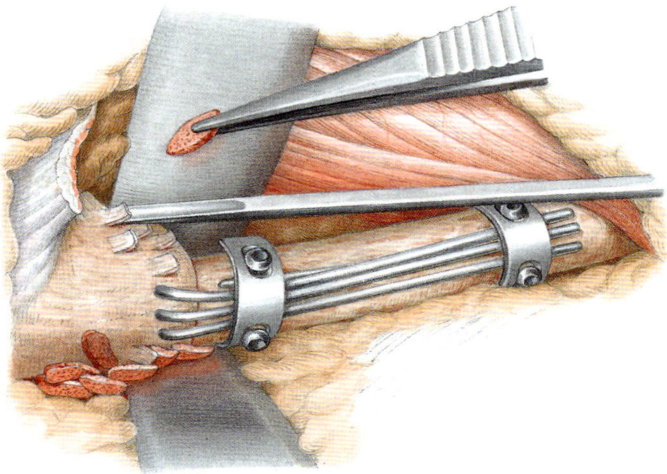

Fig. 2.**161** To help accelerate bony consolidation, the surgeon roughens the posterior and anterior surface of the two fragments, raising fine "scales" in the cortex under which fine bones chips, taken from the resected segment, are inserted.

The surgeon then reattaches the vastus lateralis by suturing it under tension to the most proximal aspect of the greater trochanter and the origin of the gluteus medius (Fig. 2.**162**). To ensure the stability of the internal fixation and preserve muscular strength, the muscle must be reattached with sufficient tension. After a suction drain has been inserted, the fascia lata is then sutured under tension (Fig. 2.**163**).

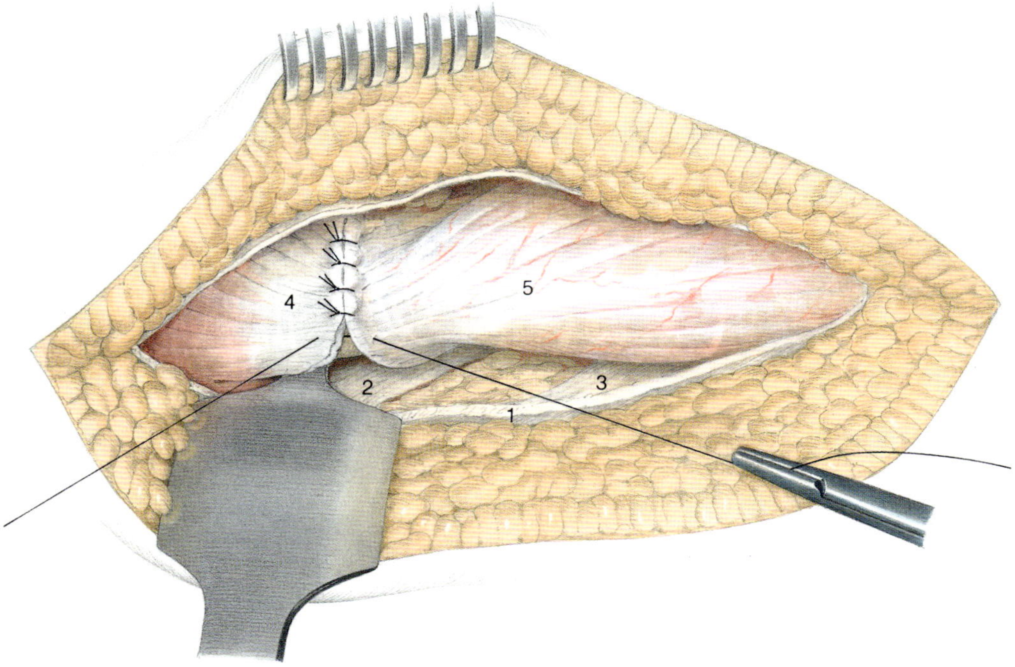

Fig. 2.**162** To restore the soft-tissue envelope, the vastus lateralis is reattached to the most proximal aspect of the greater trochanter and securely sutured to the origin of the gluteus medius.

1 Fascia lata
2 Origin of the gluteus maximus
3 Lateral intermuscular septum
4 Gluteus medius
5 Vastus lateralis

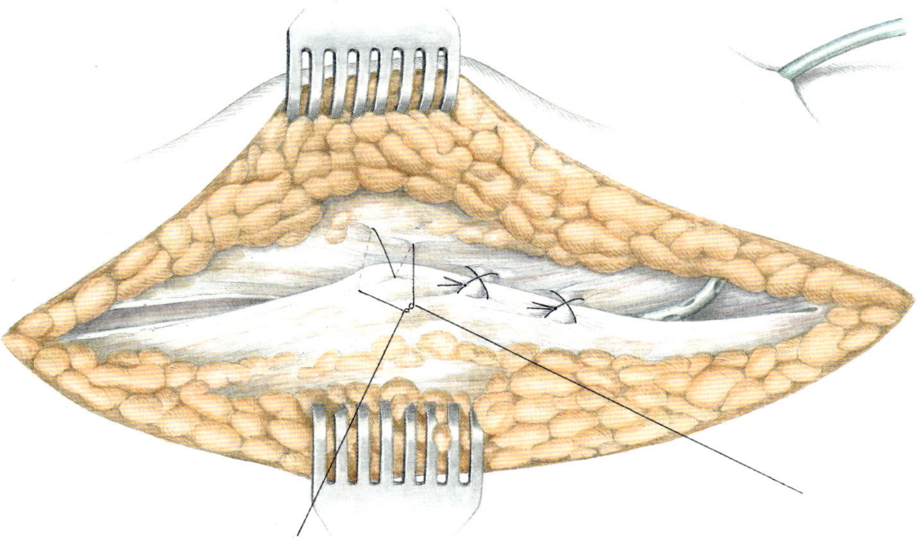

Fig. 2.**163** To further stabilize the lateral soft-tissue envelope of the hip before the incision is closed, the fascia lata is closed over a suction drain with a strong overlapping suture.

Operations on Adolescents and Young Adults

Trochanteric Advancement

Indications

For reconstructions of the proximal femur where there is a shortened femoral neck and superiorly protruding greater trochanter. The continued growth of the greater trochanter following isolated growth arrest of the femoral neck is the most common etiology. This is seen in developmentally dislocated hips, or after traumatic or inflammatory growth plate lesions produce a deformity in which the femoral neck is shortened and the greater trochanter protrudes superiorly. This results in relative lengthening of the hip abductors and subsequent loss of power in the pelvic and trochanteric musculature. This causes decreasing stability of the hip. Trochanteric advancement shifts the greater trochanter into a physiologically correct position (Fig. 2.**164**).

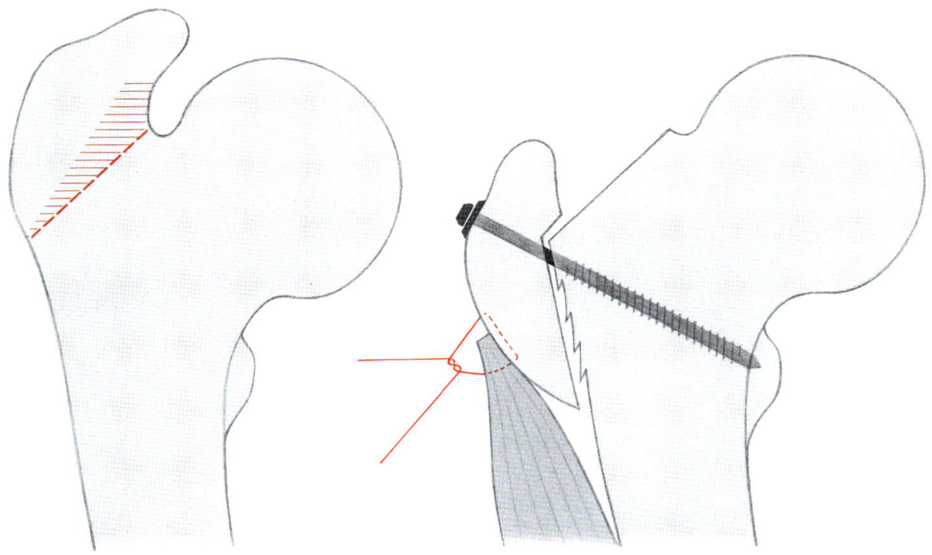

Fig. 2.**164** Principle of the trochanteric advancement. The greater trochanter is resected from the femur in an osteotomy beginning immediately superior to the trochanteric fossa and coursing superiorly and medially. After its soft-tissue attachments are mobilized, the osteotomized greater trochanter is positioned on the prepared lateral surface of the femur so that its apex is level with the center of the femoral head where it is fixed with screws. The vastus lateralis is then reattached to the tendon of the gluteus medius.

Positioning and Incision

With the patient positioned supine on a radiolucent table, a longitudinal skin incision is made that begins at the apex of the greater trochanter and courses distally (Fig. 2.**165**).

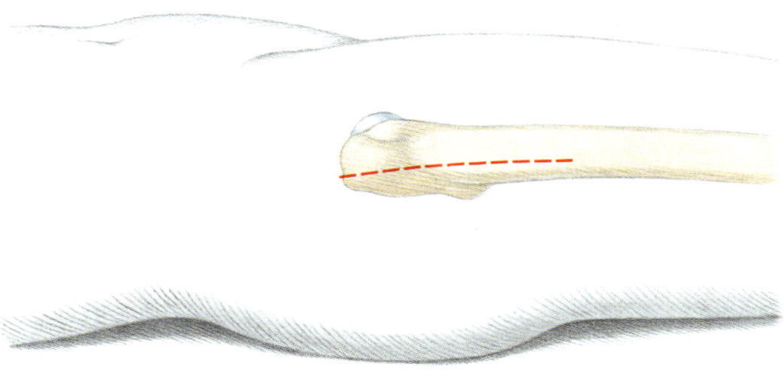

Fig. 2.**165** Positioning and incision for trochanteric advancement.

Surgical Technique

After the fascia lata above the greater trochanter is split parallel to the direction of its fibers and retracted, the origin of the vastus lateralis is dissected with an L-shaped incision immediately distal to the most proximal aspect of the greater trochanter (Fig. 2.**166**). The surgeon dissects the muscle from the lateral intermuscular septum and the femur with a periosteal elevator (Fig. 2.**167**). The vastus lateralis is lifted with an elevator inserted at the medial surface of the femur. Distal to the most proximal aspect of the greater trochanter, the surgeon inserts a marking wire aligned with the trochanteric fossa to indicate the site of the trochanteric osteotomy (Fig. 2.**168**). The position of the marker wire is verified with fluoroscopy (Fig. 2.**169**). The osteotomy should begin immediately distal to the most proximal aspect of the greater trochanter, coursing at a superior angle of 45° to the median plane and ending medially slightly superior to the trochanteric fossa (Fig. 2.**170**). The marking wire should lie approximately 3 mm proximal to the osteotomy plane to allow sufficient space for the oscillating saw. The trochanteric osteotomy is performed immediately distal and parallel to the marking wire (Fig. 2.**171**). An oscillating saw is preferable to an osteotome because it avoids damage to the trochanteric fragment even if the bone is osteopenic. This is important for the subsequent fixation of the greater trochanter. The osteotomy ends medially slightly before reaching the medial surface of the greater trochanter to avoid damaging the vascular structures located there.

The surgeon then inserts a wide chisel into the gap created by the osteotomy and lifts it superiorly to break through the me-

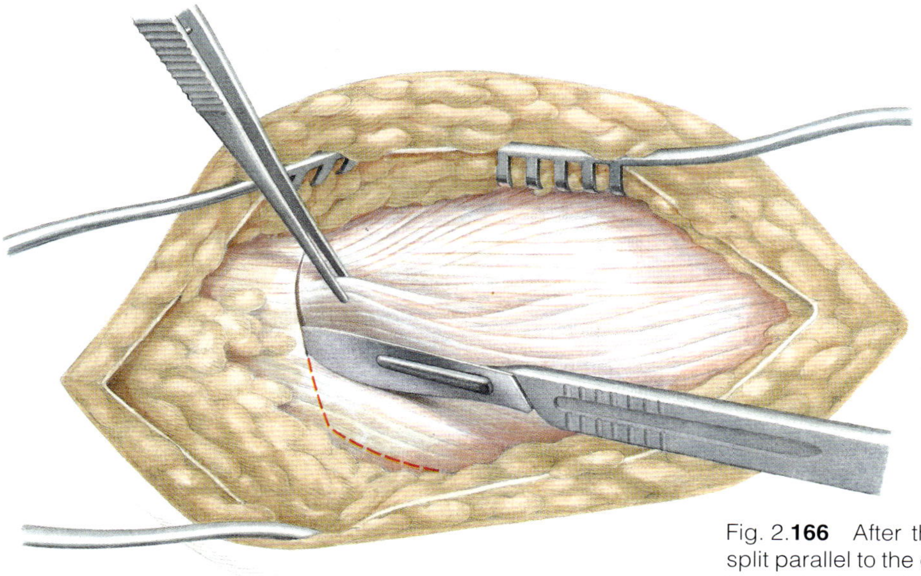

Fig. 2.**166** After the fascia lata above the greater trochanter is split parallel to the direction of its fibers and retracted, the origin of the vastus lateralis is dissected with an L-shaped incision distal to the most proximal aspect of the greater trochanter and resected from the lateral intermuscular septum.

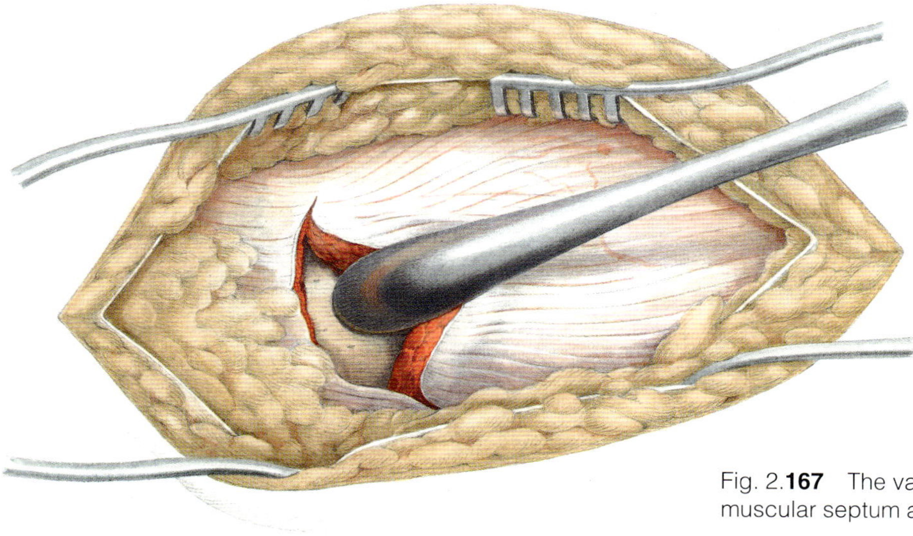

Fig. 2.**167** The vastus lateralis is dissected from the lateral intermuscular septum and the femur with a periosteal elevator.

dial cortex. The chisel is used as a lever to mobilize the medial greater trochanter, displacing it superiorly (Fig. 2.**172**). The scarred adhesions between the greater trochanter and the joint capsule (which is generally thickened) should be removed carefully so that the greater trochanter can be shifted to its corrected position without having to be forced. A narrow bone spreader is then inserted into the gap created by the osteotomy to mobilize the greater trochanter (Fig. 2.**173**).

The greater trochanter is then retracted superiorly and laterally with a narrow bone clamp, and the remaining adhesions between the greater trochanter and the joint capsule are released with curved dissection scissors (Fig. 2.**174**). The scissors should be pointed superiorly and laterally to avoid damaging the trochanteric fossa (Fig. 2.**175**). The surgeon continues to release these scarred adhesions until he feels only the elastic resistance of the pelvic and trochanteric muscles when pulling the greater trochanter and he can easily shift it into the corrected position. At this point, the surgeon may contour the osteotomy surface of the greater trochanter if required.

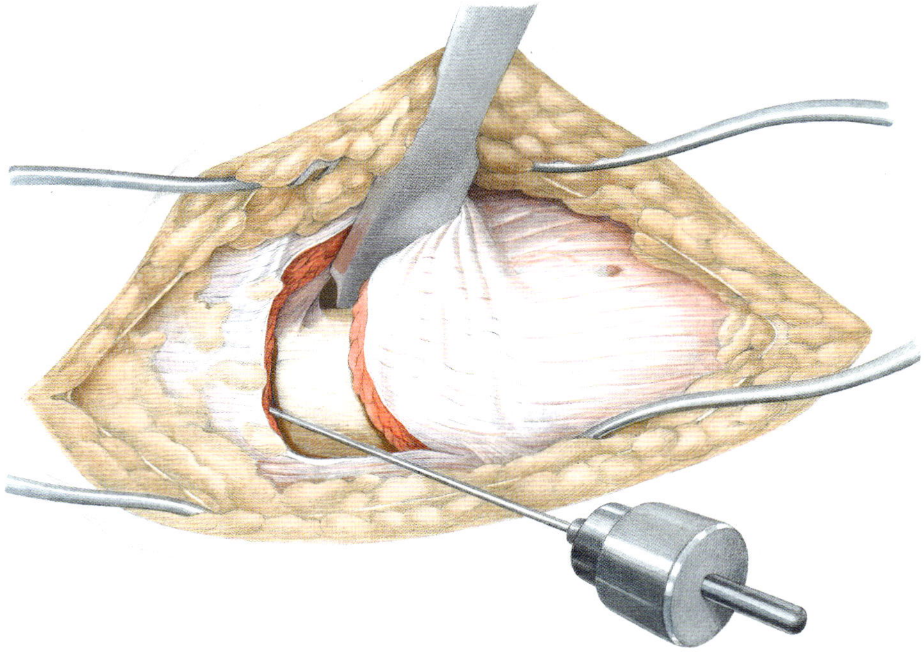

Fig. 2.**168** The vastus lateralis is lifted with an elevator. Immediately distal to the most proximal aspect of the greater trochanter, the surgeon inserts a marking wire to indicate the site of the trochanteric osteotomy.

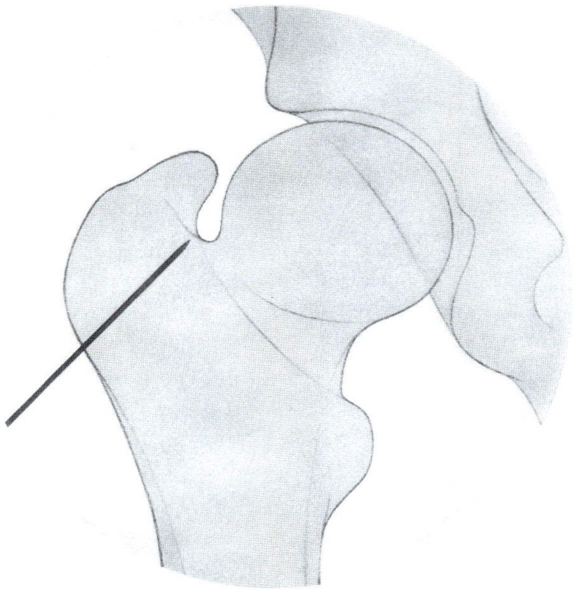

Fig. 2.**169** Verifying the position of the marker wire for the trochanteric osteotomy with fluoroscopy.

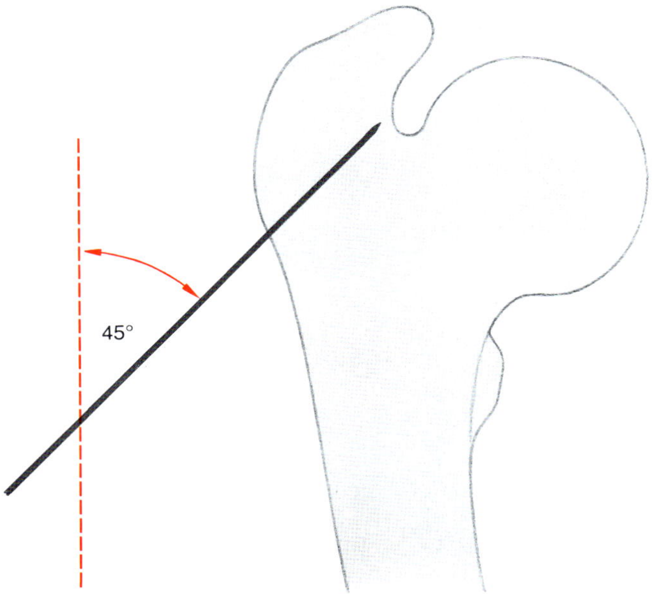

Fig. 2.**170** Desired angle of the trochanteric osteotomy.

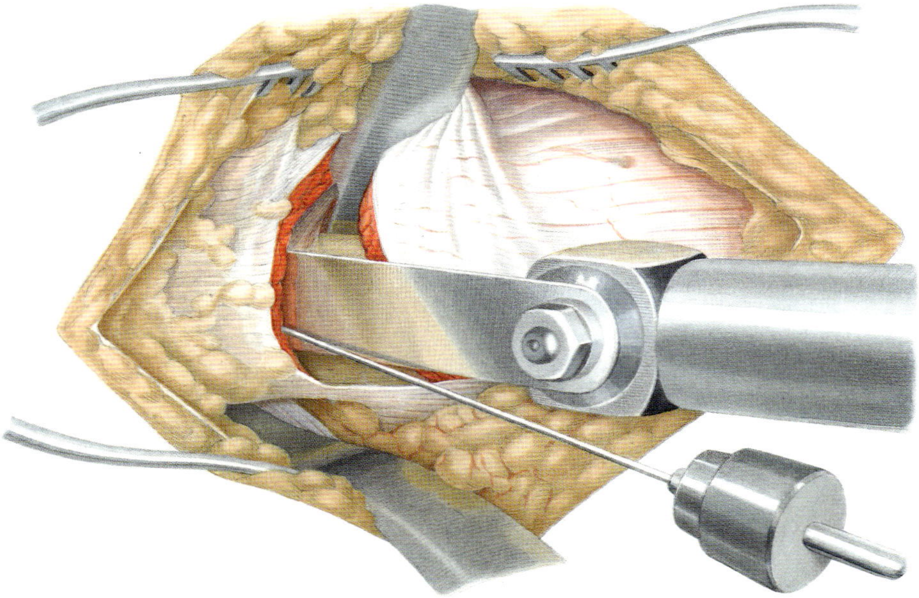

Fig. 2.**171** The trochanteric osteotomy is performed parallel to the marking wire with an oscillating saw.

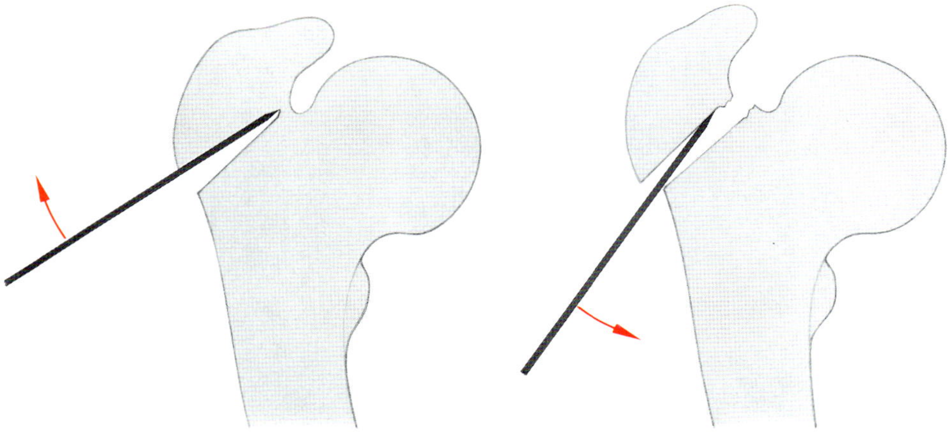

Fig. 2.**172** The trochanteric osteotomy ends medially slightly before reaching the medial surface of the greater trochanter to avoid damaging the vascular structures located there. A wide chisel inserted into the gap created by the osteotomy is used as a lever to break the narrow medial bone bridge and mobilize the greater trochanter.

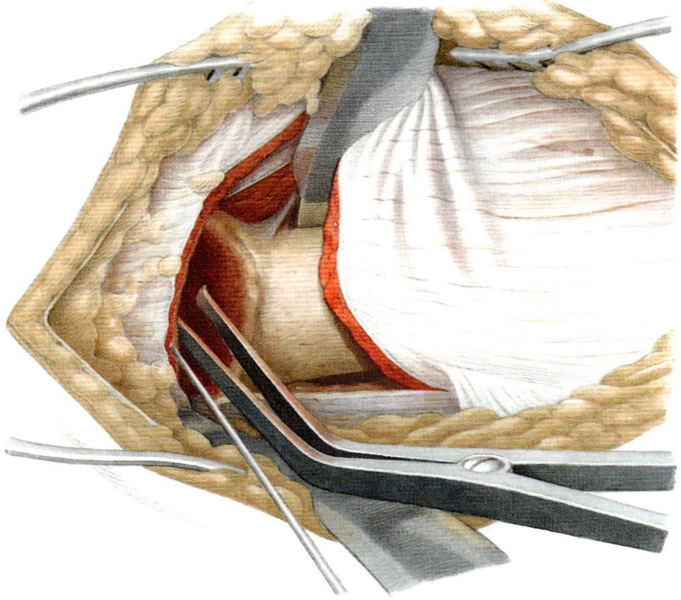

Fig. 2.**173** A bone spreader is inserted into the gap created by the osteotomy to carefully mobilize the greater trochanter.

The surgeon now prepares the lateral surface of the femur to which the greater trochanter is to be fixed. Using a narrow gouge, he or she raises "scales" in the femoral cortex to help accelerate bony consolidation (Fig. 2.**176**). The greater trochanter is now advanced on the lateral surface of the femur. It should be possible to move the greater trochanter without having to force it, provided that the adhesions have been released. If this is not the case, serious derangement can result. The trochanter is then temporarily fixed with a Kirschner wire (Fig. 2.**177**), and its position is verified with fluoroscopy.

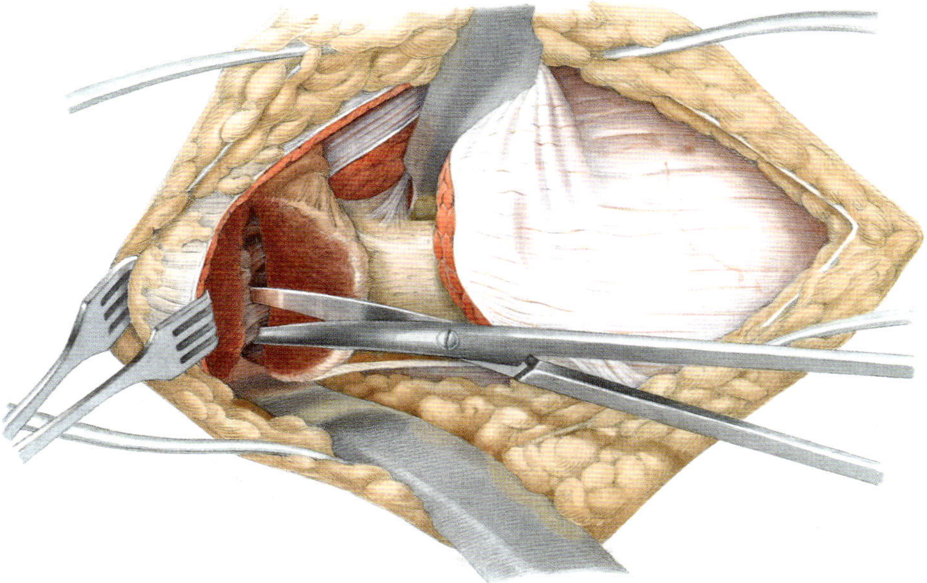

Fig. 2.**174** The scarred adhesions between the greater trochanter and the joint capsule and the medial greater trochanter are released with curved dissection scissors.

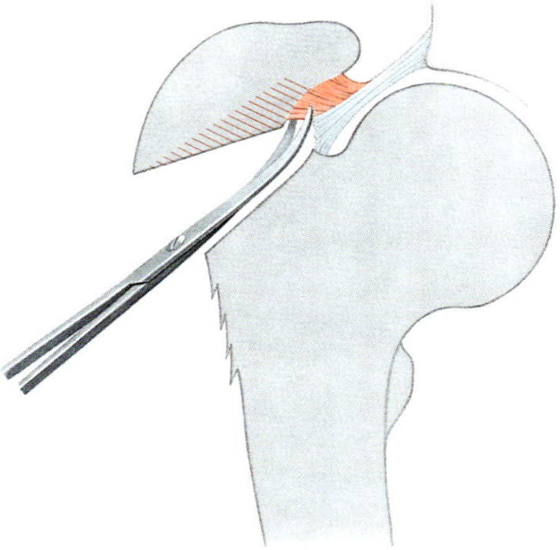

Fig. 2.**175** The scissors are pointed superiorly and laterally to avoid damaging the trochanteric fossa.

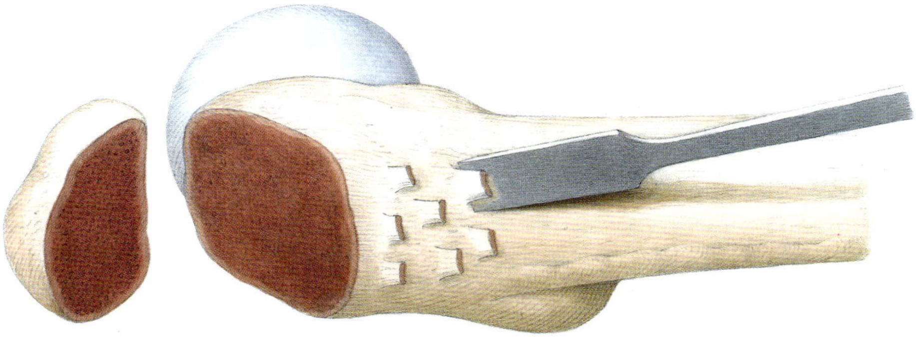

Fig. 2.**176** Preparing the lateral surface of the femur to which the greater trochanter is to be fixed. Fine "scales" are raised with a narrow gouge to help accelerate bony consolidation.

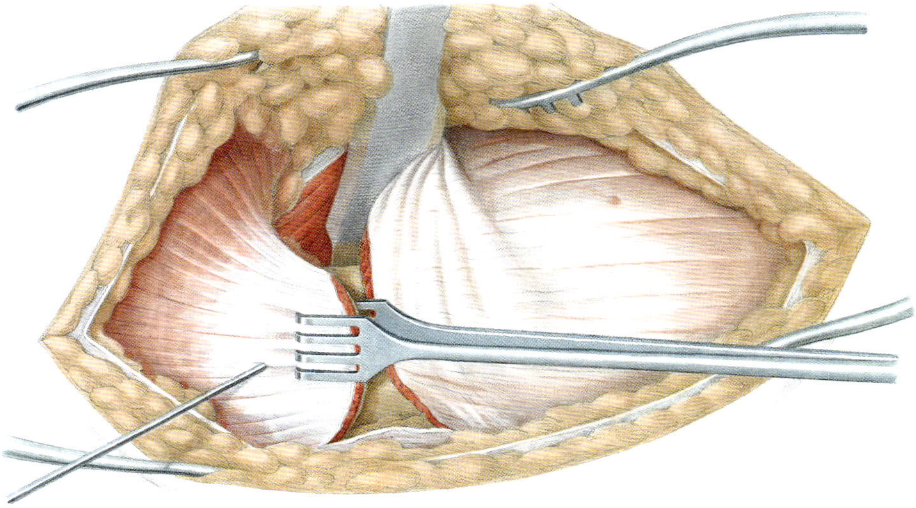

Fig. 2.**177** The greater trochanter is now advanced on the lateral surface of the femur and temporarily fixed with a Kirschner wire.

Anterior and posterior to the Kirschner wire, the tendon of the gluteus medius is incised to accommodate screws. The surgeon then inserts two screws with washers to compress the greater trochanter onto the lateral surface of the femur. The washers are placed on the surface of the bone beneath the fibers of the tendon (Fig. 2.**178**). Verify the alignment of the screws with fluoroscopy (Fig. 2.**179**). The screws are inserted medially and distally to compress the greater trochanter and the femur and to counteract the tension of the pelvic and trochanteric musculature. If Kirschner wires are to be used in place of screws (often indicated in extremely young patients), they must be inserted medially and proximally; the tension of the pelvic and trochanteric musculature will compress the greater trochanter and the lateral femur along the axis of the wires (Fig. 2.**180**).

The vastus lateralis is closed with vertical mattress sutures and securely sutured to the tendon of the gluteus medius (Figs. 2.**181** and 2.**182**). This restores the lateral soft-tissue envelope, which is crucial for the stability of the hip. The surgeon then closes the fascia lata over a suction drain with a vertical mattress suture and closes the rest of the wound in layers (Fig. 2.**32**).

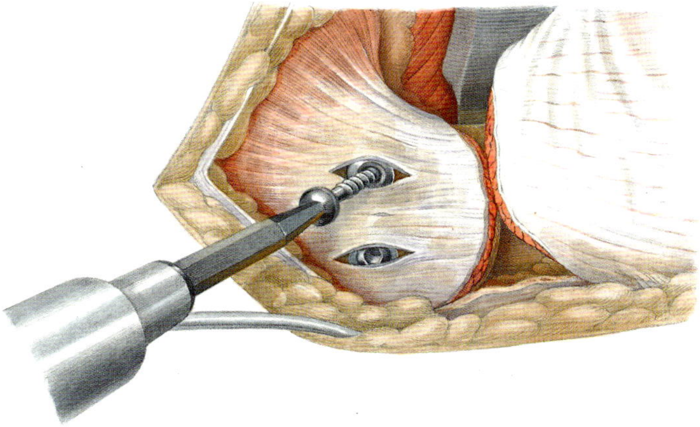

Fig. 2.**178** The tendon of the gluteus medius is incised parallel to its fibers to accommodate the screws and washers.

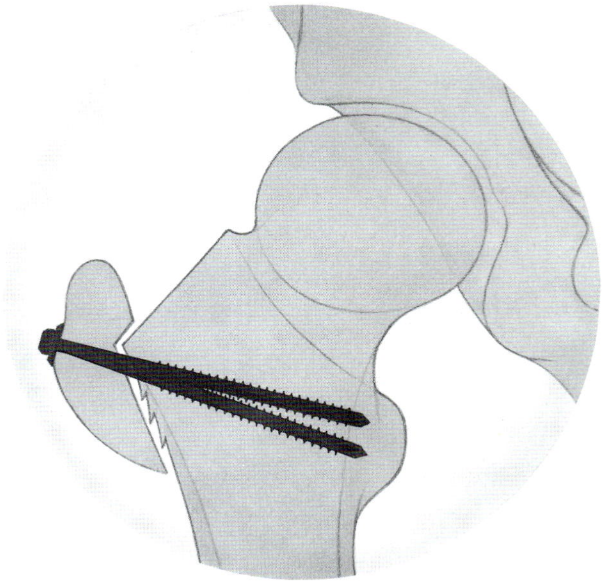

Fig. 2.**179** The corrected position of the greater trochanter is verified with fluoroscopy.

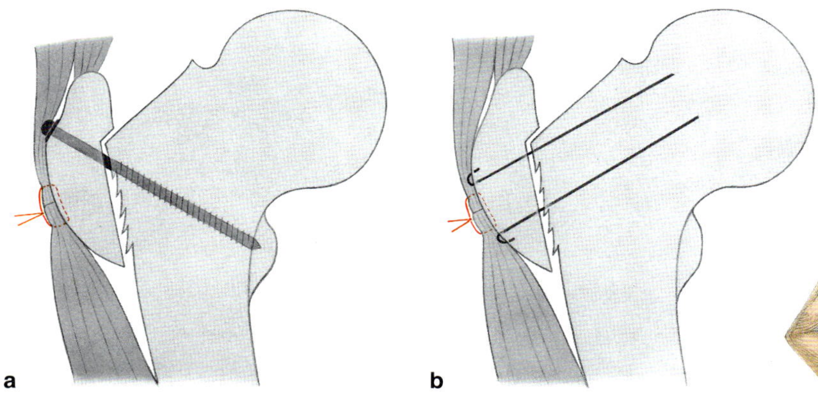

Fig. 2.**180a** and **b** If the greater trochanter is fixed with screws, they are inserted medially and distally (**a**) to compress the greater trochanter and the femur and to counteract the tension of the pelvic and trochanteric musculature. If Kirschner wires are used instead, they must be inserted medially and proximally (**b**) to allow muscular tension to compress the greater trochanter and the femur.

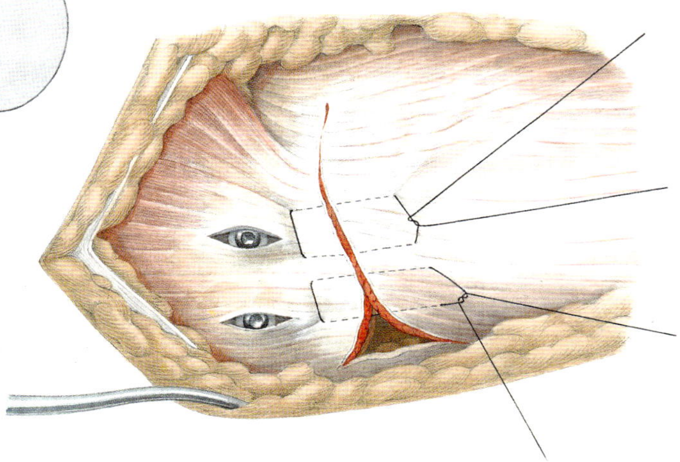

Fig. 2.**181** The vastus lateralis is reattached to restore the lateral soft-tissue envelope.

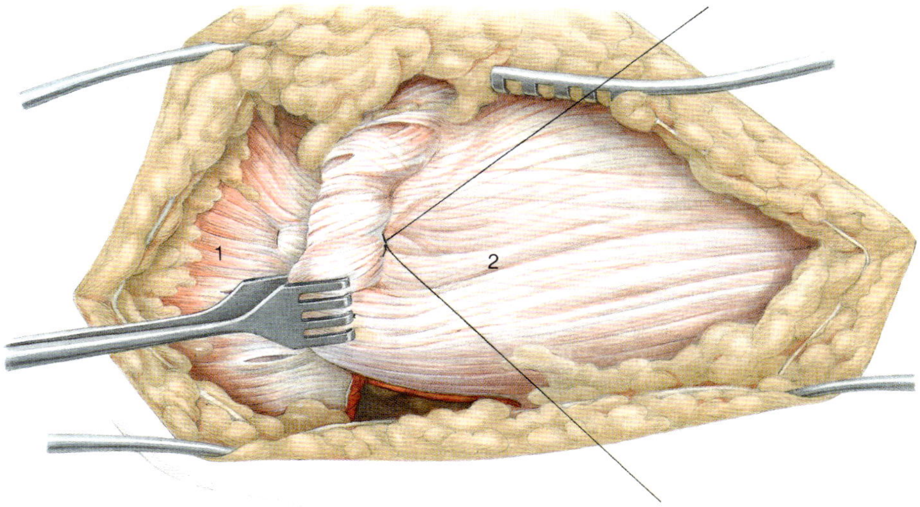

Fig. 2.**182** Retention sutures between the vastus lateralis and gluteus medius ensure proper soft-tissue tension.

1 Gluteus medius
2 Vastus lateralis

Trochanterplasty

Indications

The primary indications for trochanterplasty are growth deformities of the proximal femur with a shortened femoral neck, generally in a developmentally dislocated hip. The apex of the greater trochanter is typically at the normal level, i.e., level with the center of rotation of the hip; however, the distance between the greater trochanter and the center or rotation is less than normal. Thus the pelvic and trochanteric musculature does not have sufficient leverage to maintain adequate soft-tissue balance. An osteotomy is performed and the greater trochanter is laterally displaced so that the distance between it and the center of rotation of the hip is equal to the diameter of the femoral head.

Positioning and Incision

With the patient positioned supine on a radiolucent table, a longitudinal skin incision is made that begins over the posterior margin of the greater trochanter. The approach is identical to the one used with the intertrochanteric osteotomy except that the incision is not extended as far distally.

Technique

Surgical technique is essentially identical to that employed in trochanteric advancement. Instead of a distal shift, the osteotomized greater trochanter is shifted laterally until the proper displacement is achieved. A bone spreader is used to widen the diastasis between the lateral and medial osteotomy surfaces, after which the fragment is temporarily fixed with two Kirschner wires. Two fully threaded cancellous screws are inserted to bridge the gap created by the osteotomy and maintain the lateral shift of the greater trochanter. About 10 cm distal to the inferior cancellous screw, a cortical screw is inserted into the femoral diaphysis with its head projecting 10 mm above the surface of the bone. Then a tension banding wire is wrapped around the cortical screw and either the distal cancellous screw or both cancellous screws. Tightening the diaphyseal screw increases the tension on the wire, effectively stabilizing the lateral position of the greater trochanter (Fig. 2.**183**). The gap created by the osteotomy is filled with autologous graft. The vastus lateralis is reattached to the greater trochanter by securely suturing it to the tendon of the gluteus medius. Restoring this muscular tension is essential to stabilize the greater trochanter. The fascia lata is then closed over a suction drain with a retention suture, and the wound is closed in layers.

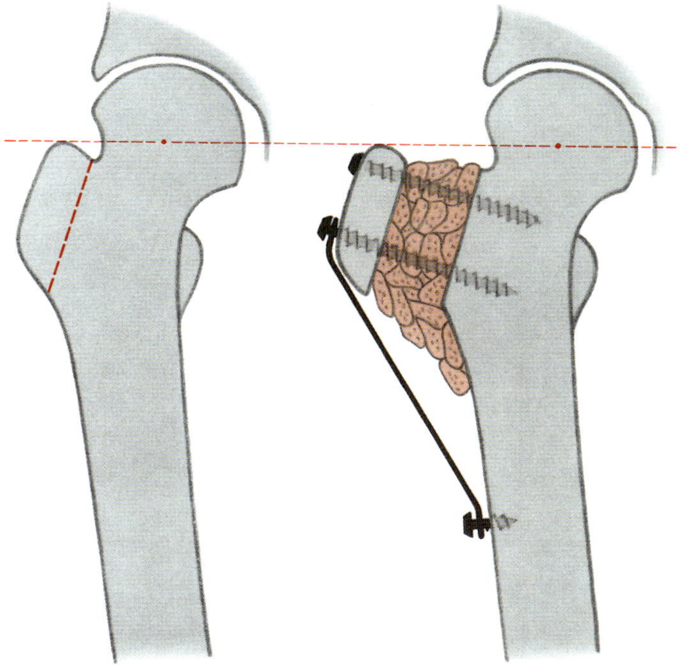

Fig. 2.**183** Trochanterplasty. The osteotomized greater trochanter is shifted laterally until the normal physiological distance is achieved between the apex of the greater trochanter and the center of rotation of the hip. The greater trochanter is fixed is this position with two cancellous screws, and the gap created by the osteotomy is filled with autologous graft. The pull of pelvic and trochanteric musculature is offset by tension banding to the femoral diaphysis.

Intertrochanteric Osteotomies Using Osteotomy Plates

Intertrochanteric Varus Osteotomy

Indications

- Surgical correction of a valgus deformity of the proximal femur. Typically the deformity occurs in a developmentally dislocated hip, but it may also be posttraumatic or the result of impaired growth of the femoral neck.
- The most frequent indication is coxa valga with anteversion and a dysplastic acetabulum in a developmentally dislocated hip; this is corrected by performing an intertrochanteric varus derotation osteotomy.
- Another major indication is osteoarthritis of the hip with a flattened acetabulum. Here, the intertrochanteric varus osteotomy pushes the femoral head deeper into the acetabulum so that stress is transferred to a larger part of the articular surface of the femoral head. This also improves the leverage of the hip musculature.

Experience has shown that intertrochanteric varus osteotomies are performed too often, and that too often the deformity is overcorrected. Overcorrection widens the hip and shortens the leg excessively, and it produces instability by excessively relieving pelvic and trochanteric soft-tissue tension. This can be avoided with careful preoperative planning. If centering the femoral head is important enough to justify accepting a deformity of the femoral neck to achieve it, then a simultaneous trochanteric advancement will preserve the functional integrity of the pelvic and trochanteric musculature. However, the surgeon should note that insufficient coverage of the femoral head cannot be corrected on the proximal femur if the acetabulum is dysplastic. For optimum results, the correction should be made at the site of the deformity.

Positioning and Incision

With the patient positioned supine, a straight longitudinal skin incision is made, which begins over the apex of the greater trochanter and courses distally (Fig. 2.**190**).

Technique

After the proximal femur is exposed through a lateral approach, a marker wire is inserted into the proximal greater trochanter and up the femoral neck to mark the direction of the seating chisel. This wire determines the degree of varus correction (Fig. 2.**184a**). A second marker wire is inserted into the capsule along the anterior surface of the femoral neck to determine the amount of anteversion (see Fig. 2.**198**). The seating chisel is then impacted distal to the trochanteric marker wire and parallel to both marker wires (Fig. 2.**184b**). The angle of the first marker wire determines the degree of the planned varus correction, and the angle of the anterior marker wire ensures that the blade will travel through the center of the femoral neck and not perforate its anterior or posterior cortex. A narrow groove is cut into the lateral cortex to mark the osteotomy site. Distal to the groove, a marker wire is inserted anteriorly at a right angle to the seating chisel, to allow the surgeon to verify the rotational correction after the osteotomy (Fig. 2.**184c**). The medial edge of the distal fragment is resected with an oscillating saw through the gap created by the osteotomy (Fig. 2.**185a**). This provides a medial contact surface for the two fragments (Fig. 2.**185b**). The seating chisel is then replaced with a condylar plate (Fig. 2.**185c**), and the fragments are compressed and secured with internal fixation (Fig. 2.**186**). The degree of derotation of the femoral neck can be verified by checking the angle between the two marker wires.

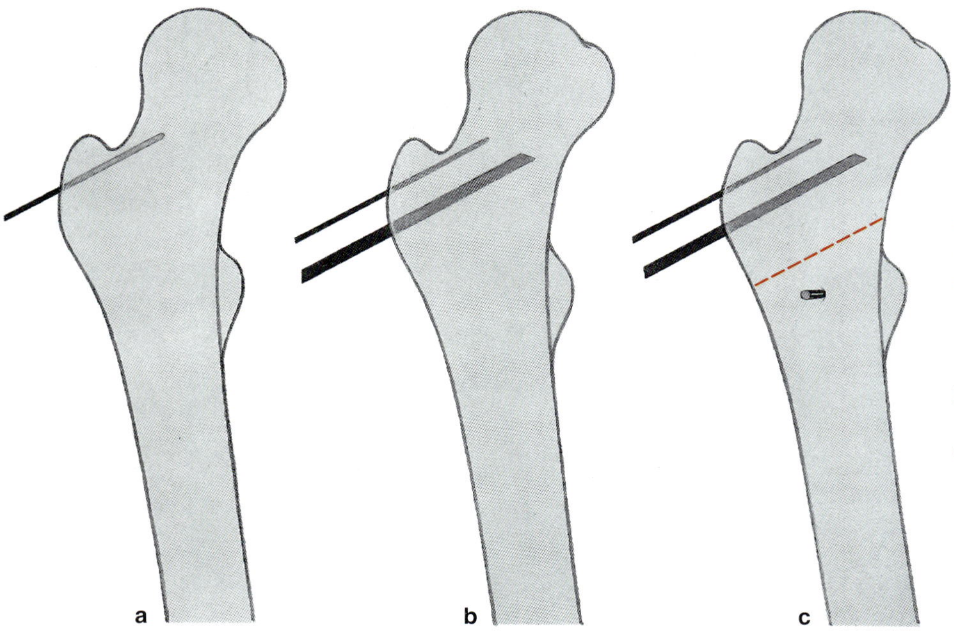

Fig. 2.**184a–c** Intertrochanteric varus osteotomy.
a A marker wire inserted into the greater trochanter determines the position of the blade of the osteotomy plate and thus the degree of varus correction.
b The seating chisel is impacted distal parallel to the marker wire.
c The site of the intertrochanteric osteotomy is marked parallel to the seating chisel. A second marker wire is inserted in the sagittal plane distal to the osteotomy. This wire is at a right angle to the seating chisel and is used as a reference for verifying the rotation.

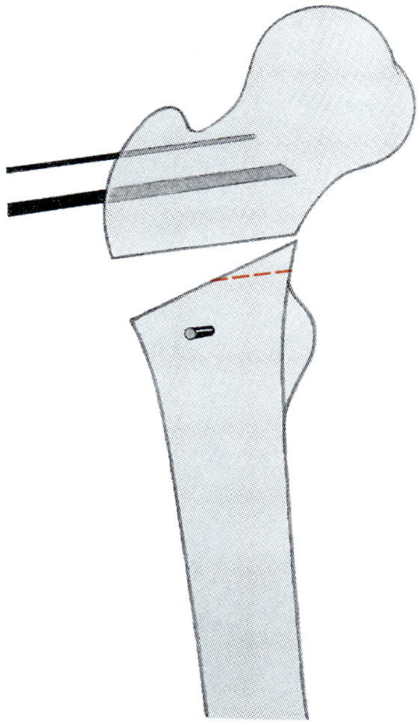

Fig. 2.**185a** The plane of the intertrochanteric osteotomy parallels the seating chisel. The seating chisel is used as a handle to make the varus correction in the position of the proximal fragment.

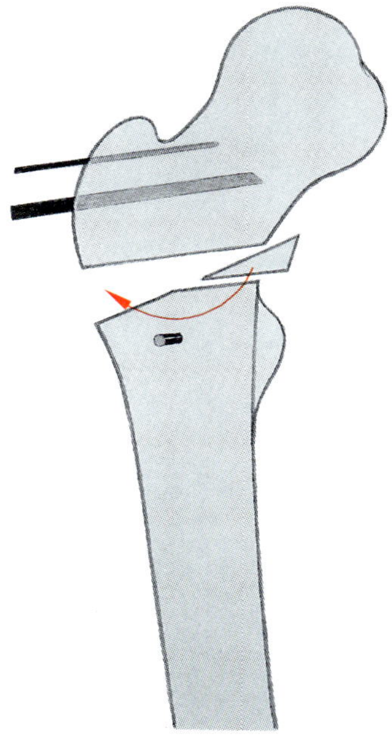

Fig. 2.**185b** Through the gap created by the osteotomy, a medial wedge is resected from the distal fragment and moved to the lateral surface of the distal fragment.

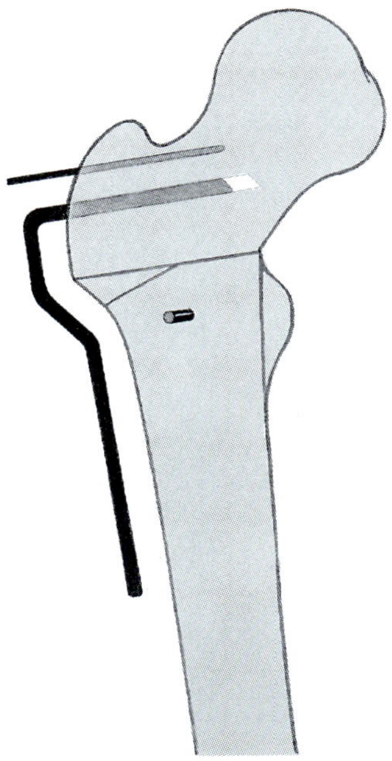

Fig. 2.**185c** The seating chisel is replaced with an osteotomy plate.

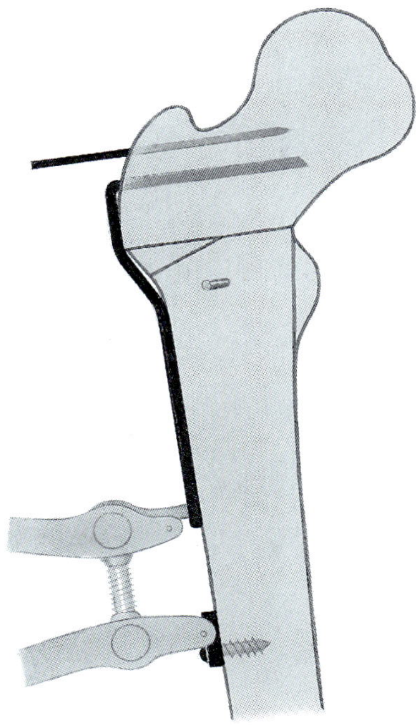

Fig. 2.**186** Interfragmentary compression is achieved with an articulated plate tensioner.

In a long femoral neck, the varus osteotomy produces greater lateral displacement of the distal fragment with a varus shift in the entire axis of the leg. The bending moment at the site of the osteotomy is also increased; this can impede stability and bony consolidation. Using a condylar plate with a larger offset (K) shifts the distal fragment medially to avoid this effect (Fig. 2.**187**).

In patients with good bone quality, the shortening effect of the intertrochanteric varus correction can be reduced or even eliminated. A transverse osteotomy is performed perpendicular to the longitudinal axis of the femur and the proximal fragment is shifted to a varus position by spreading the lateral side of the osteotomy. The gap created by the osteotomy is filled with autologous cancellous graft to ensure rapid healing. The cancellous graft may be taken from the center of the proximal and distal osteotomy surfaces with a narrow gouge or curette. The resulting bony defects and the remaining gap in the center of the osteotomy are then filled with gelatin foam. The cancellous graft is placed in the lateral side of the gap created by the osteotomy (Fig. 2.**188**).

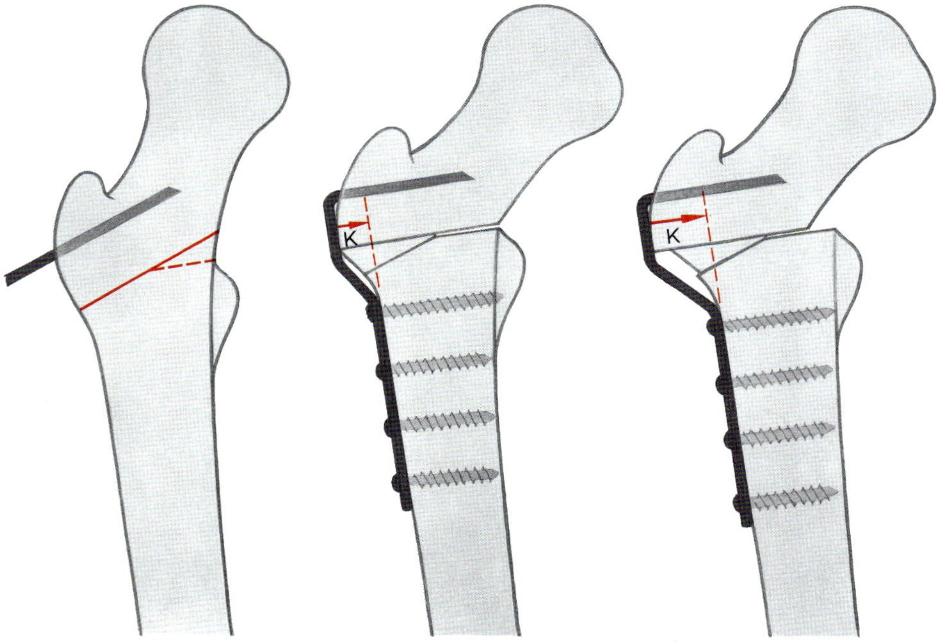

Fig. 2.**187** Shifting the distal fragment medially avoids the varus shift in the axis of the leg produced by the intertrochanteric varus osteotomy. The medial shift varies according to the offset (K) of the osteotomy plate.

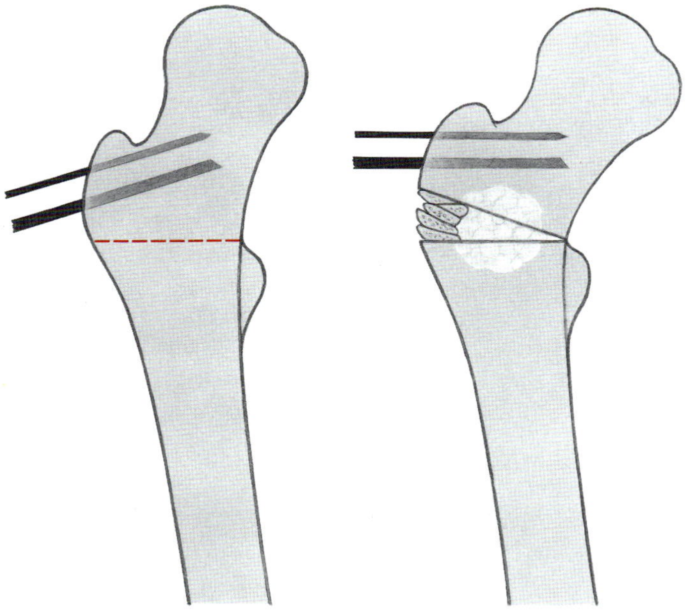

Fig. 2.**188** Transverse intertrochanteric osteotomy to reduce the decrease in leg length. The proximal fragment is shifted to a varus position without a wedge being removed. The lateral gap created by the osteotomy is filled with cancellous graft taken from the center of the osteotomy surfaces.

The intertrochanteric osteotomy shifts the greater trochanter superiorly and can result in a severe loss of pelvic and trochanteric soft-tissue tension. This can be avoided by employing M. E. Müller's technique, in which the greater trochanter is transected from the proximal fragment, left in its physiological position, and secured with internal fixation. This requires first preparing an opening for the blade of the osteotomy plate in the greater trochanter. The greater trochanter is osteotomized and mobilized as described in the section on trochanteric advancement. The femoral neck is then prepared to accommodate to the blade of the osteotomy plate and the intertrochanteric osteotomy is performed. The blade of the condylar plate is inserted through the greater trochanter and into the femoral neck fragment. The three fragments are then compressed, and the shaft of the osteotomy plate is fastened to the distal fragment with screws (Fig. 2.**189**).

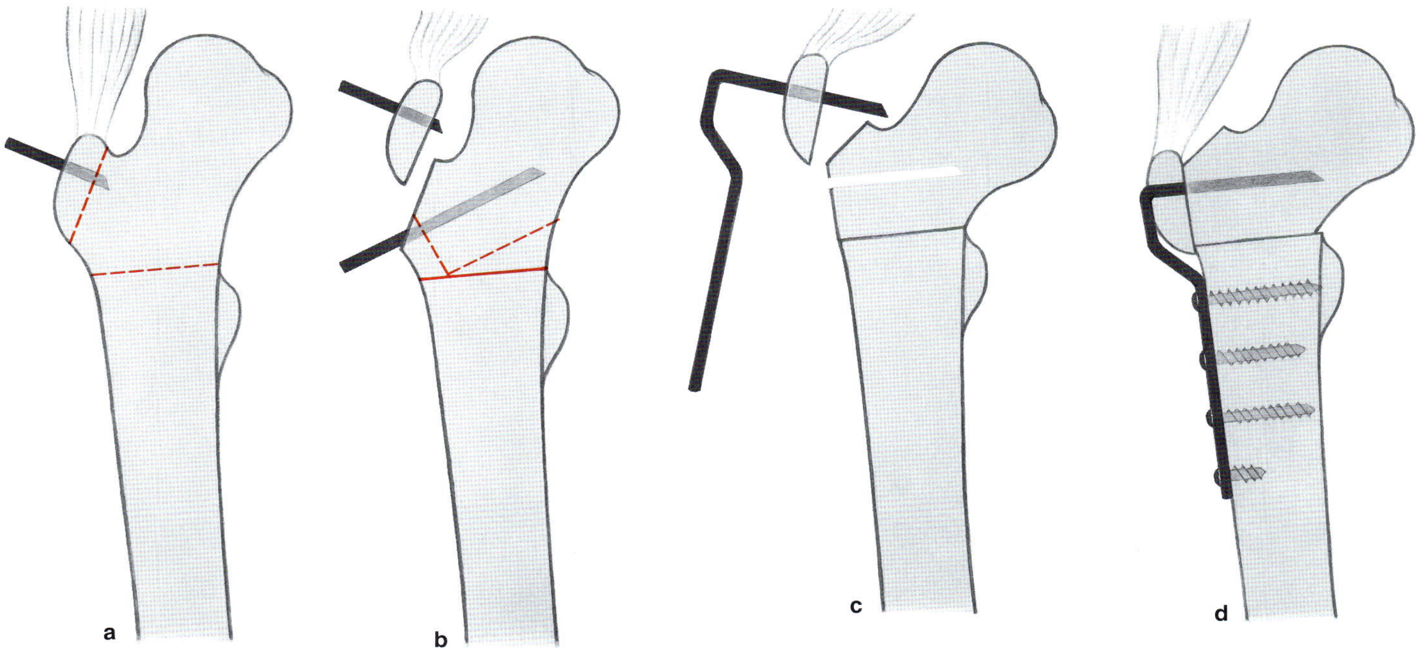

Fig. 2.**189a–d** Intertrochanteric varus osteotomy with simultaneous trochanteric advancement prevents a superior shift in position of the greater trochanter.

a First an opening for the blade of the osteotomy plate is prepared in the greater trochanter, and then the greater trochanter is osteotomized.

b The femoral neck is then prepared to accommodate to the blade of the osteotomy plate, and the seating chisel is inserted. Then the intertrochanteric osteotomy is performed and a wedge is removed.

c After the varus shift in the proximal fragment is made, the blade of the osteotomy plate is inserted through the greater trochanter and into the femoral neck fragment.

d Interfragmentary compression is achieved with an articulated plate tensioner, and the shaft of the plate is fastened to the distal fragment with screws.

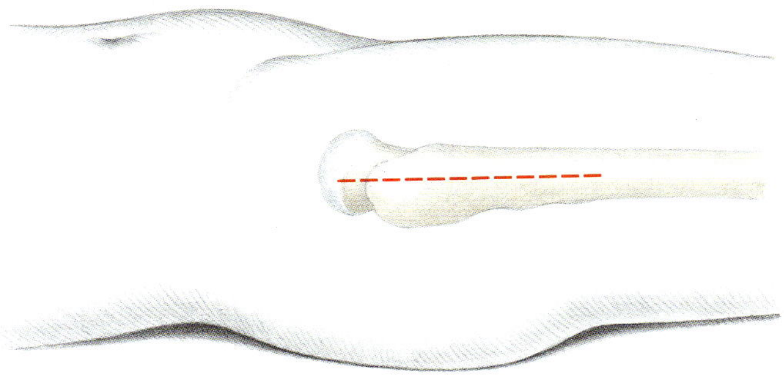

Fig. 2.**190** Positioning and incision for the intertrochanteric varus osteotomy. The patient is positioned supine for a longitudinal skin incision over the lateral hip.

After the fascia lata is split parallel to the direction of its fibers and retracted, the origin of the vastus lateralis is dissected with an L-shaped incision (Fig. 2.**191**). The surgeon dissects the muscle from the lateral intermuscular septum and the femur with a scalpel and periosteal elevator (Fig. 2.**192**). A marker wire is inserted into the bone proximal to the most proximal aspect of the greater trochanter to indicate the desired angle of correction. The position of the wire is verified with fluoroscopy. The marker wire for the varus osteotomy is inserted medially and anteriorly; after the axial correction, it lies perpendicular to the longitudinal axis of the femur (Fig. 2.**193**). The correct position of the wire is verified with fluoroscopy (Fig. 2.**194**).

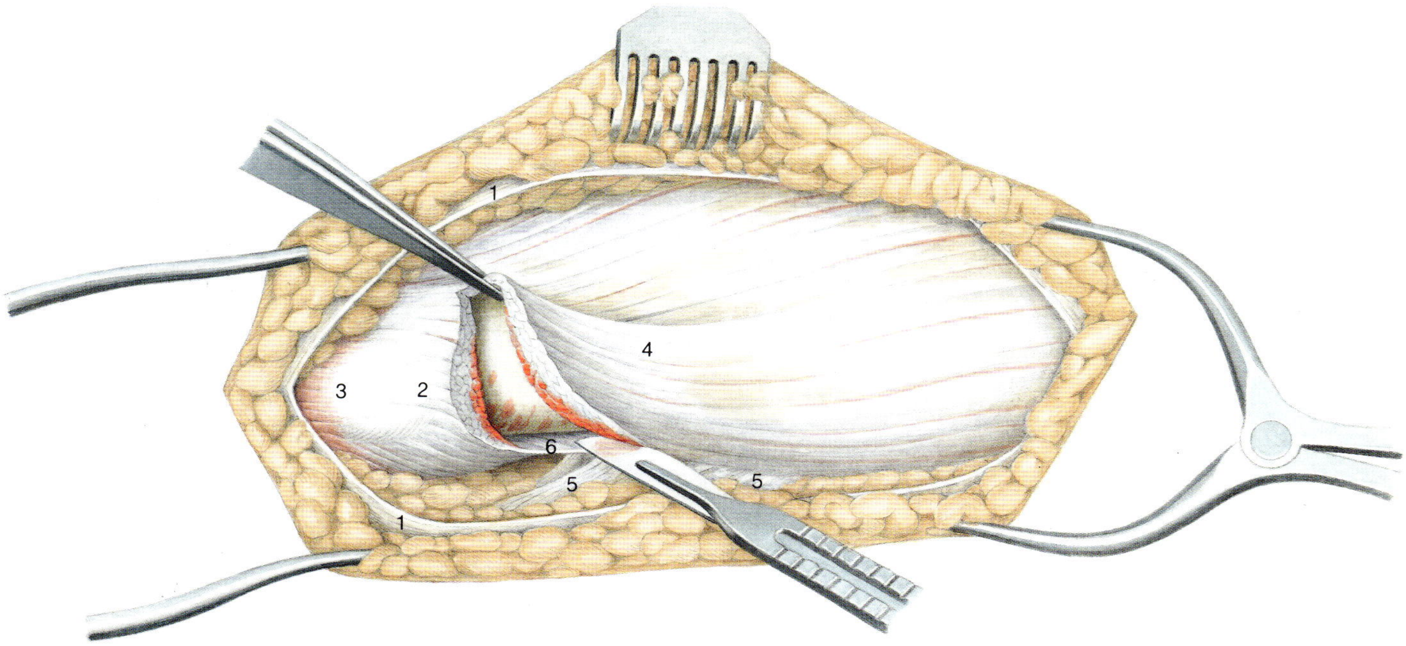

Fig. 2.**191** After the fascia lata is split parallel to the direction of its fibers and retracted, the origin of the vastus lateralis is dissected with an L-shaped incision distal to the most proximal aspect of the greater trochanter.

1 Fascia lata
2 Most proximal aspect of the greater trochanter
3 Gluteus medius
4 Vastus lateralis
5 Lateral intermuscular septum
6 Vastus lateralis fascia

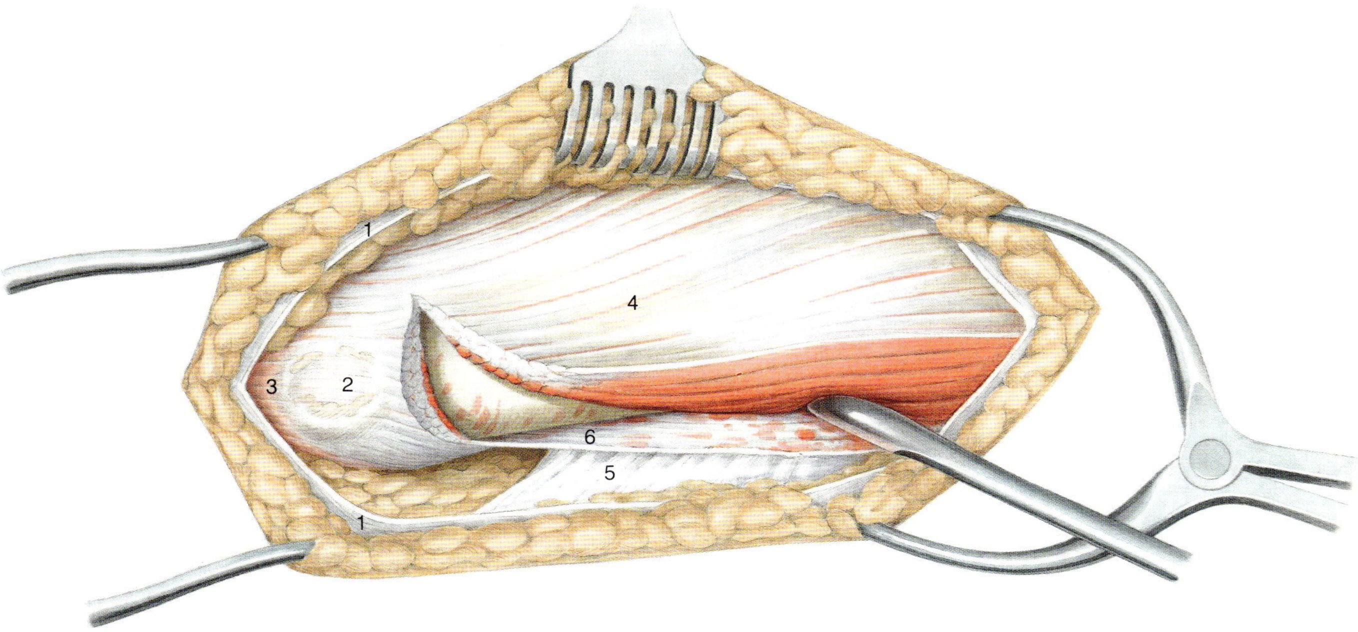

Fig. 2.**192** The vastus lateralis is dissected from the femur and the lateral intermuscular septum and retracted anteriorly.

1 Fascia lata
2 Most proximal aspect of the greater trochanter
3 Gluteus medius
4 Vastus lateralis
5 Lateral intermuscular septum
6 Vastus lateralis fascia

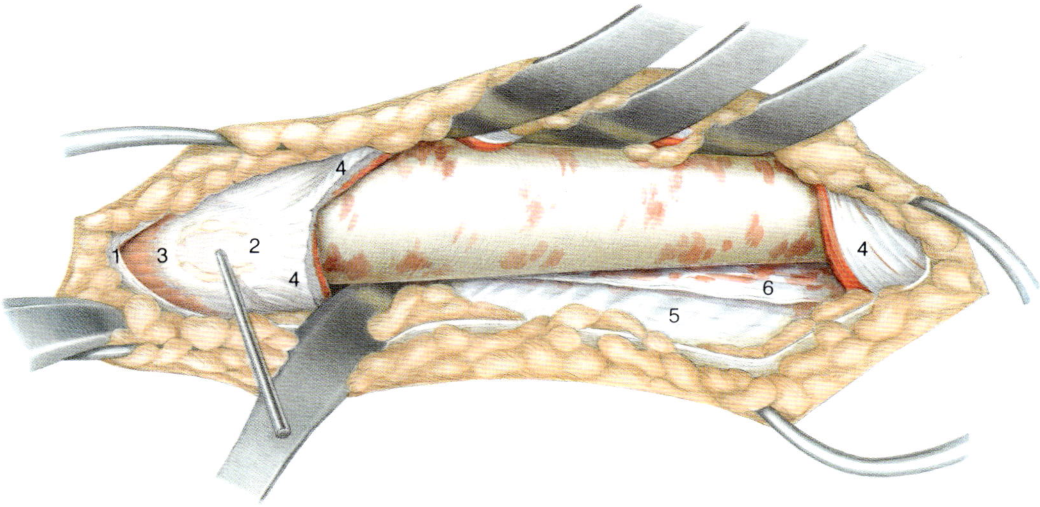

Fig. 2.**193** The vastus lateralis is lifted with elevators. A marker wire is inserted into the greater trochanter to indicate the desired angle of correction. The position of the wire is verified with fluoroscopy.

1 Fascia lata
2 Most proximal aspect of the greater trochanter
3 Gluteus medius
4 Vastus lateralis
5 Lateral intermuscular septum
6 Fascia of the vastus lateralis

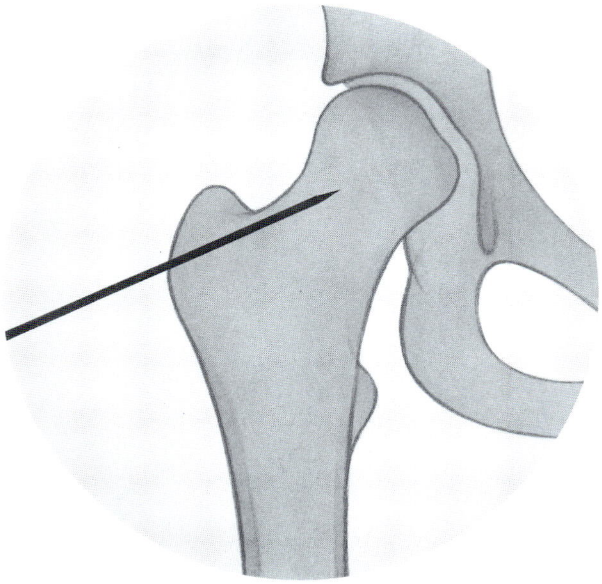

Fig. 2.**194** Verifying the correct position of the marker wire with fluoroscopy.

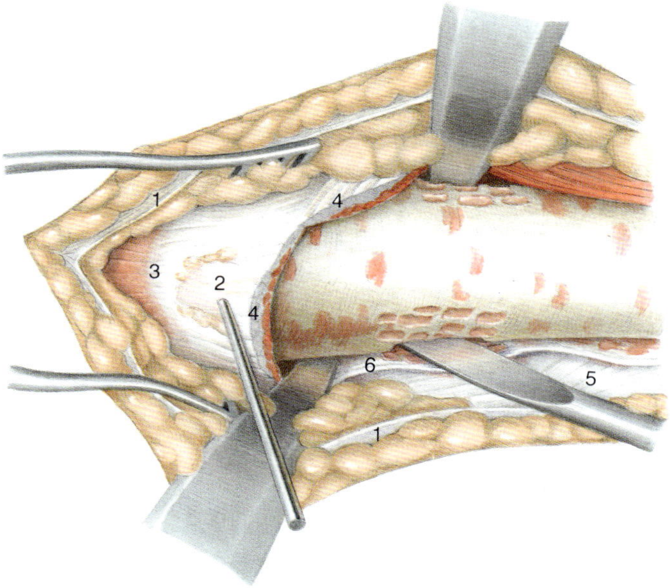

Fig. 2.**195** Decorticating the femoral cortex at the osteotomy site.

1 Fascia lata
2 Most proximal aspect of the greater trochanter
3 Gluteus medius
4 Vastus lateralis
5 Lateral intermuscular septum
6 Fascia of the vastus lateralis

The surgeon exposes the anterior and posterior femoral cortex at the osteotomy site, raising small scales that retain their periosteal attachments with a mallet and periosteal elevator. This decortication improves bony healing and prevents damage to the vascular structures on the posterior femur (Fig. 2.**195**). Elevators are then inserted anteriorly and posteriorly to protect the surrounding soft tissue. The tendinous origin of the vastus lateralis is dissected from the surface of the bone distal to the marker wire to expose the osteotomy site for the blade of the osteotomy plate (Fig. 2.**196**).

To accommodate the blade of the osteotomy plate, the surgeon drills a row of holes about 10 mm deep with a spiral drill bit immediately distal to the marker wire and parallel to it (Fig. 2.**197**). The holes are joined and widened by driving a 15-mm chisel into the surface of the bone and moving it back and forth. This prevents the relatively dull seating chisel from causing a fracture of the proximal femoral cortex. Next, a marker wire is inserted into the capsule along the anterior surface of the femoral neck to mark the anteversion of the femoral neck. This wire ensures that the seating chisel will travel through the center of the femoral neck and not perforate its anterior or posterior cortex (Fig. 2.**198**).

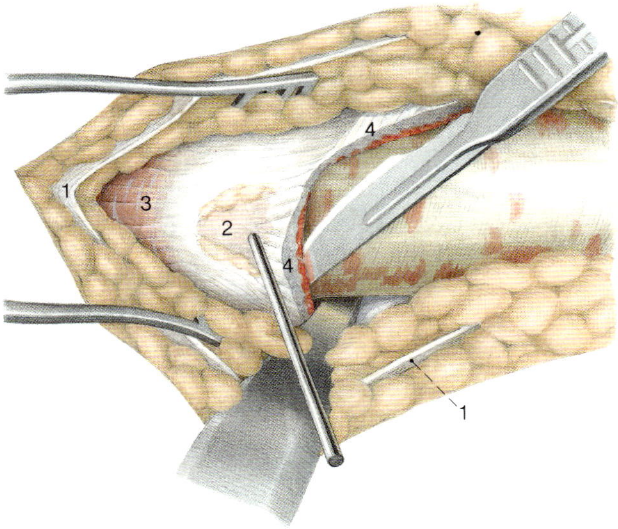

Fig. 2.**196** The tendinous origin of the vastus lateralis is dissected from the surface of the bone distal to the marker wire to expose the osteotomy site for the blade of the angled blade plate.

1 Fascia lata
2 Most proximal aspect of the greater trochanter
3 Gluteus medius
4 Vastus lateralis

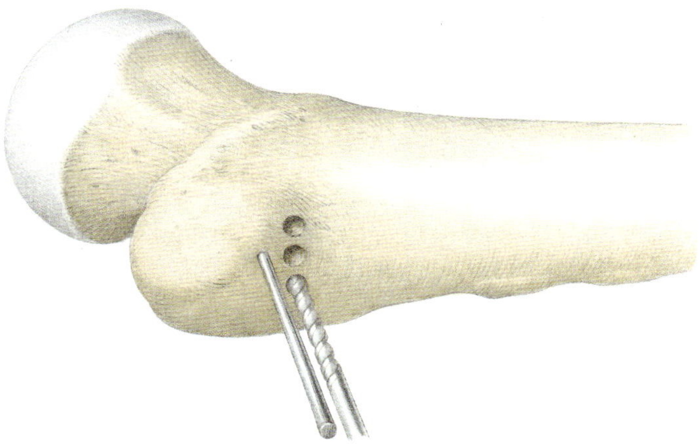

Fig. 2.**197** Holes are drilled to accommodate the blade of the angled blade plate.

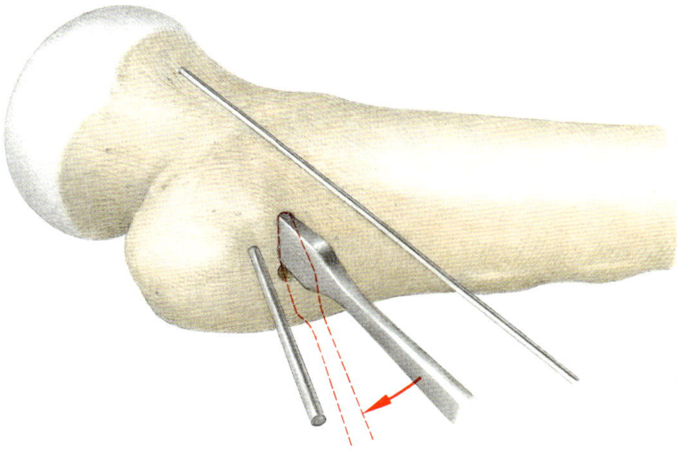

Fig. 2.**198** A 15-mm flat chisel is driven 10 mm into the surface of the bone and moved back and forth to widen the holes and prevent the seating chisel from causing a cortical fracture. A marker wire is inserted into the surface of the capsule along the anterior surface of the femoral neck to mark the anteversion of the femoral neck.

The seating chisel is driven into the slot. The seating chisel is the same width as the blade of the osteotomy plate and cuts a channel for the blade through the cancellous bone. The seating chisel is impacted parallel to the marker wire in the greater trochanter in the coronal plane, and in the transverse plane it travels parallel to the marker wire along the anterior surface of the femoral neck. Rotation of the chisel is controlled by a slotted hammer that is shaped like a tuning fork. Chisel rotation determines the final axial alignment of the osteotomy plate, which may follow the axis of the existing femur or deviate from it to allow for correcting the position of the proximal fragment (Fig. 2.**199**).

After the bone has been prepared, the slotted hammer is partially withdrawn so that the surgeon can replace it with the blade of the osteotomy plate without having to apply excessive force to the short proximal fragment. The marker wire on the anterior surface of the femoral neck is now removed.

The surgeon now measures distance from the seating chisel to the osteotomy on the femoral cortex and marks the site with an osteotome (Fig. 2.**200**). The distance between the blade and the osteotomy must be long enough so there is no risk of fracture, as this would result in severe instability.

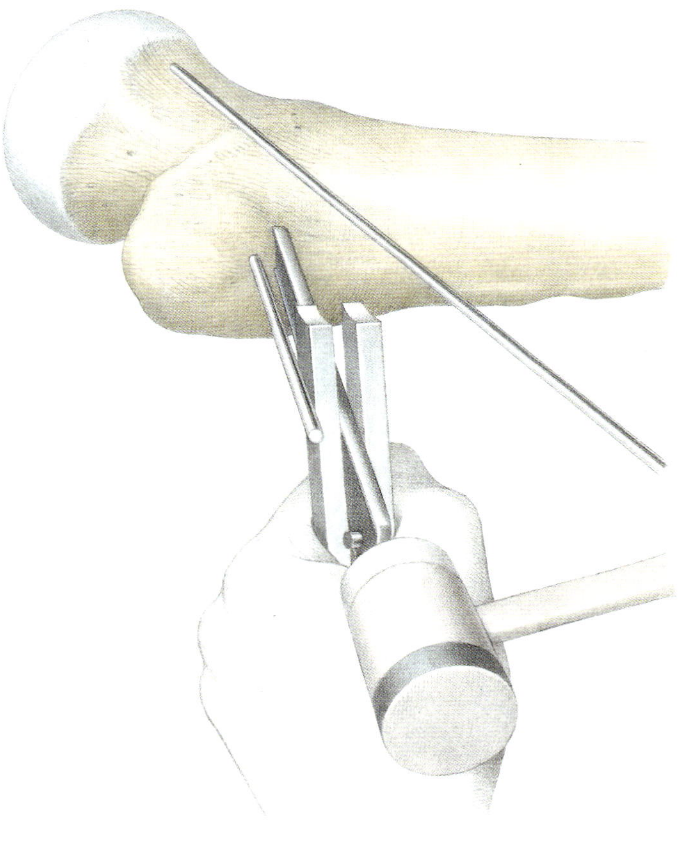

Fig. 2.**199** Driving in the seating chisel. The slotted hammer that fits over the seating chisel controls the rotation of the chisel. The seating chisel must travel parallel to the marker wire in the greater trochanter in the coronal plane to achieve the planned varus correction, and parallel to the marker wire along the femoral neck in the transverse plane to avoid a cortical fracture of the anterior or posterior femoral neck.

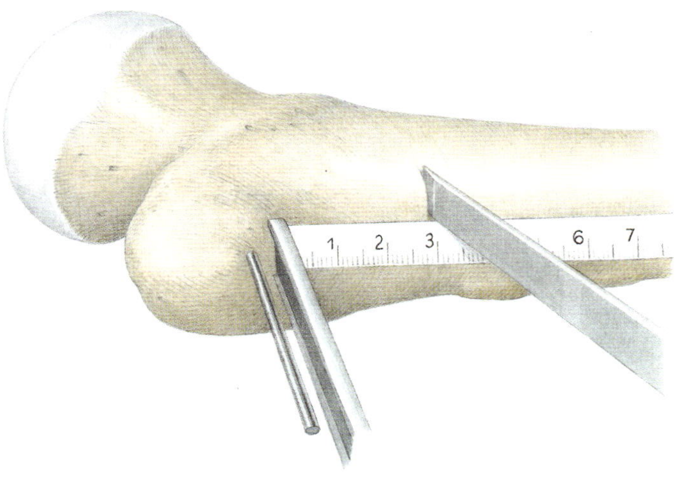

Fig. 2.**200** The seating chisel marks the planned osteotomy site on the femoral cortex.

A marker wire is inserted at the planned osteotomy site and its position is verified with fluoroscopy. Distal to the osteotomy site, a second marker wire is inserted into the anterior femur at a right angle to the seating chisel in the transverse plane. This marker wire is used to gauge rotation after the osteotomy is performed (Fig. 2.**201**). Alternatively, the surgeon may opt to insert two parallel marker wires, one proximal and one distal to the osteotomy site. The angle between these wires would then indicate the degree of rotation. The surgeon verifies the positions of the marker wires with fluoroscopy before beginning the osteotomy (Fig. 2.**202**).

The intertrochanteric osteotomy is performed at the marked site (Fig. 2.**203**). Depending on the correction planned, the osteotomy plane lies parallel to the seating chisel, and a medial wedge is removed from the distal fragment; or it lies perpendicular to the shaft of the femur, and a medial wedge is removed from the proximal fragment. In either case, the medial contact surface of the distal fragment is at a right angle to the axis of the femur; correcting the rotation of the distal fragment does not affect the axial position of the proximal fragment.

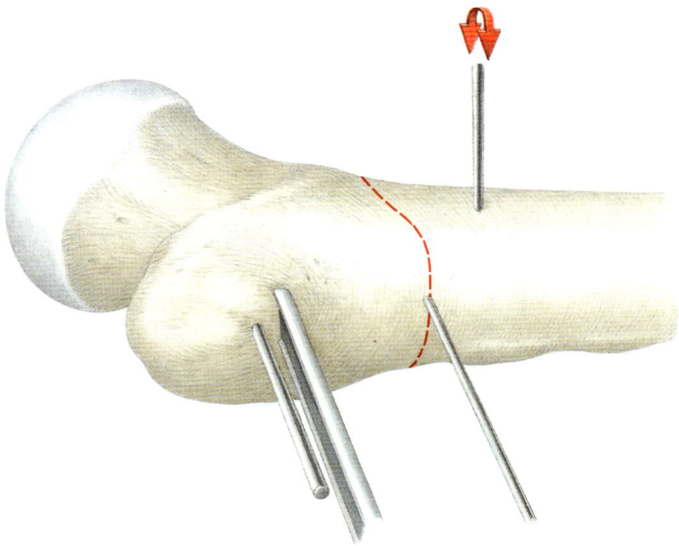

Fig. 2.**201** A marker wire is inserted at the planned osteotomy site and its position is verified with fluoroscopy. Distal to the osteotomy site, a second marker wire is inserted into the anterior femur at a right angle to the seating chisel in the transverse plane.

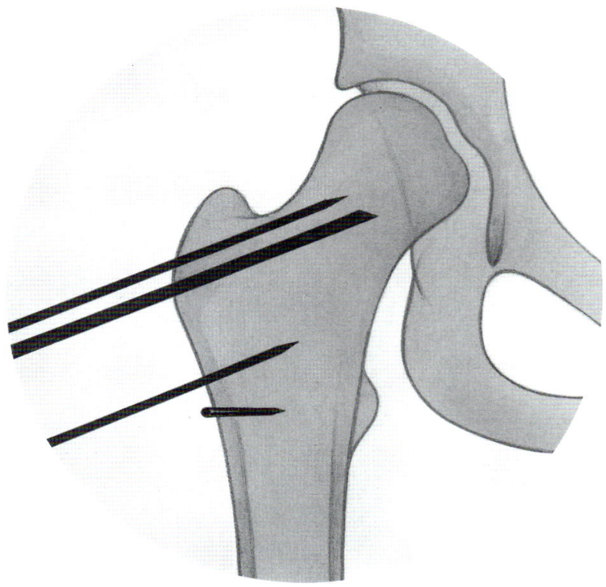

Fig. 2.**202** The positions of the seating chisel and marker wires for the intertrochanteric osteotomy are verified with fluoroscopy.

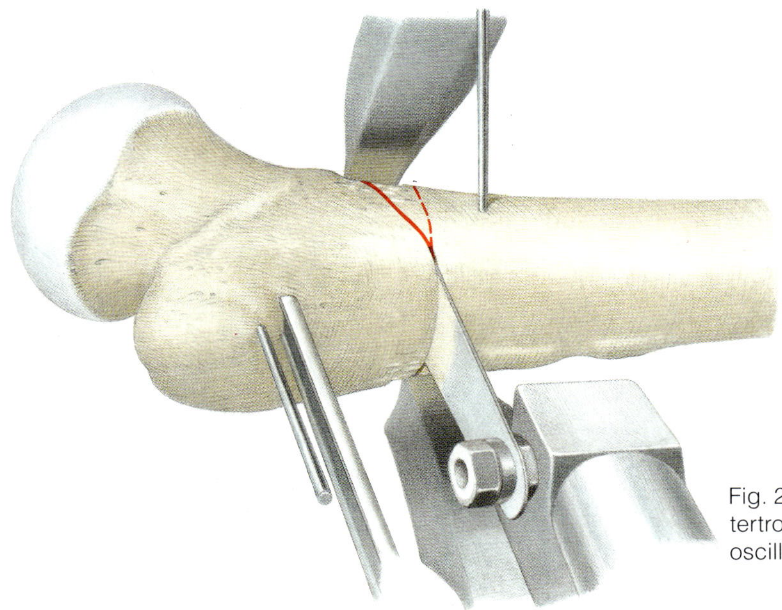

Fig. 2.**203** With elevators inserted to protect the soft tissue, the intertrochanteric osteotomy is performed at the marked site with an oscillating saw.

The surgeon now pushes the distal fragment medially with a forceps while using the seating chisel to rotate the proximal fragment into varus. This opens the osteotomy laterally and allows resection of the medial wedge (Fig. 2.**204**). A medial wedge is removed in every procedure except the transverse osteotomy shown in figure 2.**188**, where the surgeon removes autologous cancellous graft from the proximal and distal osteotomy surfaces. After the fragments are opposed, the seating chisel is removed from the proximal fragment and replaced with a condylar plate. The offset of the plate determines the medial shift of the distal fragment. The osteotomy plate is inserted into the prepared bone with the inserter-extractor parallel to the marker wire, and is driven in with a mallet. The surgeon inserts the blade 2–3 cm by hand, using a mallet only if resistance is encountered. This prevents the blade (which is relatively sharp) from deviating from the prepared channel in the cancellous bone. The shaft of the osteotomy plate is held against the distal fragment with a forceps (Fig. 2.**205**).

After verifying the rotation, the surgeon compresses the fragments with an articulated plate tensioner that engages the distal end of the plate and a screw inserted into the femoral diaphysis. Shortly before final compression is reached, the surgeon inserts the medial bone wedge into the lateral gap created by the osteotomy (Fig. 2.**206**). The shaft of the osteotomy plate is then fastened to the distal fragment with two screws, the articulated plate tensioner and the marker wires are removed, and the remaining screws are inserted into the shaft of the plate (Fig. 2.**207**). The vastus lateralis is returned to its original position, covering the femur and the osteotomy site. The muscle is reattached where it was transected (distal to the proximal aspect of the greater trochanter) with vertical mattress sutures (Fig. 2.**208**). The fascia lata is closed with retention sutures over a suction drain (see Fig. 2.**163**). Restoring fascial tension is very important for the stability of the hip.

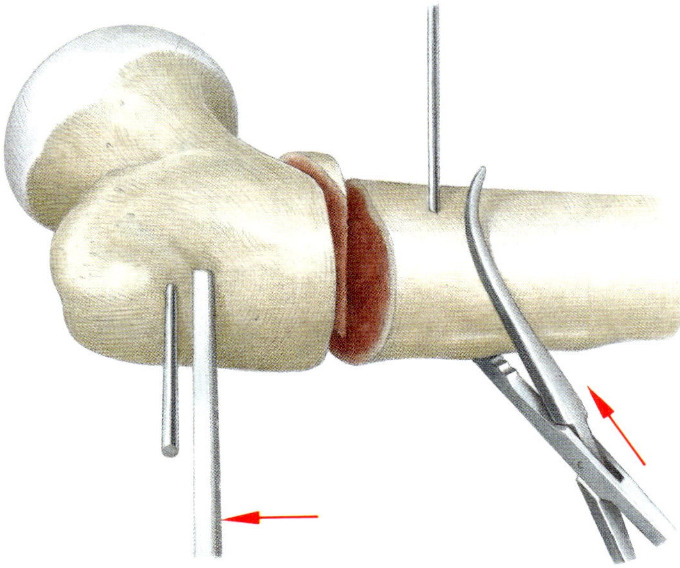

Fig. 2.**204** After the osteotomy, the distal fragment is pushed mediallyl with a forceps while the proximal fragment is rotated into varus. This opens the osteotomy laterally to allow resection of a medial wedge on the distal fragment.

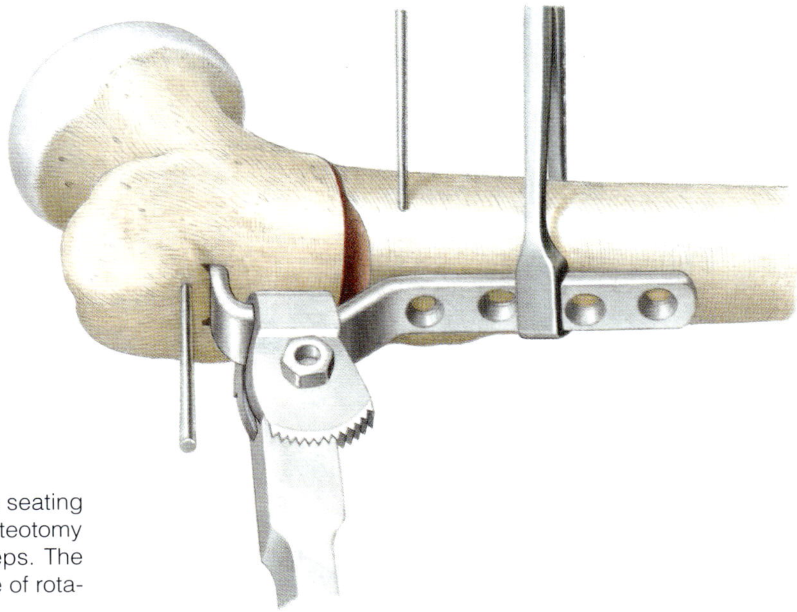

Fig. 2.**205** After the fragments have been opposed, the seating chisel is replaced with a condylar plate. The shaft of the osteotomy plate is pressed against the distal fragment with a forceps. The angle between the two marker wires indicates the degree of rotation.

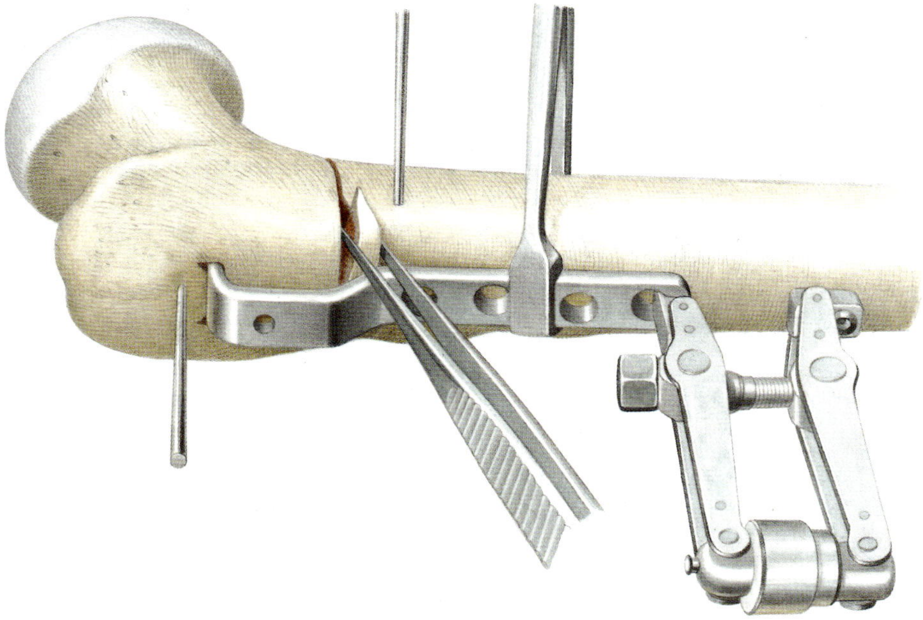

Fig. 2.**206** Interfragmentary compression is achieved with an articulated plate tensioner. Shortly before final compression is reached, the medial bone wedge is inserted into the lateral gap created by the osteotomy.

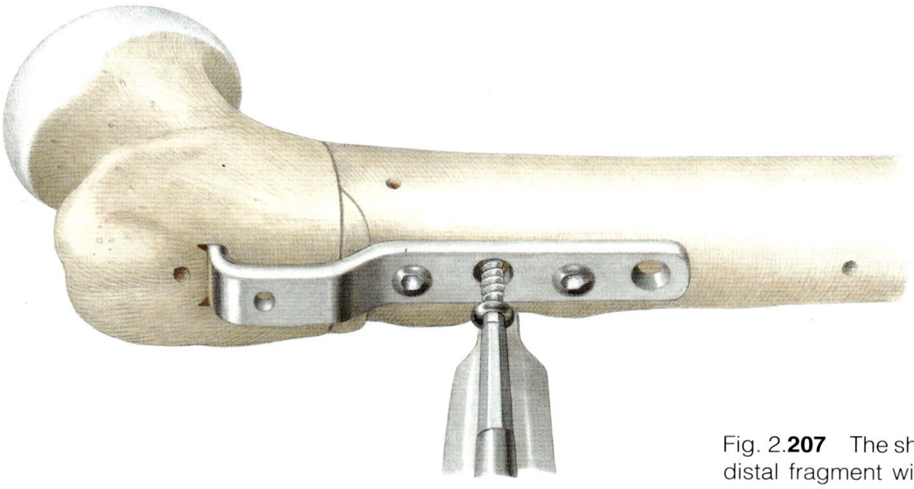

Fig. 2.**207** The shaft of the osteotomy plate is then fastened to the distal fragment with screws, and the articulated plate tensioner and marker wires are removed.

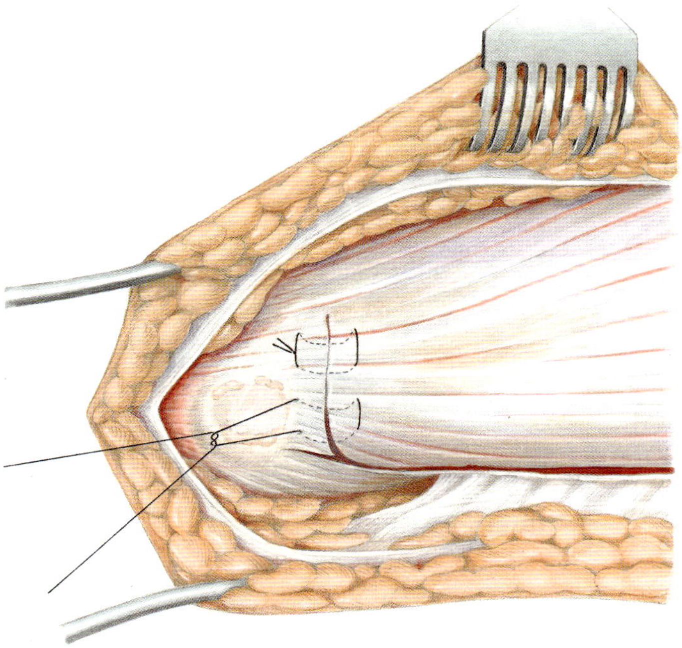

Fig. 2.**208** The vastus lateralis is reattached where it was transected (distal to the proximal aspect of the greater trochanter) with vertical mattress sutures.

Valgus Intertrochanteric Osteotomy

Indications

- Surgical correction of a varus deformity of the proximal femur resulting from trauma or growth arrest
- Improvement of joint congruity in developmentally dislocated hips where there is a shortened femoral neck and flattening of the femoral head
- Coxa plana or coxa magna following Legg–Calvé–Perthes disease or epiphyseal dysplasia

Positioning and Incision

With the patient positioned supine, a skin incision is made that courses distally from the greater trochanter on the lateral side of the hip (Fig. 2.**212**).

Technique

The procedure is performed as an intertrochanteric osteotomy to maintain the greater trochanter in its anatomic position. A hip with an extremely shortened femoral neck, where the distal margin of the femoral head projects inferiorly, may require performing the osteotomy distal to the lesser trochanter. Such cases may require advancing the iliopsoas tendon.

The intertrochanteric *wedge* osteotomy is the most common procedure for achieving a valgus correction of the femoral neck. Different internal fixation procedures may be used to stabilize the osteotomy.

When a 130° angled blade plate is used, the plane of osteotomy is inclined superiorly in the coronal plane; the varus stress on the femoral neck produces interfragmentary compression. The blade of the angled blade plate lies distal to the intersection of the stress trajectories in the femoral neck to provide the best possible support, particularly in osteopenic bone (Fig. 2.**209**).

When a condylar plate is used, the plane of osteotomy is horizontal; interfragmentary compression is achieved by prestressing the condylar plate (Fig. 2.**210**).

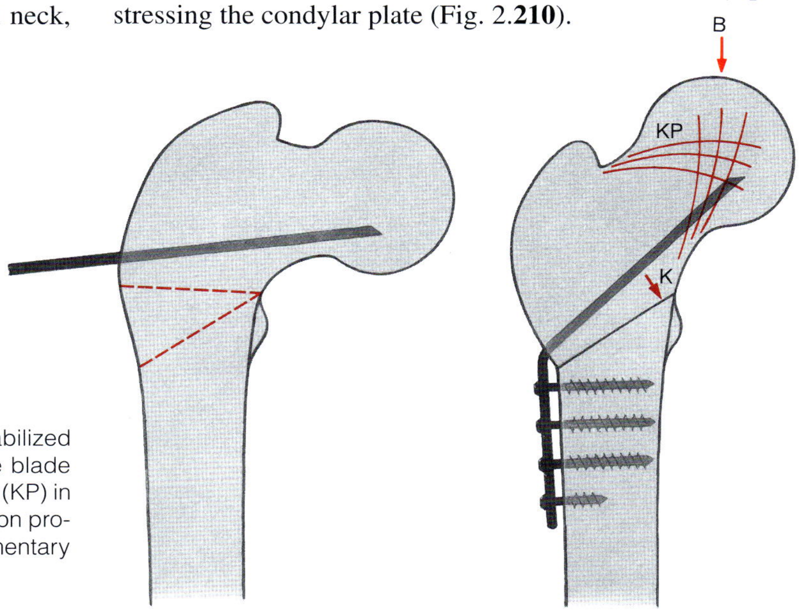

Fig. 2.**209** Valgus intertrochanteric wedge osteotomy stabilized with a 130° angled blade plate. For stability, the tip of the blade should lie beneath the intersection of the stress trajectories (KP) in the center of the femoral neck. Weight and soft-tissue tension produce varus stress on the femoral neck (B) and interfragmentary compression (K).

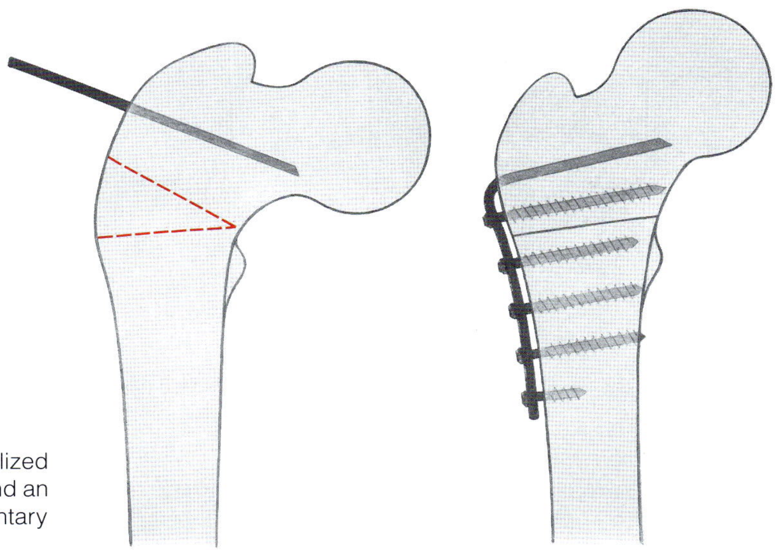

Fig. 2.**210** Valgus intertrochanteric wedge osteotomy stabilized with a condylar plate. The plane of osteotomy is horizontal, and an articulated plate tensioner is used to achieve interfragmentary compression.

A lateral shift intertrochanteric osteotomy is the most versatile valgus correction of the proximal femur. Interfragmentary compression is achieved with a condylar plate. This is particularly effective in treating severe deformities of the proximal femur with pronounced shortening of the femoral neck. Since the transverse osteotomy is performed without resecting a wedge, the proximal fragment is not weakened. The lateral shift in the distal fragment lengthens the shortened femoral neck. The lateral edge of the proximal fragment is impacted into the distal osteotomy surface for particularly stable interfragmentary integration. Even if this lateral edge must be resected to achieve a greater shift, there will still be a wide contact surface between the two fragments (Fig. 2.**211**). A technical problem associated with this procedure is that the valgus shift greatly increases the distance between the medial edges of the fragments. This requires careful resection of the hardened soft-tissue structures generally present on the medial side of the osteotomy.

All valgus osteotomies of the proximal femur result in an increase in the length of the femur. This effect is desirable when the femoral neck is shortened, yet the correction may lengthen the femur excessively and produce intra-articular compression that could damage the hip. Thus, preoperative planning should include special consideration of the lengthening effect. Intraoperative fluoroscopy can be used to effectively measure the length of the femur.

After the fascia lata above the greater trochanter is split parallel to the direction of its fibers and retracted, the vastus lateralis is dissected with an L-shaped incision immediately distal to the most proximal aspect of the greater trochanter (see Fig. 2.**191**). The surgeon dissects the vastus lateralis from the lateral intermuscular septum and the femur with a scalpel and periosteal elevator (see Fig. 2.**192**). The muscle is retracted anteriorly, and elevators are inserted to expose the bone. The leg is adducted until the femoral neck is in the desired corrected position, which is verified with fluoroscopy. This position is marked by inserting a Steinmann pin into the femoral neck proximal tot he most proximal aspect of the greater trochanter (Fig. 2.**213**). The Steinmann pin is perpendicular to the median plane and parallel to the coronal plane of the patient, i.e., parallel to the floor of the operating room. These two reference planes permit simple yet ex-

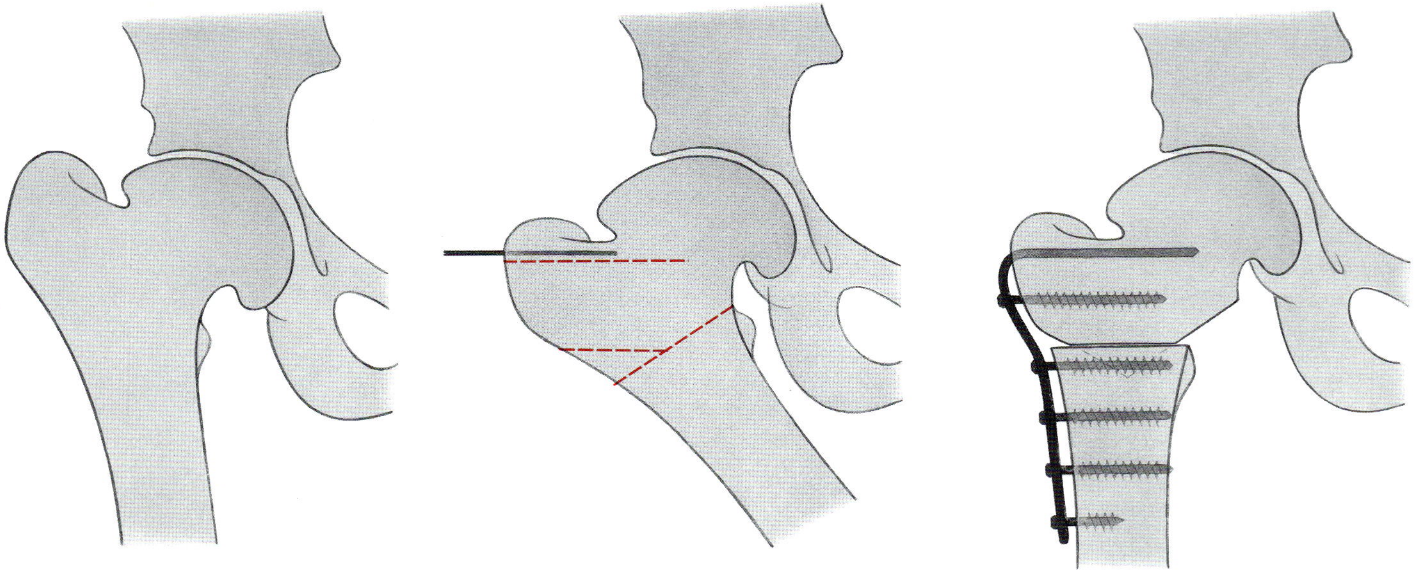

Fig. 2.**211** Lateral shift intertrochanteric valgus osteotomy. The osteotomy is stabilized with a condylar plate. Interfragmentary compression is achieved with an articulated plate tensioner. Shifting the distal fragment laterally produces a relative increase in the length of the femoral neck and increases the distance between the shaft of the femur and the vertical line through the center of rotation of the hip.

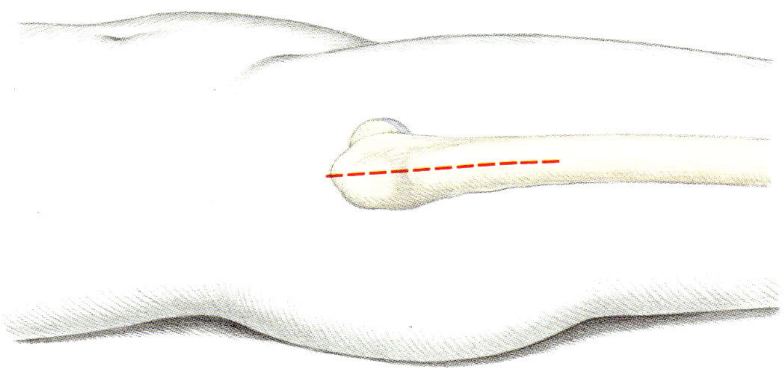

Fig. 2.**212** Positioning and Incision. A skin incision is made on the lateral side of the hip with the patient positioned supine.

tremely precise verification of the corrected position of the proximal fragment after the osteotomy. The corrected position of the femoral neck and the proper position of the Steinmann pin are verified with fluoroscopy (Fig. 2.**214**).

The surgeon exposes the anterior and posterior femoral cortex at the osteotomy site with a mallet and periosteal elevator and then inserts elevators anteriorly and posteriorly to protect the surrounding soft tissue. The tendinous origin of the vastus lateralis is dissected from the bone distal to the Steinmann pin to expose the insertion site of the blade of the condylar plate (Fig. 2.**215**).

To accommodate the blade of the condylar plate, the surgeon drills a row of holes about 10 mm deep with a spiral drill bit immediately distal to the Steinmann wire and parallel to it

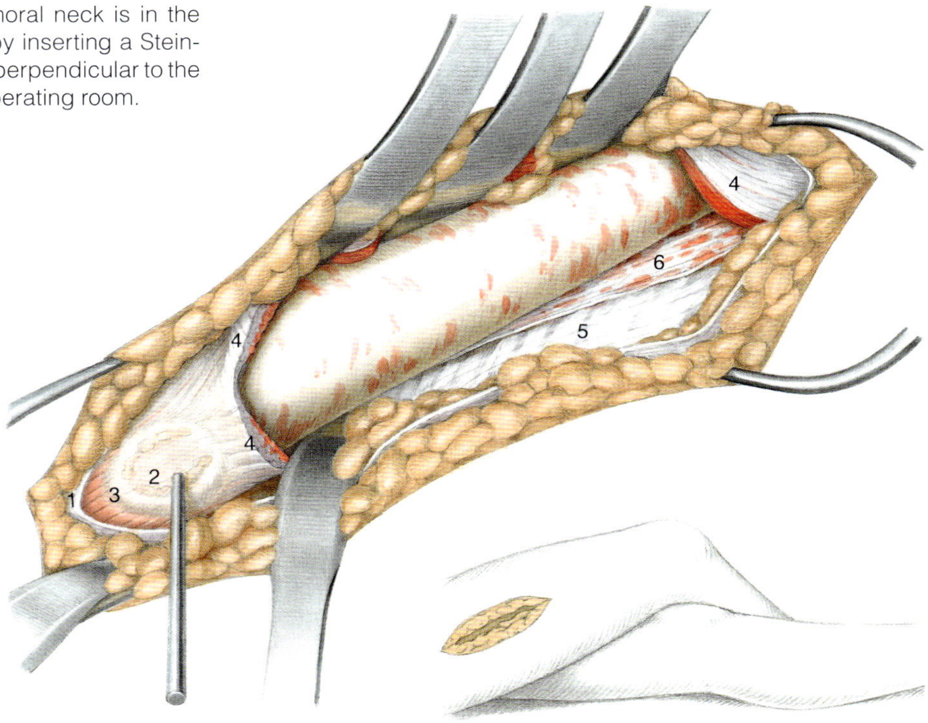

Fig. 2.**213** The leg is adducted until the femoral neck is in the desired corrected position, which is marked by inserting a Steinmann pin into the greater trochanter. The pin is perpendicular to the median plane and parallel to the floor of the operating room.

1 Fascia lata
2 Most proximal aspect of the greater trochanter
3 Gluteus medius
4 Vastus lateralis
5 Lateral intermuscular septum
6 Fascia of the vastus lateralis

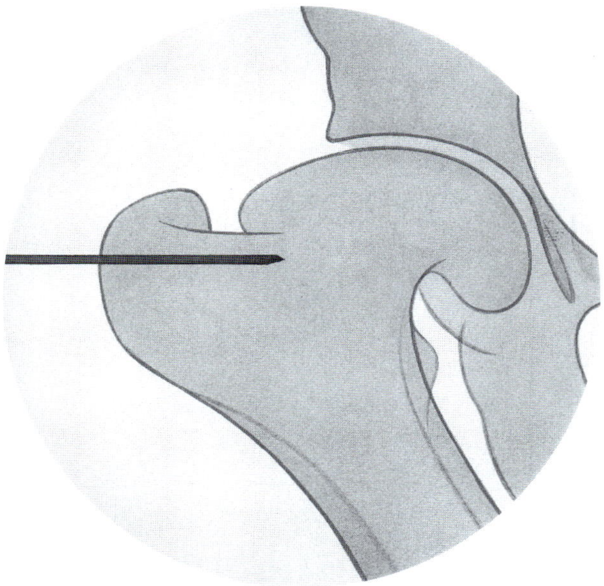

Fig. 2.**214** The corrected position of the femoral neck and the proper position of the Steinmann pin are verified with fluoroscopy.

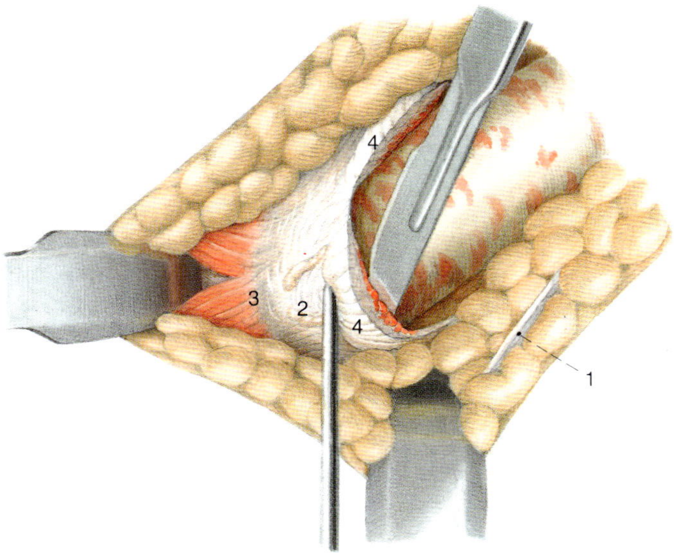

Fig. 2.**215** The tendinous origin of the vastus lateralis is dissected from the bone distal to the Steinmann pin to expose the insertion site of the blade of the condylar plate.

1 Fascia lata
2 Most proximal aspect of the greater trochanter
3 Gluteus medius
4 Vastus lateralis

(Fig. 2.**216**). The holes are joined and widened to accommodate the blade by driving a 15-mm chisel into the surface of the bone and moving it back and forth. This prevents the relatively dull seating chisel from fracturing the proximal femoral cortex (Fig. 2.**217**).

The seating chisel is driven into the slot. The seating chisel is the same width as the blade of the condylar plate and cuts a channel for the blade through the cancellous bone. The seating chisel is impacted parallel to the Steinmann wire. Rotation of the chisel is controlled by a slotted hammer that is shaped like a tuning fork. Chisel rotation determines the final axial alignment of the condylar plate, which may follow the axis of the existing femur or match that of the distal fragment after the position of the proximal fragment has been corrected. After the bone has been prepared, the slotted hammer

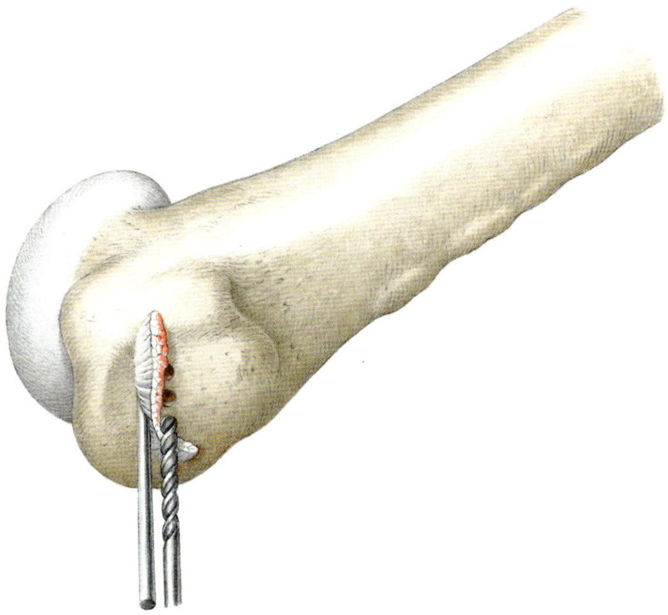

Fig. 2.**216** A row of holes are drilled in the surface of the bone to accommodate the blade of the condylar plate.

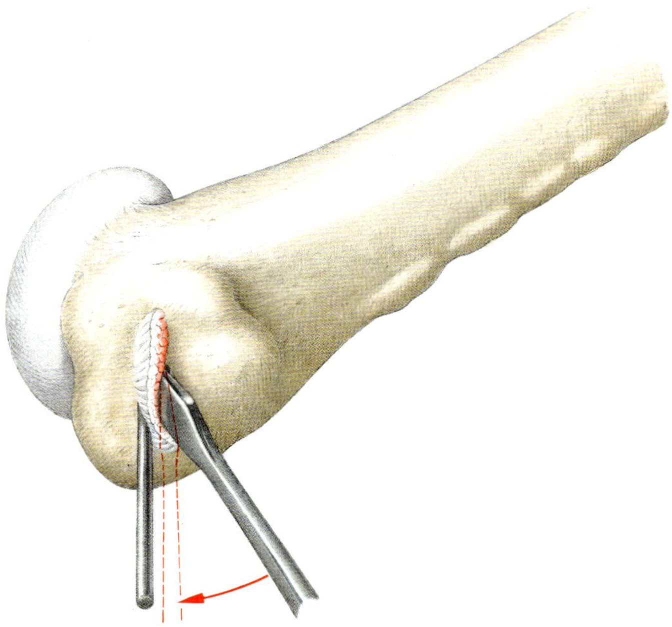

Fig. 2.**217** The holes are joined and widened to accommodate the blade by driving a 15-mm chisel about 10 mm into the surface of the bone and moving it back and forth.

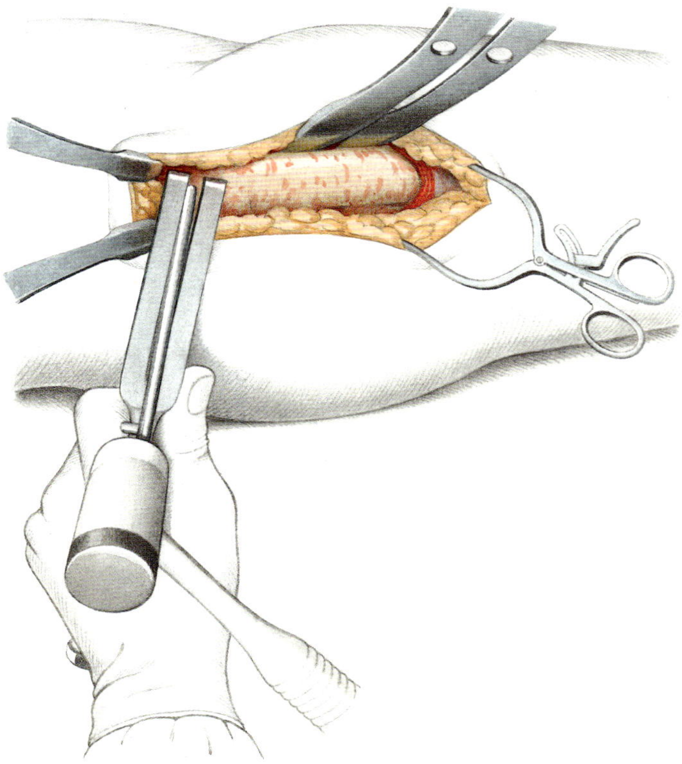

Fig. 2.**218** The seating chisel is driven into the slot parallel to the Steinmann wire. Rotation of the chisel is controlled by a slotted hammer that is shaped like a tuning fork.

is partially withdrawn so that the surgeon can replace it with the blade of the condylar plate without having to apply excessive force to the short proximal fragment (Fig. 2.**218**).

The surgeon now measures distance from the seating chisel to the osteotomy on the femoral cortex and marks the site with an osteotome (Fig. 2.**219**). A Kirschner wire is inserted at the osteotomy site. Distal to the osteotomy site, a second Kirschner wire is inserted into the anterior femur at a right angle to the seating chisel in the transverse plane. This marker wire is used to gauge rotation after the osteotomy is performed (Fig. 2.**220**). The plane of osteotomy is verified with fluoroscopy (Fig. 2.**221**).

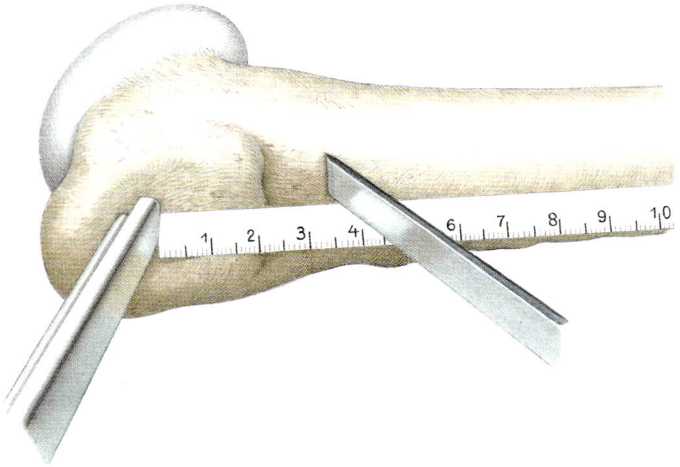

Fig. 2.**219** The distance from the seating chisel to the osteotomy is measured on the femoral cortex and the site is marked with an osteotome.

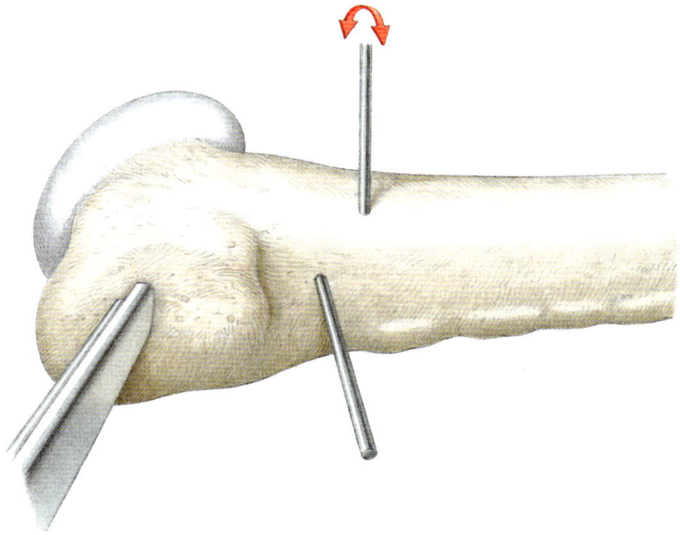

Fig. 2.**220** A marker wire is inserted at the planned osteotomy site and its position is verified with fluoroscopy. Distal to the osteotomy site, a second marker wire is inserted into the anterior femur at a right angle to gauge rotation.

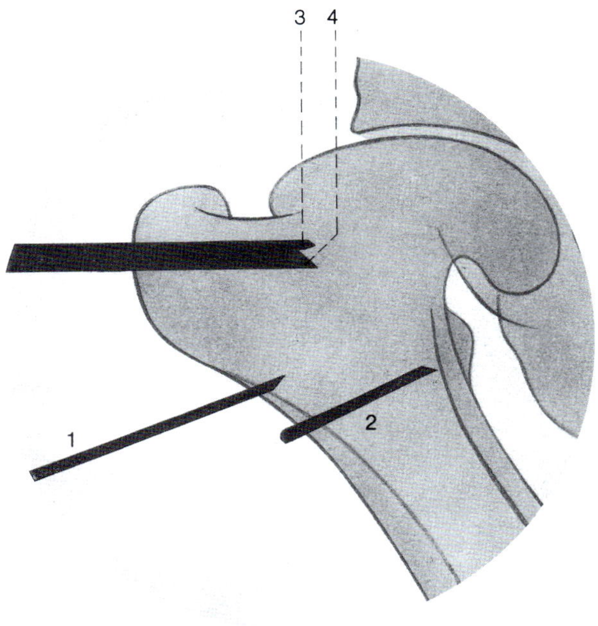

Fig. 2.**221** The position of the proximal femur and the level of the osteotomy are verified with fluroscopy.

1 Marker wire for osteotomy
2 Marker wire for gauging rotation
3 Steinmann pin for aligning seating chisel
4 Seating chisel

The osteotomy is performed at the marked site perpendicular to the distal fragment (Fig. 2.**222**). The surgeon pulls the distal fragment laterally with a forceps while using the seating chisel to rotate the proximal fragment to valgus. This presses the lateral edge of the proximal fragment into the distal osteotomy surface (Fig. 2.**223**).

After the seating chisel with the slotted hammer is removed from the proximal fragment, the condylar plate is inserted into the prepared bone with the inserter-extractor parallel to the Steinmann pin and driven in with a mallet. The surgeon inserts the blade 2–3 cm by hand, using a mallet only if re-

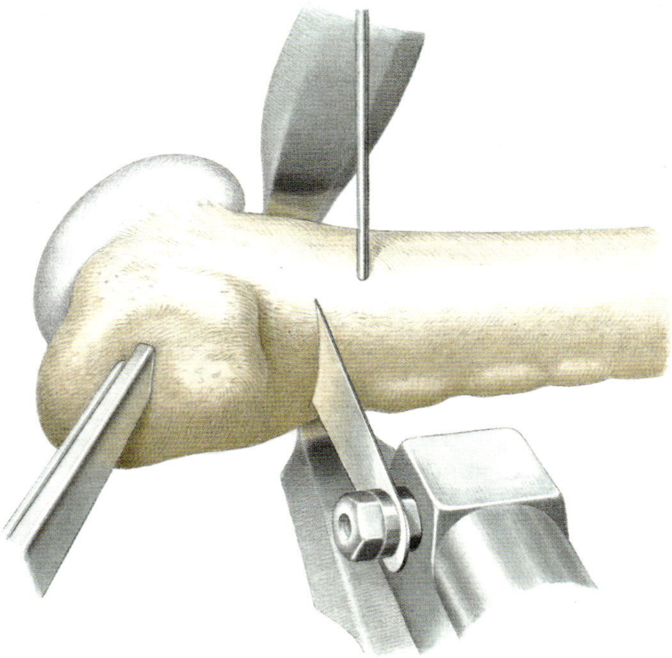

Fig. 2.**222** With elevators inserted to protect the soft tissue, the intertrochanteric osteotomy is performed perpendicular to the shaft of the femur at the marked site with an oscillating saw.

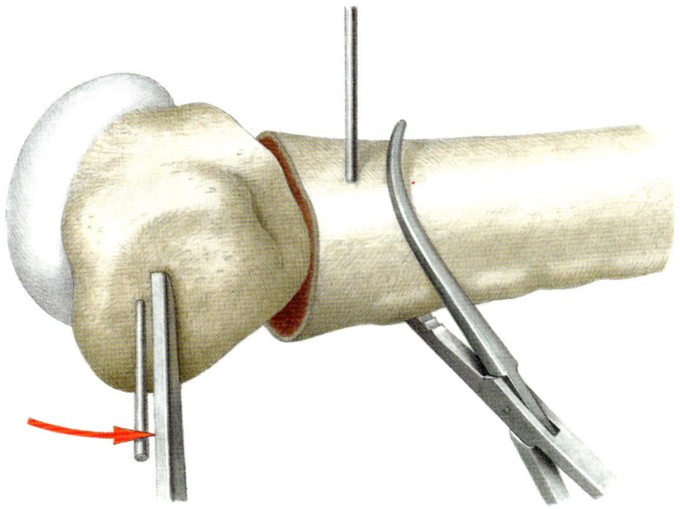

Fig. 2.**223** The distal fragment is pulled laterally with a forceps while the seating chisel is used as a handle to rotate the proximal fragment into valgus. This presses the lateral edge of the proximal fragment into the distal osteotomy surface.

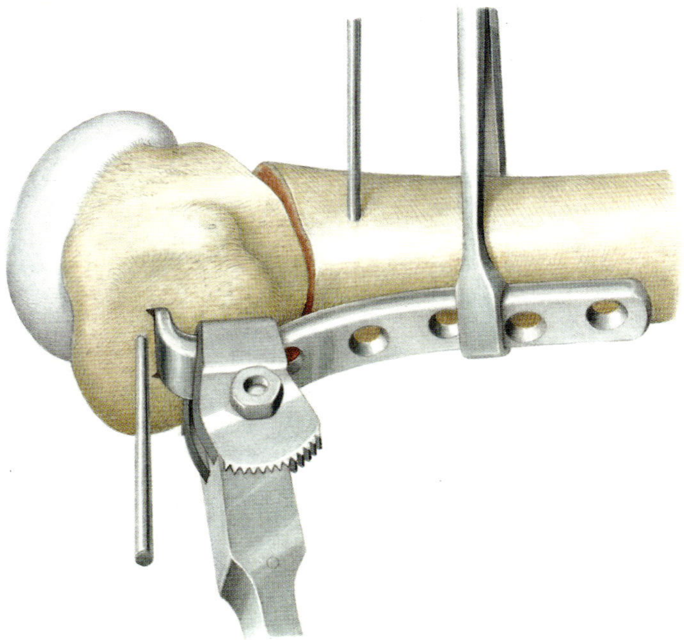

Fig. 2.**224** The seating chisel is replaced with a condylar plate, and the shaft of the plate is pressed against the distal fragment with a forceps. The angle between the Steinmann pin and the marker wire indicates the degree of rotation.

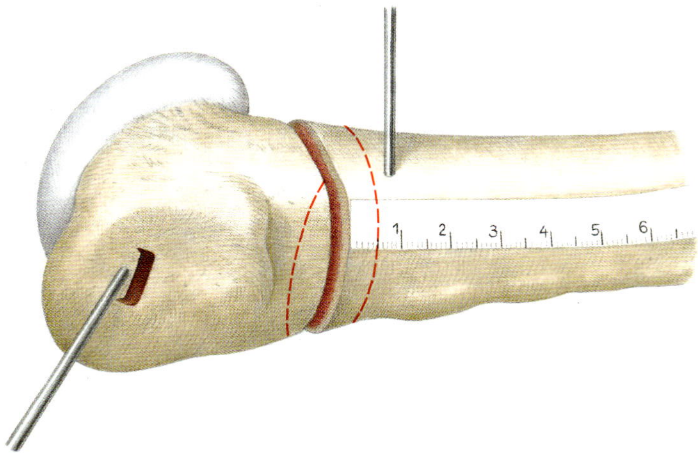

Fig. 2.**225** If intraoperative fluoroscopy reveals that the corrected femur is too long, a corresponding segment is resected at the site of the osteotomy. To do so, the surgeon releases the shaft of the plate from the distal fragment. If necessary, the blade is withdrawn from the proximal fragment as well.

sistance is encountered. This prevents the blade (which is relatively sharp) from deviating from the prepared channel in the cancellous bone. With the fragments in the corrected position, the shaft of the condylar plate is held against the distal fragment with a forceps (Fig. 2.**224**). The angle between the Steinmann pin in the proximal fragment and the Kirschner wire in the distal one indicates the degree of rotation. Intraoperative fluoroscopy is then used to verify the position of the fragments and measure the length of the femur. If the corrected femur is too long, the shaft of the condylar plate is released from the distal fragment to mobilize the fragments again. The lateral edge of the proximal fragment and a corresponding segment of the distal fragment may be resected to achieve the proper length (Fig. 2.**225**). The lesser trochanter should be left intact. When this second osteotomy has been completed, the fragments and the shaft of the condylar plate are opposed again.

The bony wedge that was previously removed may be inserted between the lateral surface of the proximal fragment and the condylar plate; interfragmentary compression is achieved with an articulated plate tensioner (Fig. 2.**226**). The shaft is fixed to the distal fragment with two screws, the articulated plate tensioner and the marker wires are removed, and the remaining screws are inserted into the shaft of the plate (Fig. 2.**227**).

The vastus lateralis is returned to its original position, covering the femur and the osteotomy site. The muscle is reattached where it was transected (distal to the proximal aspect of the greater trochanter) with vertical mattress sutures (Fig. 2.**208**). The fascia lata is closed with retention sutures over a suction drain (see Fig. 2.**163**). Restoring the original fascial tension is very important for the stability of the hip.

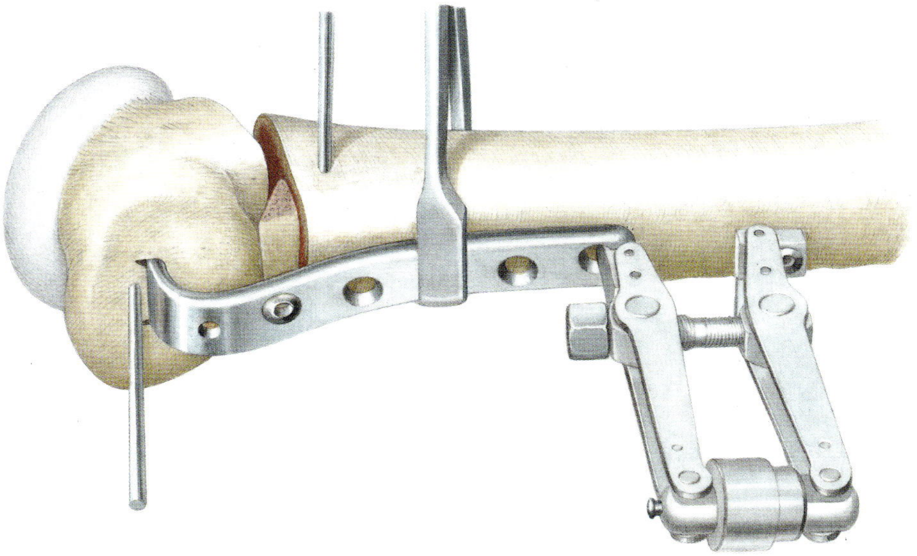

Fig. 2.**226** The blade of the condylar plate is now fastened to the proximal fragment with a screw. The fragments are opposed again, and the shaft of the condylar plate is pressed against the distal fragment. Bone graft is inserted into the lateral gap created by the osteotomy, and interfragmentary compression is achieved with an articulated plate tensioner.

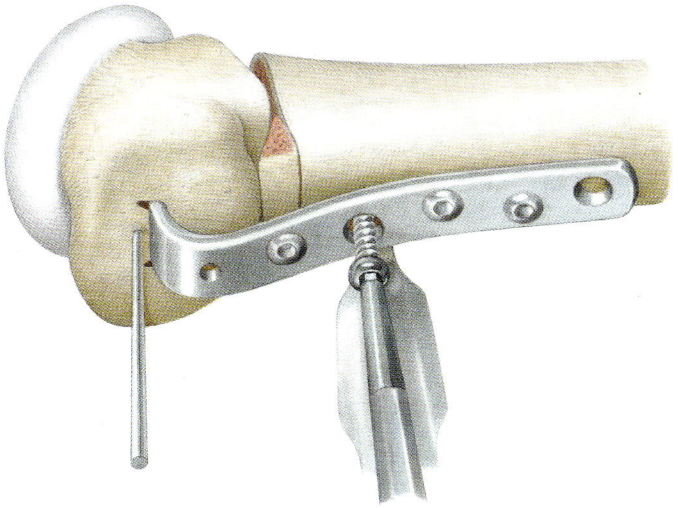

Fig. 2.**227** When fastening the shaft to the distal fragment, first insert the screws in the section of the shaft in direct contact with the bone. Only then should the most proximal screw in the distal fragment be inserted because here the shaft is not in contact with the bone. Inserting the screws in the opposite order will draw the distal fragment toward the shaft of the plate with resulting malalignment.

Intertrochanteric Extension Osteotomy

Indications

The procedure is indicated for surgical correction of a flexion deformity of the proximal femur or a fixed flexion contracture of the hip. Occasionally, an extension osteotomy is indicated to decompress segmental necrosis of the posterior femoral head.

Positioning and Incision

With the patient positioned supine, a skin incision is made that courses distally from the apex of the greater trochanter on the lateral side of the hip.

Technique

The osteotomy can be performed as a simple extension osteotomy or in combination with a varus correction, valgus correction, or rotation. The planes of the various osteotomies and the position of the channel for the blade of the condylar plate determine the resulting correction. Shifting the distal fragment in the direction of the correction prevents axial deformation of the femur at the osteotomy site and restores normal or near normal anatomy. It also greatly simplifies any future total joint arthroplasty.

The proximal femur is exposed in the same manner as in an intertrochanteric varus osteotomy. If necessary, the anterior joint capsule is exposed and resected.

After the vastus lateralis is dissected from its origin, the slot (KS) is prepared for the blade of the condylar plate (Fig. 2.**228**). The angle between the slot and the axis of the femur is the correction angle (i.e., after the extension osteotomy, the slot will be perpendicular to the shaft of the femur). If varus, valgus, or rotational corrections are planned, these components should be considered when planning the position of the slot. The slot must lie in the posterior section of the greater trochanter, so that the shaft of the condylar plate will lie along the axis of the femur after the distal fragment is shifted posteriorly.

After preparing the slot, the surgeon carefully drives the seating chisel into the blade channel with a mallet. To prevent cortical fracture, the seating chisel is impacted carefully. The surgeon should recheck the planned correction angle before final impaction of the seating chisel, using the slotted hammer as a handle to correct its position (Fig. 2.**229**). The intertrochanteric osteotomy is then performed at the superior margin of the lesser trochanter. The plane of osteotomy must lie perpendicular to the axis of the femur to prevent rotational corrections of the distal fragment from affecting the axial position of the proximal fragment.

Next, the surgeon makes the axial correction. This is best performed on the distal fragment to avoid dislodging the seating chisel (Fig. 2.**230**). Using the seating chisel to hold the proximal fragment, the surgeon brings the distal fragment into extension and makes any additional corrections the deformity may require (adduction, abduction, or rotation). The distal fragment is also shifted posteriorly to minimize the axial deformation of the proximal femur. This is important for two reasons: (1) The axis of the shaft of the femur should not be far from the bearing line (the vertical line beneath the center of rotation of the hip), and (2) minimizing the axial deformation of the femur greatly simplifies any future total joint arthroplasty.

For particularly stable interfragmentary integration, the posterior edge of the proximal fragment is impacted into the distal osteotomy surface. If the bone quality will not permit this, a small wedge is resected from the posterior edge of the proximal fragment parallel to the distal osteotomy surface. After the correction is made, the anterior edge of the proximal fragment projects relatively far into the surrounding soft tissue. This edge is resected and inserted into the posterior gap between the two fragments, thus restoring the physiological femoral contour.

The seating chisel is replaced with a condylar plate, which is fastened to the distal fragment with screws to achieve interfragmentary compression (Fig. 2.**231**). After reattaching the vastus lateralis and closing the fascia lata with retention sutures, the surgeon closes the wound in layers.

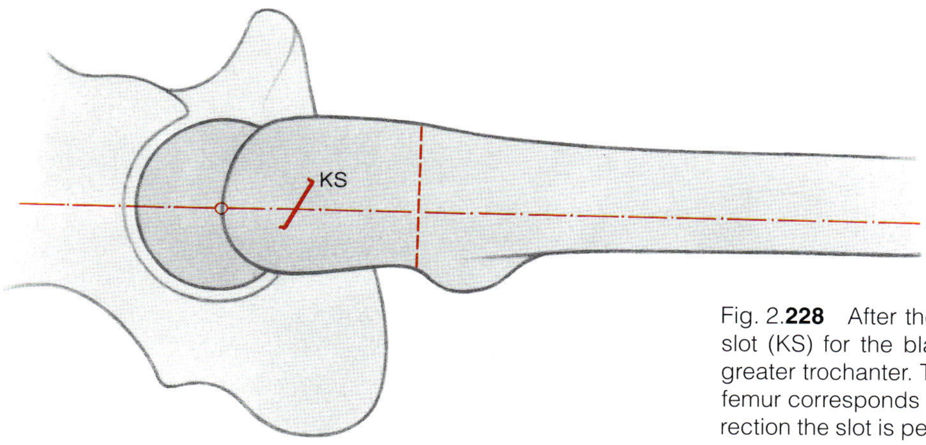

Fig. 2.**228** After the lateral surface of the femur is exposed, the slot (KS) for the blade of the condylar plate is prepared in the greater trochanter. The angle between the slot and the axis of the femur corresponds to the planned correction angle. After the correction the slot is perpendicular to the shaft of the femur.

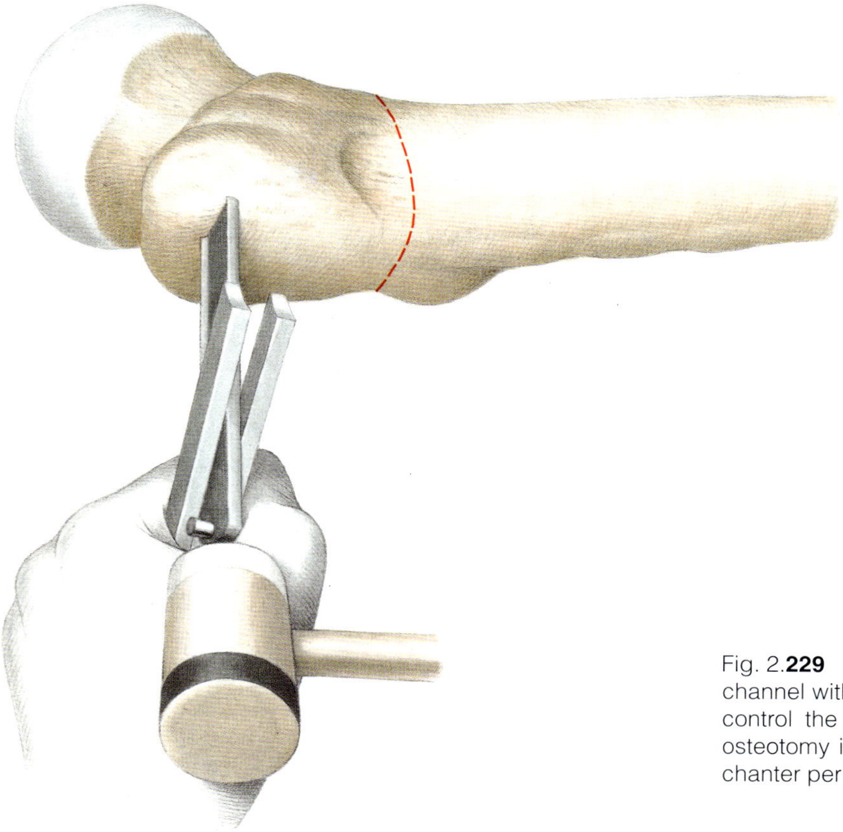

Fig. 2.**229** The seating chisel is carefully driven into the blade channel with a mallet. The slotted hammer is used as a handle to control the position of the seating chisel. the intertrochanteric osteotomy is performed at the superior margin of the lesser trochanter perpendicular to the axis of the femur.

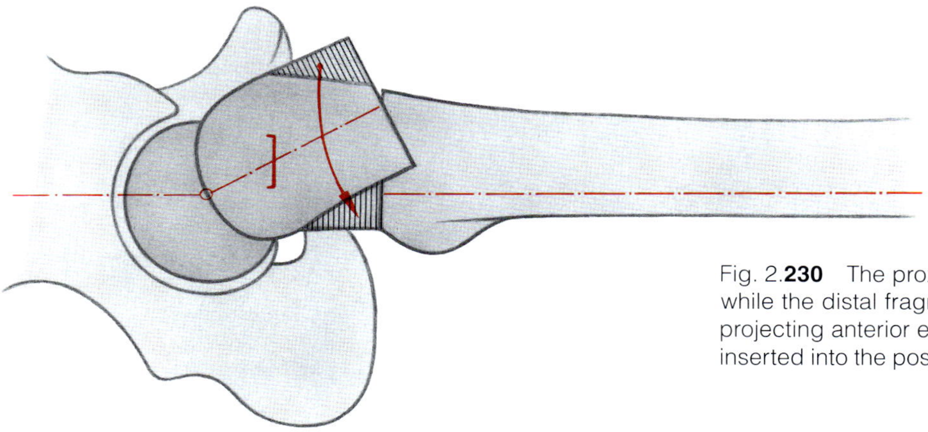

Fig. 2.**230** The proximal fragment is held with the seating chisel. while the distal fragment is extended and shifted posteriorly. The projecting anterior edge of the proximal fragment is resected and inserted into the posterior gap between the two fragments.

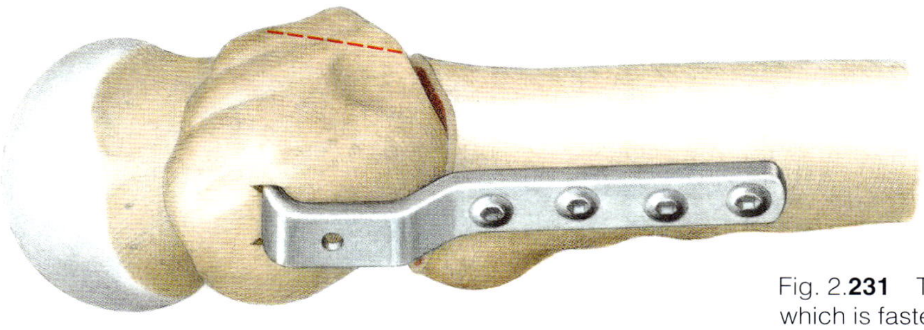

Fig. 2.**231** The seating chisel is replaced with a condylar plate, which is fastened to the distal fragment with screws to achieve interfragmentary compression.

Intertrochanteric Flexion Osteotomy with Anterior Capsulectomy

Indications

- Primarily in the surgical treatment of segmental necrosis of the femoral head in younger patients. The necrotic site can be rotated anteriorly out of area of greatest force transfer.
- Deformities of the femoral head resulting from growth arrest.
- Posttraumatic or arthritic deformities where preoperative radiographic examination reveals that opposition of the posterosuperior femoral head with the superior acetabulum would improve joint congruity.

Positioning and Incision

With the patient positioned supine, a skin incision is made that courses distally from the apex of the greater trochanter on the lateral side of the hip.

Technique

The osteotomy can be performed as a simple flexion osteotomy or in combination with a varus correction, valgus correction, or rotation. The planes of the various osteotomies and the position of the channel for the blade of the condylar plate determine the resulting correction. Shifting the distal fragment in the direction of the correction prevents axial deformation of the femur at the osteotomy site and restores normal or near normal anatomy, greatly simplifying any future total joint arthroplasty.

The proximal femur is exposed in the same manner as in an intertrochanteric varus osteotomy. The anterior joint capsule is always exposed and resected as far as the acetabular labrum; the flexion osteotomy rotates the proximal fragment into an extended position, placing tension on the anterior joint capsule with the powerful iliofemoral ligament. The extensive capsulectomy is necessary to prevent a capsular flexion contracture of the hip.

After the vastus lateralis is dissected from its origin, the soft tissue is retracted from the anterior capsule and as far as the anterior margin of the acetabulum and held with a short, sharp-tipped elevator impacted in the anterior margin of the acetabulum. The surgeon performs a partial capsulectomy, completely exposing the acetabular labrum over a 4-cm section of the capsule circumference. Now the slot (KS) is prepared for the blade of the condylar plate (Fig. 2.**232**). The angle between the slot and the axis of the femur is the correction angle (i.e., after the flexion osteotomy, the slot will be perpendicular to the shaft of the femur). If other corrections, such as varus, valgus, or rotational corrections are planned, these components should be considered when planning the position of the slot. The slot must lie in the anterior section of the greater trochanter, so that the shaft of the condylar plate will lie along the axis of the femur after the distal fragment is shifted anteriorly.

After preparing the slot, the surgeon carefully drives the seating chisel into the blade channel with a mallet. To prevent cortical fracture, the seating chisel is impacted carefully. The surgeon should recheck the planned correction angle before final impaction of the seating chisel, using the slotted hammer as a handle to correct its position (Fig. 2.**233**). Then the intertrochanteric osteotomy is performed at the superior margin of the lesser trochanter. The plane of osteotomy must lie perpendicular to the axis of the femur to prevent rotational corrections of the distal fragment from affecting the axial position of the proximal fragment.

Now the surgeon makes the axial correction. This is best performed on the distal fragment to avoid dislodging the seating

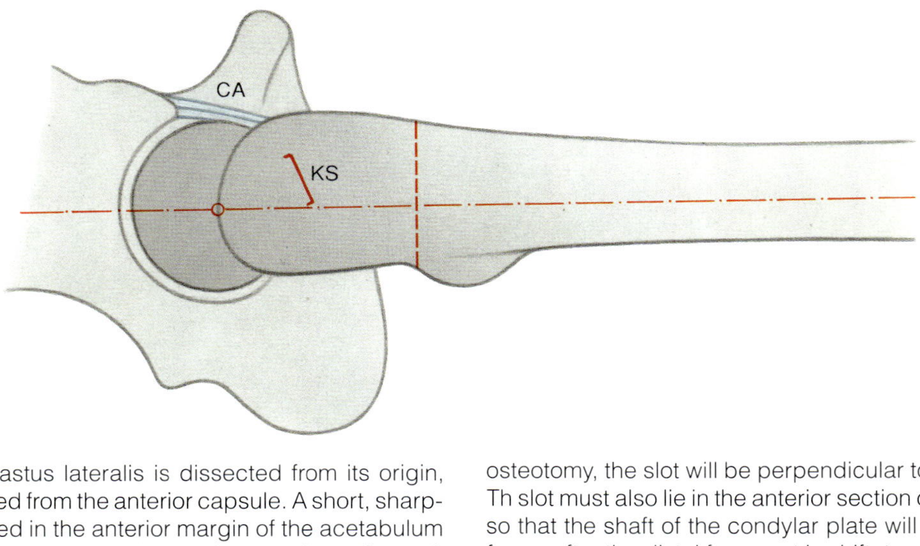

Fig. 2.**232** After the vastus lateralis is dissected from its origin, the soft tissue is retracted from the anterior capsule. A short, sharp-tipped elevator impacted in the anterior margin of the acetabulum is used to lift the soft tissue. A partial capsulectomy is performed, completely exposing the acetabular labrum over a 4-cm section of the capsule circumference. Then the slot (KS) is prepared for the blade of the condylar plate. The angle between the slot and the axis of the femur is the correction angle (i.e., after the flexion osteotomy, the slot will be perpendicular to the shaft of the femur). Th slot must also lie in the anterior section of the greater trochanter, so that the shaft of the condylar plate will lie along the axis of the femur after the distal fragment is shiftet anteriorly

KS Slot for blade of condylar plate
CA Hip joint capsule

chisel. The surgeon uses the seating chisel to hold the proximal fragment while bringing the distal fragment into flexion and making any additional corrections the deformity may require, such as adduction, abduction, or rotation (Fig. 2.**234**). The distal fragment is also shifted anteriorly to minimize the axial deformation of the proximal femur. This prevents the axis of the femur from deviating too far from the bearing line (the vertical line beneath the center of rotation of the hip). Minimizing the axial deformation of the femur also greatly simplifies any future total joint arthroplasty.

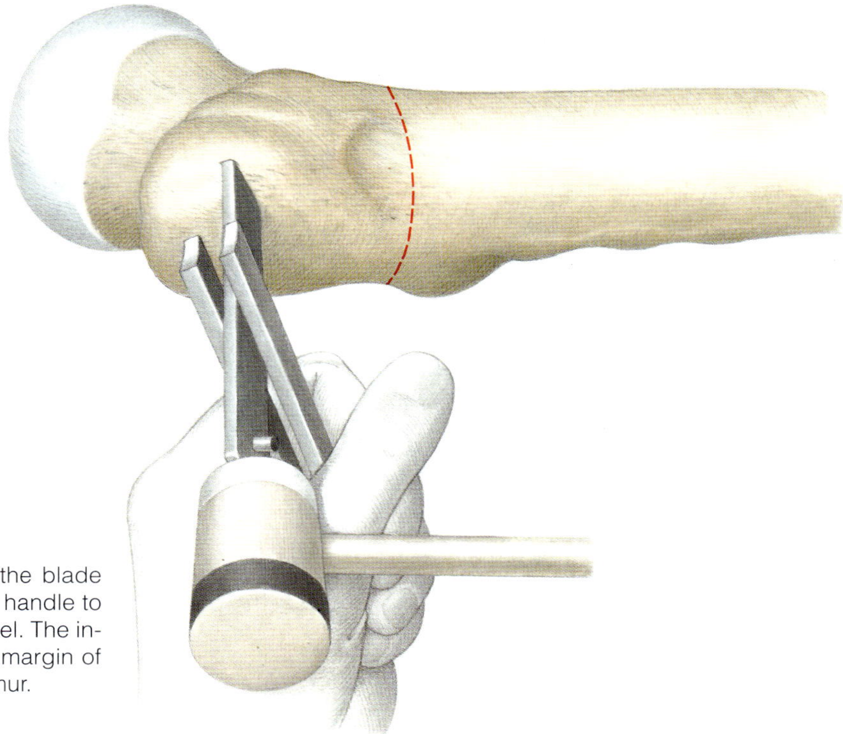

Fig. 2.**233** The seating chisel is carefully driven into the blade channel with a mallet. The slotted hammer is used as a handle to control the rotation and axial position of the seating chisel. The intertrochanteric osteotomy is performed at the superior margin of the lesser trochanter perpendicular to the axis of the femur.

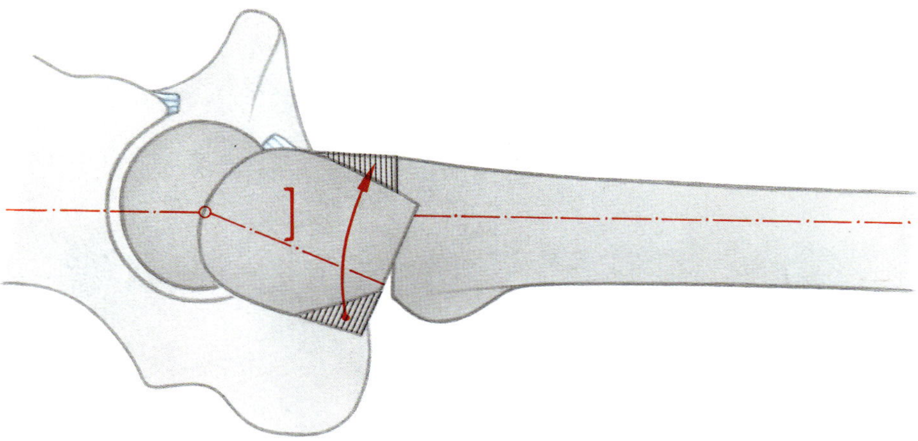

Fig. 2.**234** The axial correction should not be performed on the proximal fragment to avoid damaging the blade channel. The proximal fragment is held with the seating chisel while the distal fragment is brought into flexion, and any additional corrections, such as adduction, abduction, or rotation are made. The distal fragment is also shifted anteriorly to minimize the axial deformation of the proximal femur. Taking care to avoid damaging the vascular supply to the femoral neck, the surgeon restores the physiological contour of the posterior femur by resecting the projecting posterior edge of the proximal fragment and inserting it into the anterior gap between the two fragments.

For particularly stable interfragmentary integration, the posterior edge of the proximal fragment is impacted into the distal osteotomy surface. If the bone quality will not permit this, a small wedge is resected from the anterior edge of the proximal fragment parallel to the distal osteotomy surface. After the correction is made, the posterior edge of the proximal fragment projects relatively far into the surrounding soft tissue. Taking care to avoid damaging the vascular supply to the posterior femoral neck, the surgeon resects this edge and inserts it into the anterior gap between the two fragments, thus restoring the physiological femoral contour.

The seating chisel is replaced with a condylar plate, which is fastened to the distal fragment with screws to achieve interfragmentary compression (Fig. 2.**235**). After reattaching the vastus lateralis and closing the fascia lata with retention sutures, the surgeon closes the wound in layers.

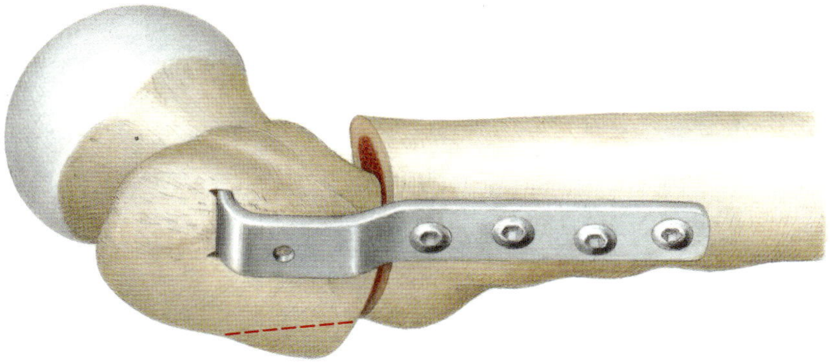

Fig. 2.**235** The seating chisel is replaced with a condylar plate, which is fastened to the distal fragment with screws to achieve interfragmentary compression.

Intertrochanteric Rotation/Derotation Osteotomy

Indications

This osteotomy is generally indicated for surgical correction of rotational deformity of the femoral neck proximal to the lesser trochanter. The topographical relationship between the axis of the femoral neck and the position of the lesser trochanter is altered; whereas the lesser trochanter and the insertion of the iliopsoas tendon remain in a physiological position with respect to the knee and the femur, there is a pathologic deviation in the axis of the femoral neck. An intertrochanteric rotation osteotomy corrects this deformity. While a subtrochanteric rotation osteotomy would also correct the defective position of the femoral neck, it would rotate the lesser trochanter away from its physiological position.

The classic indication for an intertrochanteric derotation osteotomy is pathologic anteversion of the femoral neck in a developmentally dislocated hip. This procedure is often combined with a varus osteotomy at the same site if the anteversion is accompanied by a valgus deformity.

An intertrochanteric rotation osteotomy is indicated in pathologic retroversion of the femoral neck, such as occurs in coxa vara or protrusion of the acetabulum.

Even diaphyseal or distal rotational deformities of the femur are often corrected in the proximal femur because the bone heals well, the damage to the thigh musculature is minimal, and the procedure is more conservative than a more distal osteotomy. Here the same internal fixation is used, yet the osteotomy is performed distal to the lesser trochanter so that it remains in its physiological position after the rotational correction.

Positioning and Incision

As with every intertrochanteric osteotomy, the patient is positioned supine, and a skin incision is made that courses distally from the apex of the greater trochanter on the lateral side of the hip.

Technique

If a simple rotational correction is required, a transverse osteotomy is performed perpendicular to the axis of the femur and the two fragments are rotated toward one another. The osteotomy is stabilized with a condylar plate. If the rotation is combined with a correction in the coronal or sagittal plane, a wedge must be resected or the fragments shifted as in a lateral shift intertrochanteric osteotomy. The osteotomy of the distal fragment must lie perpendicular to the axis of the femur to prevent rotational corrections of the distal fragment from affecting the axial position of the femoral neck.

The approach to the proximal femur is identical to the one used in an intertrochanteric varus osteotomy.

After the proximal femur is exposed, a marker wire is inserted into the greater trochanter to indicate the direction of the blade of the condylar plate. Fluoroscopy can be used to verify the position of the wire. If a simple rotational correction is required, the angle between the blade and the femur is 95°. The marker wire and blade are always centered on the axis of the femoral neck in the horizontal plane. After preparing the channel for the blade and inserting the seating chisel, the surgeon inserts marker wires proximal and distal to the planned osteotomy plane to gauge rotation. The angle between two wires indicates the degree of the planned rotational correction. After the correction, the two wires are parallel.

After the osteotomy has been performed, the seating chisel is replaced with a condylar plate. The shaft of the plate is pressed against the distal fragment. Since the channel for the blade was prepared at an angle of 95°, the 90°condylar plate will result in a slight varus shift in the femoral neck. The two fragments are opposed at the medial edge of the osteotomy, whereas there is a slight gap at its lateral edge. When an articulated plate tensioner is applied to achieve interfragmentary compression, the angle of the condylar plate is opened to 95°, the neck-shaft angle femoral neck returns to its original position, and the lateral gap created by the osteotomy is forced closed. This provides the medial support of the fragments required for stable internal fixation. If this initial overcorrection were omitted applying interfragmentary compression would open the angle of the condylar plate to 95°, but it would also open a gap at the medial edge of the osteotomy and compromise stability (Fig. 2.**236**).

After the shaft of the osteotomy plate is fastened to the distal fragment, the marker wires are removed. The wound is closed in the same manner as an intertrochanteric varus osteotomy.

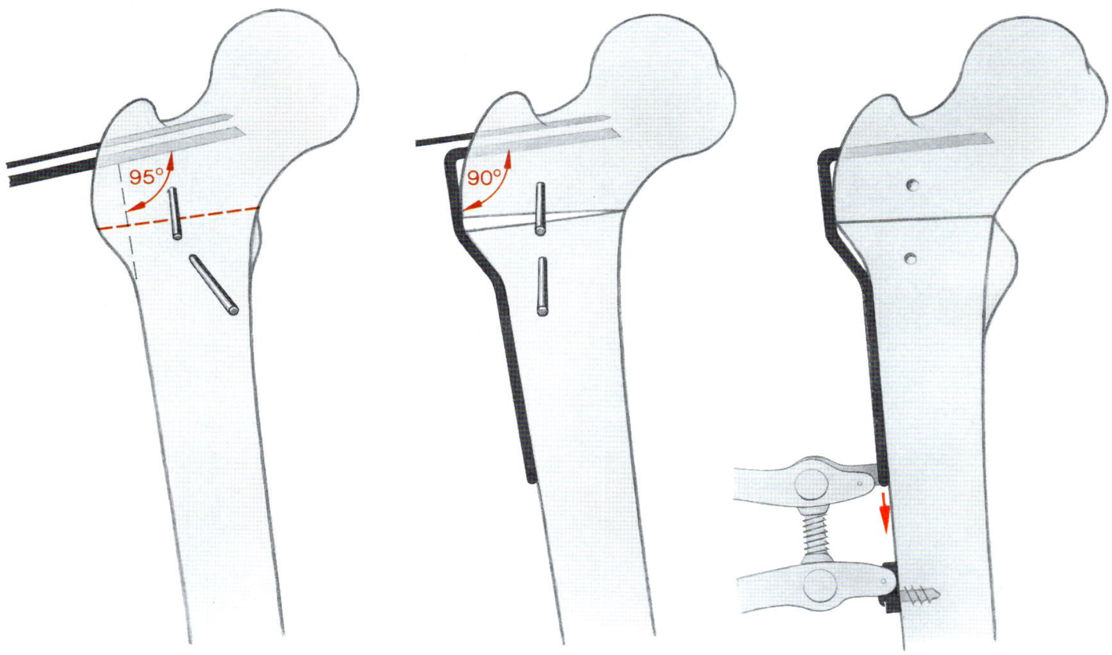

Fig. 2.**236** A marker wire is inserted into the greater trochanter and up the femoral neck. Then the seating chisel is inserted parallel to the wire at a 95° angle to the shaft of the femur. Marker wires are inserted proximal and distal to the planned osteotomy in the sagittal plane to gauge rotation. The angle between two wires indicates the degree of the planned rotational correction. After the correction, the two wires are parallel. After the blade of the condylar plate has been inserted, there is a slight gap at the lateral edge of the osteotomy. When interfragmentary compression is applied, the lateral gap is forced closed. This provides the medial support of the fragments required for stable internal fixation.

Intertrochanteric Shortening Osteotomy

Indications

This osteotomy is primarily indicated for surgical correction of an excessively long femur. The condition may be posttraumatic or the result of growth stimulation due to systemic disease. This procedure may also be used to correct a contralateral leg length differential in tall patients in whom the decrease in body height would not be readily apparent. To minimize loss of muscular tension and alteration of body proportions, the segmental osteotomy should not exceed 6 cm.

Positioning and Incision

With the patient positioned supine, a lateral approach to the proximal femur is made through a straight longitudinal skin incision on the lateral side of the hip.

Technique

The procedure is performed as an intertrochanteric osteotomy to shorten the femur by removing a segment corresponding to the desired correction length. The proximal osteotomy surface is angled to maintain the lesser trochanter in its anatomic position (Fig. 2.**237**). The large area of the contact between the two fragments increases the stability of the internal fixation and promotes bony consolidation. The intertrochanteric osteotomy lies in the region of the origin of the quadriceps femoris where muscular function produces the least degree of tissue displacement. This procedure results in significantly smaller loss of muscular tension than a supracondylar osteotomy.

The relatively large proportion of the cancellous bone in the proximal osteotomy surface is a further advantage of this site.

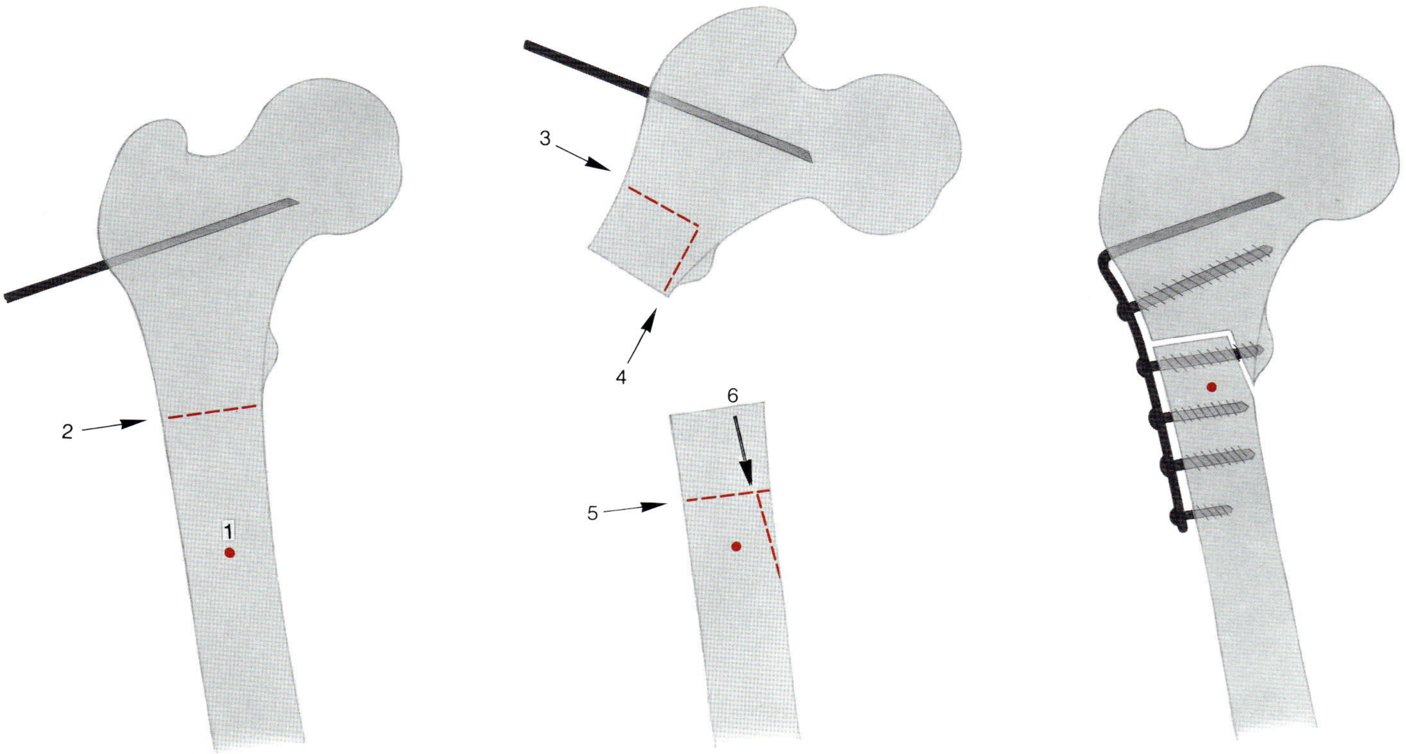

Fig. 2.**237** To shorten the femur, an intertrochanteric osteotomy is performed, and a segment corresponding to the desired correction length is removed. The angled proximal osteotomy surface maintains the lesser trochanter in its anatomic position. A segment is removed from the femur and the fragments are opposed. An osteotomy plate is implanted and interfragmentary compression is applied for internal fixation of the osteotomy.

1 Marking on the preoperative drawing to determine the length of the resected segment
2 Subtrochanteric osteotomy
3 Intertrochanteric osteotomy stops short of the posterior cortex
4 Longitudinal osteotomy to resect the proximal portion of the segment leaves the lesser trochanter intact
5 Subtrochanteric transverse osteotomy to resect the distal portion of the segment
6 Medial bone wedge is resected from the distal fragment to accommodate the lesser trochanter

After a longitudinal skin incision has been made on the lateral side of the hip (Fig. 2.**238**), the fascia lata is split parallel to the direction of its fibers and retracted. The vastus lateralis is dissected with an L-shaped incision immediately distal to the most proximal aspect of the greater trochanter (see Fig. 2.**191**). The surgeon carefully dissects the muscle fibers from the outer surface of the femur with a periosteal elevator. The fascia of the vastus lateralis is split in the direction of its fibers where it joins the lateral intermuscular septum. Now the musculature is dissected from the lateral intermuscular septum as well, and the femur is exposed (see Fig. 2.**192**).

Using intraoperative fluoroscopy, the surgeon inserts four marker wires into the lateral femur (Fig. 2.**239** and 2.**240**). The most proximal wire marks the site of the blade channel for the osteotomy plate. The second wire marks the proximal end of the osteotomy. The third wire indicates the distal margin of the lesser trochanter, and the fourth one marks the level of the distal osteotomy. The segment is resected between the second and fourth wire; the distance between these wires corresponds to the length of bone resected (in this example, 35 mm).

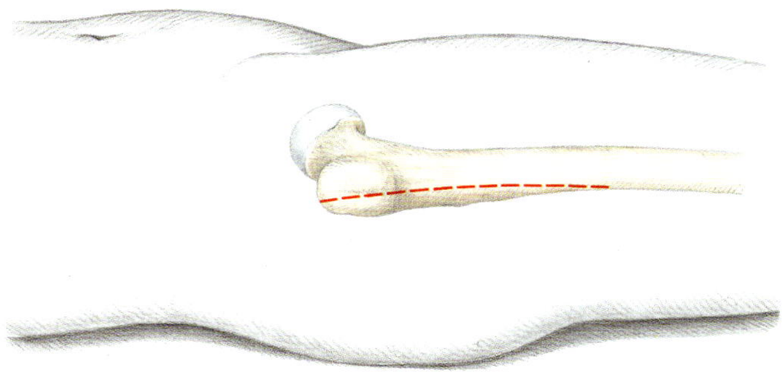

Fig. 2.**238** A longitudinal skin incision is made beginning at the greater trochanter and coursing distally.

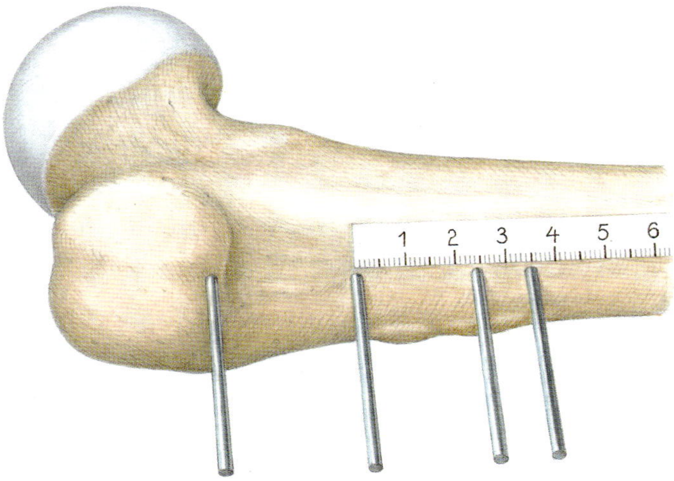

Fig. 2.**239** Four marker wires are inserted into the lateral femur. The most proximal wire marks the site of the blade channel for the osteotomy plate. The second wire marks the proximal end of the osteotomy. The third wire indicates the distal margin of the lesser trochanter, and the fourth one marks the level of the distal osteotomy.

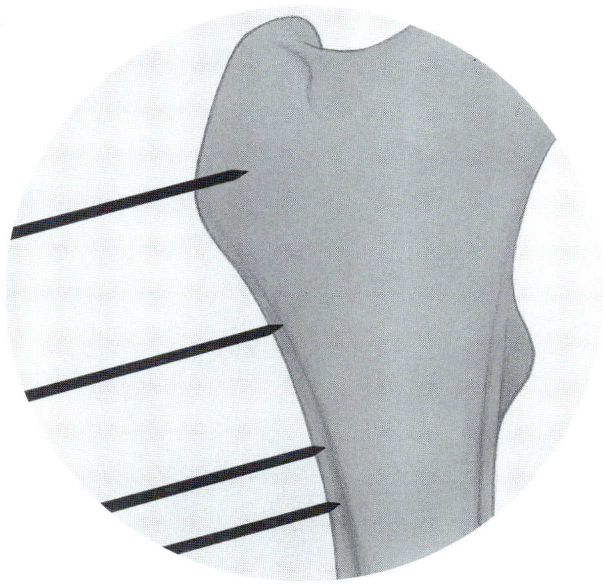

Fig. 2.**240** The correct position of the marker wires is verified with fluoroscopy.

The most proximal marker wire is left in place to mark the direction of the blade of the osteotomy plate. The remaining wires are removed, and the cortex is notched with a chisel at their insertion sites. Distal to the osteotomy site, a marker wire is inserted into the distal fragment in the sagittal plane to gauge rotation. This wire is perpendicular to the marker wire for the blade channel (Fig. 2.**241**). The proximal stump of the origin of the vastus lateralis is carefully dissected from the surface of the bone to expose the site of the blade channel.

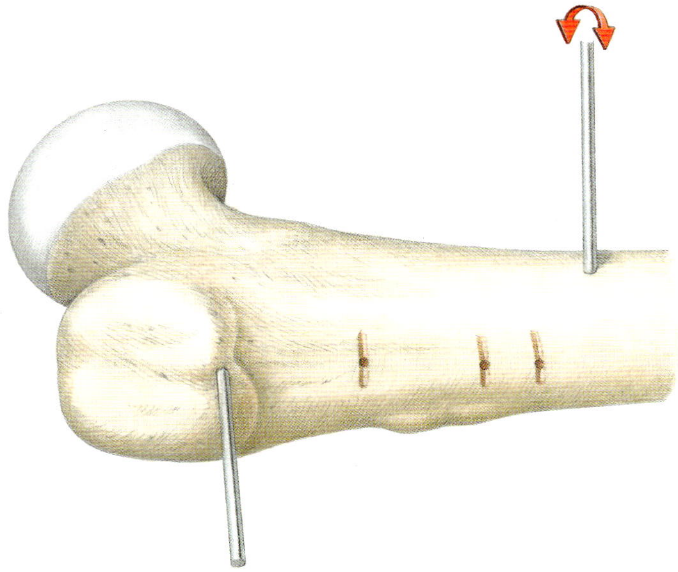

Fig. 2.**241** The most proximal marker wire is left in place to mark the direction of the blade of the osteotomy plate. The remaining wires are removed and the cortex is notched with a chisel at their insertion sites. Distal to the osteotomy site, a marker wire is inserted into the distal fragment in the sagittal plane to gauge rotation. This wire is perpendicular to the marker wire for the blade channel.

To accommodate the blade of the condylar plate, the surgeon drills a row of holes (Fig. 2.**242**). The holes are joined and widened to accommodate the blade by driving a chisel into the surface of the bone and moving it back and forth. This prevents the blade from fracturing the proximal femoral cortex (Fig. 2.**243**).

The seating chisel is impacted into the prepared slot parallel to the marker wire. Rotation and axial alignment of the chisel are controlled by a slotted hammer (Fig. 2.**244**). The surface of the seating chisel must be perpendicular to the longitudinal axis of the femur so that the plate shaft will be in contact with the surface of the bone parallel to the axis of the femur after the osteotomy.

The surgeon decorticates the posterior femoral cortex at the osteotomy site with a mallet and periosteal elevator (Fig. 2.**245**). The soft tissue is raised in a subperiosteal dissection, preventing damage to the vascular structures. The surgeon also raises small scales, which retain their periosteal attachments. This “fish scaling” improves bony healing. Elevators are then inserted posteriorly to protect the surrounding soft tissue during the osteotomy.

The first saw cut is made perpendicular to the longitudinal axis of the femur at the distal margin of the lesser trochanter (Fig. 2.**246**). Irrigation is used to prevent thermal necrosis at the osteotomy sites.

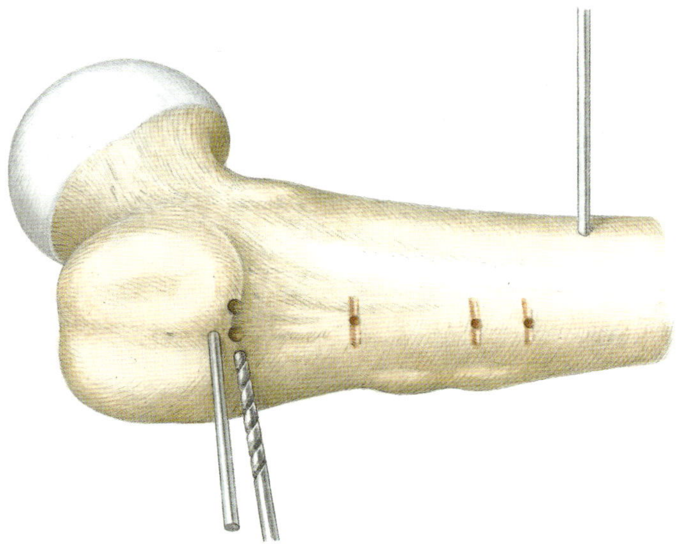

Fig. 2.**242** A row of closely spaced holes are drilled in the surface of the bone.

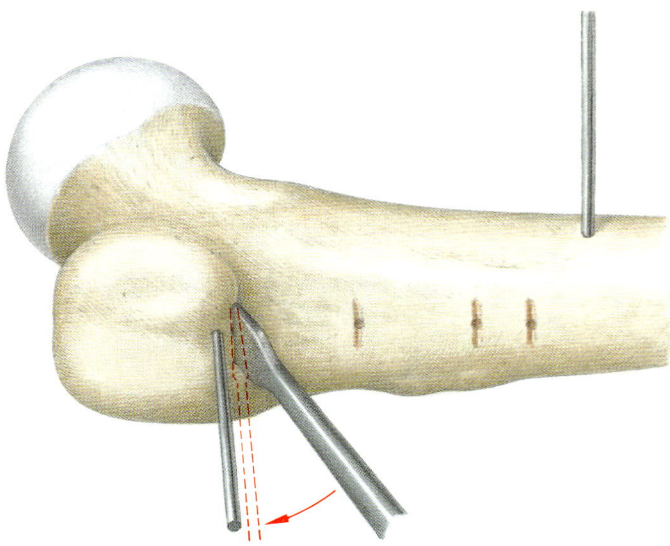

Fig. 2.**243** The holes are joined and widened by driving a chisel into the surface of the bone and moving it back and forth. This prevents the blade from fracturing the proximal femoral cortex.

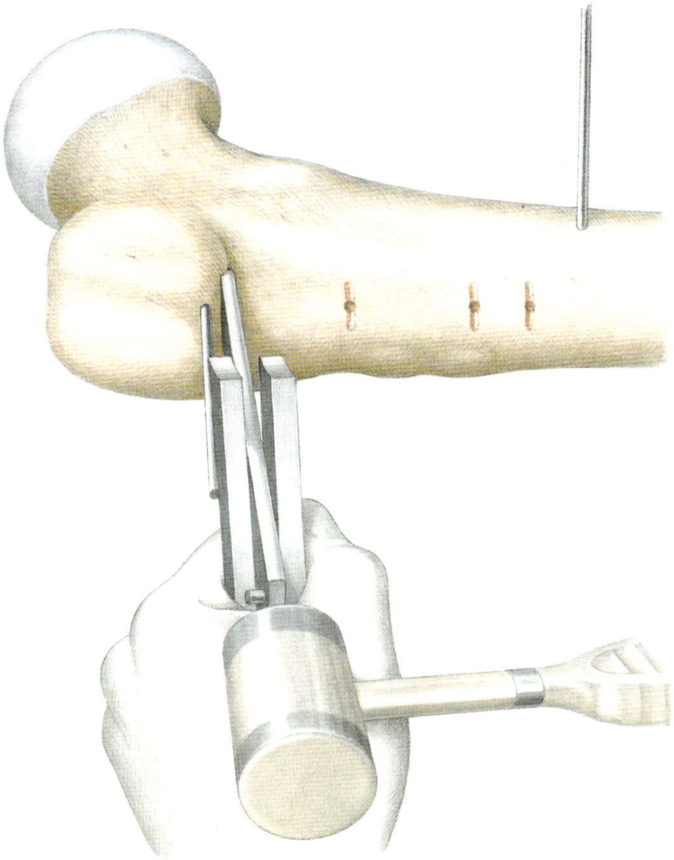

Fig. 2.**244** The seating chisel is impacted into the prepared slot parallel to the marker wire. The slottes hammer controls the rotation and axial alignment of the chisel.

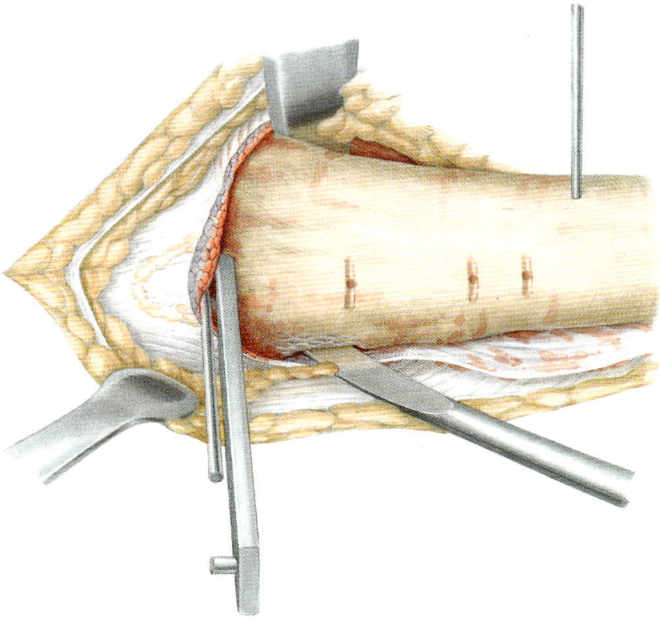

Fig. 2.**245** A mallet and periosteal elevator are used to decorticate the posterior femoral cortex at the osteotomy site.

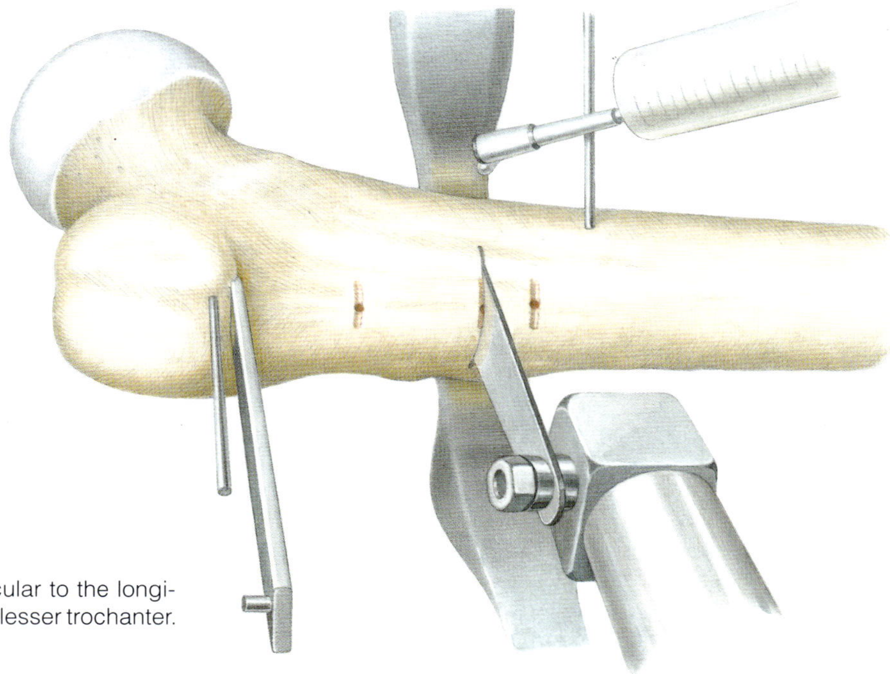

Fig. 2.**246** The first saw cut is made perpendicular to the longitudinal axis of the femur at the distal margin of the lesser trochanter.

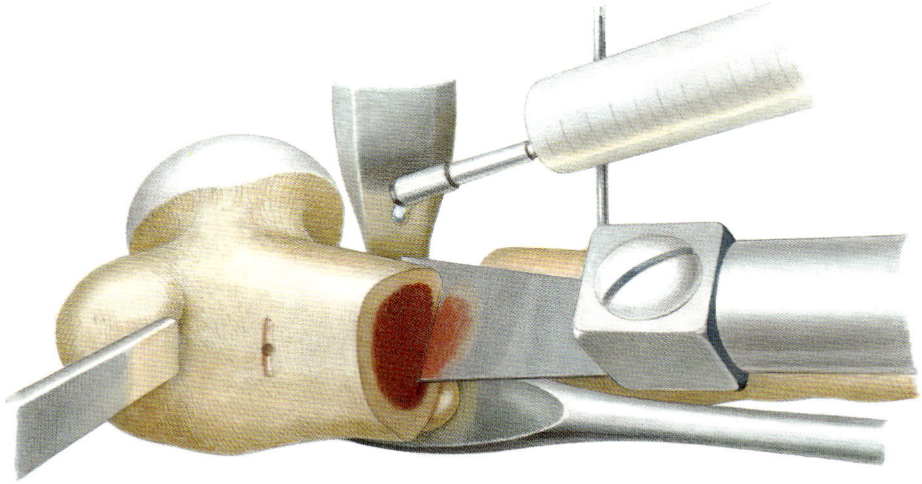

Fig. 2.**247** Spreading the osteotomy, shifting the distal fragment medially, and abducting the proximal fragment exposes the entire lesser trochanter and the proximal osteotomy site. First, a longitudinal osteotomy is performed, which begins at the base of the lesser trochanter and courses proximally, avoiding the lesser trochanter and the medial cortex. The lesser trochanter must remain in its posteromedial position.

The surgeon then spreads the osteotomy, shifting the distal fragment medially, and abducting the proximal fragment to expose the entire lesser trochanter and the proximal osteotomy site (Fig. 2.**247**). Two osteotomies perpendicular to each other are performed on the proximal fragment to remove the proximal portion of the segment. The longitudinal osteotomy begins at the base of the lesser trochanter and courses proximally parallel to the axis of the femur, avoiding the lesser trochanter and the medial cortex (Fig. 2.**247**). The lesser trochanter must remain in its posteromedial position. The proximal transverse osteotomy is performed perpendicular to the previous osteotomy. Both osteotomies are directly inspected (Fig. 2.**248**). If soft tissue prevents complete exposure, the surgeon may insert a loose saw blade into the first osteotomy for better orientation. When both osteotomies meet, the proximal portion of the segment is completely resected (Fig. 2.**249**). It is then released from its soft-tissue attachments and removed, revealing the vertical osteotomy surface with the lesser trochanter.

A transverse osteotomy is performed at the marked site on the distal fragment, and the distal portion of the segment is removed (Fig. 2.**250**). This completes resection of the entire segment.

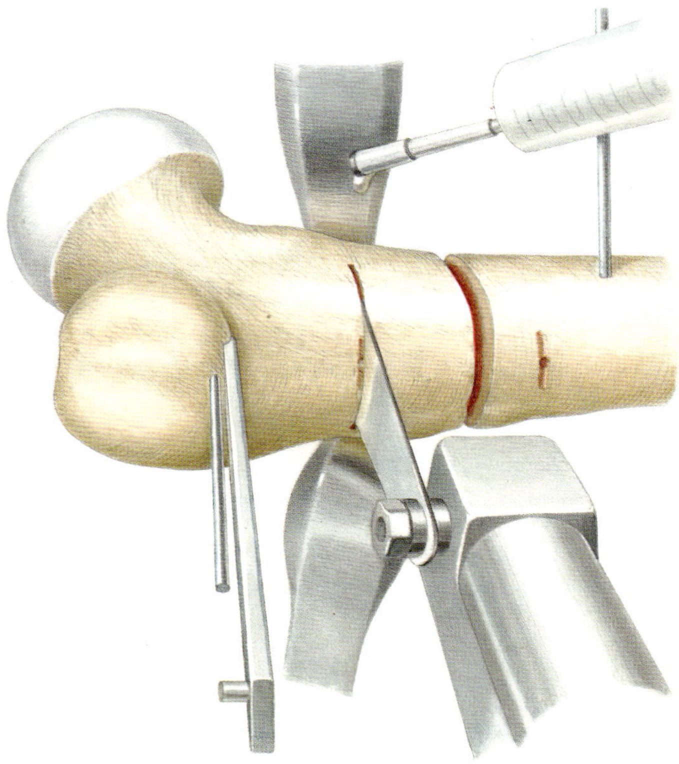

Fig. 2.**248** The proximal transverse osteotomy is performed perpendicular to the previous longitudinal osteotomy.

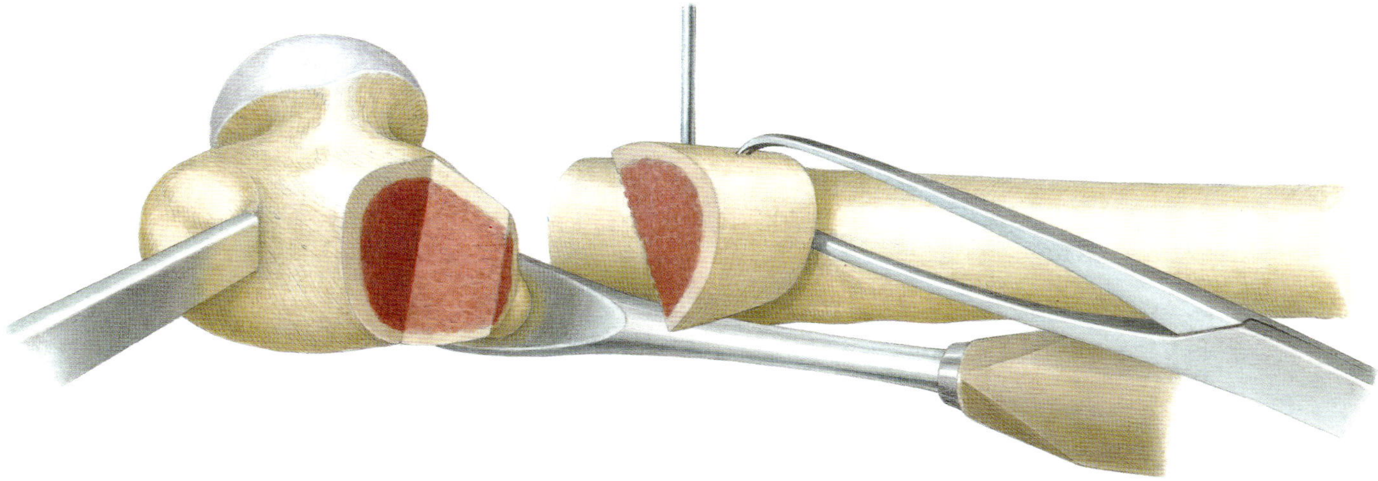

Fig. 2.**249** When both osteotomies meet, the proximal portion of the segment is completely resected and can be removed.

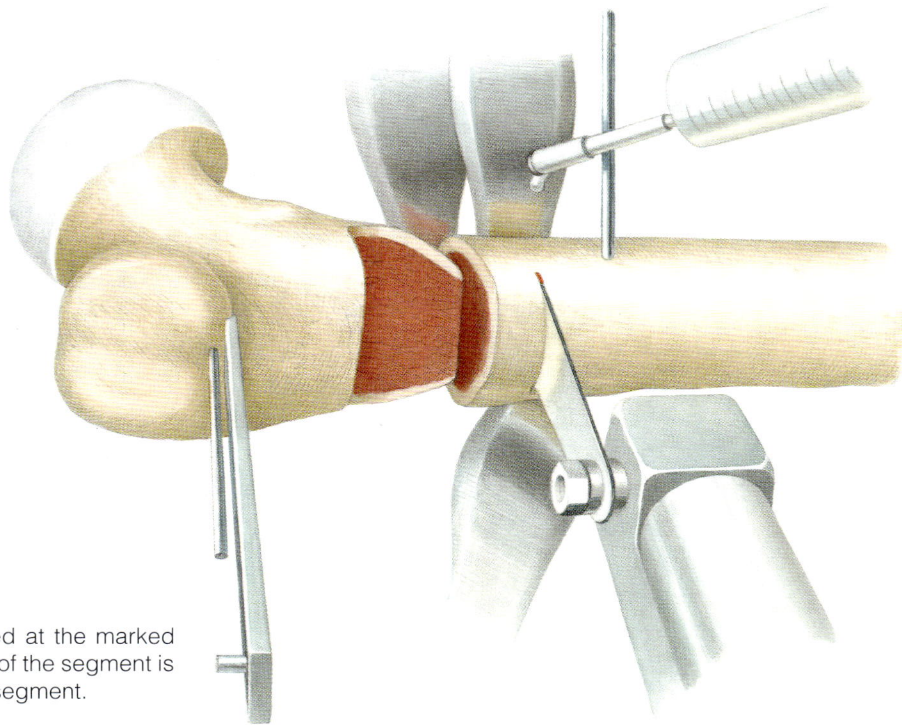

Fig. 2.**250** A transverse osteotomy is performed at the marked site on the distal fragment, and the distal portion of the segment is removed. This completes resection of the entire segment.

A posteromedial wedge is resected from the distal fragment to match the posteromedial tongue with the lesser trochanter projecting from the proximal fragment (Fig. 2.**251**). Both fragments can now be brought into direct opposition.

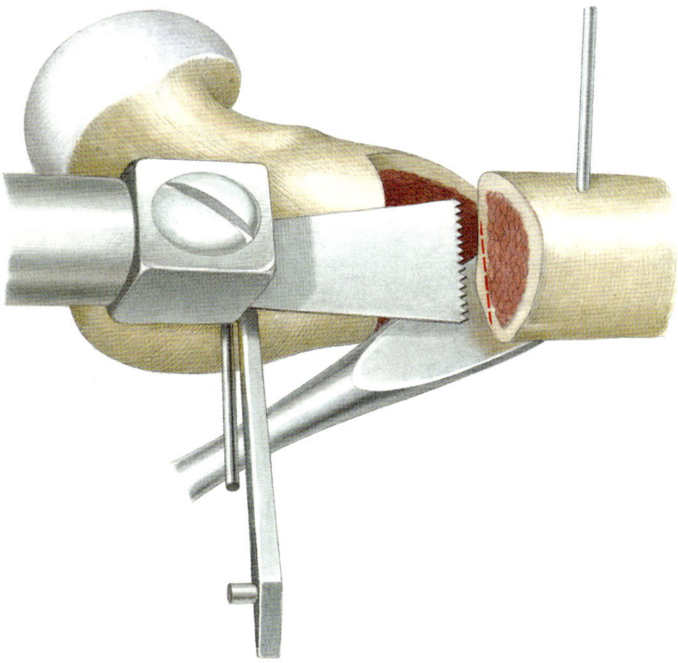

Fig. 2.**251** A posteromedial wedge is resected from the distal fragment to match the posteromedial tongue with the lesser trochanter projecting from the proximal fragment. Both fragments can now be brought into direct opposition.

The seating chisel is now removed from the proximal fragment, and the osteotomy plate is carefully inserted into the prepared bone by hand to prevent the sharp blade from deviating from the prepared channel in the cancellous bone (Fig. 2.**252**). After final impaction of the blade, the shaft of the osteotomy plate is fixed with a screw.

The shortened distal and proximal fragments are now opposed. The posteromedial bony tongue of the proximal fragment with the lesser trochanter and the shaft of the osteotomy plate fit snugly against the prepared distal fragment. The marker wires should now be perpendicular, indicating proper rotational alignment. Finally, the shaft of the osteotomy plate is held against the distal fragment with a forceps. The surgeon compresses the fragments with an articulated plate tensioner that engages the distal screw hole of the plate. The compression presses the distal fragment against the proximal one (Fig. 2.**253**). The shaft of the plate is fastened to the distal fragment with screws, and the articulated plate tensioner is removed.

The vastus lateralis is reattached to the proximal stump of its origin with vertical mattress sutures (see Fig. 2.**208**). Restoring the soft-tissue envelope formed by the vastus lateralis and gluteus medius is crucial for the muscular stability of the hip and knee. Soft-tissue coverage of internal fixation assures early healing of osteotomy sites. The fascia lata is closed with retention sutures over a suction drain (see Fig. 2.**163**). Fascial tension is also important for the stability of the hip. The wound is closed in layers.

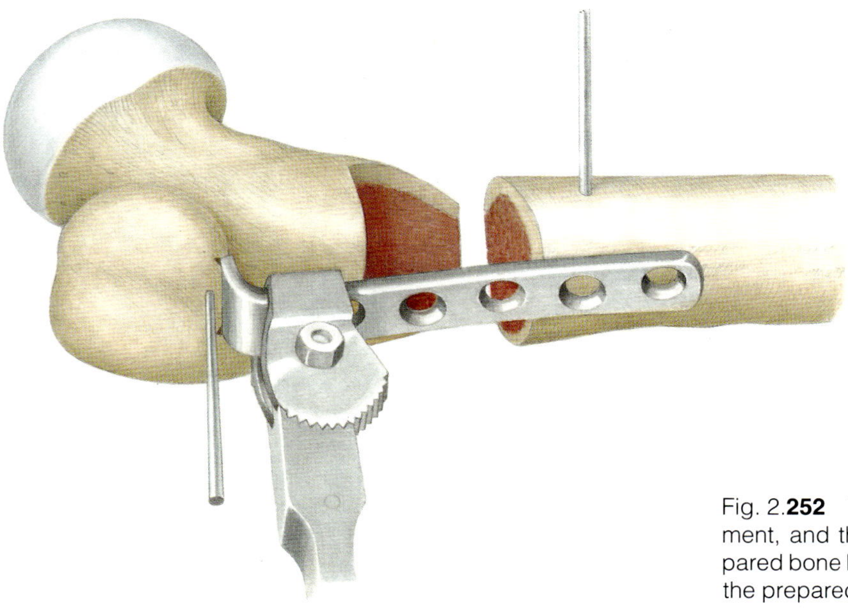

Fig. 2.**252** The seating chisel is removed from the proximal fragment, and the osteotomy plate is carefully inserted into the prepared bone by hand to prevent the sharp blade from deviating from the prepared channel in the cancellous bone.

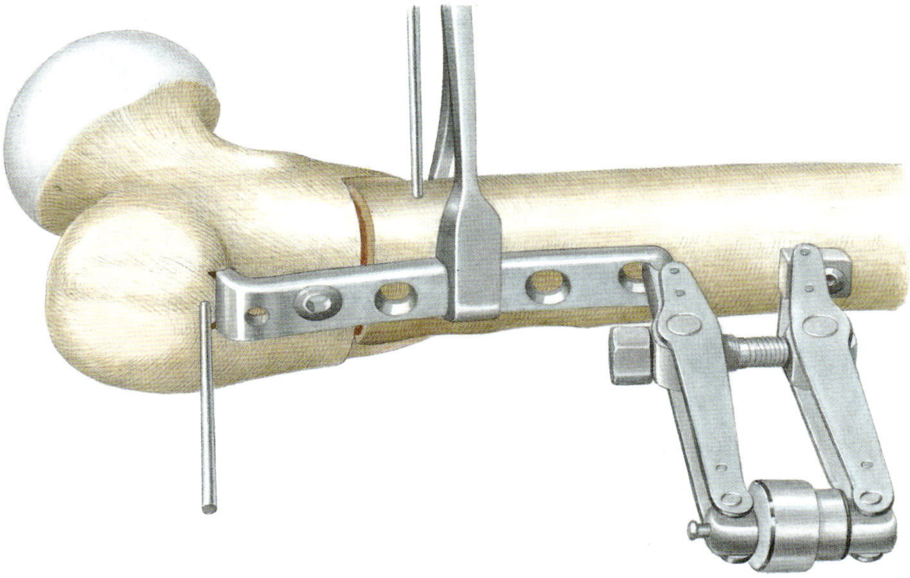

Fig. 2.**253** The shortened distal and proximal fragments are opposed. The posteromedial bony tongue of the proximal fragment with the lesser trochanter and the shaft of the osteotomy plate fit snugly against the prepared distal fragment. The marker wires should now be perpendicular, indicating proper rotational alignment. Interfragmentary compression is achieved with an articulated plate tensioner.

Intertrochanteric Osteotomy for Treatment of a Slipped Capital Femoral Epiphysis

Indications

An intertrochanteric osteotomy can be used restore function to a joint in which the capital femoral epiphysis has slipped between 20° and 45° . A slip of less than 20° does not generally require correction; a slip exceeding 45° cannot be satisfactorily treated with an intertrochanteric osteotomy, and is an indication for a subcapital osteotomy.

Positioning and Incision

Wih the patient positioned supine, a longitudinal skin incision is made which courses distally from the apex of the greater trochanter on the lateral side of the hip.

Technique

In a slipped capital femoral epiphysis, the epiphysis generally migrates medially and posteriorly on the femoral neck (Fig. 2.**254**). This produces articular incongruity in which the articular surface of the femoral head migrates inferiorly and posteriorly and the anterosuperior shelf of the femoral neck

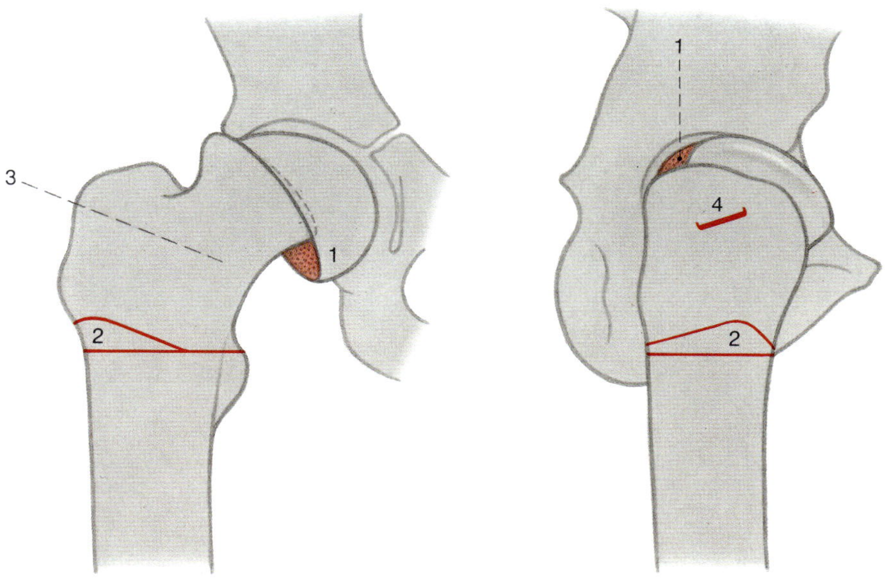

Fig. 2.**254** In a slipped capital femoral epiphysis, the epiphysis generally slips medially and posteriorly with respect to the femoral neck. An intertrochanteric osteotomy in which an anterolateral wedge is removed can correct the deformity.

1 Slipped capital epiphysis
2 Anterolateral wedge
3 Direction of the blade of the plate in the coronal plane
4 Direction of the blade channel in the lateral view.

presses against the margin of the acetabulum. The leg moves into compensatory external rotation when the hip is flexed. An intertrochanteric wedge osteotomy can restore the articular surface of the femoral head to a normal position in the acetabulum. The base of the wedge must be perpendicular to the direction of subluxation. An isolated inferior slip is corrected with a valgus osteotomy with removal of a lateral wedge; an isolated posterior slip is corrected with a flexion osteotomy with removal of an anterior wedge.

To treat the typical inferior and posterior slip, these two corrections must be combined; the base of the wedge must lie anterolaterally (Fig. 2.**254**). The angle of the wedge and the position of the base of the wedge are precisely measured in preoperative planning. The simplest method is to take a radiograph with the leg in adduction and external rotation so that the capital epiphysis is brought into its reduced position in the acetabulum. The degree of adduction determines the angle of the wedge for the intertrochanteric osteotomy, and the degree of external rotation determines the angle of the position of the base of the wedge. For example, if the femoral head is in an ideal position at 35° adduction and 25° external rotation, the angle of the wedge will be 35° and the center of the base of the wedge will be internally rotated 25° with respect to the axis of the knee joint.

The intertrochanteric osteotomy must be planned so that the resected wedge only includes about two-thirds of the cross section of the bone. This creates a large area of interfragmentary contact without sacrificing excessive leg length. Realigning the proximal fragment opens a medial gap extending across one-third of the bone cross section, but this is well tolerated. A wedge resection extending across the entire section of the bone would maximize contact at the osteotomy site, but it would also maximize leg length reduction.

The distal osteotomy surface must be perpendicular to the shaft of the femur so that after the alignment of the femoral neck is corrected, rotational malalignment can be eliminated without changing the position of the proximal fragment. Finally, the distal fragment must be shifted anteriorly to prevent axial deformation of the femur (Fig. 2.**255**). This is necessary for centering the shaft of the condylar plate on the distal fragment and preventing a deformity that could complicate future total joint arthroplasty.

A longitudinal skin incision is made that courses distally from the apex of the greater trochanter on the lateral side of the hip (see Fig. 2.**256**). The fascia lata is split and retracted, revealing the vastus lateralis. The anterior margin of the gluteus medius is conservatively detached from its insertion on the greater trochanter to provide access to the anterior surface of the hip and the joint capsule (see Fig. 2.**27**). The pericapsular fat is retracted from the anterior surface of the joint capsule with a sharp periosteal elevator, exposing the entire anterior capsule (see Fig. 2.**28**).

The reflected origin of the rectus femoris is now visible in the deep layer. Elevators are inserted on the superior and inferior sides of the femoral neck, providing broad exposure of the joint capsule (see Fig. 2.**29**). With the leg in external rotation, the surgeon performs a capsulotomy and an anterior capsulectomy. The surgeon dissects the reflected origin of the rectus femoris and lifts the muscle with its reflected origin using a short, sharp-tipped elevator impacted in the pubis. The iliopsoas tendon is now visible in the deep layer beneath the medial femoral neck (Fig. 2.**256**).

An intertrochanteric osteotomy for treatment of a slipped capital femoral epiphysis almost invariably includes an osteotomy that allows flexion of the distal fragment and extension of the proximal fragment. This invariably necessitates resection of the iliofemoral ligament to prevent a flexion contracture of the hip. The capsulectomy broadly exposes the hip joint and allows a reliable evaluation of the deformity and the correction. The acetabular labrum is visible at the margin of the acetabulum. The femoral neck lies immediately lateral to it. The anterior surface of the femoral neck is

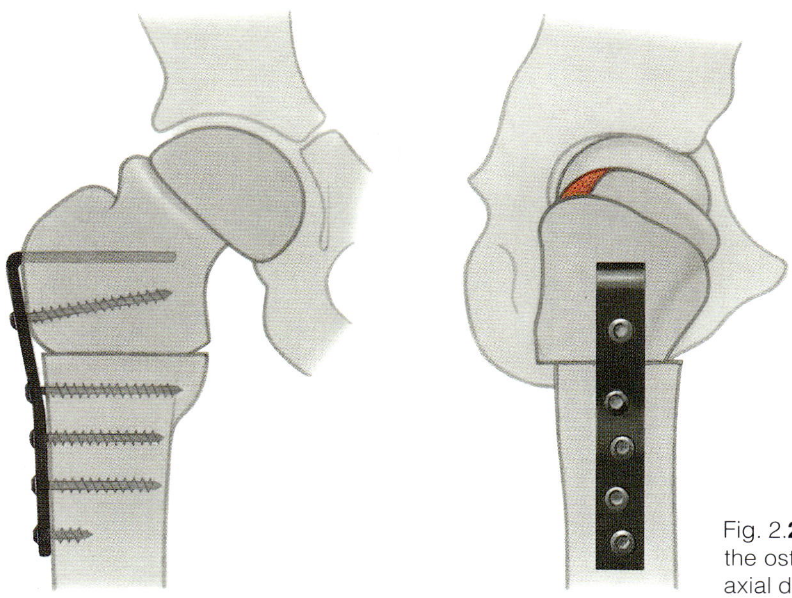

Fig. 2.**255** Position of the fragments and the internal fixation after the osteotomy. The distal fragment is shifted anteriorly to prevent axial deformation of the femur.

covered with white periosteum; immediately medial to it is the dislocation site. This surface is covered with thin translucent scar tissue and presses against the acetabular labrum. The femoral head has shifted posteriorly and inferiorly on the femoral neck and is covered by the labrum. When the leg is placed in extreme external rotation, the anterosuperior margin of the femoral neck moves away from the slippage area and the anterior margin of the slipped femoral head comes into view.

With the leg in extreme internal rotation, the vastus lateralis is dissected with an L-shaped incision immediately distal to the most proximal aspect of the greater trochanter (see Fig. 2.**191**). The surgeon dissects the muscle from the lateral intermuscular septum and the femur with a scalpel and periosteal elevator (see Fig. 2.**192**) and retracts it anteriorly with elevators to expose the femur. The leg is adducted and externally rotated to bring the femoral head into the desired position in the acetabulum, and the position is verified with fluoroscopy. A marker wire is inserted into the greater trochanter and the femoral neck horizontally (i.e., parallel to the floor) and perpendicular to the median plane (see Fig. 2.**213**). The marker wire should be inserted a few millimeters proximal to the planned slot for the blade of the condylar plate to serve as a landmark. The surgeon exposes the anterior and posterior femoral cortex at the osteotomy site, raising "fish scales" with a mallet and periosteal elevator. Anterior and posterior elevators are then inserted to protect the soft tissue. The tendinous origin of the vastus lateralis is dissected from the bone distal to the marker wire to expose the insertion site of the blade of the condylar plate (see Fig. 2.**215**). To accommodate the blade, the surgeon drills a row of holes about 10 mm deep with a spiral drill bit immediately distal to the marker wire and parallel to it (Fig. 2.**257**). The planned rotation of the channel and the flexion component of the intertrochanteric osteotomy determine the alignment of the holes.

The holes are joined and widened to accommodate the blade by driving a 15-mm chisel into the surface of the bone and moving it back and forth. This prevents the relatively dull

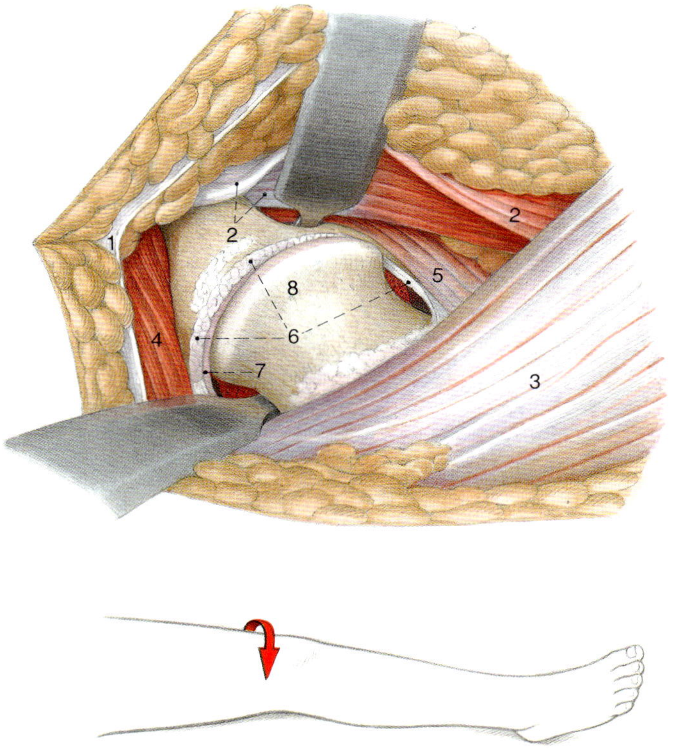

Fig. 2.**256** With the leg in external rotation, an anterior capsulectomy is performed. The reflected origin of the rectus femoris is dissected, and the musle with its reflected origin is retracted with a short, sharp-tipped elevator impacted in the pubis. The iliopsoas tendon is now visible in the deep layer beneath the medial femoral neck.

1 Fascia lata
2 Rectus femoris
3 Vastus lateralis
4 Gluteus medius
5 Iliopsoas
6 Hip joint capsule
7 Acetabular labrum
8 Anterior margin of the femoral metaphysis

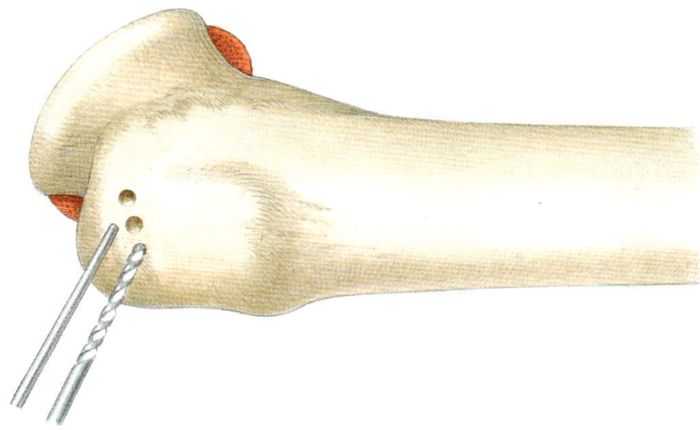

Fig. 2.**257** To accommodate the blade of the condylar plate, a row of holes about 10 mm deep is drilled with a spiral drill bit immediately distal to the marker wire and parallel to it. The rotation of the channel (i.e., the flexion component of the intertrochanteric osteotomy) determines the alignment of the holes.

seating chisel from fracturing the proximal femoral cortex (Fig. 2.**258**). The seating chisel is driven into the slot. The seating chisel is the same width as the blade of the condylar plate and cuts a channel for the blade through the cancellous bone. The seating chisel is impacted parallel to the marker wire. Rotation of the chisel is controlled by a slotted hammer that is shaped like a tuning fork. Chisel rotation determines the final axial alignment of the condylar plate that will follow the axis of the femur after the flexion correction has been made (Fig. 2.**259**). After the bone has been prepared, the slotted hammer is partially withdrawn so that the surgeon can replace it with the blade of the condylar plate without having to apply excessive force to the short proximal fragment.

The surgeon now measures distance from the seating chisel to the osteotomies on the femoral cortex and marks the sites with an osteotome (Fig. 2.**260**). The distal osteotomy plane is perpendicular to the shaft of the femur. The proximal osteotomy plane parallels the plane of the seating chisel and ends where it intersects the distal osteotomy plane. By stopping short of the medial cortex, the proximal osteotomy creates a wedge that only extends across part of the cross section of the bone, thus sacrificing less bone stock.

A marker wire for fluoroscopy is inserted proximal to the osteotomy sites. Distal to the osteotomy sites, an additional marker wire is inserted into the femur in the sagittal plane to gauge rotation. This wire is perpendicular to the marker wire for the blade channel (Fig. 2.**261**). The osteotomies are performed parallel to the two marker wires at the marked sites.

The surgeon grips the distal fragment and shifts it anteriorly with a forceps while using the seating chisel to rotate the proximal fragment into valgus extension. (Like the respec-

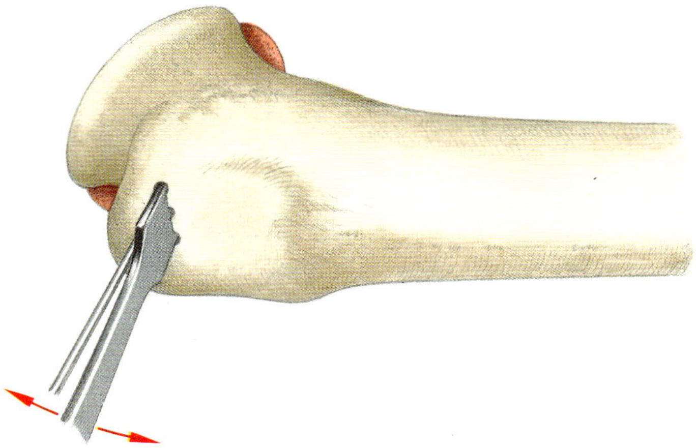

Fig. 2.**258** The holes are joined and widened to accommodate the blade by driving a 15-mm chisel into the surface of the bone and moving it back and forth. This prevents the relatively dull seating chisel from fracturing the proximal femoral cortex.

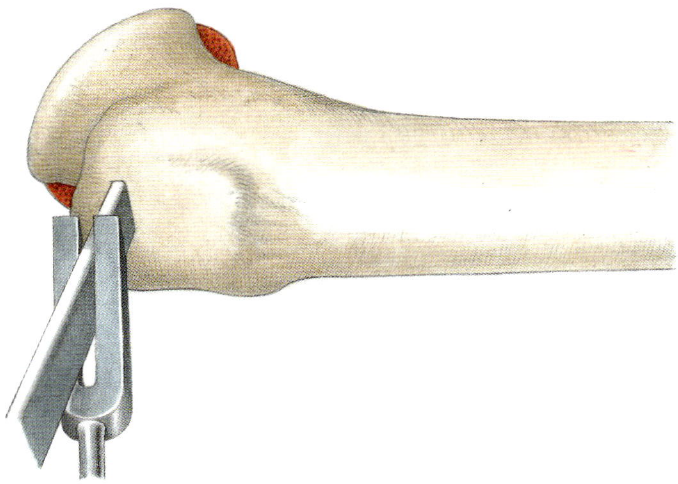

Fig. 2.**259** The seating chisel is driven into the slot. It is the same width as the blade of the condylar plate and cuts a channel for the blade though the cancellous bone.

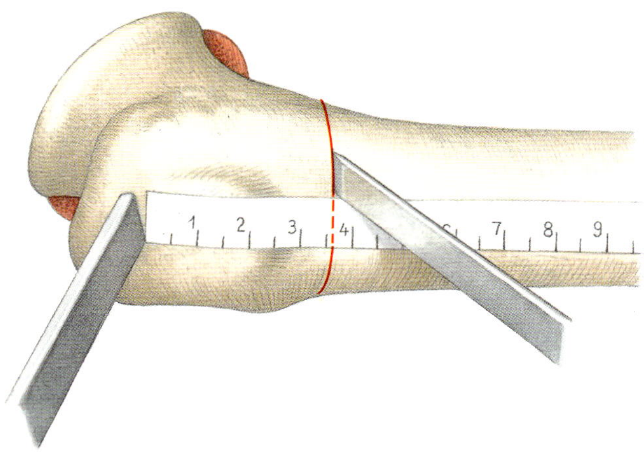

Fig. 2.**260** The distance from the seating chisel to the osteotomies is measured on the femoral cortex, and the sites are marked with an osteotome. The distal osteotomy plane is perpendicular to the shaft of the femur. The proximal osteotomy plane parallels the plane of the seating chisel.

tive fractures, the directions of correction in the osteotomies of the proximal femur are defined according to the direction of correction of the distal fragment. Thus, a flexion osteotomy corrects the distal fragment in the direction of flexion, and the proximal fragment is placed in extension, and vice versa.) The correction opposes the osteotomy surfaces of the two fragments (Fig. 2.**262**).

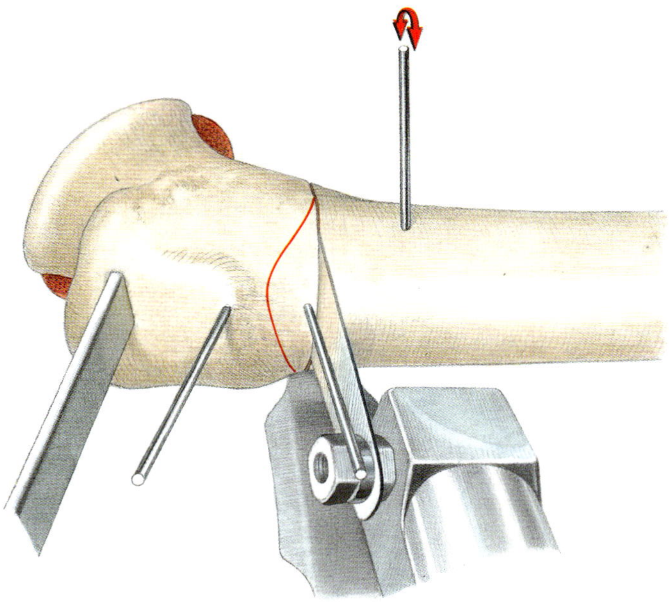

Fig. 2.**261** A marker wire for fluoroscopy is inserted proximal to the osteotomy sites. Distal to the osteotomy sites, an additional marker wire is inserted into the femur in the sagittal plane to gauge rotation. This wire is perpendicular to the marker wire for the blade channel in the transverse plane.

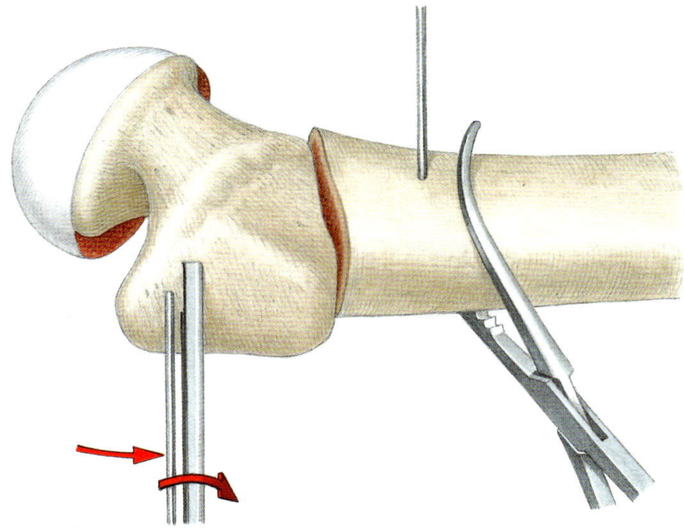

Fig. 2.**262** After the osteotomies are performed, the distal fragment is gripped and shifted anteriorly with a forceps while the seating chisel is used to rotate the proximal fragment into valgus extension. The correction opposes the osteotomy surfaces of the two fragments.

After the seating chisel and slotted hammer are removed from the proximal fragment, the condylar plate is inserted into the prepared bone with the inserter-extractor parallel to the marker wire and driven in with a mallet (Fig. 2.**263**). The surgeon inserts the blade 2–3 cm by hand, using a mallet only if resistance is encountered. This prevents the blade (which is relatively sharp) from deviating from the prepared channel in the cancellous bone. With the fragments in the corrected position, the shaft of the condylar plate is held against the distal fragment with a clamp. The angle between the marker wire in the proximal fragment and the marke wire in the distal fragment indicates the degree of rotation. The rotation must now be evaluated. If maximum internal rotation is less than 10°, then the further internal rotation of the distal fragment is indicated. The osteotomy perpendicular to the axis of the femur allows the surgeon to easily make this correction without changing the alignment of the proximal fragment. The correction is verified with fluoroscopy.

Interfragmentary compression is achieved with an articulated plate tensioner (Fig. 2.**264**). After the plate shaft has been fastened to the distal fragment, the two fragments shuold be opposed at the medial edge of the proximal osteotomy, whereas there should be about a 2 mm gap at its lateral edge, which gradually closes as interfragmentary compression is applied (Fig. 2.**265**). This provides the medial buttress opposite the condylar plate that is crucial for bony healing. The shaft of the condylar plate is then fastened to the distal fragment with screws, the articulated plate tensioner and the marker wires are removed, and the remaining screws are inserted into the shaft of the plate.

The vastus lateralis is returned to its original position, covering the femur and the osteotomy site. The muscle is reattached where it was transected (distal to the proximal aspect of the greater trochanter) with vertical mattress sutures (see Fig. 2.**208**). A subfascial suction drain is placed and the anterior margin of the gluteus medius is reattached (see Fig. 2.**31**). The fascia lata is closed with retention sutures (see Fig. 2.**163**). Restoring the original fascial tension is important for the stability of the hip.

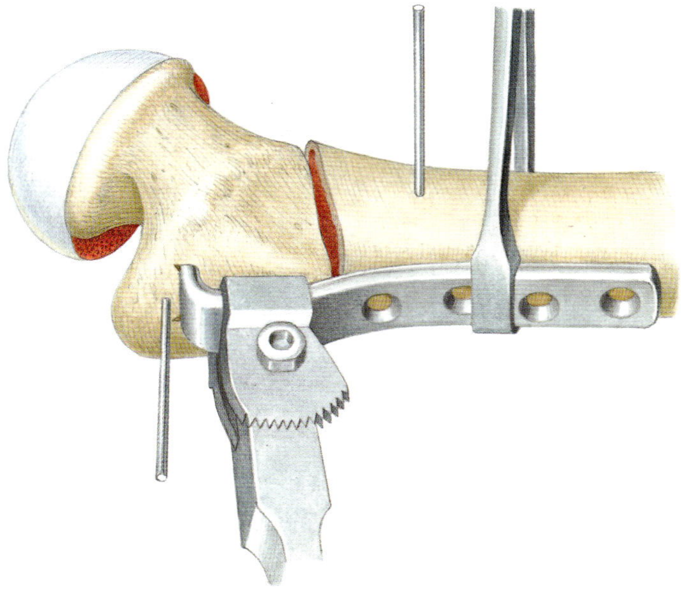

Fig. 2.**263** The seating chisel is replaced with a condylar plate. The shaft of the plate is pressed against the distal fragment with a forceps.

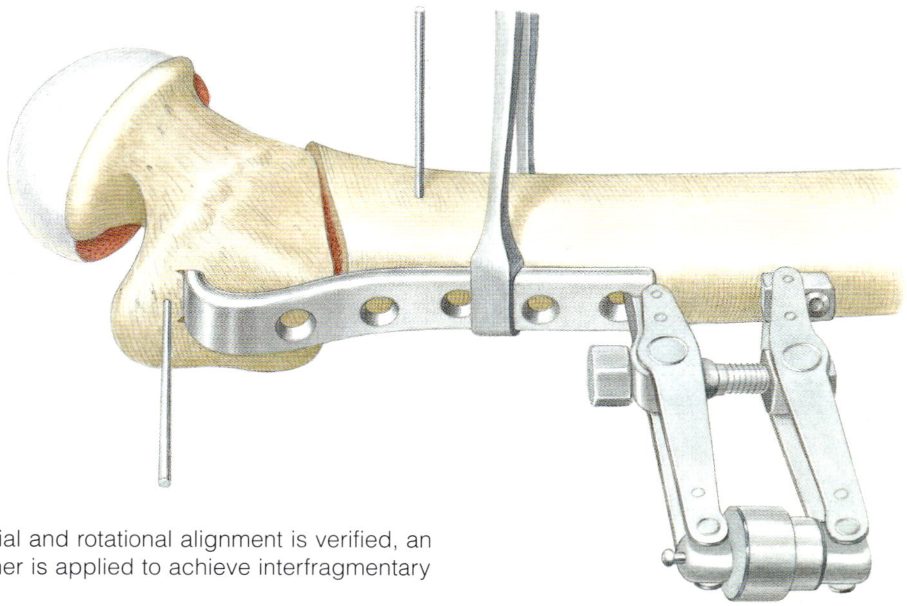

Fig. 2.**264** After the axial and rotational alignment is verified, an articulated plate tensioner is applied to achieve interfragmentary compression.

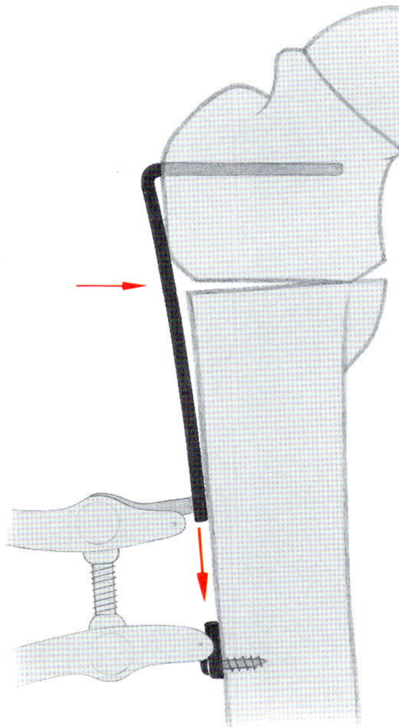

Fig. 2.**265a** After the fragments have been prepared and the condylar plate applied, the medial edges of the fragments are in contact and there is about a 2-mm gap between their lateral edges.

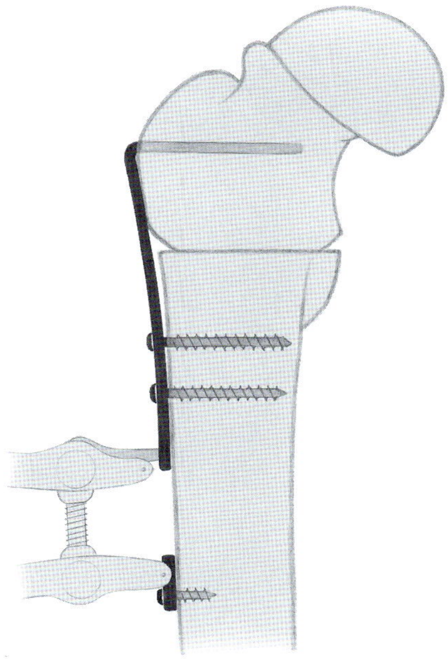

Fig. 2.**265b** The lateral gap gradually closes as interfragmentary compression is applied. This provides the medial support of the fragments that is crucial for stable internal fixation.

Intertrochanteric Osteotomy for Treatment of Femoral Neck Nonunions

Indications

The intertrochanteric valgus osteotomy is primarily indicated in young patients for surgical correction of a steeply inclines nonunion of the femoral neck where the femoral head remains vascularized. In children, pseudarthrosis of the femoral neck is rare, but an osteotomy may be indicated even when the femoral head is avascular because remaining cartilage reserves offer better prospects of regeneration. Total hip arthroplasty is the treatment of choice in older patients.

Occasionally, a fresh femoral neck fracture may require osteotomy if medial comminution jeopardizes the support of the fragments required for stable internal fixation.

According to Pauwels, rapid bony consolidation will occur after a valgus osteotomy is performed to bring a steeply inclined nonunion (Pauwels III) into a more horizontal position. The force vectors are now perpendicular to the plane of the nonunion; what were previously shear forces acting along the plane of the nonunion now become compressive forces which, together with internal fixation, act to stabilize the nonunion.

Positioning and Incision

With the patient supine, a longitudinal skin incision is made that courses distally from the anterior margin of the greater trochanter on the lateral side of the hip and permits exposure of the anterior capsule if required.

Surgical Technique

Preoperative planning is essential to ensure correct alignment of the nonunion plane. The position of the osteotomy plate and the alignment of the osteotomy planes must be determined so that the planned correction can be easily achieved.

The surgical approach is identical to the one used in an intertrochanteric varus osteotomy. After the proximal femur is exposed, a marker wire is inserted into the femoral neck to indicate the direction of the blade of the osteotomy plate. The position of the wire is verified with fluoroscopy. Distal to this wire, the surgeon prepares the blade channel by drilling holes, which are then joined and widened with a chisel (see varus osteotomy). The seating chisel is then inserted parallel to the marker wire. Using fluoroscopy, the surgeon inserts two marker wires to indicate the site of the intertrochanteric osteotomy to remove the lateral wedge. These two marker wires are also used to gauge rotation. The two osteotomies are performed between the two wires and parallel to them, and the wedge between the osteotomy planes is removed. The implant of choice for stabilizing the osteotomy is a 120° osteotomy plate (Fig. 2.**266**).

The seating chisel is replaced with a 120° osteotomy plate. The tip of the blade should lie immediately beneath the center of the femoral head. The liens of force on the femoral head and neck intersect in the center of the femoral head. In response to these forces, the trabeculae of cancellous bone are thicker here than elsewhere. The condensation of the trabeculae provide particularly strong support for implants. The remaining bony bridge to the medial femoral cortex is also now resected.

The femoral neck is aligned in an upright position, and the shaft of the osteotomy plate is pressed against the distal fragment. This can result in a lateral shift in the proximal fragment across the diagonal distal osteotomy surface, which is useful for interfragmentary compression. Since the angle of the blade of the 120° osteotomy plate is too steep to compress the fragments in the manner of a condylar plate, interfragmentary compression is achieved by shifting the fragments laterally (Fig. 2.**267**). When the proper lateral shift has been achieved, a screw is inserted into the most inferior hole in the shaft and tightened. Then the screws in the proximal part of the shaft are fastened. This displaces the proximal fragment medially and presses it against the osteotomy surface, providing very effective interfragmentary compression. After the osteotomy plate has been fastened, the marker wire is removed from the proximal fragment. If required, it can be replaced with a partially threaded screw. The screw provides additional compression to further stabilize the nonunion. However, the threads should not penetrate the superior layers of the femoral head. This avoids damaging the vascular

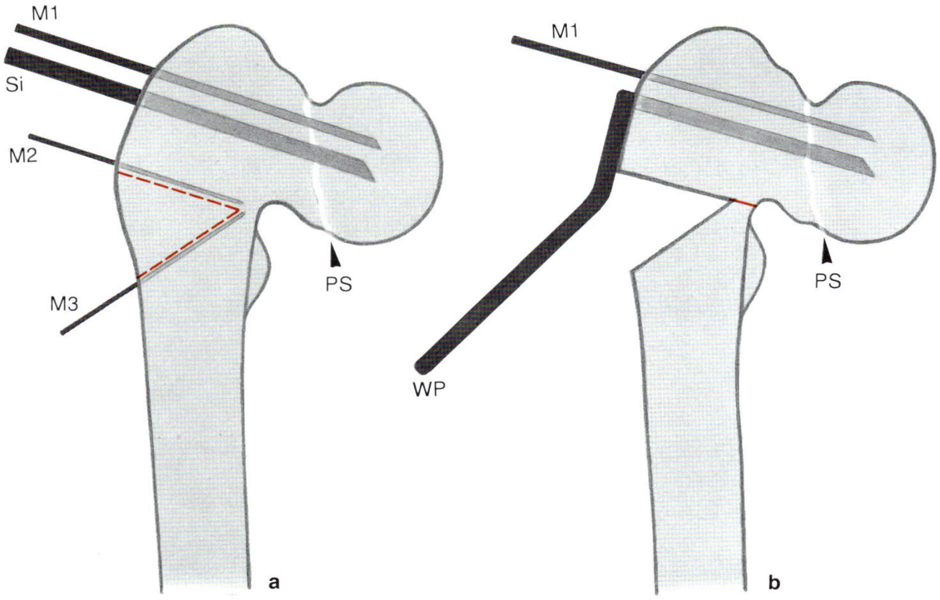

Fig. 2.**266a** and **b** Intertrochanteric valgus corrective osteotomy.

a A marker wire (M1) is insertead into the femoral neck to indicate the direction of the blade. The blade channel is prepared distal to this wire and parallel to it, and the seating chisel is impacted. The tip of the seating chisel (Si) lies distal to the center of the femoral head and bridges the pseudarthrosis (PS). Two marker wires (M2, M3) are inserted to indicate the wedge to be resected.

b The seating chisel is replaced with a 120° osteotomy plate (WP).

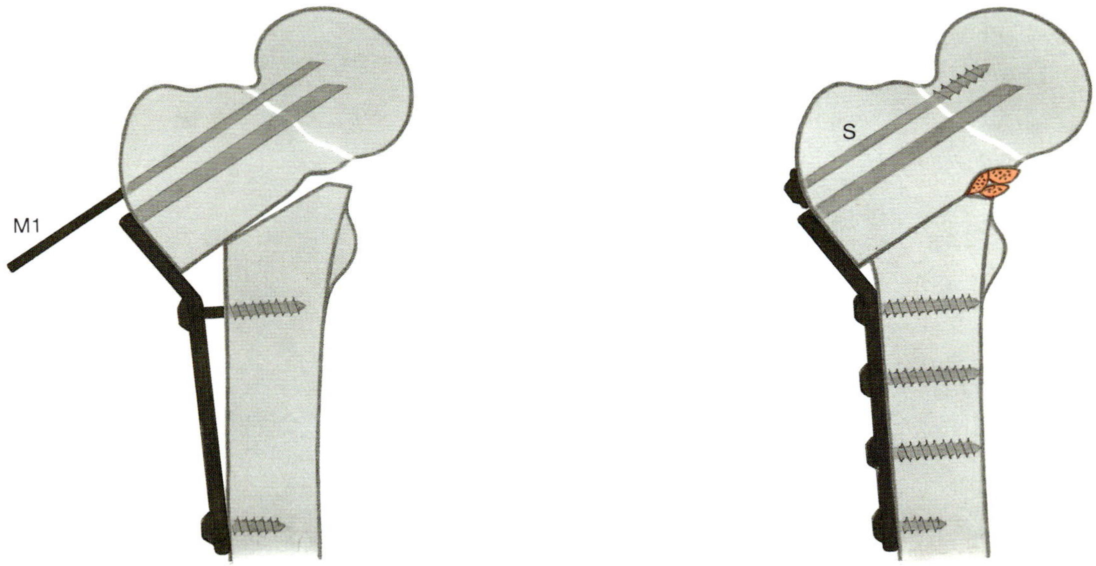

Fig. 2.**267a** The proximal fragment is aligned in a slightly overcorrected upright position and shifted laterally about 6 mm. The distal end of the plate shaft is now in contact with the distal fragment and is fastened with a screw. Then a screw is inserted into the proximal shaft of the plate, which draws the distal fragment toward the plate.

Fig. 2.**267b** Shifting the proximal fragment medially reduces the valgus overcorrection and provides interfragmentary compression at the osteotomy site. Now the remaining screws are inserted into the plate. Marker wire 1 is replaced with a screw (S). Autologous cancellous graft taken from the resected wedge is inserted into the medial side of the osteotomy.

supply to this vital area. A washer should be used to prevent sinking the head of the screw into the soft cortical bone of the greater trochanter. Autologous cancellous graft taken from the resected wedge is inserted into the medial side of the osteotomy to accelerate bony consolidation. Finally, the vastus lateralis is reattached to the greater tochanter and securely sutured to the tendon of the gluteus medius. The fascia lata is closed with retention sutures. Restoring this soft-tissue envelope accommodates the tensile forces acting on the lateral hip, reduces the bending stress on the proximal femur, and stabilizes the osteotomy.

Intertrochanteric Double Osteotomy with and without Extension of the Femoral Neck

Indications

- Severe deformation of the proximal femur, primarily distinguished by shortening of the femoral neck and a superiorly protruding greater trochanter.
- Additional associated deformities such as anteversion, retroversion, varus deformity, or valgus deformity of the femoral neck are also corrected with the intertrochanteric double osteotomy.
- Finally, the femoral neck can be rotated around its longitudinal axis to improve joint congruity. Lengthening the femoral neck in this procedure will necessarily result in an increase in leg length.

An intertrochanteric double osteotomy should not be used solely for leg lengthening if correction of the proximal femur is not indicated. Leg length can be increased with less complicated procedures.

Positioning and Incision

With the patient supine, a straight longitudinal skin incision is made on the lateral side of the hip.

Surgical Technique

The intertrochanteric double osteotomy combines trochanteric advancement with an intertrochanteric osteotomy. The osteotomies produce three fragments that can be corrected independently of each other (Fig. 2.**268**). The distal fragment is shifted laterally and the intermediate fragment is rotated into valgus, thereby lengthening the femoral neck. If the valgus correction were not made, the femur shaft would only be shifted laterally without an increase in leg length. The surgeon can also correct anteversion or retroversion at the site of the intertrochanteric osteotomy, and a flexion or extension correction can be made by rotating the femoral neck around its longitudinal axis. Finally, the greater trochanter is brought into the corrected position and secured on the lateral side of the osteotomy. The gaps and crevices created by the osteotomy are filled with graft.

In preoperative planning, the anatomy of the contralateral proximal femur is used as a template for the correction unless

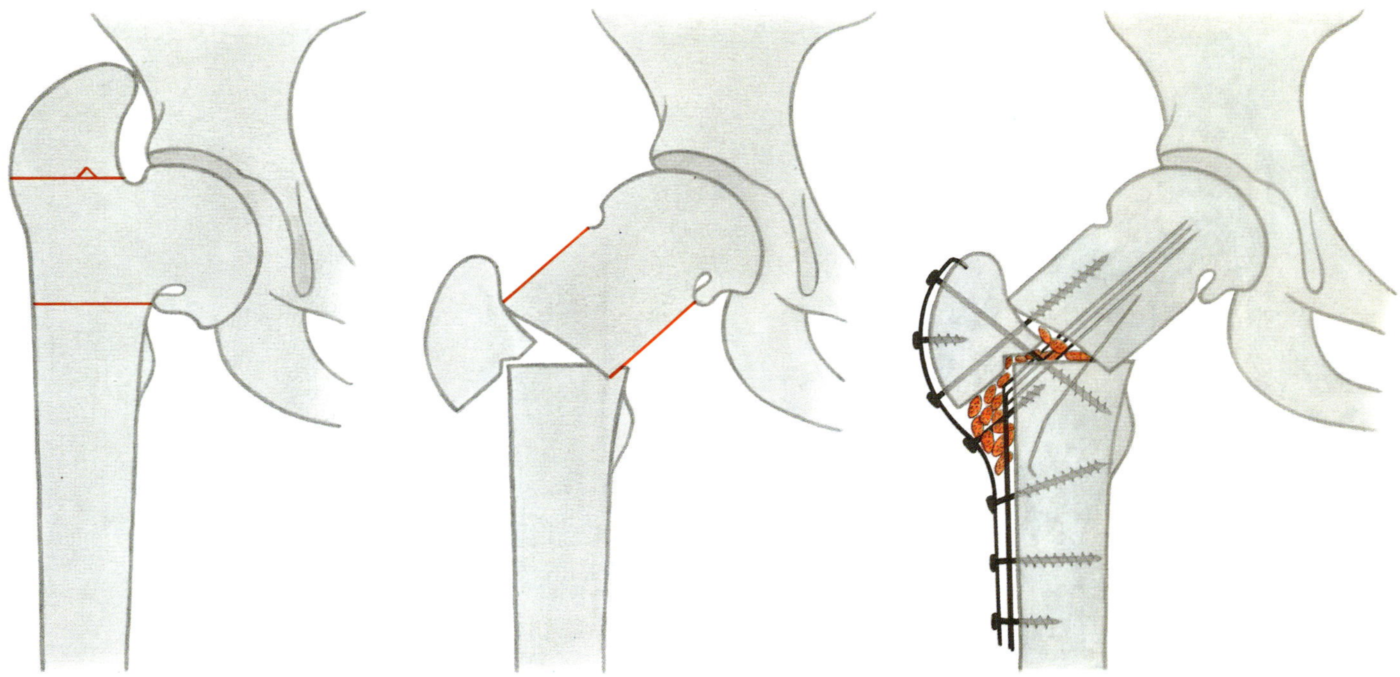

Fig. 2.**268** Principle of the intertrochanteric double osteotomy. A trochanteric advancement is combined with an intertrochanteric osteotomy to produce three fragments that can be corrected independently of each other. The intermediate fragment is rotated into valgus, lengthening the femoral neck.

there is a marked deformity here, too. The rule of thumb is that the greater trochanter should be level with the center of rotation of the femoral head, and the distance between the two should be equal to the diameter of the femoral head.

Despite the fact that the intertrochanteric double osteotomy involves extensive corrections with three independent fragments, secure internal fixation can be achieved if the fragments are stabilized at their contact surfaces and medial support is provided. Three Kirschner wires bridge the osteotomy to stabilize the proximal and distal fragments, and tension banding using a semitubular plate bent to fit the surface of the bone is applied over the greater trochanter. The pathoanatomy does not generally permit the safe use of large implants. When closing the wound, the surgeon must reattach the vastus lateralis to the greater trochanter under tension and close the fascia lata with a retention suture. These two tensile structures are crucial to the stability of the proximal femur.

After a longitudinal skin incision has been made on the lateral side of the hip, the fascia lata is split parallel to the direction of its fibers and retracted. An L-shaped incision is then made in the vastus lateralis immediately distal to the most proximal aspect of the greater trochanter. The muscle is dissected from the lateral intermuscular septum and the femur is exposed. Elevators are inserted to lift the muscle. A thick marker wire is inserted into the apex of the greater trochanter (Fig. 2.**269**). Using this wire as a reference point, the surgeon measures the distances to the osteotomies on the femoral cortex and marks the sites with an osteotome.

At the most proximal aspect of the greater trochanter, the origin of the vastus lateralis and a thin flake of bone are raised like a fish scale to facilitate reattaching the muscle during closure (Fig. 2.**270**). The dissected origin of the vastus lateralis is lifted with a narrow elevator. Fine Kirschner wires are inserted at the marked osteotomy sites to provide fluoroscopic landmarks. Three 2.5-mm Kirschner wires are inserted into the femoral neck. These are used to move the fragment into position after the osteotomy and later in internal fixation (Fig. 2.**271**). At this stage, the surgeon must decide whether the femoral neck should be rotated around its longitudinal axis to achieve a flexion or extension correction. In a simple varus or valgus correction, the Kirschner wires are arranged in a line perpendicular to the shaft of the femur. If a flexion correction is planned, the line is inclined superiorly; if an extension correction is planned, it is inclined inferiorly. In either case, the line of Kirschner wires will be perpendicular to the distal fragment after the correction (see intertrochanteric flexion and extension osteotomy with plate fixation).

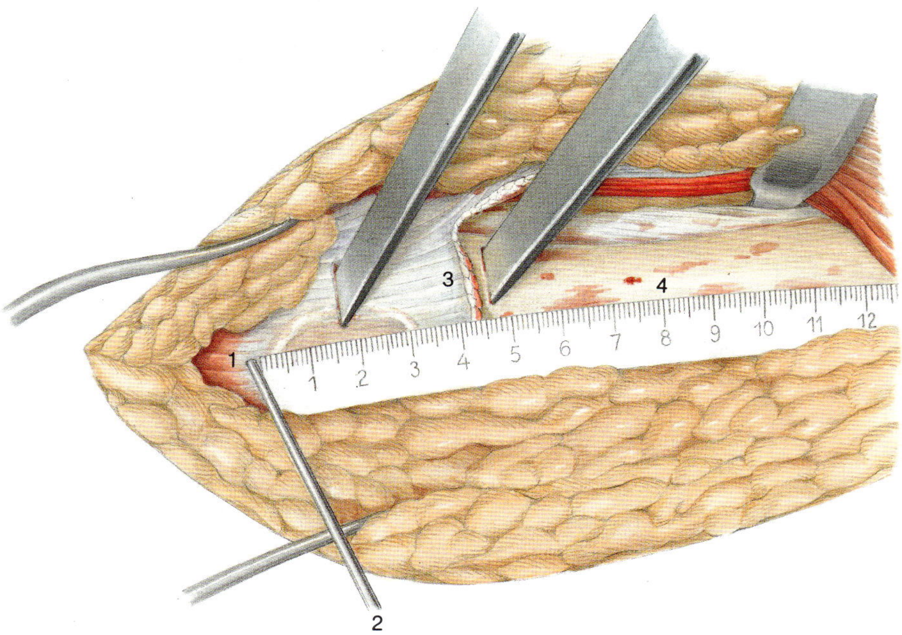

Fig. 2.**269** Intertrochanteric double osteotomy performed on the right hip. After the fascia lata is split parallel to its fibers and retracted and the vastus lateralis is dissected, a marker wire is inserted into the apex of the greater trochanter. This wire is used as a reference point for measuring the distances to the osteotomy sites on the femoral cortex, which are then marked with an osteotome.

1 Gluteus medius
2 Marker wire in the apex of the greater trochanter
3 Vastus lateralis
4 Femur

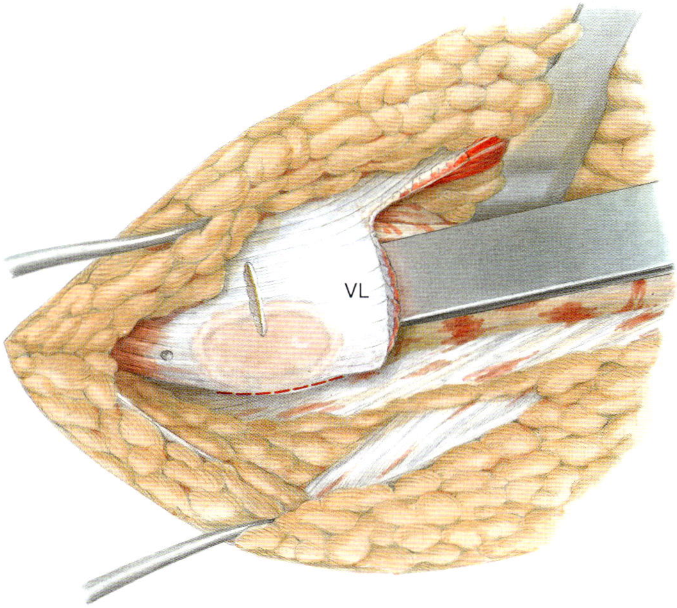

Fig. 2.**270** The origin of the vastus lateralis (VL) and a thin bone flake are raised like a fish scale to facilitate reattaching the muscle during closure.

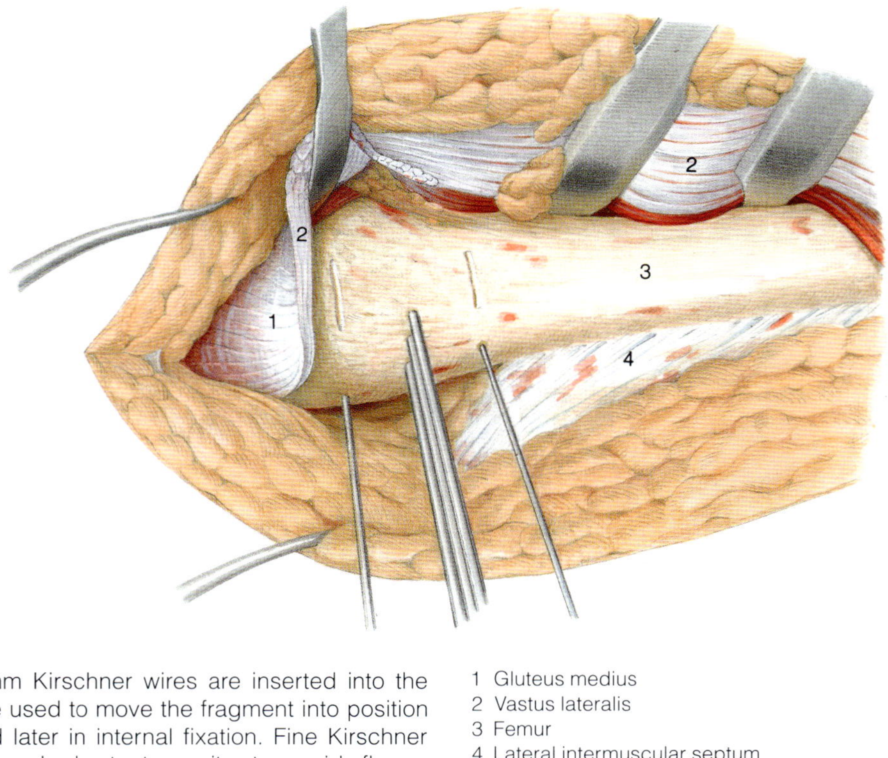

Fig. 2.**271** Three 2.5-mm Kirschner wires are inserted into the femoral neck. These are used to move the fragment into position after the osteotomy and later in internal fixation. Fine Kirschner wires are inserted at the marked osteotomy sites to provide fluoroscopic landmarks.

1 Gluteus medius
2 Vastus lateralis
3 Femur
4 Lateral intermuscular septum

The position of the wires is verified with fluoroscopy (Fig. 2.**272**). The surgeon exposes the cortex at the osteotomy sites with a mallet and periosteal elevator and inserts elevators to protect the surrounding soft tissue (Fig. 2.**273**).

First the osteotomy of the greater trochanter is performed parallel to the proximal marker wire with an oscillating saw. The osteotomy stops short of the medial cortex to avoid damaging the vascular supply to the trochanteric fossa (Fig. 2.**274**). The surgeon then inserts a wide chisel into the gap created by the osteotomy and lifts it superiorly to spread the osteotomy and break through the medial cortex. The chisel is used as a lever to mobilize the greater trochanter, separating it from its medial soft-tissue attachments and displacing it superiorly.

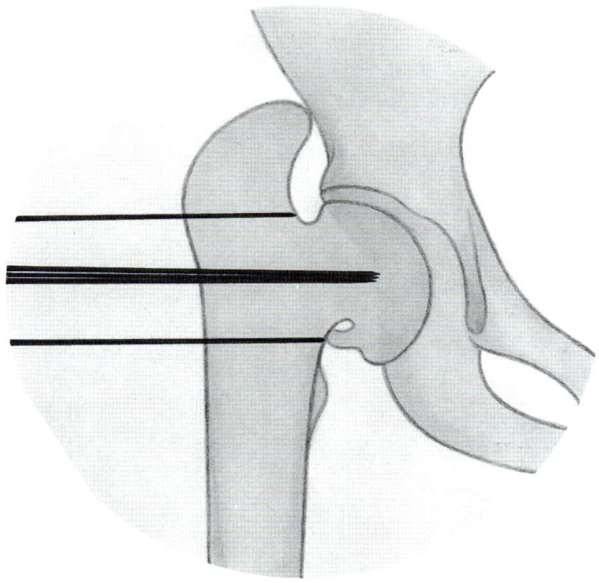

Fig. 2.**272** The positions of the Kirschner wires are verified with fluoroscopy.

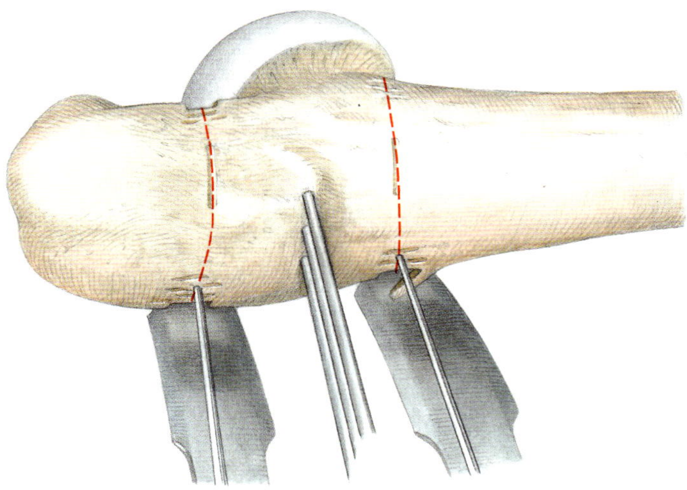

Fig. 2.**273** The cortex at the osteotomy sites is exposed with a mallet and periosteal elevator, and elevators are inserted to protect the surrounding soft tissue.

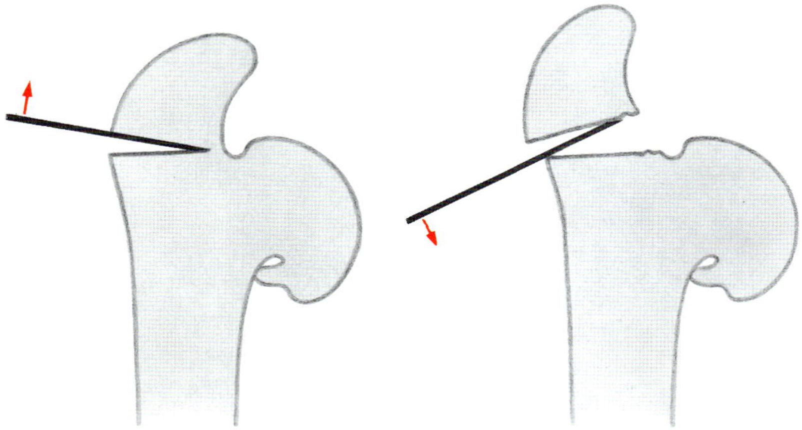

Fig. 2.**274** The osteotomy of the greater trochanter stops short of the medial cortex to avoid damaging the vascular supply to the trochanteric fossa. A wide chisel inserted into the gap created by the osteotomy is used as a lever to spread the osteotomy and break through the medial cortex. The chisel is used as a lever to mobilize the greater trochanter, separating it from its medial soft-tissue attachments and displacing it superiorly.

The greater trochanter is then retracted superiorly and laterally with a fine-toothed forceps. If hardened adhesions are present, a bone spreader can be inserted in the gap created by the osteotomy to help mobilize the greater trochanter. The scarred adhesions between the greater trochanter and the joint capsule (which is generally thickened) should be removed carefully so that the greater trochanter can be shifted to its corrected position without having to be forced. The scarred adhesions on the medial surface of the greater trochanter are released with curved dissection scissors. The scissors should be pointed superiorly and laterally to avoid damaging the trochanteric fossa (Fig. 2.**275**). These scarred adhesions are released until the surgeon feels only the elastic resistance of the pelvic and trochanteric muscles when pulling the greater trochanter and it can be easily shifted into the corrected position.

Now the intertrochanteric osteotomy is performed perpendicular to the shaft of the femur parallel to the distal marker wire. The gap created by the intertrochanteric osteotomy can be spread by using the three Kirschner wires to rotate the intermediate fragment into varus. The surgeon opens the gap created by the osteotomy with a bone spreader and releases the medial soft-tissue adhesions with dissecting scissors (Fig. 2.**276**). Since a shortened femoral neck is always accompanied by fibrotic tissue in the vicinity of the lesser trochanter and joint capsule, this stage of the procedure requires extreme caution.

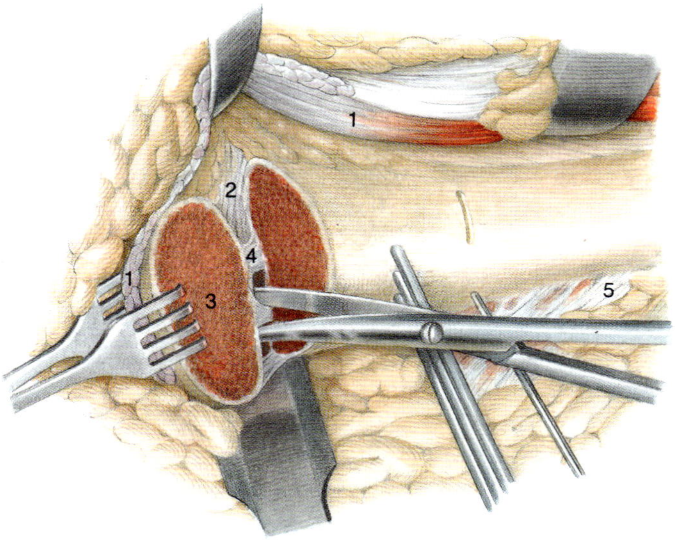

Fig. 2.**275** The greater trochanter is then retracted superiorly and laterally with a forceps. The scarred adhesions between the greater trochanter and the joint capsule (which is generally thickened) should be removed carefully so that the greater trochanter can be shifted to its corrected position without having to be forced. The curved dissection scissors should be pointed superiorly and laterally to avoid damaging the trochanteric fossa. These scarred adhesions are released until the surgeon feels only the elastic resistance of the pelvic and trochanteric muscles when pulling the greater trochanter.

1 Vastus lateralis
2 Hip joint capsule
3 Greater trochanter
4 Scarred adhesions
5 Lateral intermuscular septum

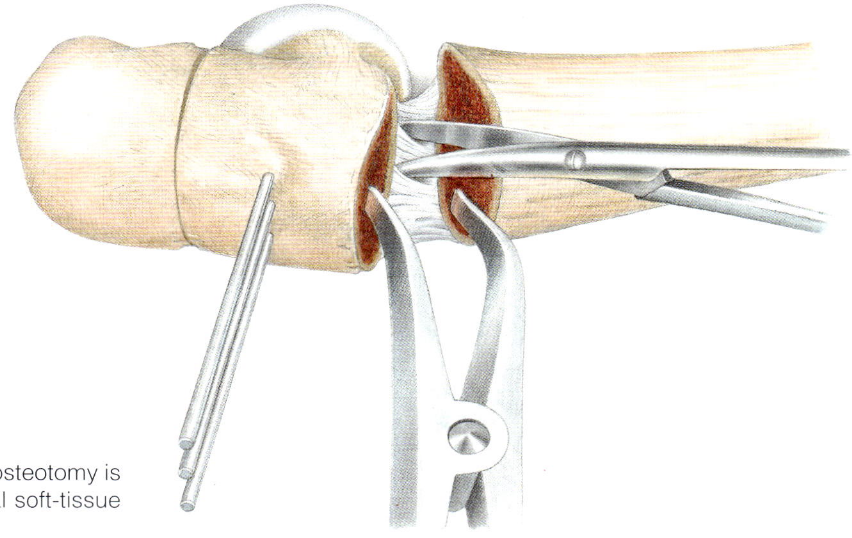

Fig. 2.**276** The gap created by the intertrochanteric osteotomy is opened with a bone spreader and the scarred medial soft-tissue adhesions are released with dissecting scissors.

The distal fragment also has adhesions, particularly on its medial and posterior aspects, which interfere with the lateral shift and the leg length correction. On rare occasions, the tension of the iliopsoas tendon requires resecting the lesser trochanter and reattaching it on the distal and medial edge of the intermediate fragment. Generally, the tension of the iliopsoas tendon is due to a fibrotic tendon sheath, and careful resection of this sheath will greatly relieve tension. The soft-tissue adhesions are dissected off the medial and posterior aspects of the distal fragment until the fragment is sufficiently mobilized (Fig. 2.**277** and 2.**278**). The three Kirschner wires are used to rotate the intermediate fragment of the femoral neck into an ideal valgus position while the distal fragment is pulled laterally with a reduction forceps until the lateral edge of the intermediate fragment and the medial edge of the distal fragment are close together (Fig. 2.**279**). Now the surgeon corrects the anteversion of the femoral neck and the rotation of the knee joint.

Solid contact between the intermediate and the distal fragments on the medial side of the osteotomy is necessary to ensure a stable construct. To provide this construct, the two fragments are fixed by a 1.8-mm diagonal Kirschner wire, which is inserted into a hole drilled in the cortex of the distal fragment and passes through this contact point (Fig. 2.**280**). If the bone is osteopenic, two diagonal wires may be required. The diagonal Kirschner wire is first bent superiorly close to the surface of the bone with a bending iron and then rotated distally with a forceps until it lies flat on the surface of the bone. If the wire does not lie completely flat, it can be rotated back and bent a bit more. To secure the wire, the surgeon can bend the free end into a hook and press it into a shallow hole drilled in the cortex (Fig. 2.**281**).

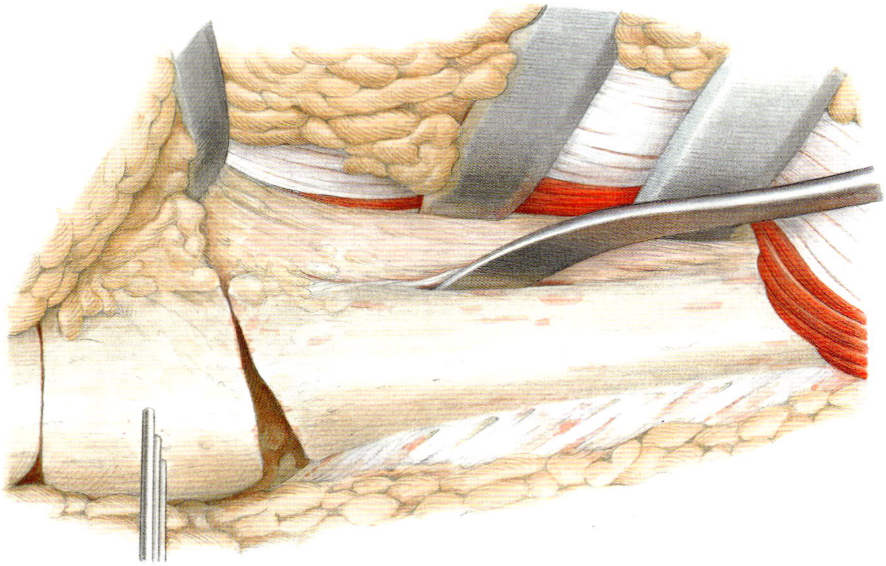

Fig. 2.**277** The soft tissue is dissected from the medial femur with a periosteal elevator.

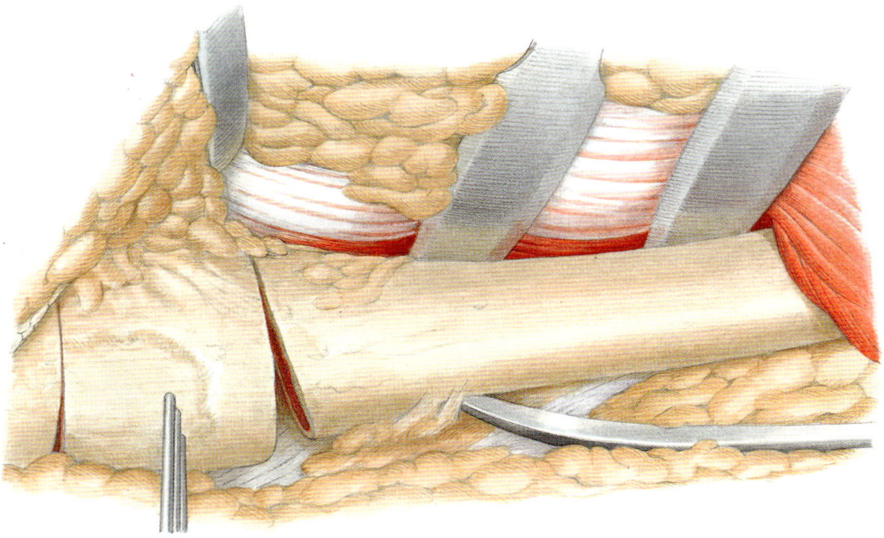

Fig. 2.**278** Elevators are inserted along the medial surface of the femur to lift the vastus lateralis. The soft-tissue adhesions, including the lateral intermuscular septum, are dissected off the posterior surface of the distal fragment until the fragment is sufficiently mobilized.

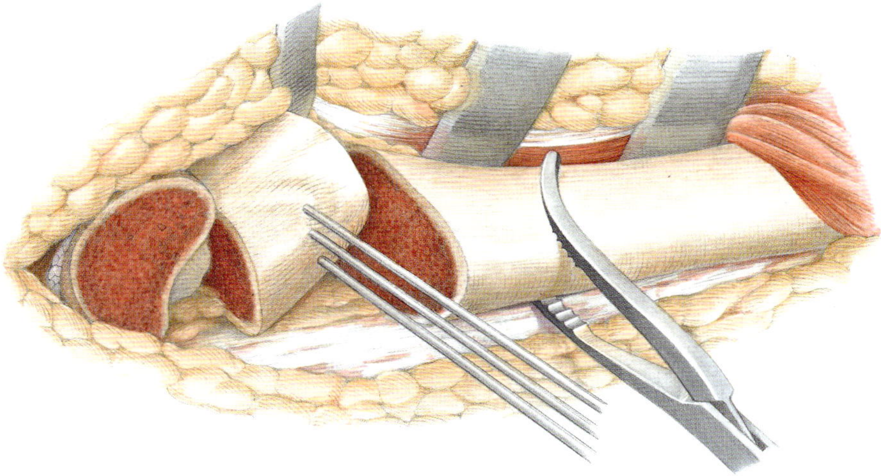

Fig. 2.**279** The distal fragment is pulled laterally with a reduction forceps until the lateral edge of the intermediate fragment and the medial edge of the distal fragment close together. If a valgus correction of the intermediate fragment is required, the three Kirschner wires are used to rotate the intermediate fragment of the femoral neck into the desired position.

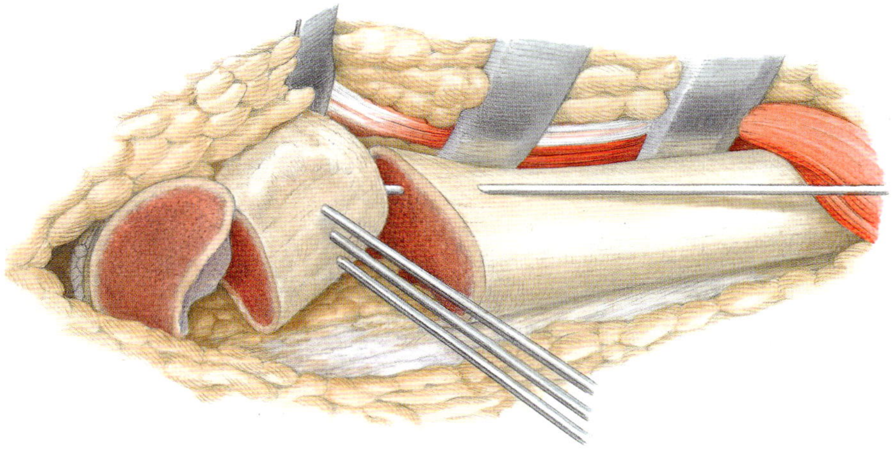

Fig. 2.**280** Solid contact between the intermediate and the distal fragments on the medial side of the osteotomy is necessary to ensure the medial support of the fragments required for stable internal fixation. To provide this support, the two fragments are fixed by a diagonal Kirschner wire that passes through this contact point.

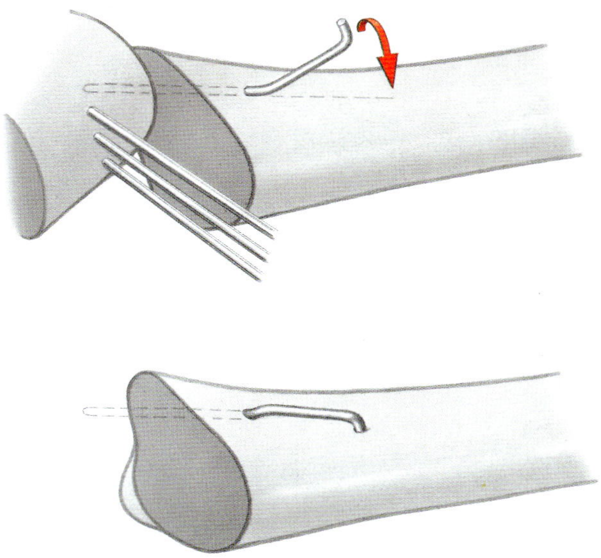

Fig. 2.**281** The free end of the diagonal Kirschner wire is bent superiorly close to the surface of the bone with a bending iron and then rotated distally with a forceps until it lies flat on the surface of the bone. The free end of the wire can be bent into a hook and pressed into a shallow hole drilled in the cortex.

One after the other, the thick Kirschner wires in the femoral neck are bent distally with a bending iron until they are at an angle of 25° to the surface of the distal fragment. For the internal fixation to be stable, there must be enough distance between the wires and the surface of the distal fragment to create sufficient tension when the wires are pressed to the surface of the bone. The Kirschner wires are then pressed against the distal fragment with a holding forceps (Fig. 2.**282**). Finally, the greater trochanter is brought into the corrected position and fixed with a Kirschner wire (Fig. 2.**283**).

The surgeon now fits a hook-shaped semitubular plate over the Kirschner wire projecting from the greater trochanter, placing its distal end over the three Kirschner wires (Fig. 2.**284**). This fabricated implant consists of a semitubular plate in which the most proximal screw hole has been modified to form a sharpened bifurcate hook that can be impacted into the origin of the gluteus medius. The plate is not initially in contact with the bone at the center of the osteotomy; only later is it brought into contact when the remaining screws are inserted to achieve interfragmentary compression. The surgeon verifies the position of the fragments and implants with fluoroscopy before completing internal fixation (Fig. 2.**285**).

Now the hooked plate is successively fastened to the three fragments. First a cancellous screw is inserted into the most proximal screw hole. This tightens the plate against the greater trochanter and presses the greater trochanter against the intermediate femoral neck fragment (Fig. 2.**284**). When the screws are inserted into the distal fragment, the Kirschner wires are pressed together with a forceps so that the semitubular plate covers them and fastens them in place. The Kirschner wire is now removed from the greater trochanter. The screws in the distal fragment press the plate agains the surface of the bone and compress the fragments. The biggest advantage of this type of internal fixation over using an osteotomy plate is that it can be specifically adapted to conditions at the osteotomy site. It also avoids the risk of fracturing the fragments, which is always present when the wide blade of an osteotomy plate is inserted into small bone segments. After completing internal fixation, the surgeon fills the gaps between the three fragments with graft (Fig. 2.**286**).

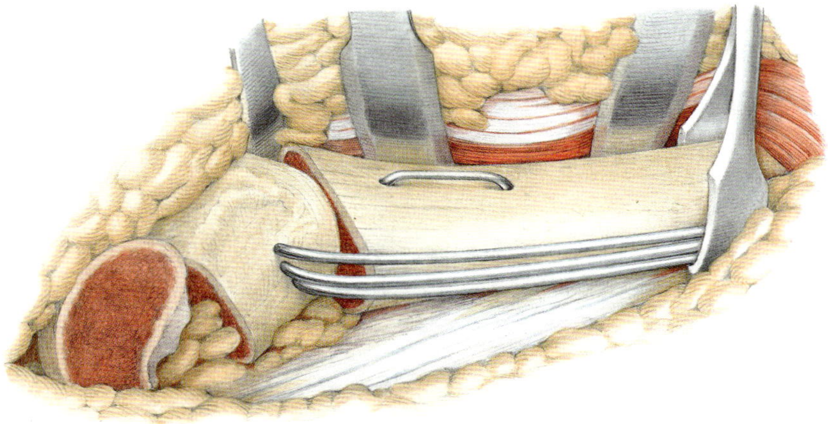

Fig. 2.**282** The three wires in the femoral neck are bent distally until they are at an angle of 25° to the surface of the distal fragment. The wires are then pressed against the distal fragment with a holding forceps.

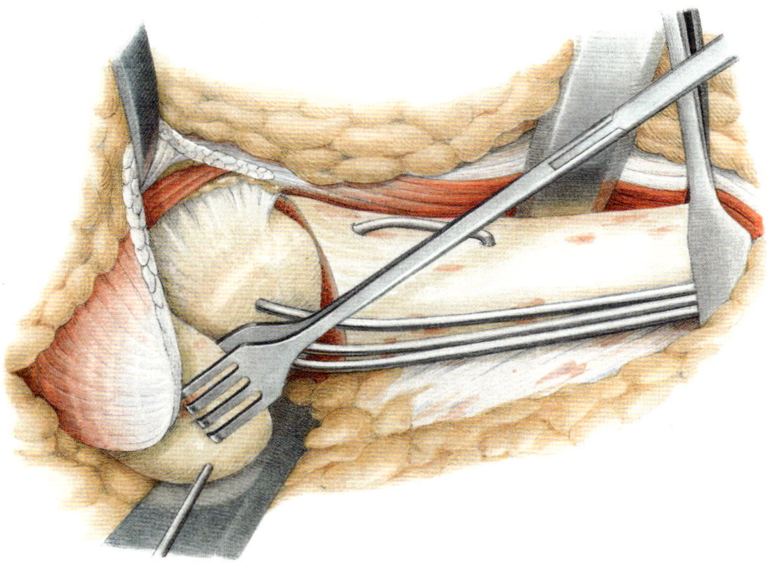

Fig. 2.**283** The greater trochanter is brought into the corrected position on the lateral edge of the intermediate fragment and fixed with a Kirschner wire.

Fig. 2.**284** A implant fabricated from a semitubular plate is fit over the Kirschner wire projecting from the greater trochanter. The hooked proximal end is impacted into the greater trochanter and fastened with a cancellous screw, which is inserted through the most proximal screw hole and engages the greater trochanter and femoral neck. The distal end of the plate covers the three Kirschner wires and is fastened to the bone with screws. As the screws are being inserted, the Kirschner wires are pressed together with a forceps so that they remain under the semitubular plate.

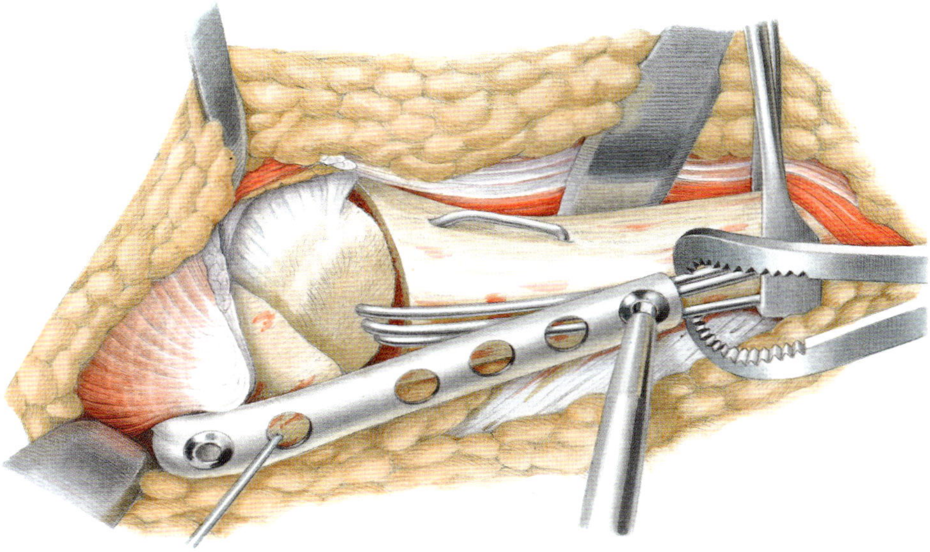

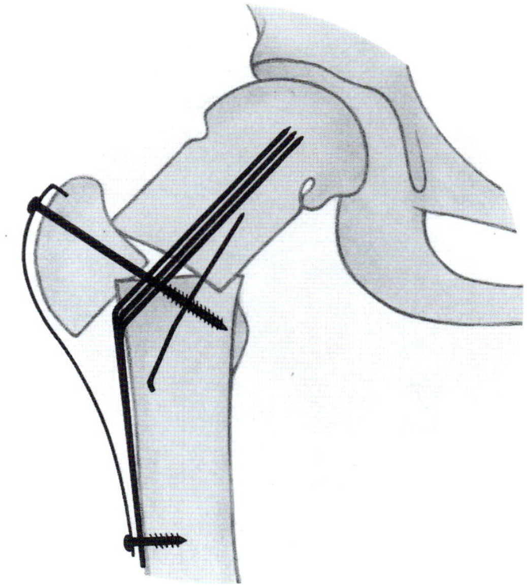

Fig. 2.**285** Before all the screws are inserted, the position of the fragments and implants is verified with fluoroscopy to permit making any necessary changes. The plate is not initially in contact with the bone at the center of the osteotomy; this occurs only when the remaining screws are inserted to achieve interfragmentary compression.

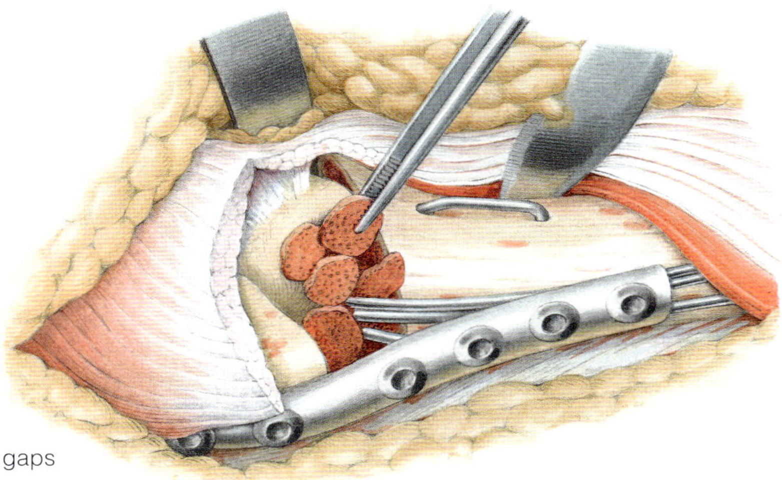

Fig. 2.**286** After internal fixation has been completed, the gaps between the three fragments are filled with graft.

The origin of the vastus lateralis with the attached bone flake is folded back onto the greater trochanter, where it partially covers the internal fixation implants. The vastus lateralis is reattached with vertical mattress sutures (Fig. 2.**287**). The fascia lata is closed with retention sutures over a suction drain (see Fig. 2.**32**). Proper tension of the vastus lateralis and fascia lata is important for the stability of the internal fixation. Although the increase in leg length generally increases the tension in these soft-tissue structures, the surgeon should give careful consideration to this aspect when suturing the soft tissue.

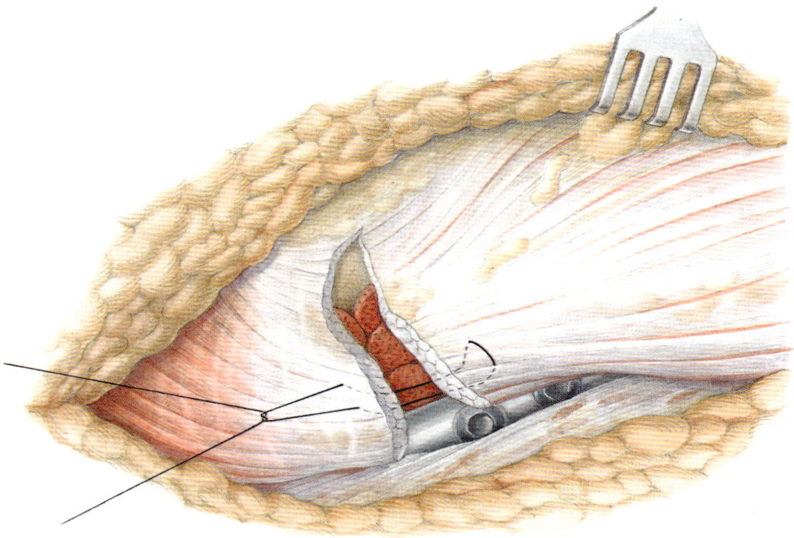

Fig. 2.**287** The origin of the vastus lateralis is reattached under tension with vertical mattress sutures.

Stabilizing a Slipped Capital Femoral Epiphysis with Kirschner Wire or Screw Fixation

Indication

History of loosening of the epiphysis on the femoral neck or slipped capital femoral epiphysis.

Clinical Considerations

With a slipped capital femoral epiphysis, there is a high risk that the epiphysis of the "healthy" contralateral hip will also slip. To prevent this, the contralateral capital femoral epiphysis is stabilized with internal fixation.

Positioning and Incision

With the patient supine, a straight longitudinal skin incision is made on the lateral side of the hip.

Surgical Technique

In young patients in whom significant axial growth is still expected, the epiphysis is stabilized with Kirschner wires. This prevents slippage and minimizes the risk of physeal arrest. In the course of further growth, the epiphysis may grow past the ends of the Kirschner wires so that it is no longer stabilized. If this occurs, the Kirschner wires should be replaced with longer ones.

In patients nearing the end of growth, significant further axial growth of the femoral neck is not to be expected. In these patients, the epiphysis can be stabilized with screw fixation, which soon leads to bony epiphysiodesis. The screws are inserted in the same manner as the Kirschner wires.

A relatively short longitudinal skin incision is made on the lateral side of the hip (Fig. 2.**288**). After the fascia lata is split parallel to the direction of its fibers and retracted, the surgeon inserts three Kirschner wires into the femoral neck through incisions in the vastus lateralis distal to the most proximal aspect of the greater trochanter. The positions of the wires are verified with fluoroscopy, and they are advanced as far as the femoral head (Fig. 2.**289**). The Kirschner wires extend through the femoral neck, fanning out evenly over the cross section of the femoral head in both the transverse and coronal planes. Fluoroscopy should be used to monitor the direction of the Kirschner wires when they are inserted (Fig. 2.**290 a** and **b**). Wires inserted from the middle of the lateral surface of the femur can only engage the anterior part of the femoral head.

In a slipped capital femoral epiphysis, the epiphysis generally migrates medially and posteriorly. The Kirschner wires or screws on the greater trochanter must be inserted in such a manner that they extend diagonally through the femoral neck and are aligned perpendicular to the femoral head. Generally, the best point of insertion will lie on the anterior aspect of the greater trochanter (Fig. 2.**291 a** and **b**). Implants inserted from the middle of the lateral surface of the femur will only engage the femoral head anteriorly.

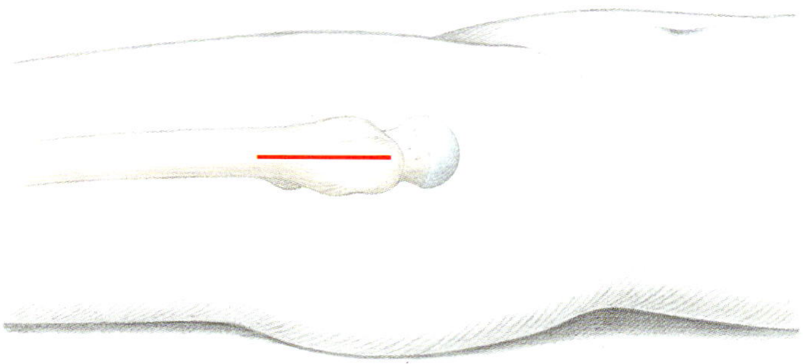

Fig. 2.**288** Stabilization of a slipped capital femoral epiphysis in the left hip. The short longitudinal skin incision on the lateral side of the hip courses distally from the apex of the greater trochanter.

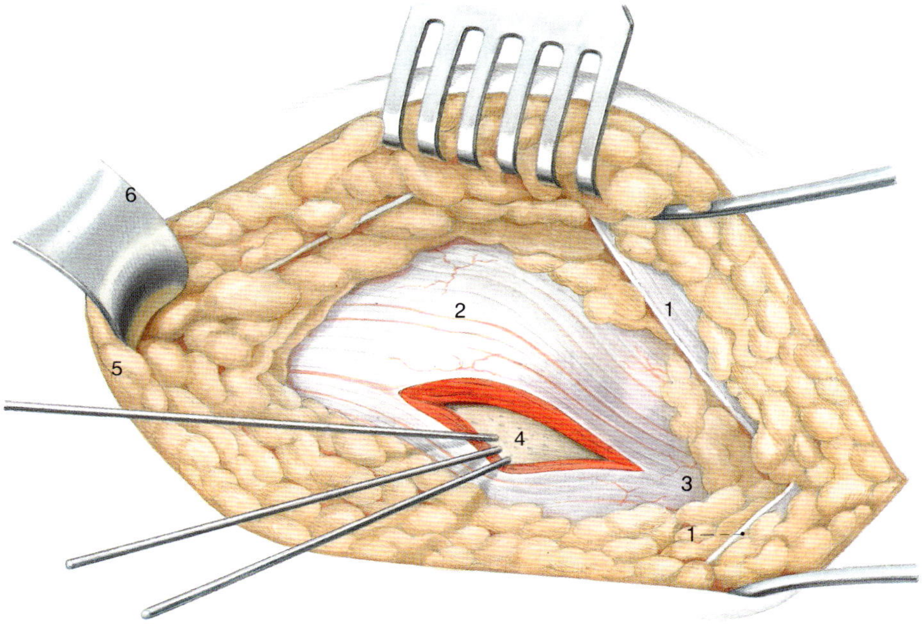

Fig. 2.**289** After the fascia lata is split parallel to the direction of its fibers and retracted, three Kirschner wires are inserted into the femoral neck through incisions in the vastus lateralis distal to the most proximal aspect of the greater trochanter. The positions of the wires are verified with fluoroscopy, and they are advanced as far as the femoral head.

1 Fascia lata
2 Vastus lateralis
3 Most proximal aspect of the greater trochanter
4 Femur

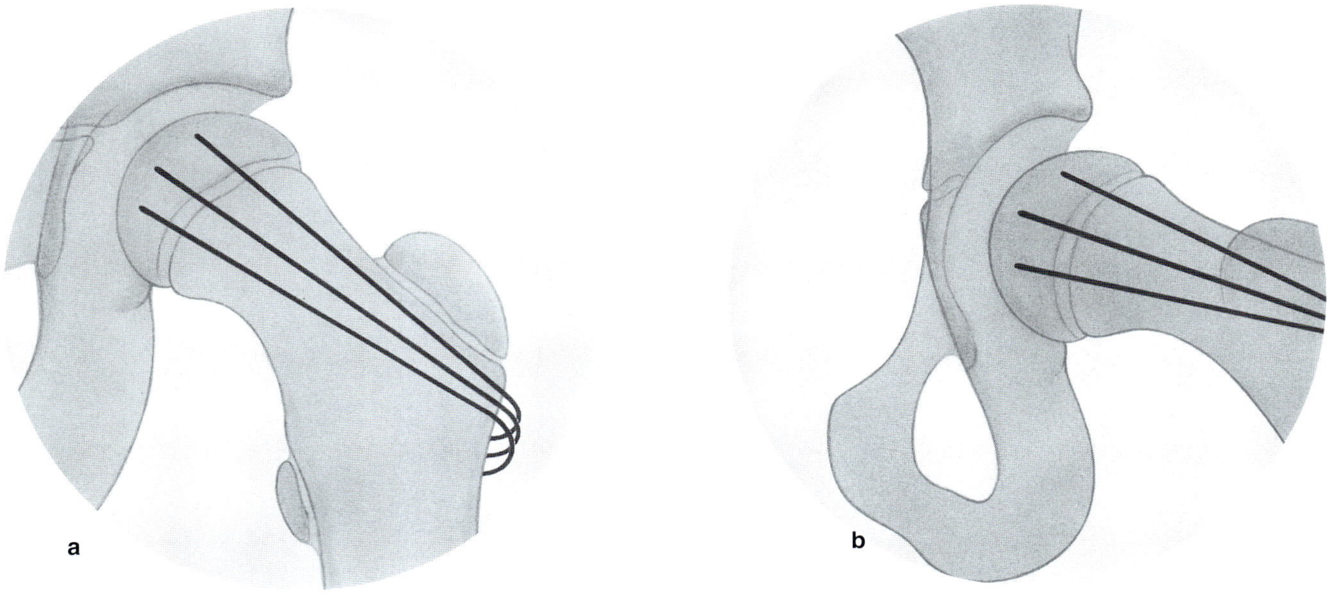

Fig. 2.**290 a** and **b** The Kirschner wires fan out evenly over the cross section of the femoral head.

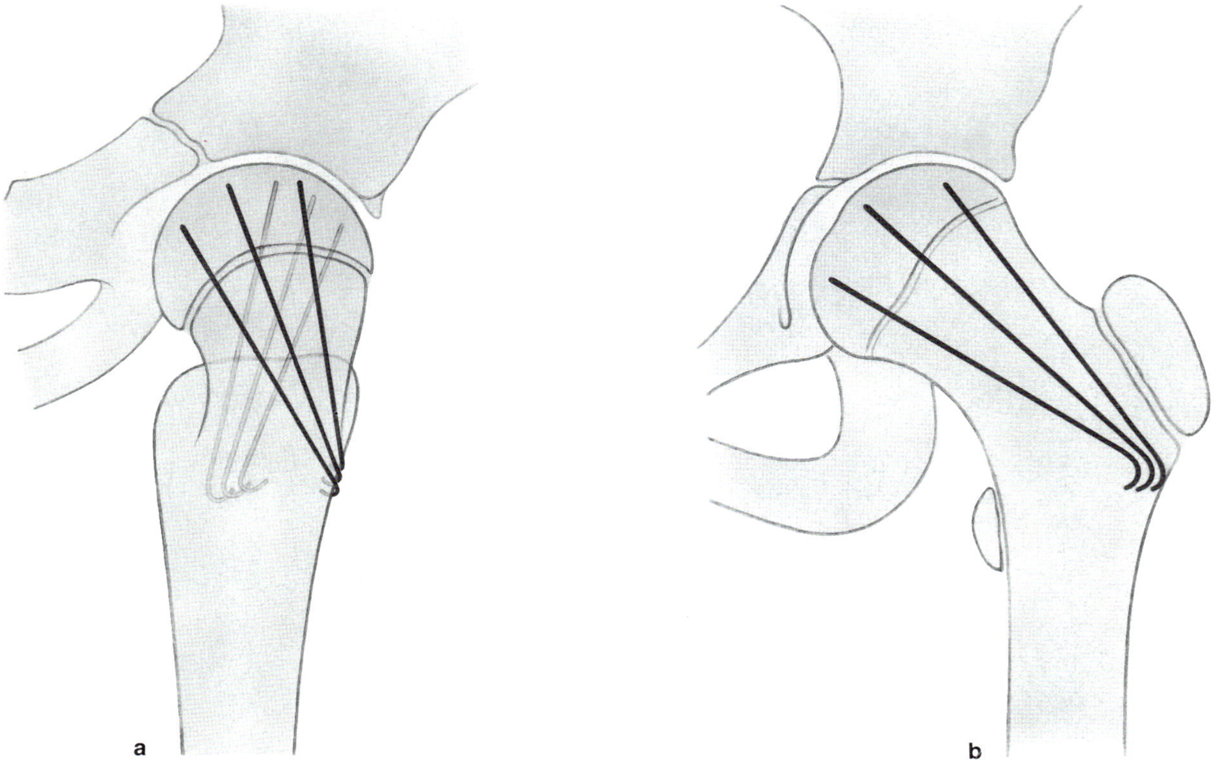

Fig. 2.**291 a** and **b** In a dislocation of the femoral head, the point of entry of the Kirschner wires must be chosen so that the wires travel diagonally through the femoral neck into the femoral head. Wires inserted from the middle of the lateral surface of the femur can only engage the anterior part of the femoral head.

The projecting ends of the Kirschner wires are bent into large hooks whose curvature projects above the surface of the bone in the incision in the vastus lateralis. This makes it easier to remove them later (Fig. 2.**292**). If the ends of the wires are simply bent to lie parallel to the surface of the bone, they will be covered with bone within a short period of time. Removing the implants may leave a defect in the femoral cortex, which could lead to fracture. Closure is begun by suturing the gap in the vastus lateralis. The surgeon then closes the fascia lata with a secure vertical mattress suture, overlapping the lips of the wound (Fig. 2.**293**).

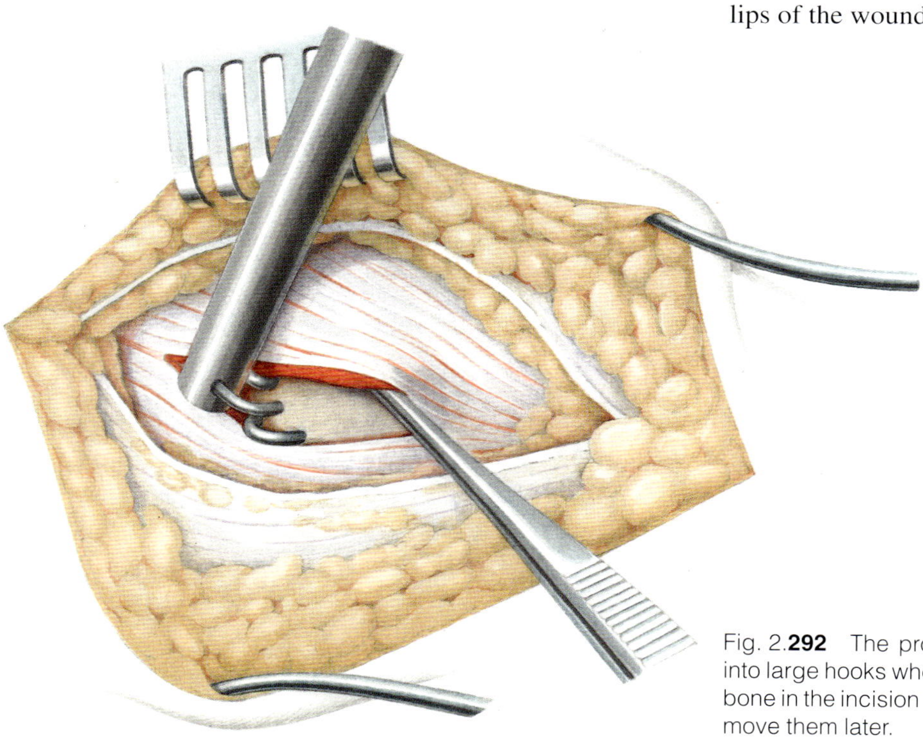

Fig. 2.**292** The projecting ends of the Kirschner wires are bent into large hooks whose curvature projects above the surface of the bone in the incision in the vastus lateralis. This makes it easier to remove them later.

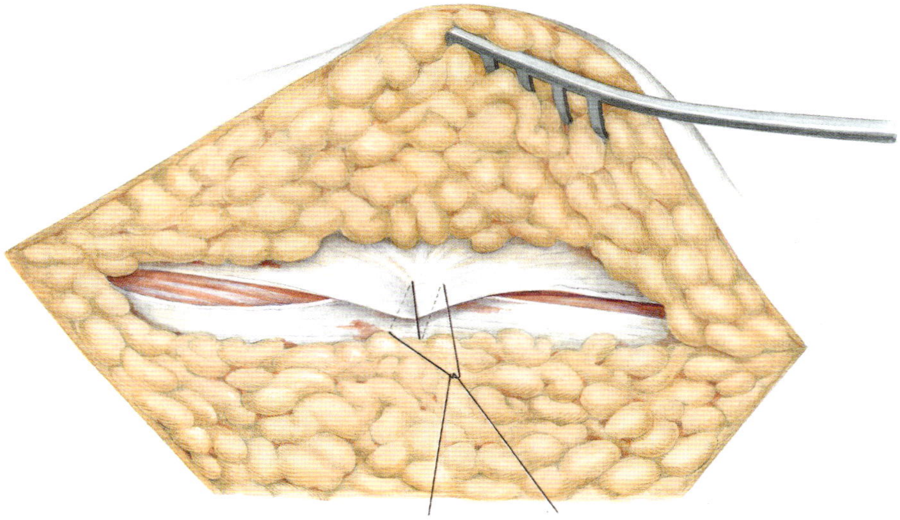

Fig. 2.**293** After the gap in the muscle is closed, the fascia lata is closed with a secure vertical mattress suture, overlapping the lips of the wound.

Subcapital Osteotomy of the Femoral Neck for a Slipped Capital Femoral Epiphysis

Indication

Severe slipped capital femoral epiphysis in which the femoral head partially projects from the acetabulum posteriorly and inferiorly, and the stump presses anterosuperiorly against the margin of the acetabulum, producing the typical external rotation deformity of the leg.

Clinical Considerations

Strictly speaking, the subcapital osteotomy is a late open reduction of an acute condition where the slip area is not yet covered with bone. If the condition is chronic and there is bony consolidation, an osteotomy would involve a high risk of necrosis of the femoral head.

Positioning and Incision

With the patient supine, a longitudinal skin incision is made that courses distally from the apex of the greater trochanter on the lateral side of the hip.

Surgical Technique

After exposing the hip joint with an anterior capsulectomy, the surgeon shortens the stump of the femoral neck by sparingly removing a wedge-shaped segment from the proximal femoral neck. The base of the wedge is anterior and superior. The apex on the posterior surface of the femoral neck is resected to prevent compression of vascular structures. After preparing the base of the slipped capital femoral epiphysis, the surgeon carefully reduces the fracture and then stabilizes it with screw fixation.

A lateral incision is made (see Fig. 2.**26**), and the fascia lata is split and retracted. The anterior margin of the gluteus medius is conservatively detached from its insertion on the greater trochanter to provide access to the anterior surface of the hip joint capsule (see Fig. 2.**27**). The pericapsular fat is retracted from the anterior surface of the joint capsule with a sharp periosteal elevator, exposing the entire anterior capsule (see Fig. 2.**28**). The reflected origin of the rectus femoris is now visible in the deep layer. Elevators are inserted on the superior and inferior sides of the femoral neck, providing broad exposure of the joint capsule. The surgeon performs a capsulotomy and an anterior capsulectomy (Fig. 2.**294**), and dissects the reflected origin of the rectus femoris.

The capsulectomy broadly exposes the hip joint. The acetabular labrum is visible in the deep layer. The stump of the femoral neck lies immediately lateral to it. The anterior surface of the femoral neck is covered with white periosteum; immediately medial to it is the dislocation site. The red surface of the bone surface is exposed and presses against the acetabular labrum. The femoral head has shifted posteriorly on the femoral neck and is covered by the labrum.

In the lateral plane, the epiphysis lies on the posterior surface of the femoral neck. A beak-shaped bony layer soon forms between the slipped epiphysis and the posterior surface of the femoral neck. The slipped head pushes the femoral neck anteriorly with respect to the acetabulum (Fig. 2.**295**).

In the subcapital osteotomy, a wedge-shaped segment (Fig. 2.**296 a**) is resected from the femoral neck. This is done to shorten the femoral neck and permit reduction without applying excessive tension to the posterior soft tissue and vascular structures. The posterior beak-shaped bony layer (Fig. 2.**296 b**) is also resected to prevent it from compressing vascular structures inferiorly after the fracture has been reduced. After the stump of the femoral neck has been prepared in this manner, the surgeon carefully extends, abducts, and internally rotates the leg, and gently restores the epiphysis to its anatomic position. The correction is stabilized with three screws (Fig. 2.**297**).

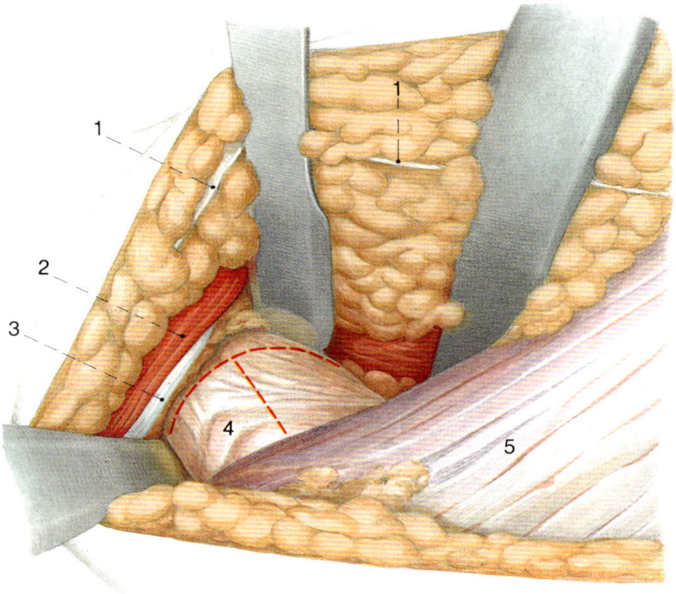

Fig. 2.**294** Elevators are inserted on the superior and inferior sides of the femoral neck. The reflected origin of the rectus femoris is now visible in the deep layer. An anterior capsulectomy is performed and the iliofemoral ligament is resected (indicated by dotted line). The reflected origin of the rectus femoris is dissected.

1 Fascia lata
2 Gluteus medius
3 Reflected origin of the rectus femoris
4 Hip joint capsule
5 Vastus lateralis

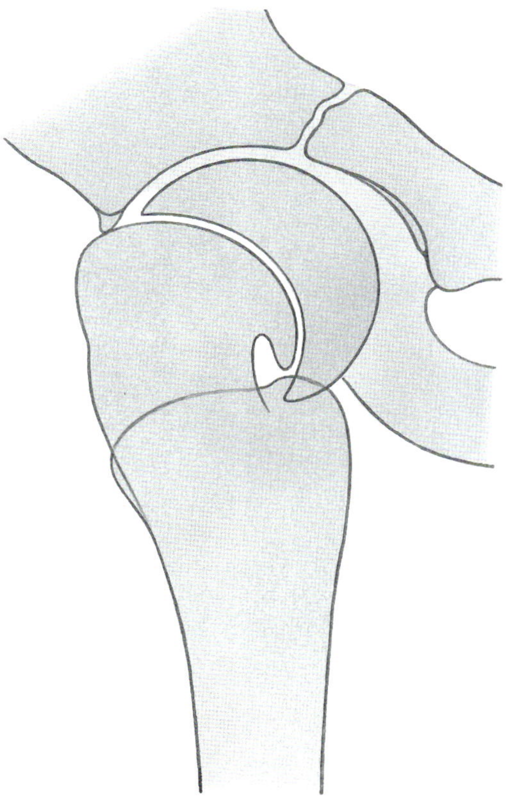

Fig. 2.**295** In the lateral plane, the epiphysis lies on the posterior surface of the femoral neck. A beak-shaped bony layer soon forms between the slipped epiphysis and the posterior surface of the femoral neck.

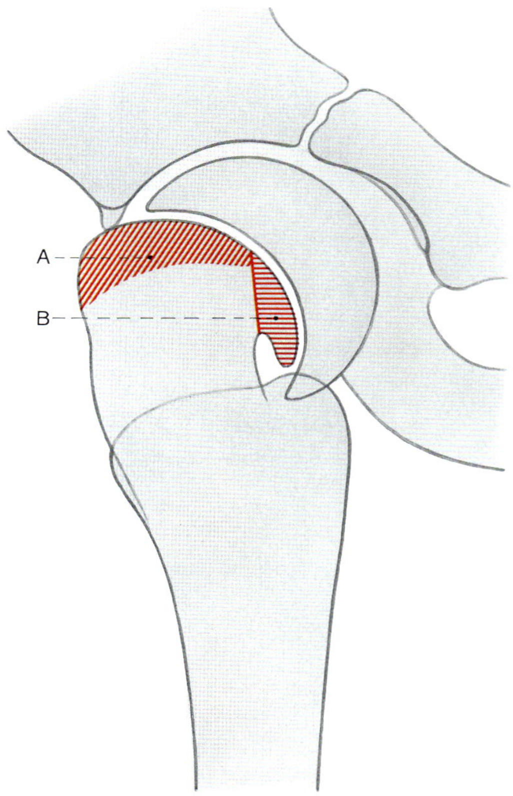

Fig. 2.**296** In preparation for reduction, a wedge-shaped bone segment (A) is resected from the femoral neck. This is done to shorten the femoral neck and permit reduction without applying excessive tension to the posterior soft tissue and vascular structures. The posterior beak-shaped bony layer (B) is also resected to prevent it from compressing vascular structures inferiorly after the fracture has been reduced.

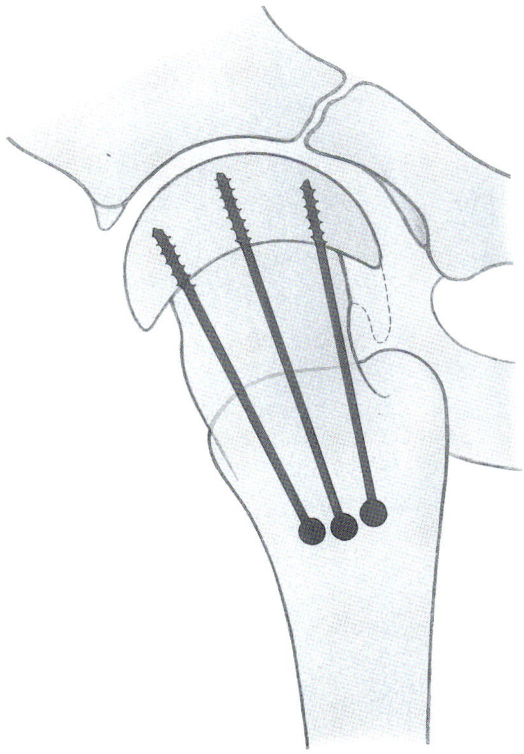

Fig. 2.**297** After the stump of the femoral neck has been prepared, the epiphysis is gently restored to its anatomic position with the leg carefully extended, abducted, and internally rotated. The correction is stabilized with three screws.

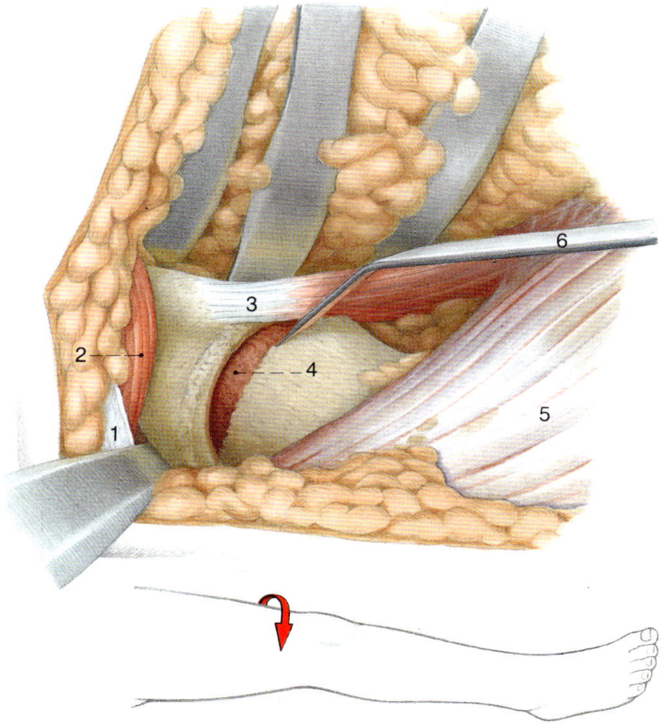

Fig. 2.**298** With the leg in external rotation, a wedge-shaped segment is removed from the stump of the femoral neck with an angled osteotome.

1 Fascia lata
2 Gluteus medius
3 Direct origin of the rectus femoris
4 Slip area on the femoral neck
5 Vastus lateralis
6 Angled osteotome

With the leg in external rotation, a wedge-shaped segment is removed from the stump of the femoral neck (Fig. 2.**298**). The surgeon then increases the external rotation and resects the beak-shaped bony layer on the posterior surface of the femoral neck with an angled osteotome (Fig. 2.**299**). With the leg slightly extended, abducted, and internally rotated, the surgeon gently restores the femoral head to its anatomic position. The cross section of the osteotomized femoral neck is smaller than that of the femoral head, so that the anterior margin of the femoral head projects beyond the femoral neck when the fracture is reduced and proper axial alignment is achieved (Fig. 2.**300**).

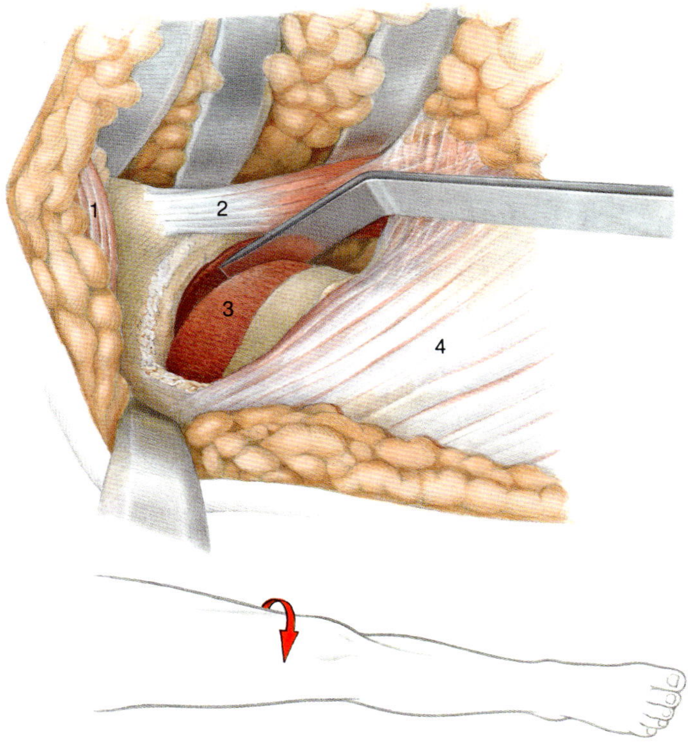

Fig. 2.**299** The external rotation of the leg is increased and the beak-shaped bony layer on the posterior surface of the femoral neck is resected with an angled osteotome.

1 Gluteus medius
2 Rectus femoris
3 Stump of femoral neck
4 Vastus lateralis

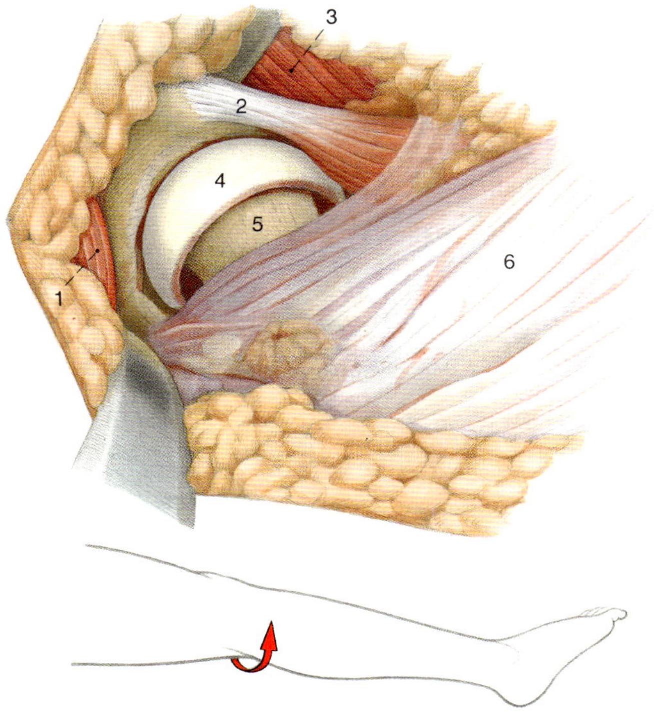

Fig. 2.**300** With the leg slightly extended, abducted, and internally rotated, the femoral head is gently restored to its anatomic position. The cross section of the osteotomized femoral neck is smaller than that of the femoral head, so that the anterior margin of the femoral head projects beyond the femoral neck when the fracture is reduced and proper axial alignment is achieved.

1 Gluteus medius
2 Reflected origin of the rectus femoris
3 Iliopsoas
4 Femoral head
5 Femoral neck
6 Vastus lateralis

When the internal rotation is increased, the femoral head migrates under the acetabular labrum into the acetabulum while the greater trochanter appears in the deep layer of the wound. To aid orientation, the leg is internally rotated until the femoral neck lies in the horizontal plane, i.e., parallel to the floor of the operating room. The vastus lateralis is incised parallel to its fibers 2 cm distal to the most proximal aspect of the greater trochanter. A Kirschner wire is inserted parallel to the floor through this incision in the muscle into the femoral neck and advanced into the femoral head. This stabilizes the femoral head sufficiently to verify its position and assess the hip's range of motion with fluoroscopy. Now the femoral head is fixed with screws (Fig. 2.**301**). The surgeon now inserts the screws next to the Kirschner wire, using the wire as a marker to indicate the axis of the femoral neck. If the Kirschner wire is left in place as part of the fixation, the surgeon generally inserts two partially threaded cancellous screws, or three if the wire is removed. The screws are aligned so that they are uniformly distributed over the cross section of the femoral head (Fig. 2.**302** and 2.**303**).

A subfascial drain is placed and taken to suction. The anterior margin of the gluteus medius is reattached (see Fig. 2.**31**). The fascia lata is closed with retention sutures.

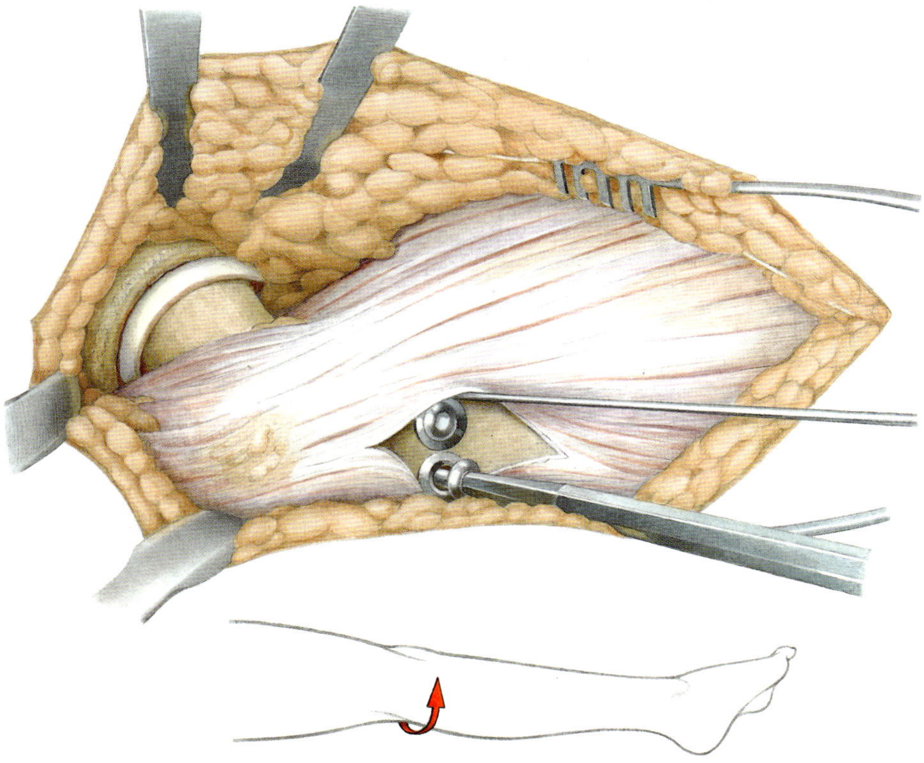

Fig. 2.**301** When the internal rotation is increased, the femoral head migrates under the acetabular labrum into the acetabulum while the greater trochanter appears in the deep layer of the wound. For better orientation, the leg is internally rotated until the femoral neck lies in the horizontal plane, i.e., parallel to the floor of the operating room. The vastus lateralis is incised parallel to its fibers 2 cm distal to the most proximal aspect of the greater trochanter. A Kirschner (parallel to the floor) wire is inserted through this incision in the muscle into the femoral neck and advanced into the femoral head. After the position of the wire and the hip's range of motion are verified with fluoroscopy, the femoral head is fixed with screws. The screws are inserted next to the Kirschner wire, which is used as a marker to indicate the axis of the femoral neck.

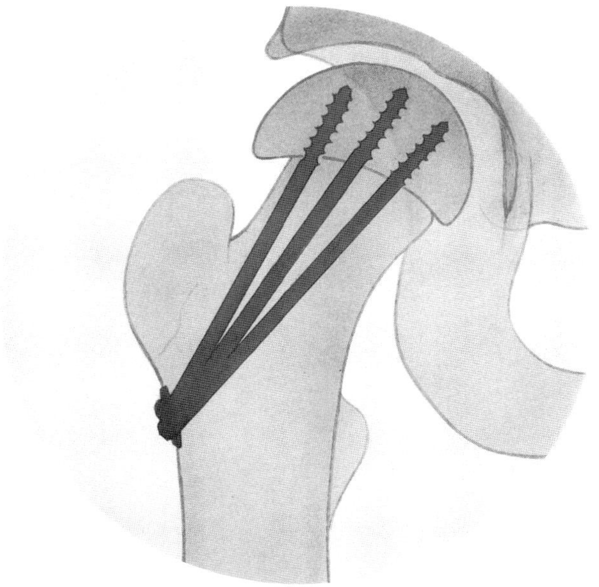

Fig. 2.**302** Verifying alignment of the screws in the sagittal plane with fluoroscopy. The crews are aligned so that they are uniformly distributed over the cross section of the femoral head.

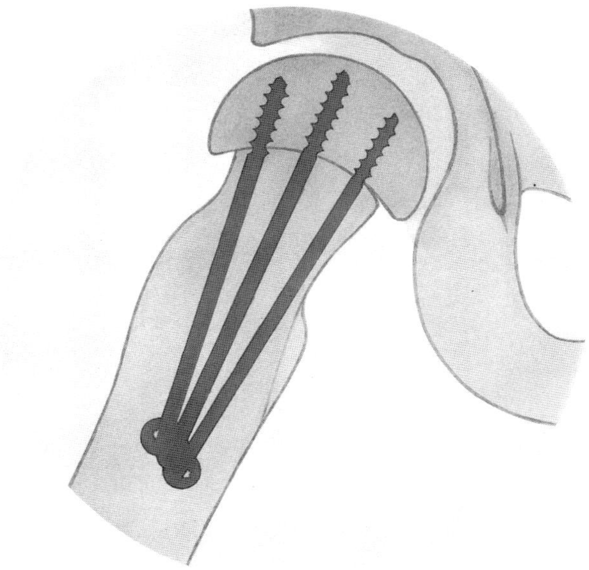

Fig. 2.**303** Verifying alignment of the screws in the lateral plane with fluoroscopy. The screws should be aligned so that they are uniformly distributed in the lateral plane as well.

Subtrochanteric Supporting Osteotomies

Indication

Surgical treatment of degenerative hip disorders that result in proximal femoral shortening. Common etiologies include septic or tuberculous coxitis or condition after removal of a total hip arthroplasty without reimplantation.

Clinical Considerations

This condition is accompanied by severe instability. The femur lacks support in the acetabulum, while the pelvic and trochanteric muscles lack a buttress against which they can develop torque between the pelvis and femur to stabilize the hip. The superior migration of the proximal femur results in a decrease in leg length, which exacerbates the effect of the muscular instability of the hip.

The subtrochanteric supporting osteotomy creates a buttress between the femur and the pelvis, preventing the femur from moving superiorly when weight is applied to the hip and permitting the pelvic and trochanteric musculature to develop stabilizing tension.

Positioning and Incision

With the patient supine, a longitudinal skin incision is made that courses distally from the apex of the greater trochanter on the lateral side of the hip.

Surgical Technique

The surgeon creates an artifical femoral neck by performing a subtrochanteric valgus osteotomy (approximately 90°) and shifting the distal fragment laterally. This femoral neck presses against the pelvis, stabilizing both the femur and the ilium and providing a buttress from the pelvic and trochanteric musculature. Best results are achieved when the apophysis of the lesser trochanter is inserted into the acetabulum prior to cessation of growth because the apophysis can develop into a substitute femoral head.

The initial stage of the procedure is identical to an intertrochanteric osteotomy. The fascia lata is split parallel to the direction of its fibers and retracted. An L-shaped incision is then made in the vastus lateralis immediately distal to the most proximal aspect of the greater trochanter. The muscle is dissected from the lateral intermuscular septum and the femur. Elevators are inserted to lift the muscle, exposing the femur. The leg is then externally rotated to expose the lesser trochanter. A rentention suture is placed on the iliopsoas tendon. Then the surgeon transects the tendon, taking care to avoid damaging the apophysis of the lesser trochanter (Fig. 2.**304**).

The gluteus medius is split parallel to its fibers, and the leg is placed in extreme adduction. Now the apex of the greater trochanter is exposed. The slot for the blade of the condylar plate is prepared according to the preoperative plan, and the seating chisel is impacted. The transverse osteotomy is then performed perpendicular to the axis of the femur at the distal margin of the lesser trochanter (Fig. 2.**305**).

The seating chisel is used to rotate the proximal fragment further into valgus, which shifts the lesser trochanter into the scarred acetabulum. In rare cases, the lesser trochanter will not be far enough medial and the surgeon will have to resect the scar tissue from the acetabulum. The distal fragment is brought from adduction back to a middle position and is pushed laterally beneath the decorticated bone of what was

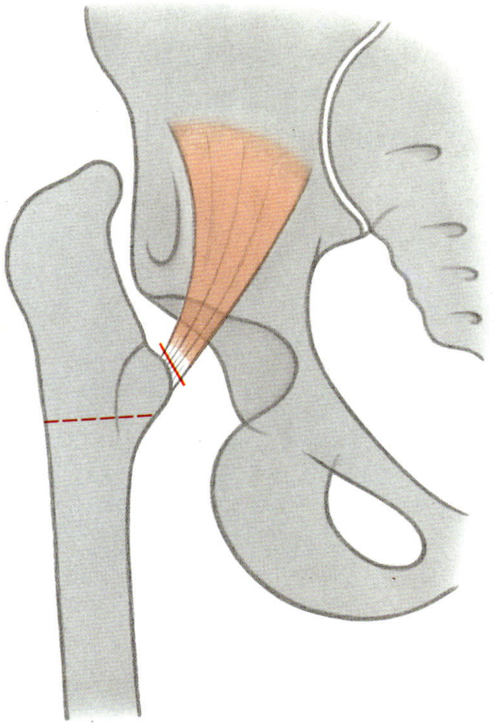

Fig. 2.**304** In the subtrochanteric osteotomy, the proximal femur segment and the acetabulum are exposed through an anterolateral approach. With the leg in external rotation, a retention suture is placed on the iliopsoas tendon and the tendon is transected at the lesser trochanter.

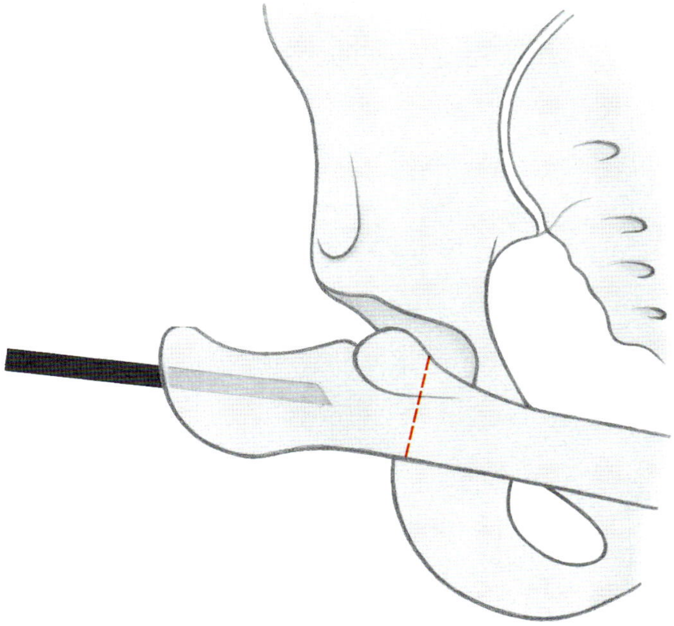

Fig. 2.**305** The gluteus medius is split parallel to its fibers, and the leg is placed in extreme adduction. Now the apex of the greater trochanter is exposed. The slot for the blade of the condylar plate is prepared according to the preoperative planning, and the seating chisel is impacted. The transverse osteotomy is then performed perpendicular to the axis of the femur at the distal margin of the lesser trochanter.

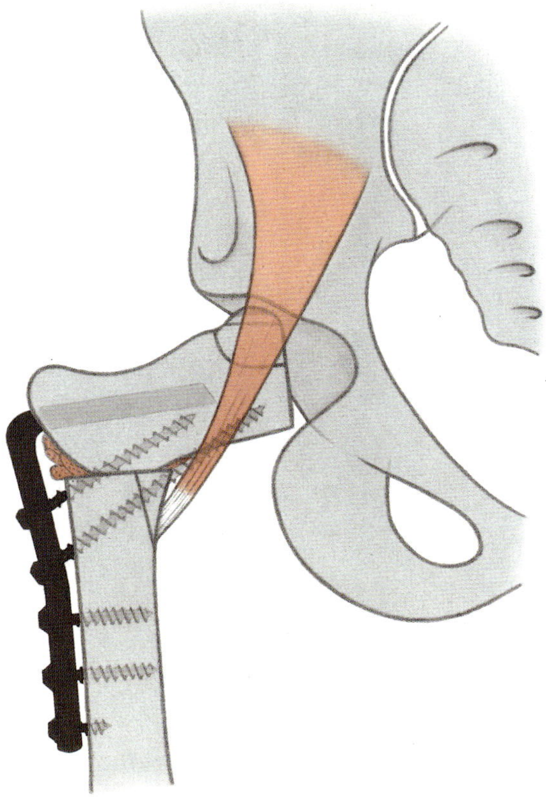

the lateral surface of the greater trochanter. Here, it is temporarily secured with Kirschner wires. The seating chisel is replaced with a condylar plate, which is fastened to the two fragments with screws to achieve interfragmentary compression (Fig. 2.**306**). The Kirschner wires are removed, the iliopsoas tendon is sutured to the decorticated edge of the distal fragment, and the gaps at the contact surface between the two fragments are filled with graft.

Fig. 2.**306** The seating chisel is used to rotate the proximal fragment further into valgus, which shifts the lesser trochanter into the scarred acetabulum. In rare cases, the lesser trochanter will not be far enough medial and the surgeon will have to resect the scar tissue from the acetabulum. The distal fragment is brought from adduction back to a middle position, and is pushed laterally beneath the decorticated bone of what was the lateral surface of the greater trochanter, where it is temporarily secured with Kirschner wires. The seating chisel is replaced with a condylar plate, which is fastened to the two fragments with screws to achieve interfragmentary compression. The Kirschner wires are removed, the iliopsoas tendon is sutured to the decorticated edge of the distal fragment, and the gaps at the contact surface between the two fragments are filled with graft.

Weight bearing will result in articulation between the proximal fragment and the acetabulum, which radiographically resembles an anatomical hip joint. Impressive remodelling can be achieved, particularly in young patients in whom the apophysis of the lesser trochanter is still growing (Fig. 2.**307**). The artificial femoral neck also simplifies any future total joint arthroplasty.

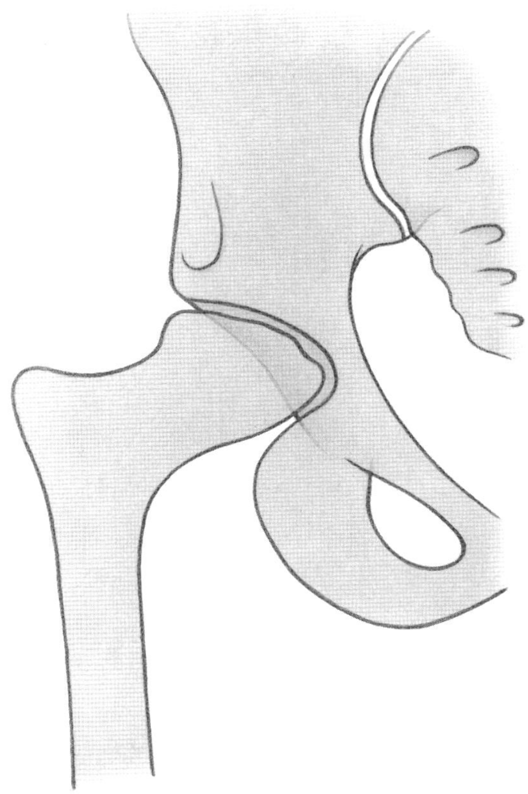

Fig. 2.**307** Weight bearing will result in articulation between the proximal fragment and the acetabulum, which radiographically resembles an anatomical hip joint.

Arthrodesis

Indications

Arthrodesis is indicated primarily in the surgical treatment of severe painful degeneration of the hip joint accompanied by a deformity or weight-bearing instability where conservative treatment cannot improve the condition, and joint-preserving procedures have been unsuccessful.

Clinical Considerations

The decision to perform arthrodesis is easier to make if the patient already suffers from painful partial immobility and has learned to cope with this loss of motion. These patients regard the elimination of pain and the correction of the deformity as benefits that outweigh the loss of residual motion.

Arthrodesis provides a hip that remains stable and free of pain for decades, yet it does this at the cost of completely eliminating hip motion. In addition to being a handicap in numerous situations, arthrodesis places abnormal stresses on the knee and spinal column. The handicap is greater in taller patients, who have difficulties sitting in a car or in low chairs.

Recent progress in total joint arthroplasty has greatly narrowed the range of indications for arthrodesis. Today, arthrodesis is primarily a procedure used in younger patients. However, it can be indicated in older patients if total joint arthroplasty is contraindicated by a septic disorder. Arthrodesis is not always the first step in treating a severe hip disorder, even where it might be warranted. Due to personal and occupational considerations, total joint arthroplasty may be preferable to arthrodesis for the individual patient, especially since it remains an option even if total arthroplasty proves unsuccessful.

The same applies in the case of a severe condition in both hips. Arthrodesis on both sides is not an option, but arthrodesis of one hip and total joint arthroplasty of the other may be considered in young patients. However, since it is not possible to foretell which arthroplasty will fail first, the best solution is double total hip arthroplasty. Arthrodesis can then be performed on the hip in which the implant fails first. Naturally, a contingent approach of this sort requires sufficient understanding on the part of the patient.

The surgeon must remember that problems with the knee joint on the same side or the spine may necessitate taking down the arthrodesis in the distant future. For this reason, important anatomical structures should be preserved when the arthrodesis is performed.

Positioning and Incision

With the patient positioned supine, a transverse roll 15 cm in diameter under both knees will maintain the required hip flexion during surgery (Fig. 2.**308**). Both legs are prepped and draped to permit free movement so that leg length can be compared intraoperatively. The surgeon stands at the foot of the operating table, lifts both the patient's feet until the legs are extended, and examines the legs from above with the feet 5 cm apart. This permits reliable assessment of leg length when applying internal fixation (Fig. 2.**309**).

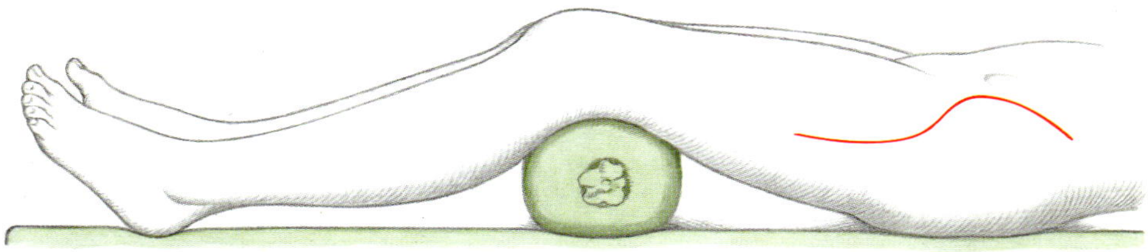

Fig. 2.**308** Arthrodesis of the left hip. The patient is positioned supine with a transverse roll 15 cm in diameter under both knees to maintain the required hip flexion during surgery. Both legs are prepped and draped to permit free movement, so that leg length can be compared when internal fixation is applied.

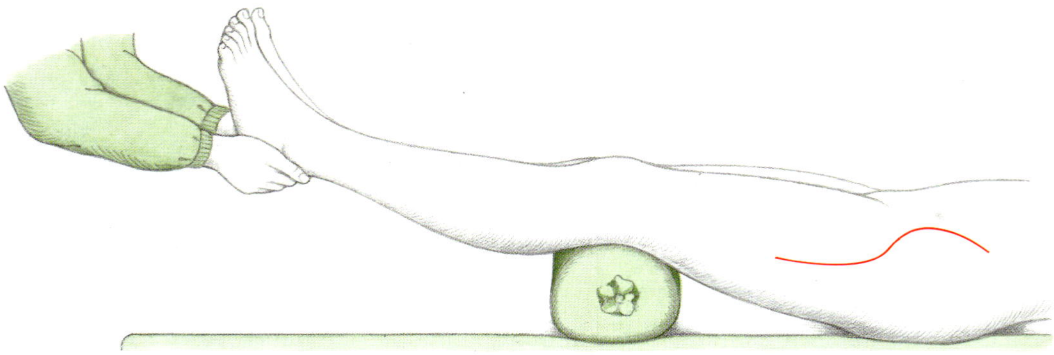

Fig. 2.**309** To compare leg length, the surgeon stands at the foot of the operating table and lifts both the patient's feet until the legs are extended and no longer in contact with the surface of the roll. Examining the legs from above, with the feet 5 cm apart, permits reliable assessment of leg length when applying internal fixation.

Surgical Technique

In hip arthrodesis, the cartilage is resected from the articular surfaces and the joint is bridged with internal fixation. This eliminates the need to immobilize the patient and facilitates rapid bony consolidation. The hip should be fused in 15° flexion to minimize interferene with movement. This position is a good compromise because it makes it easier for the patient to sit while the lordosis of the lumbar spinal column remains within acceptable tolerances. While a greater degree of flexion would make it easier for the patient to sit on low chairs, it would increase both the inclination of the pelvis and the lordosis of the lumbar spinal column, severely handicapping the patient's ability to stand and walk. The lesser degree of flexion is better for younger patients who are more physically active in an erect posture. Over several decades, the degree of flexion increases as a result of the physiological bone changes that occur with aging. This benefits older patients, who are primarily sedentary. Optimum position in the coronal plane is 7° adduction with leg length equal and the feet about 5 cm apart. In patients younger than 15 years, a neutral position is preferred because as the bone grows, the hip will spontaneously assume an adducted position. Fifteen degrees of external rotation is optimum.

The hip and proximal femur are exposed through an anterolateral approach to the hip made through an S-shaped skin incision that permits resection of the articular cartilage and internal fixation between the ilium and the femur. After the skin incision is made and the lips of the wound are retracted, the fascia lata is split along the iliac crest from proximal to distal, and the anterior margin of the tensor fasciae latae is split as far as the lateral surface of the vastus lateralis. The surgeon retracts the tensor fasciae latae laterally and then ligates and transects the ascending branch of the lateral femoral circumflex artery (Fig. 2.**310**).

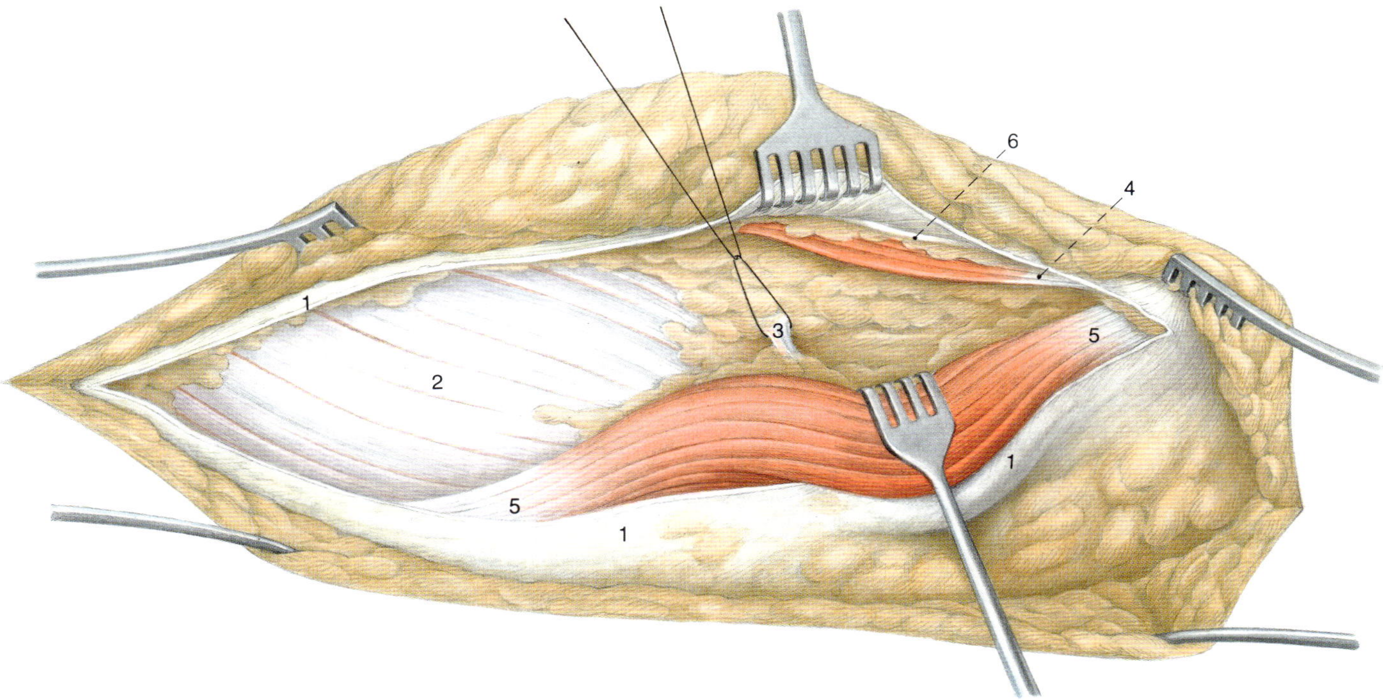

Fig. 2.**310** The hip and proximal femur are exposed through an anterolateral approach to the hip made through an S-shaped skin incision that permits resection of the articular cartilage and internal fixation between the ilium and the femur. The fascia lata is split along the iliac crest from proximal do distal, and the anterior margin of the tensor fasciae latae is split as far as the lateral surface of the vastus lateralis. The tensor fasciae latae is retracted laterally, and the ascending branch of the lateral femoral circumflex artery is ligated and transected.

1 Fascia lata
2 Vastus lateralis
3 Lateral femoral circumflex artery
4 Sartorius
5 Tensor fasciae latae
6 Lateral femoral cutaneous nerve

The surgeon subperiosteally dissects the tensor fasciae latae from the outer surface of the ilium, retracting the muscle laterally and posteriorly to expose the outer surface of the greater trochanter (Figs. 2.**311** and 2.**312**). A braod sharp-tipped elevator is impacted in the posterior surface of the greater trochanter, and the vastus lateralis is dissected from the lateral intermuscular septum and the most proximal aspect of the greater trochanter (Fig. 2.**312**).

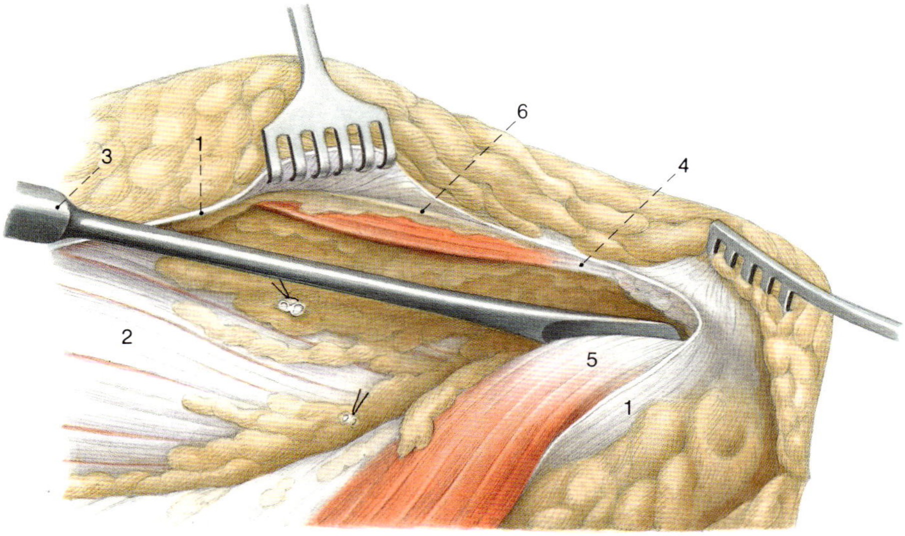

Fig. 2.**311** The tensor fasciae latae is subperiosteally dissected from the outer surface of the ilium and retracted laterally and posteriorly to expose the outer surface of the greater trochanter.

1 Fascia lata
2 Vastus lateralis
3 Periosteal elevator
4 Sartorius
5 Tensor fasciae latae
6 Lateral femoral cutaneous nerve

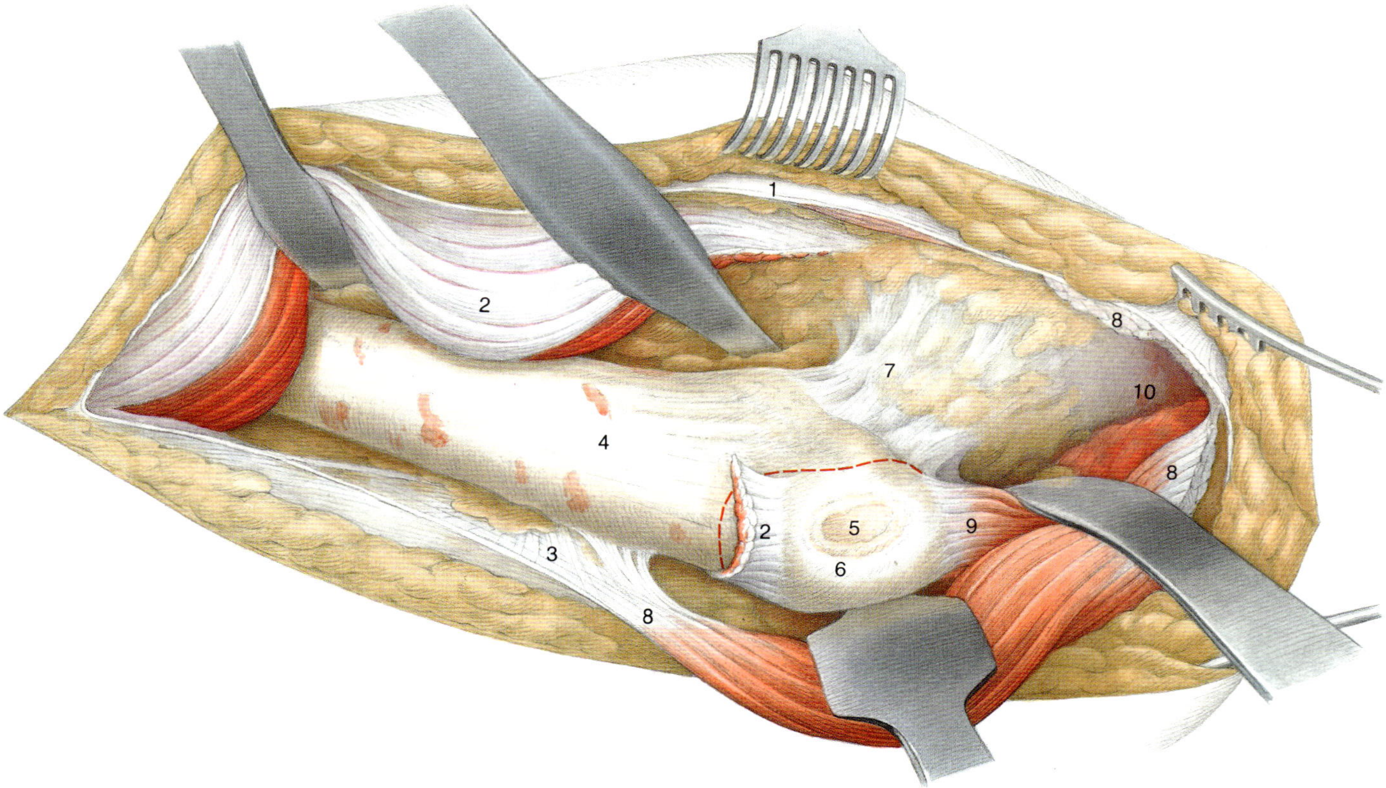

Fig. 2.**312** A broad sharp-tipped elevator is impacted in the posterior surface of the greater trochanter, and the tensor fasciae latae is retracted posteriorly. The vastus lateralis is dissected from the lateral intermuscular septum and from the femur distal to the most proximal aspect of the greater trochanter. Then it is lifted with elevators to expose the joint capsule. An elevator is inserted between the capsule and the gluteus medius. An osteotomy (dotted red line) is performed at the base of the greater trochanter. The osteotomy curves toward the superior margin of the femoral neck, continuing the line of the lateral surface of the femur. The capsule is then resected.

1 Fascia lata
2 Vastus lateralis
3 Lateral intermuscular septum
4 Femur
5 Greater trochanter
6 Most proximal aspect of the greater trochanter
7 Hip joint capsule
8 Tensor fasciae latae
9 Gluteus medius
10 Iliac wing

Further dissection of the vastus lateralis exposes the anterior surface of the shaft of the femur and the femoral neck. An elevator is inserted on the medial side of the femoral neck to medially retract the soft tissue. A second elevator is inserted on the superior side of the femoral neck. Now the surgeon osteotomizes the greater trochanter with a flat osteotome. The osteotomy curves toward the superior margin of the femoral neck, continuing the line of the lateral surface of the femur (Fig. 2.**312**). The greter trochanter and its soft-tissue attachments are then retracted superiorly. These soft-tissue structures must be carefully preserved to ensure stability in the event that total joint arthroplasty may be indicated in the future to remobilize the hip. The surgeon now resects the scarred capsule and the periarticular scar tissue until the capsule is broadly exposed.

With the leg adducted and externally rotated, the surgeon carefully dislocates the hip. This should be done gently to avoid fracturing the femur. Since arthrodesis of the hip is generally indicated only in the presence of severe degeneration, remaining periarticular or intra-articular scar tissue may interfere with dislocation. In such cases, the surgeon can only dislocate the hip gradually while progressively resecting the scar tissue.

When the joint has been completely dislocated, the entire acetabulum is exposed. Elevators insert into the obturator foramen and posterior to the posterior acetabular margin are used to retract the surrounding soft-tissue structures distally and the proximal femur posteriorly, providing broader exposure of the acetabulum.

Now the articular cartilage is resected, and the articular surfaces are prepared. Stability is improved by shaping the articular surfaces to form a square peg and a square hole, providing interference fit. If interference fit around the entire circumference cannot be achieved because of a bony defect, then at least the superior segment of the joint segment should have horizontal contact surfaces that provide stable medial support for the lateral internal fixation.

Resection of the cartilage and preparation of the bone begins in the acetabulum. The surgeon should resect bone sparingly to minimize size discrepancies between the femoral head and the acetabulum. The anterior acetabulum is osteotomized to form a flat vertical surface (Fig. 2.**313**), then the superior part of the acetabulum is osteotomized to form a flat horizontal surface. Then cartilage and scar tissue are resected from the remaining parts of the acetabulum, and the floor of the acetabulum is deepened until bleeding cancellous bone is visible across the entire osteotomy surface.

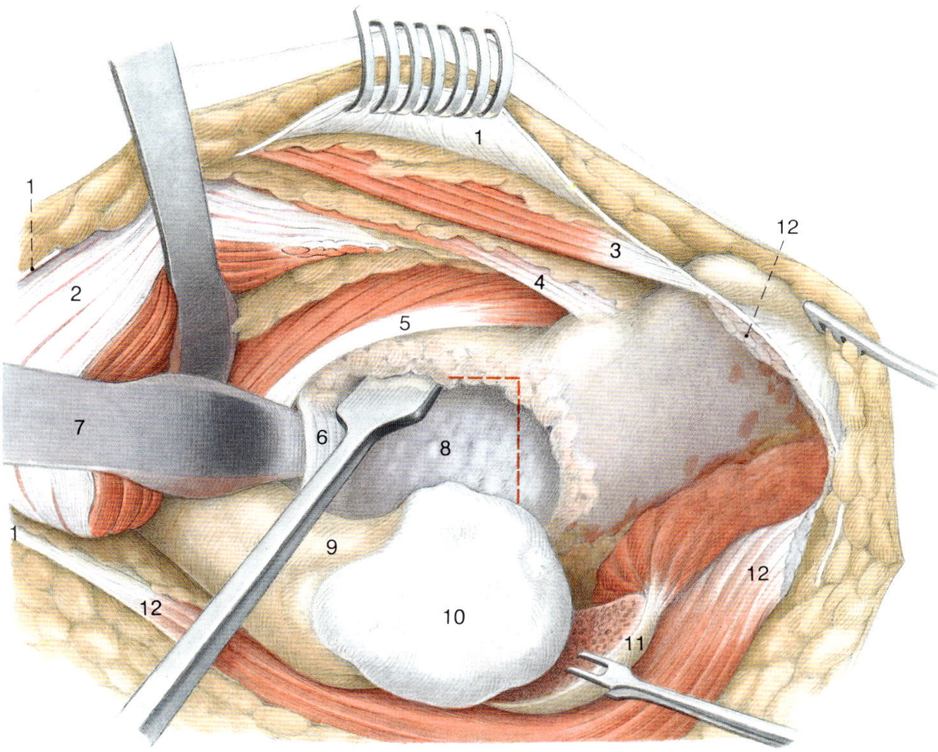

Fig. 2.**313** The greater trochanter and ist soft-tissue attachments are retracted superiorly. With the leg adducted and externally rotated, the hip is dislocated. The articular cartilage is resected and the acetabulum is osteotomized to form a square hole for the best interference fit that bone quality permits.

1 Fascia lata
2 Vastus lateralis
3 Sartorius
4 Rectus femoris
5 Iliopsoas
6 Transverse acetabular ligament
7 Elevator inserted into the obturator foramen
8 Acetabulum
9 Femoral neck
10 Femoral head
11 Greater trochanter
12 Tensor fasciae latae

With the leg externally rotated 90°, a broad sharp-tipped elevator is inserted beneath the femur to lift the proximal femur and retract posterior soft-tissue attachments, providing broad exposure of the femoral head. Using an osteotome, the surgeon now resects the cartilage from the femoral head and shapes it to form a square peg (Fig. 2.**314**). Bone stock (including osteophytes) is resected sparingly to achieve the best possible interference fit in the acetabulum. While shaping the bone, the surgeon repeatedly inserts femoral head into the prepared acetabulum to check the fit.

After resecting the cartilage and preparing the articular surfaces, the surgeon reinserts the femoral head into the acetabulum and flexes, adducts, and externally rotates the femur 15°, respectively. By deepening the acetabulum and resecting the medial segment of the femoral head, the surgeon can shift the proximal femur medially until only a slight lateral offset remains (Fig. 2.**315a**), which can easily be bridged with internal fixation. A so-called cobra head plate is applied to the outer surface of the femur and ilium. Since this plate must match the surface contour well, it may be necessary to resect bone distal to the trochanteric osteotomy site or use bending irons to contour the plate. The cobra head plate is temporarily fixed in the corrected position with Kirschner wires to prevent it from slipping when the screws are inserted. First the proximal blade of the plate is fixed superior to the roof of the acetabulum with two screws, and an articulated plate tensioner is attached to the distal end (Fig. 2.**315b** and **c**). As tension is increased, the femoral head is first pressed into the acetabulum, and then the femur gradually returns from extreme adduction to the desired position of 7° adduction (Fig. 2.**316**). At this stage, the surgeon again checks the flexion, adduction, and external rotation of the femur because now any necessary corrections can be made easily. Checking leg length is especially important, as this also determines the desired adduction. The surgeon stands at the foot of the operating table and takes both the patient's feet in his hands (Fig. 2.**317**), lifting both feet until the knees are extended and no longer in contact with the surface of the roll. The height of the roll keeps the hips at proper flexion. Equal leg length with the feet 5 cm apart provides the desired slight degree of adduction. If there was an existing anatomic difference in leg length, the appropriate adjustment should be made now. This very simple procedure is far more reliable than measuring the angles between the iliac crests and the femur.

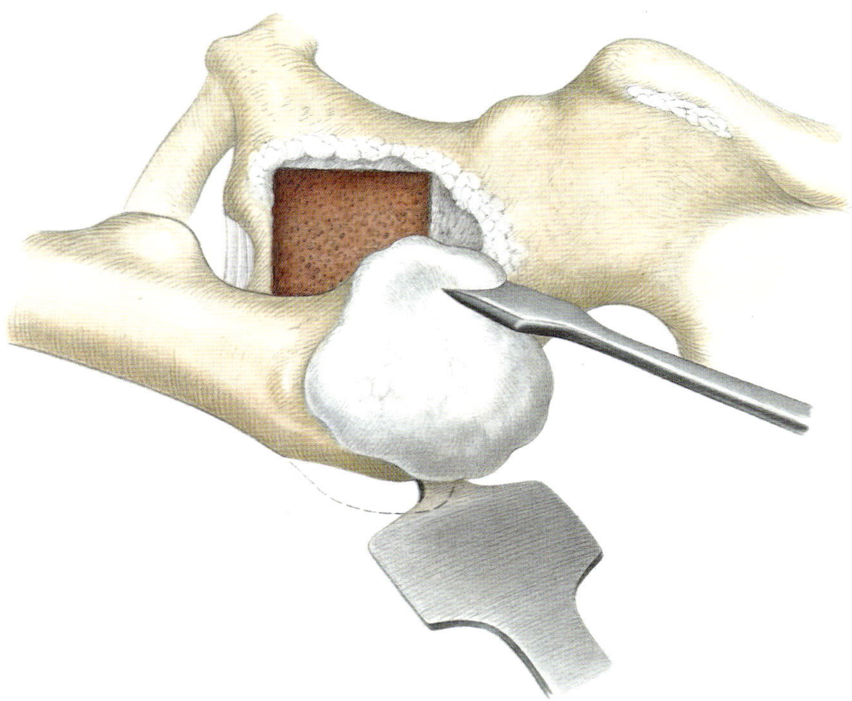

Fig. 2.**314** With the leg externally rotated 90°, a broad elevator is inserted beneath the femur to lift the proximal femur and retract posterior soft-tissue attachments, providing broad exposure of the femoral head. An osteotome is used to resect the cartilage from the femoral head and shape it to form a square peg.

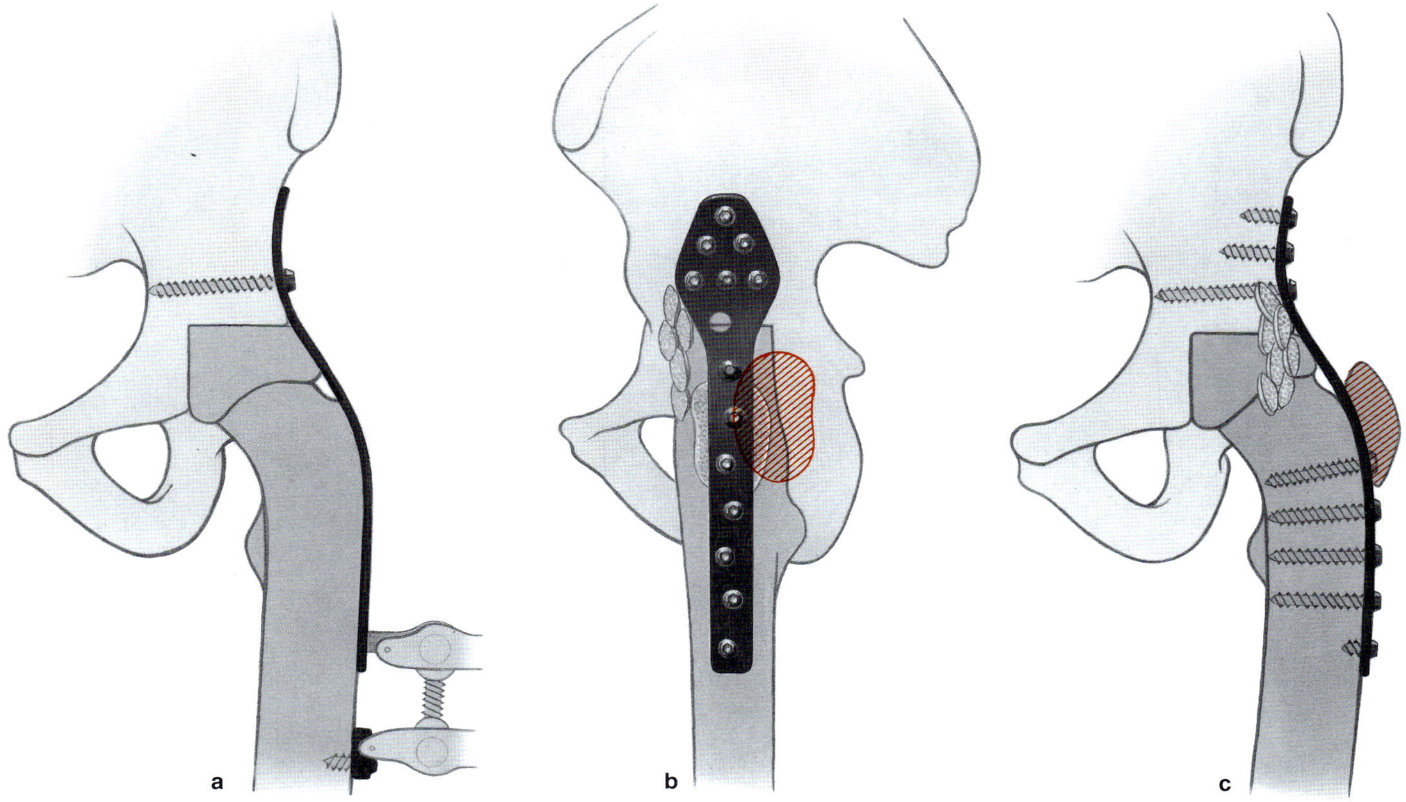

Fig. 2.**315 a–c** After the resection of the cartilage and preparation of the articular surfaces, the femoral head is reinserted into the acetabulum and the femur is flexed, adducted, and externally rotated 15°, respectively. A cobra head plate is applied to the outer surface of the femur and ilium, which must match the surface contour well. First the proximal blade of the cobra head plate is fixed superior to the roof of the acetabulum with two screws, then an articulated plate tensioner is attached to the distal end of the plate (**a**). After interfragmentary compression is applied and all screws have been inserted, the hip is filled with graft and the greater trochanter is returned to its physiological position (**b** and **c**).

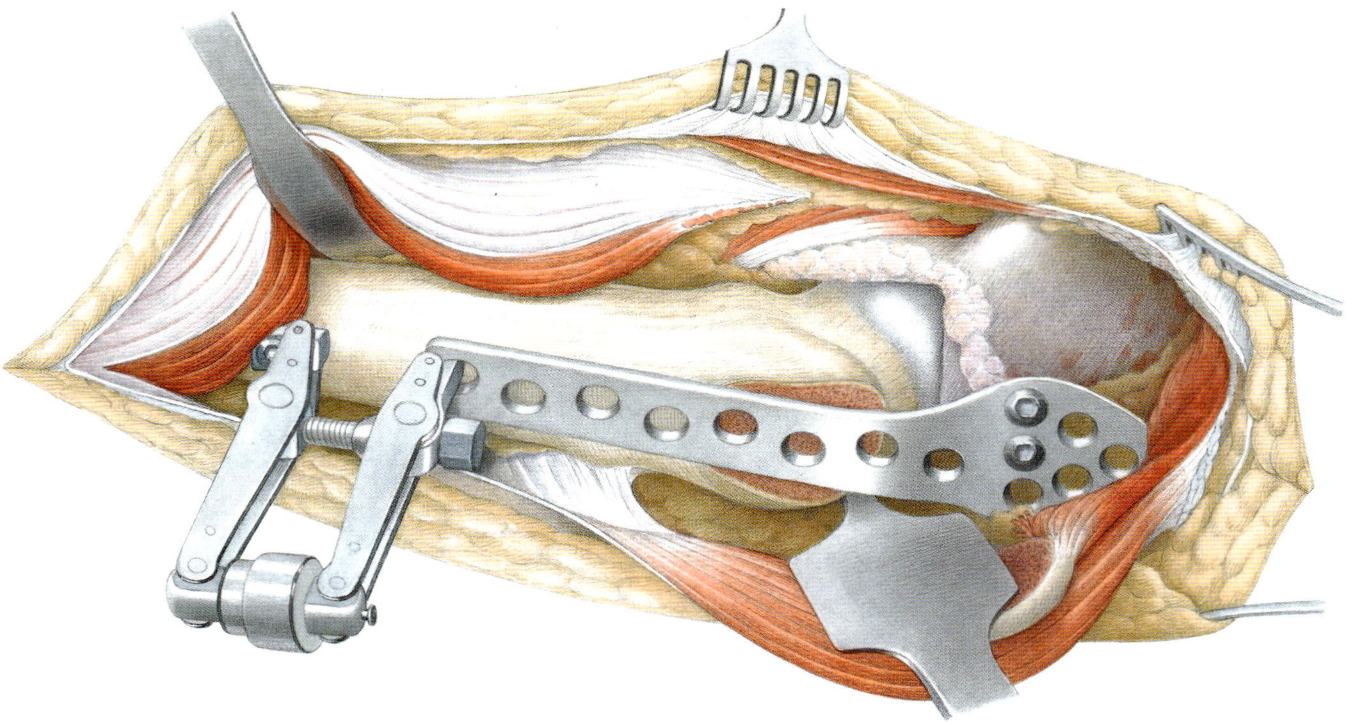

Fig. 2.**316** The proximal blade of the cobra head plate is fixed first superior to the roof of the acetabulum with two screws, and an articulated plate tensioner is attached to the distal end. Interfragmentary compression is applied gradually, and the femoral head is pressed into the acetabulum.

Now all the screws ae inserted in the proximal blade of the cobra head plate. Compression is increased slightly with the articulated plate tensioner; this does not result in any significant change in the position of the femur (Fig. 2.**317**). Finally, the shaft of the plate is fastened to the femur, and the articulated plate tensioner is removed. A short screw is inserted in the most distal screw hole so that the rigidity of the construct increases gradually from distal to proximal.

The hip is filled with graft taken when the surfaces were being prepared. Now the greater trochanter is returned to its original position along with its soft-tissue attachments; its anterior half covers the cobra head plate. The vastus lateralis is reattached to the greater trochanter under tension (Fig. 2.**318**). The surgeon places a deep suction drain, reattaches the dissected pelvic and trochanteric musculature to the iliac crest (Fig. 2.**319**), and closes the fascia lata with retention sutures. Then the wound is closed in layers.

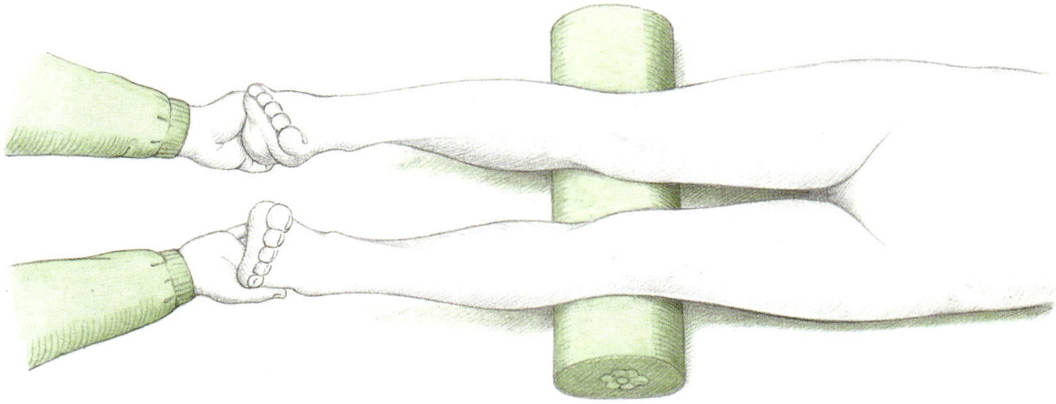

Fig. 2.**317** When interfragmentary compression is applied, the leg position should be checked again because now any necessary corrections can be made easily. The surgeon stands at the foot of the operating table and takes both the patient's feet in his hands, lifting both feet until the knees are extended and no longer in contact with the surface of the roll. The height of the roll keeps the hips at proper flexion. Equal leg length with the feet 5 cm apart provides the desired slight degree of adduction.

References

Bauer R, Kerschbaumer F, Poisel S. Operative Zugangswege in Orthopädie und Traumatologie. Stuttgart: Thieme; 1986.

Chiari K. Ergebnisse mit der Beckenosteotomie als Pfannendachplastik. Orthop. 1956; 87:14.

Ganz R, Klaue K, Mast JW. A new periacetabular osteotomy of the treatment of hip dysplasias: technique and primary results. Clin Orthop. 1988; 232:26.

Müller ME. Die hüftnahen Femurosteotomien. 2nd ed. Stuttgart: Thieme; 1971.

Müller ME, Allgöwer M, Schneider R, Willenegger H. Manual der Osteosynthese. 3rd ed. Berlin: Springer; 1992.

Pauwels F. Atlas zur Biomechanik der gesunden und kranken Hüfte. Berlin: Springer; 1973.

Schneider R. Die Arthrodese des Hüftgelenks mit Kreuzplatte und Beckenosteotomie. Bern: Huber; 1976.

Steel HH. Triple osteotomy of the innominate bone. J Bone Jt Surg 1973; 55:343.

Sutherland DH, Greenfield R. Double innominate osteotomy. J Bone Jt Surg. 1977; 55:1082.

Tachdjian MO. Pediatric Orthopedics. Philadelphia: Saunders; 1990.

Wagner H, Holder J. Treatment of osteoarthritis of the hip by corrective osteotomy of the greater trochanter. In: Schatzker J, ed. The Intertrochanteric Osteotomy. Berlin: Springer; 1984.

Wagner H. Die Verschiebeosteotomie als Korrekturprinzip. In: Hierholzer G, Müller KH, eds. Korrekturosteotomien nach Traumen an der unteren Extremität. Heidelberg: Springer; 1984.

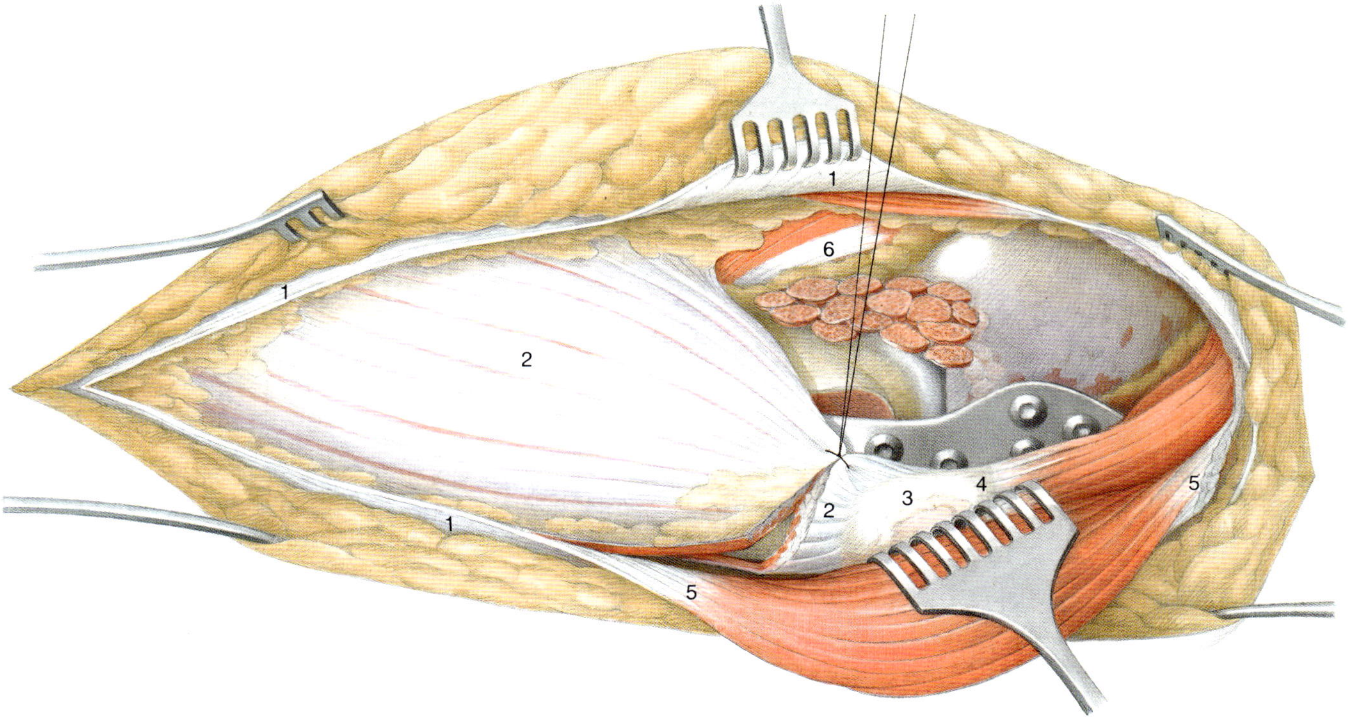

Fig. 2.**318** After the plate has been completely fastened and the hip has been filled with graft, the greater trochanter is returned to its original position. The vastus lateralis is reattached to the greater trochanter under tension.

1 Fascia lata
2 Vastus lateralis
3 Greater trochanter
4 Gluteus medius
5 Tensor fasciae latae
6 Iliopsoas

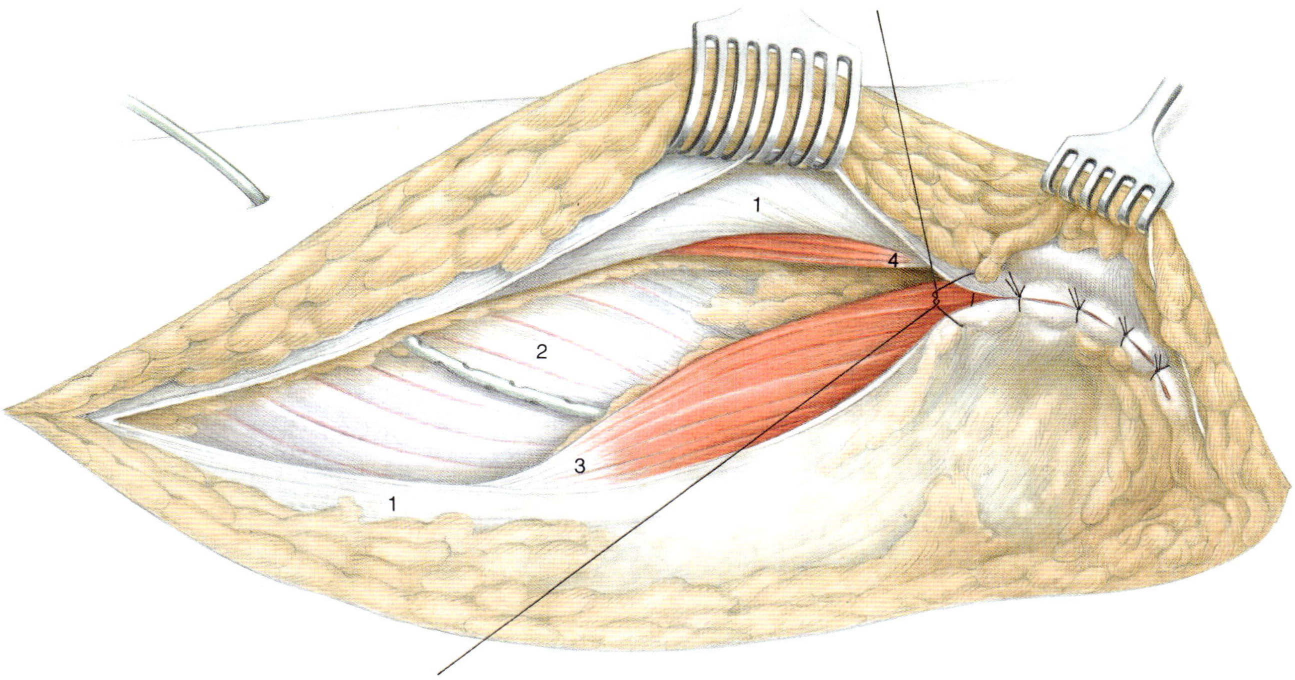

Fig. 2.**319** A deep suction drain is placed, the tensor fasciae latae is reattached, and the fascia lata is closed with retention sutures. The wound is then closed in layers.

1 Fascia lata
2 Vastus lateralis
3 Tensor fasciae latae
4 Sartorius

3 Primary Total Hip Arthroplasty

F. Kerschbaumer

Introduction

For clarity, we have divided the chapter on total hip arthroplasty into separate sections on acetabular components and femoral components. The section on acetabular implants describes the surgical procedure for the cementless threaded acetabular cup and the cemented polyethylene acetabular cup. The section on femoral components describes the technique for cemented and cementless straight-stem implants and the implantation of custom cementless femoral components. Our treatment of the subject is limited to a few implant models with which we have personal experience.

Preoperative Planning

Preoperative planning is generally simple. Clinical examination reveals the difference in leg length and the presence of possible flexion/adduction or external rotation contractures. A plain pelvic radiograph (Fig. 3.**1a**) and a prosthetic template are used to determine the size of the acetabular cup.

The template is inclined 45° so that the inferior margin of the acetabular cup is level with the acetabular teardrop. The center of the acetabular cup (PM) is marked, and the contour of the acetabular cup is traced on the radiograph (Fig. 3.**1b**). The surgeon then superimposes the stem template on the femur to determine the probable size of the femoral component. The center of the prosthetic head (KM) should be approximately level with the apex of the greater trochanter (Fig. 3.**1c**). Ideally, points PM and KM should align. When leg length has been equalized, they are at the same height.

The surgeon now traces the contours of the femur and femoral component on the acetate sheet and marks the height of the shoulder of the implant in relation to the apex of the greater trochanter. The osteotomy plane is also marked on the femoral neck. Now the surgeon moves the acetate sheet medially until points PM and KM are aligned and traces the contours of the pelvis and the acetabular cup (Fig. 3.**1d**).

Special Cases

Precise preoperative planning of the femoral component is difficult with *external roation* and *flexion contractures.* Here, the surgeon can determine the approximate size by superimposing the femoral implant template on the radiograph of the contralateral femur.

When severe *coxa vara* or a previous varus osteotomy makes it difficult to achieve axial alignment, the surgeon should consider performing a trochanteric osteotomy. In the preoperative planning, it must also be considered that a leg-length difference may be desirable when a unilateral varus osteotomy has been performed, whereas a difference in leg length is best avoided when treating primary coxa vara with total hip arthroplasty.

In *coxa valga,* the plane of osteotomy on the femoral neck is higher than normal. Since the center of the prosthetic head (KM) is higher than the greater trochanter, a longer stem will be required.

In *juvenile chronic polyarthritis* or *ankylosing spondylitis* with stiffening of the joint, the surgeon should plan a double osteotomy of the femoral neck parallel to the plane of the rim of the acetabulum and at the customary site, about 1 – 1.5 cm superior to the lesser trochanter. The knee should be included in the preoperative clinical and, if necessary, radiological examinations; valgus malalignment of the knee is often encountered in patients suffering from chronic polyarthritis. Implants with a valgus neck-shaft angle (greater than 135°) and only a slight offset (lateral displacement) should not be used in these patients. Implants with lateral displacement should be used in these patients to avoid increased stress in the lateral knee joint and subsequent pain.

Preoperative planning for patients with arthritic hip dysplasia or developmentally dislocated hips will be discussed later in the section on dysplastic acetabular cups.

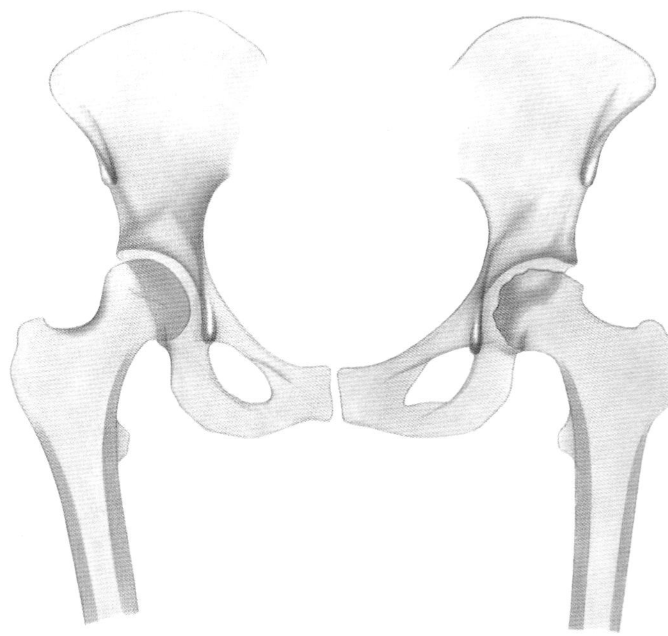

Fig. 3.**1a** Preoperative plain pelvic radiograph showing osteoarthritis of the left hip

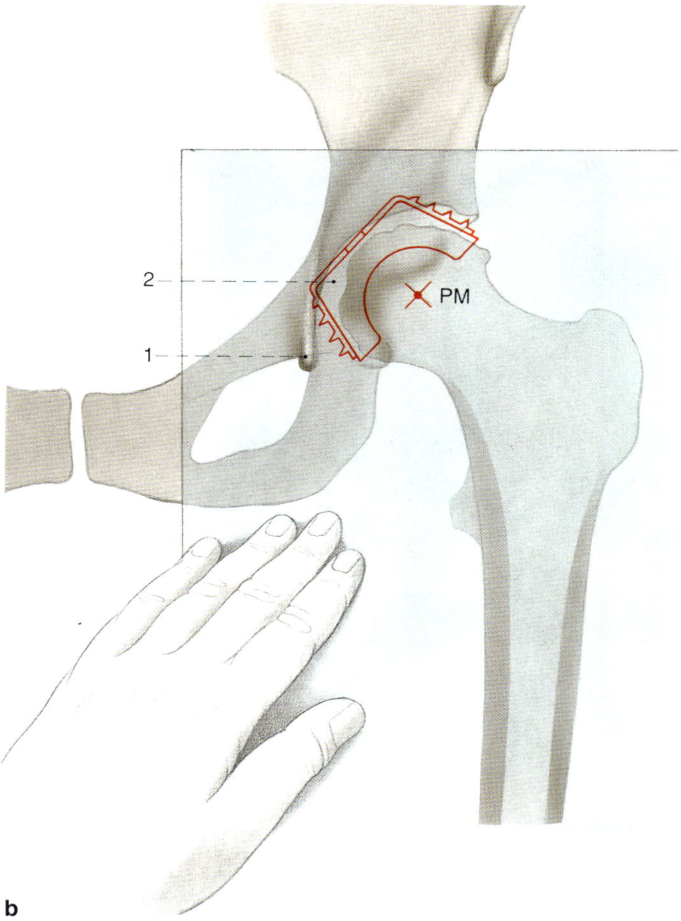

b

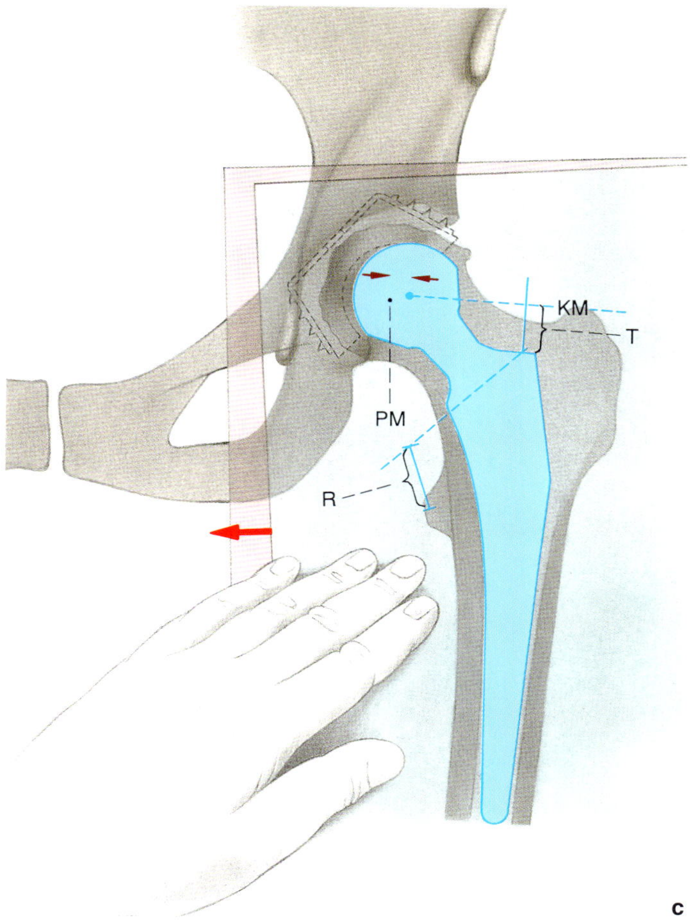

c

Fig. 3.**1 b** When the size of the acetabular cup has been determined, the radiograph is superimposed on the template for the acetabular cup and rotated until the cup is in an anatomically correct position. Then the center of the acetabular cup (PM) is marked, and the outline of the acetabular cup is traced on the radiograph.

1 Acetabular teardrop
2 Acetabular cup template
PM Center of the acetabular cup

Fig. 3.**1 c** The stem template is superimposed on the femur in the radiograph to determine the size of the femoral component. Then the contours of the femoral shaft and the implant are traced on a superimposed acetate sheet.

PM Center of the acetabular cup
KM Center of the prosthetic head
T Distance from greater trochanter to shoulder of the implant
R Distance from lesser trochanter to plane of osteotomy

Fig. 3.**1 d** The acetate sheet is moved medially until points PM and KM are aligned, and the contours of the pelvis and the acetabular cup are traced. The drawing is now complete.

PM Center of the acetabular cup
KM Center of the prosthetic head
T Distance from greater trochanter to shoulder of the implant
R Distance from lesser trochanter to plane of osteotomy

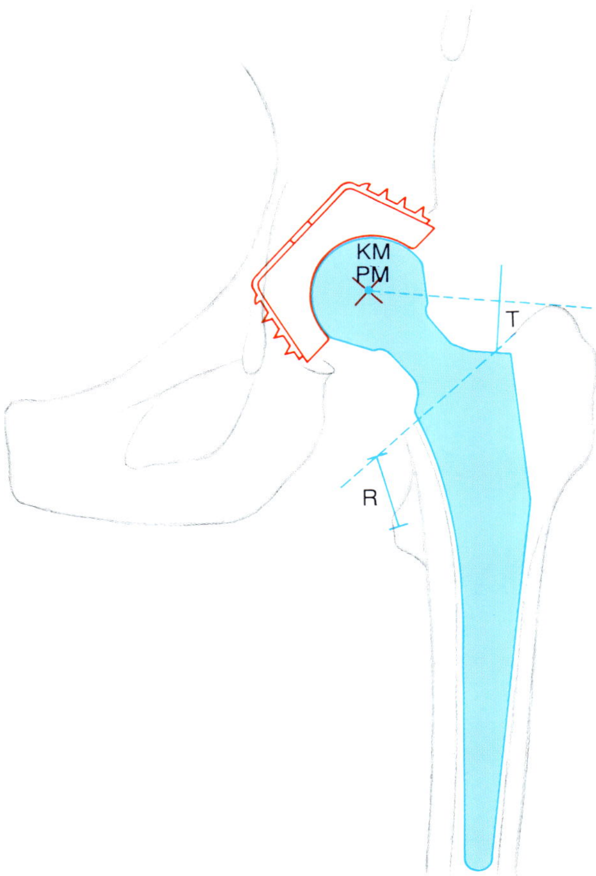

d

Cemented Acetabular Cup

Indications

- Osteoarthritis of the hip
- Medial dislocated femoral neck fracture in older patients
- Osteoporosis accompanied by osteoarthritis
- Arthritic hip dysplasia

The cemented acetabular cup is used primarily in older patients with osteoporosis or chronic polyarthritis. Metal spacer rings are indicated where there are extensive bony defects or when osteoporosis is present.

Positioning and Incision

The patient is positioned supine or in a lateral position according to the approach. The following section describes the surgical technique for a transgluteal approach with the patient supine (see Chapter 1: Approaches). The leg is prepped and draped to permit free movement. The inguinal region should remain accessible in case a tenotomy of the adductors is required after the prosthesis is implanted. The abdomen and thorax should also be prepared and draped to permit retroperitoneal exposure of the internal iliac artery if pelvic bleeding occurs. The patient is placed on a radiolucent operating table to facilitate intraoperative fluoroscopy.

Surgical Technique

After the capsule has been incised, two narrow Hohmann retractors are inserted around the femoral neck. With the leg externally rotated, traction is applied to dislocate the hip. If necessary, a so-called "corkscrew" can be used (Fig. 3.**2**). After resecting osteophytes on the anterior femoral neck, we osteotomize the femoral neck using an oscillating saw, inserting two Hohmann retractors to protect soft tissue (Fig. 3.**3**). The plane of osteotomy lies at ay 45° angle to the axis of the femoral shaft and is generally 1 – 1.5 cm proximal to the lesser trochanter. In a fracture of the femoral neck, the fragments of the femoral head are first removed, and then the neck is cut with the oscillating saw.

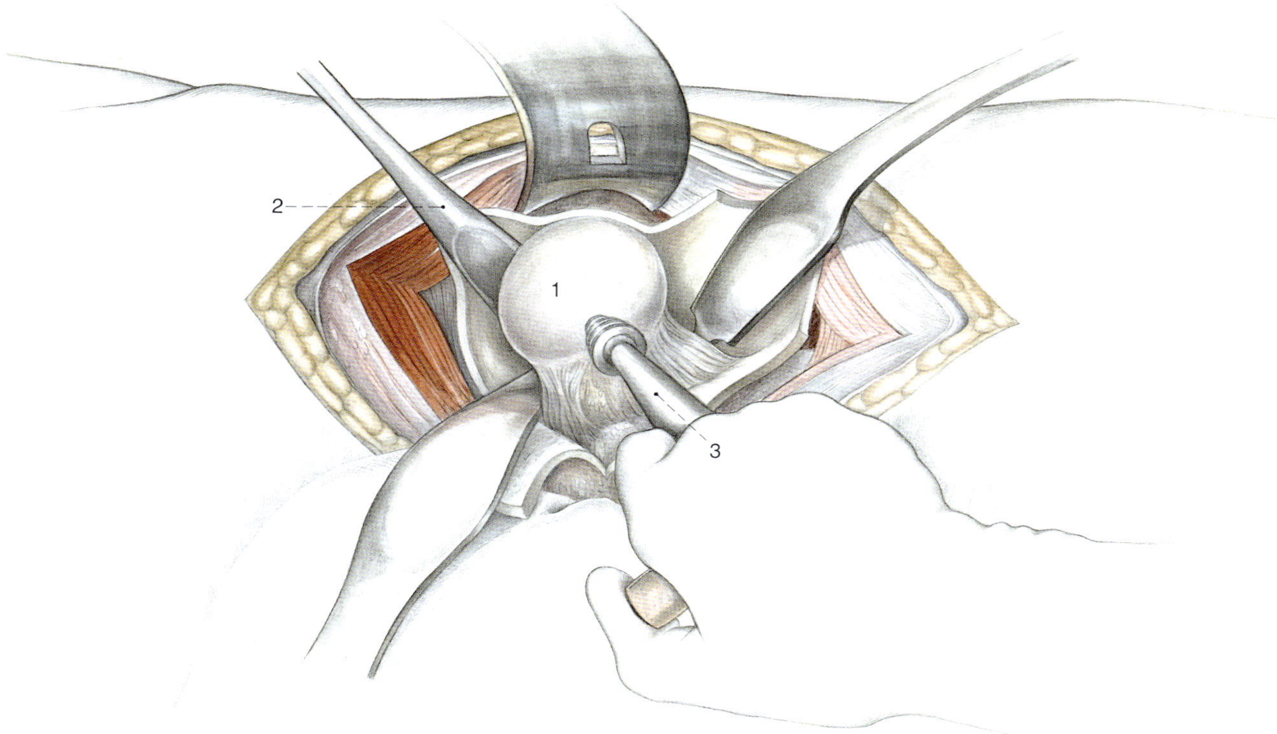

Fig. 3.**2** Dislocating the hip using a "corkscrew" and a hip skid.

1 Femoral head
2 Hip skid
3 Corkscrew

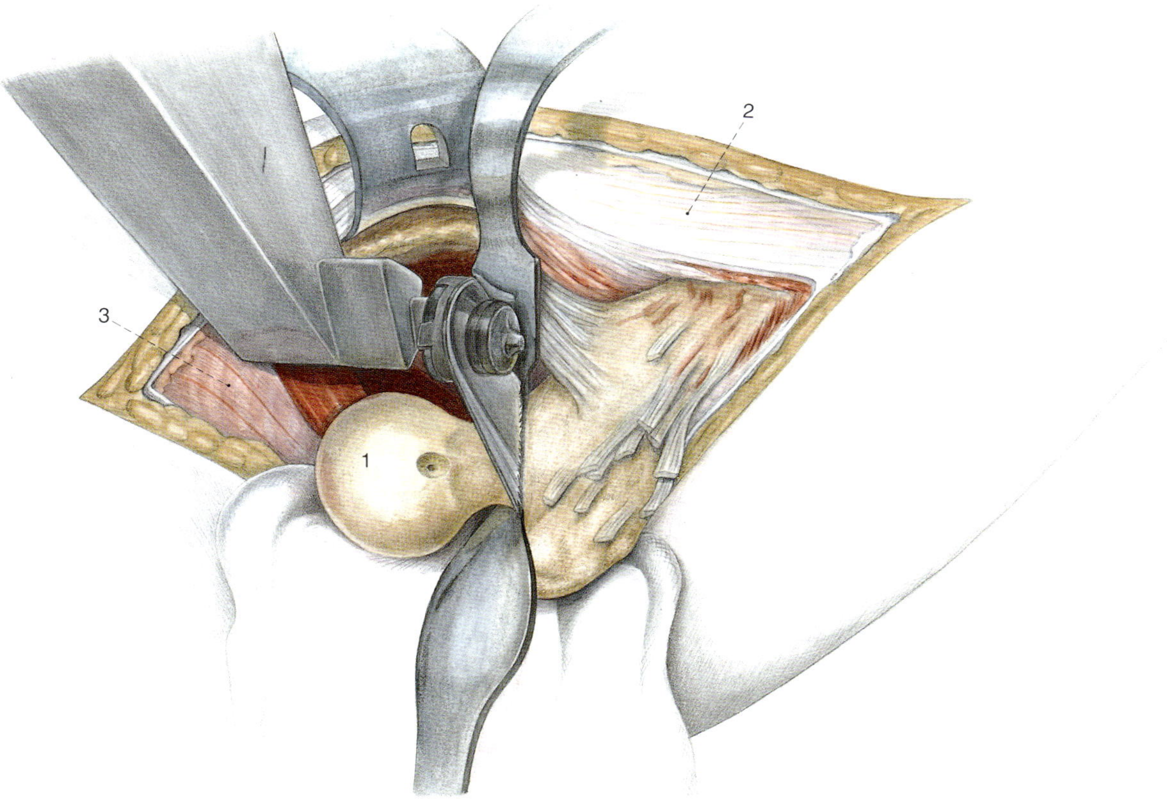

Fig. 3.**3** Osteotomy of the femoral neck according to preoperative planning. With collarless straight-stem implants, the plane of osteotomy lies at a 45° angle to the femoral shaft. Two Hohmann retractors are inserted around the femoral neck to protect soft tissue.

1 Femoral head
2 Vastus lateralis
3 Gluteus medius

The anterior circumference of the flaps of the incised capsule is exposed, and the psoas musculature and iliopsoas tendon are transected with a periosteal elevator and dissection scissors (Fig. 3.**4**). The taut fascia connecting the superior capsule to the gluteus minimus must also be dissected. Next either a partial or total capsulectomy is performed (Fig. 3.**5**). A total capsulectomy is preferable where contracture is present and in revision surgery. If soft tissue is not contracted, the posteroinferior capsule can be left intact. In any case, broad exposure of the entire circumference of the acetabulum is required. The surgeon locates the cotyloid notch and transverse acetabular ligament and inserts a narrow Hohmann retractor around it. A femoral retractor is used to expose the posteroinferior acetabular margin (Fig. 3.**6**).

A Müller elevator may also be impacted into the ischium for this purpose.

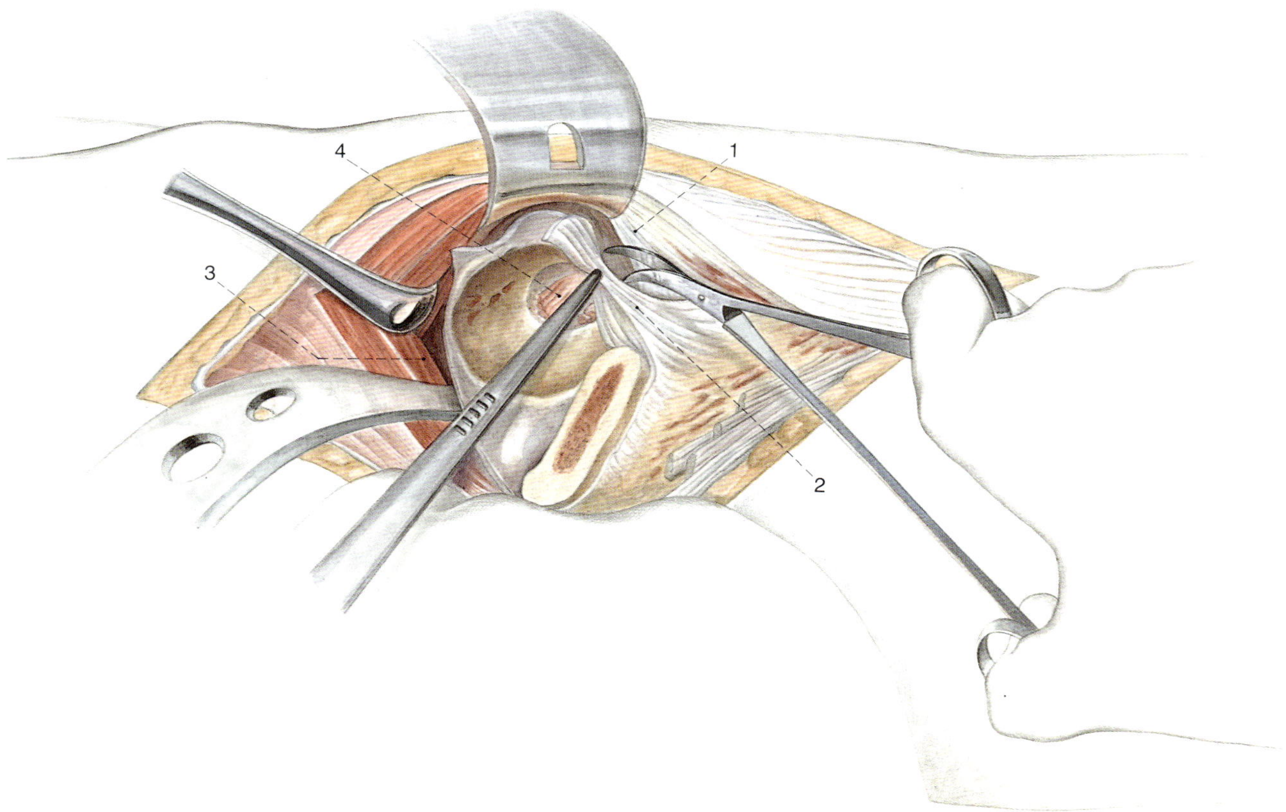

Fig. 3.**4** Releasing the hip capsule from its soft-tissue attachments. Dissection between the iliopsoas tendon and anterior capsule, and between the posterosuperior capsule and gluteus minimus.

1 Iliopsoas tendon
2 Joint capsule
3 Gluteus minimus
4 Acetabular fossa

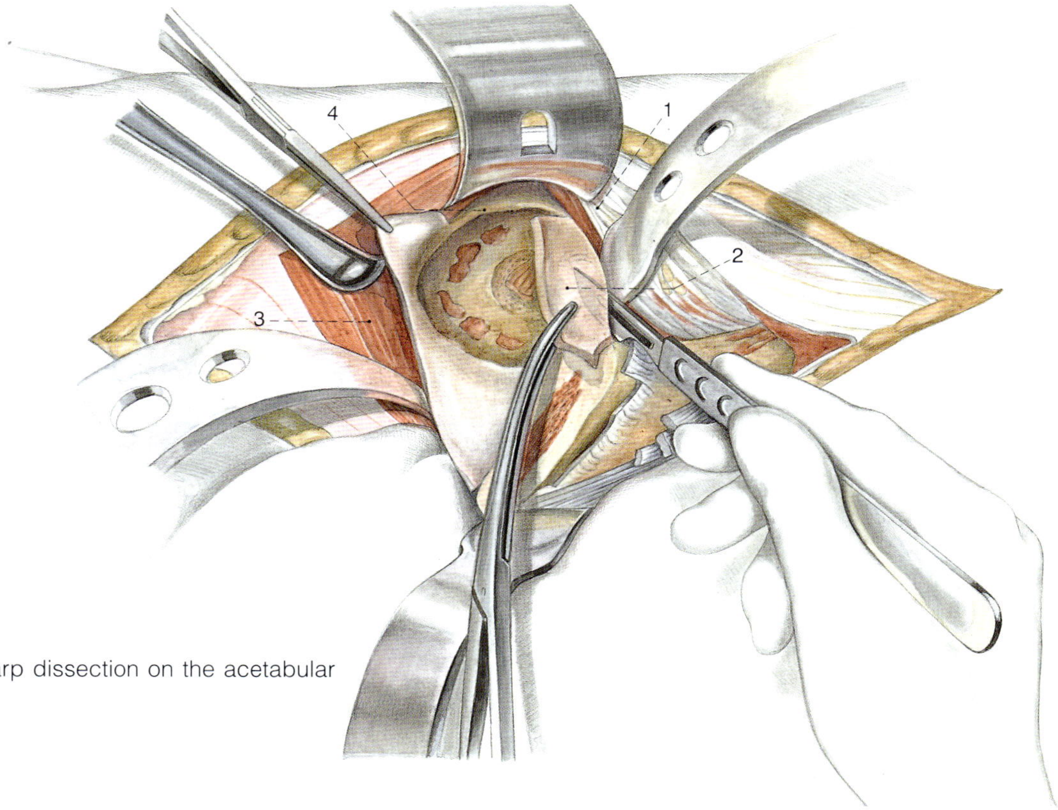

Fig. 3.**5** Capsulectomy with sharp dissection on the acetabular margin and femur.

1 Iliopsoas tendon
2 Joint capsule
3 Gluteus minimus
4 Anterior margin of the acetabulum

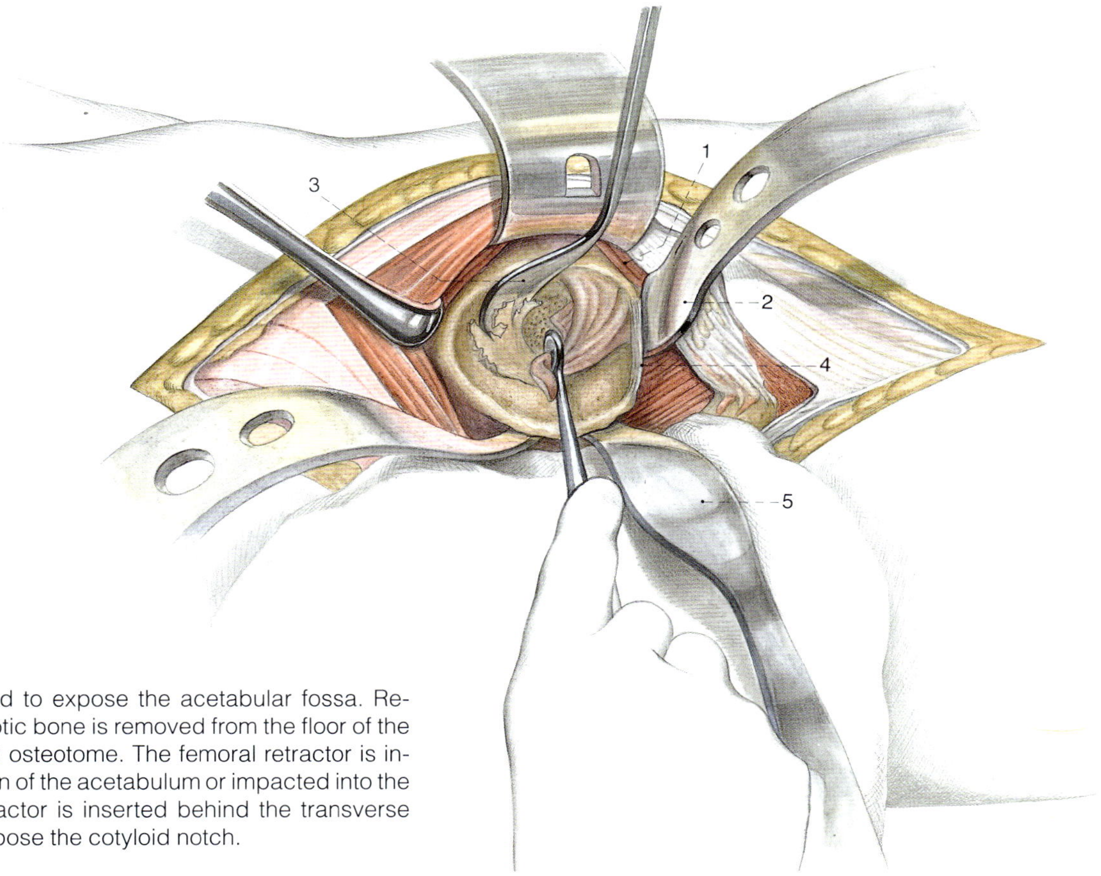

Fig. 3.**6** A curette is used to expose the acetabular fossa. Residual cartilage and sclerotic bone is removed from the floor of the acetabulum with a curved osteotome. The femoral retractor is inserted at the inferior margin of the acetabulum or impacted into the ischium. A Hohmann retractor is inserted behind the transverse acetabular ligament to expose the cotyloid notch.

1 Iliopsoas
2 Hohmann retractor behind the transverse acetabular ligament
3 Osteotome
4 Transverse acetabular ligament
5 Femoral retractor

The soft tissue is dissected from the floor of the acetabulum and the acetabular fossa with a curette. In patients with severe chronic osteoarthritis with sclerotic bone, subluxation of the hip, and a "double floor" of the acetabulum, the acetabulum should be deeply excavated with a curved osteotome. A small acetabular reamer (44 mm) is used in normal bone. We use this reamer to clean the floor of the acetabulum. It is not initially inserted parallel to the plane of the rim of the acetabulum, but perpendicular to the longitudinal axis of the body. We use progressively larger reamers to prepare the floor of the acetabulum, taking care not to remove the subchondral bone layer on the roof of the acetabulum (Fig. 3.**7**). When a 50 mm polyethylene cup is used, the surgeon should ream the acetabulum to 52–54 cm.

To ensure a good base for the cement, the surgeon continues reaming until bleeding bone becomes visible on the sclerotic roof of the acetabulum, being careful to prevent the reamer from wandering superiorly and anteriorly. This is best done by stabilizing the powered shaft by hand with a Teflon grip (Fig. 3.**7**). The products of reaming are kept for filling cysts in the roof of the acetabulum. Verify the correct parallel orientation of the largest reamer, i.e., inclined 45° with 10–20° of anteversion (Fig. 3.**8a**).

After removing the reamings from the floor of the acetabulum, we insert a trial cup 2–4 mm smaller than the last reamer used. We use a cup positioner (Fig. 3.**8b** and **c**) to align the acetabular cup (inclined 45° with 10–20° of anteversion). The surgeon must ensure that the patient's pelvis is level to avoid underestimating the anteversion of the acetabular cup. If the anterior superior iliac spine on the affected side is higher than that of the contralateral side, then the operating table should be inclined before proceeding. Now the surgeon can also determine the depth of the acetabular cup. Projecting osteophytes are removed (Fig. 3.**9**).

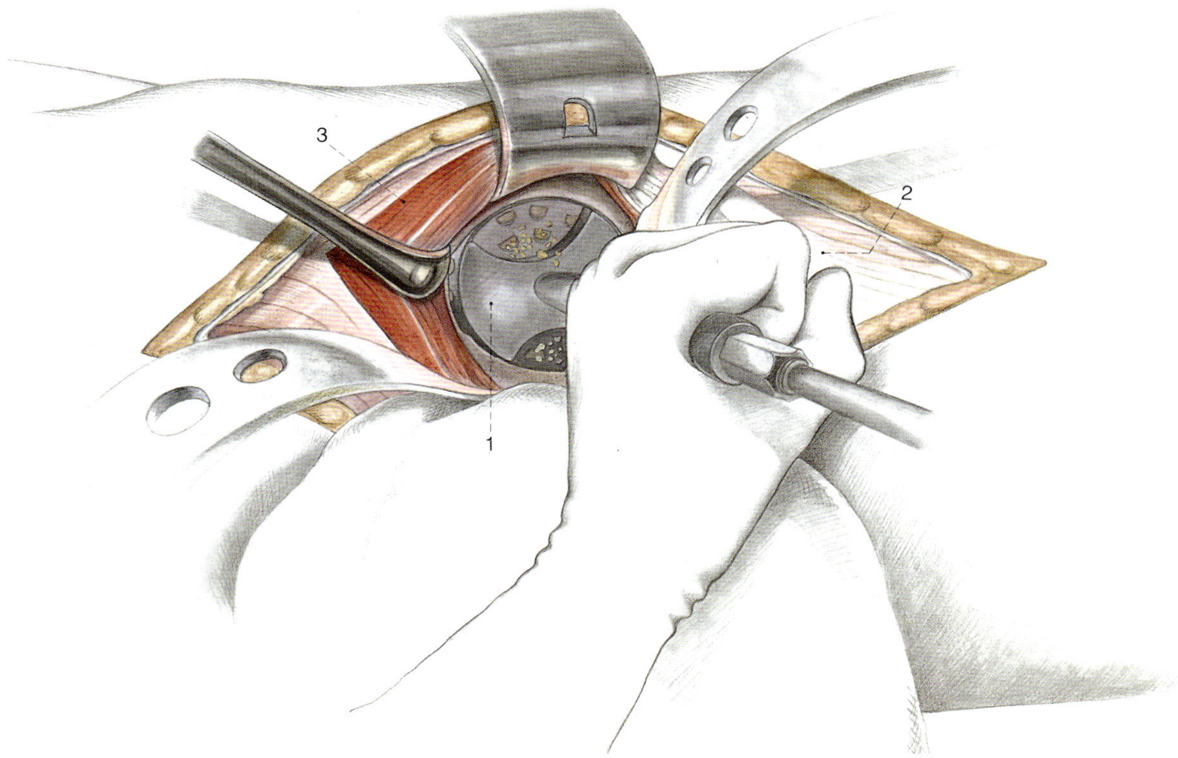

Fig. 3.**7** A powered acetabular reamer with successively larger heads is used to prepare the acetabulum. After initially inserting the smallest head medially, the surgeon reams parallel to the plane of the rim of the acetabulum.

1 Acetabular reamer
2 Vastus lateralis
3 Gluteus medius

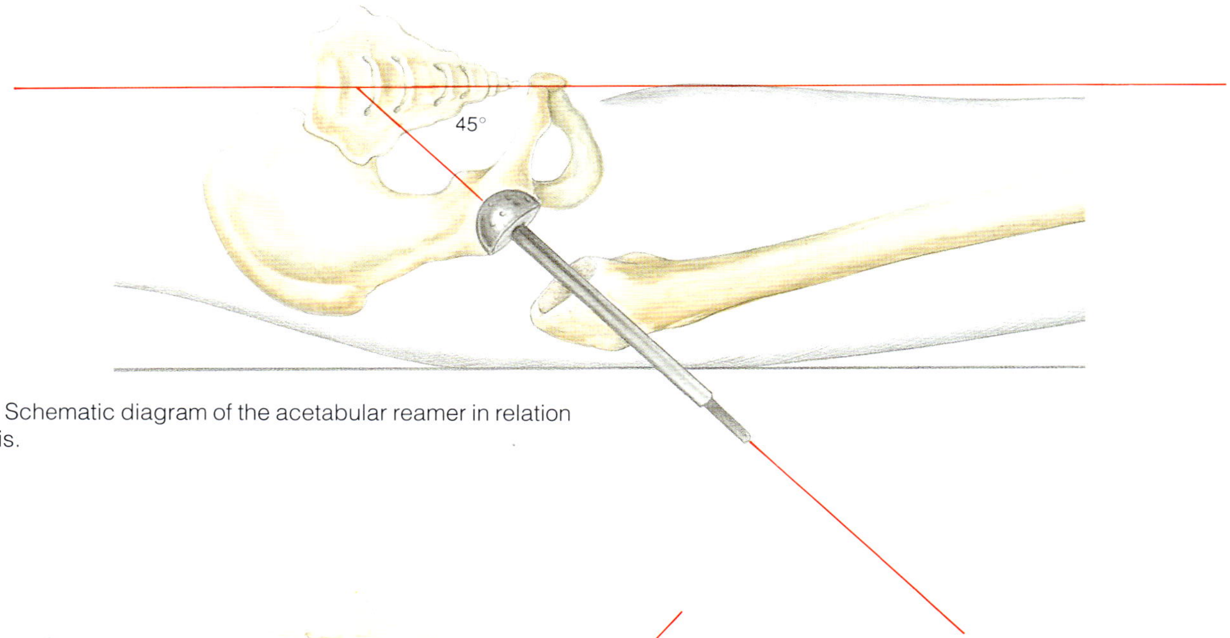

Fig. 3.**8a** Schematic diagram of the acetabular reamer in relation to the pelvis.

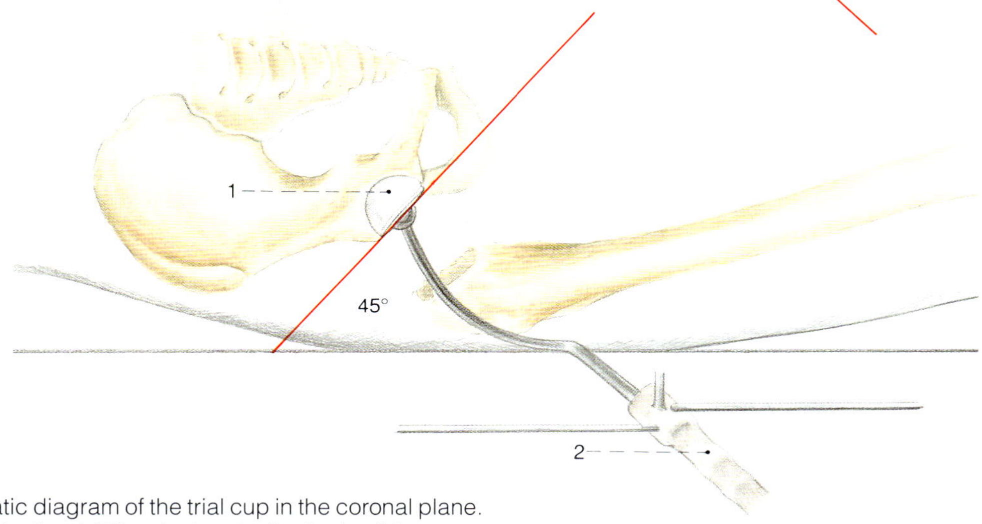

Fig. 3.**8b** Schematic diagram of the trial cup in the coronal plane. Note that the cup is inclined 45° to the longitudinal axis of the operating table. The bars of the cup positioner are parallel to the edge of the table. The transverse axis of the pelvis should be perpendicular to the longitudinal axis of the operating table.

1 Trial cup
2 Cup positioner

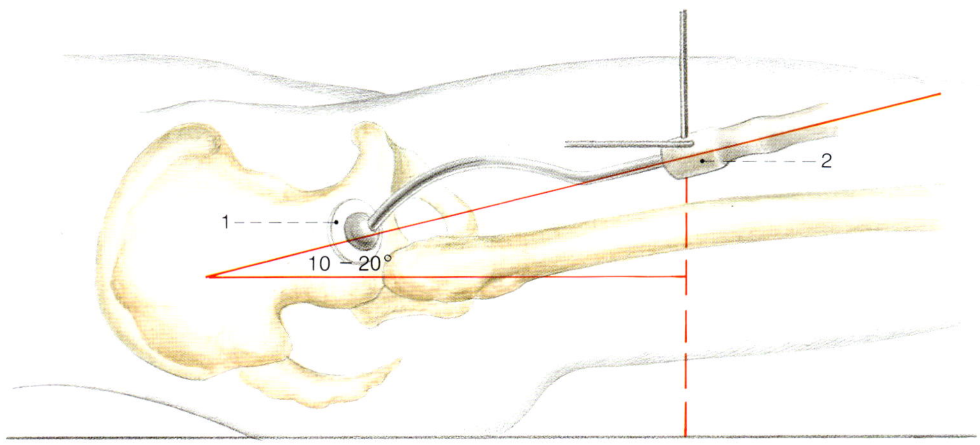

Fig. 3.**8c** Schematic diagram of the position of the trial cup in the sagittal plane. The trial cup should have 10–20° of anteversion. The vertical bar of the cup positioner is perpendicular to the operating table.

1 Trial cup
2 Cup positioner

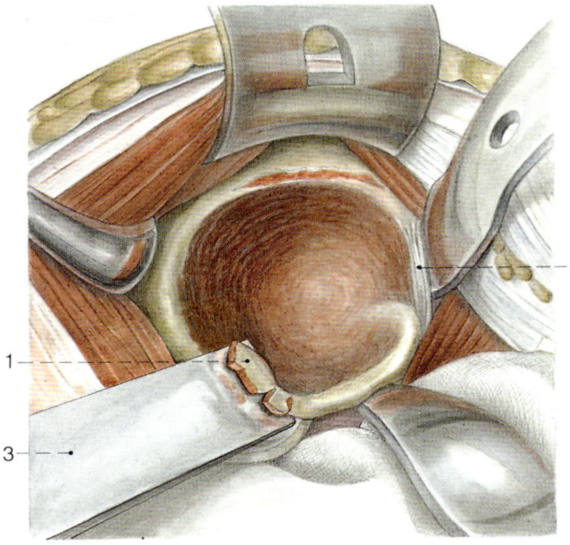

Fig. 3.**9** Projecting osteophytes are removed with an osteotome.

1 Posterior osteophyte
2 Transverse acetabular ligament
3 Osteotome

The surgeon now drills three or four holes in the roof of the acetabulum parallel to the lines of force with a calibrated 6 mm drill bit (Fig. 3.**10**). The holes are cleaned with a sharp curette, and the acetabulum is thoroughly irrigated to completely remove all residual reamings. The acetabulum is then packed with thrombin-impregnated compresses. While the acetabulum is drying, the cement is mixed and prepared for implantation. Cooled precompressed cement should be used. When the thrombin-impregnated compresses have been removed, the cement is pressed against the sides and floor of the acetabulum with a curette or swab (Fig. 3.**11**). We insert the polyethylene acetabular cup into the acetabulum by hand or with an inserter, keeping it as horizontal as possible (Fig. 3.**12a**). This permits deep insertion into the acetabulum while allowing excess cement to escape. Then we tilt the inserter to achieve the desired cup angle of 45° to horizontal and 10–20 ° anteversion (Fig. 3.**12b**).

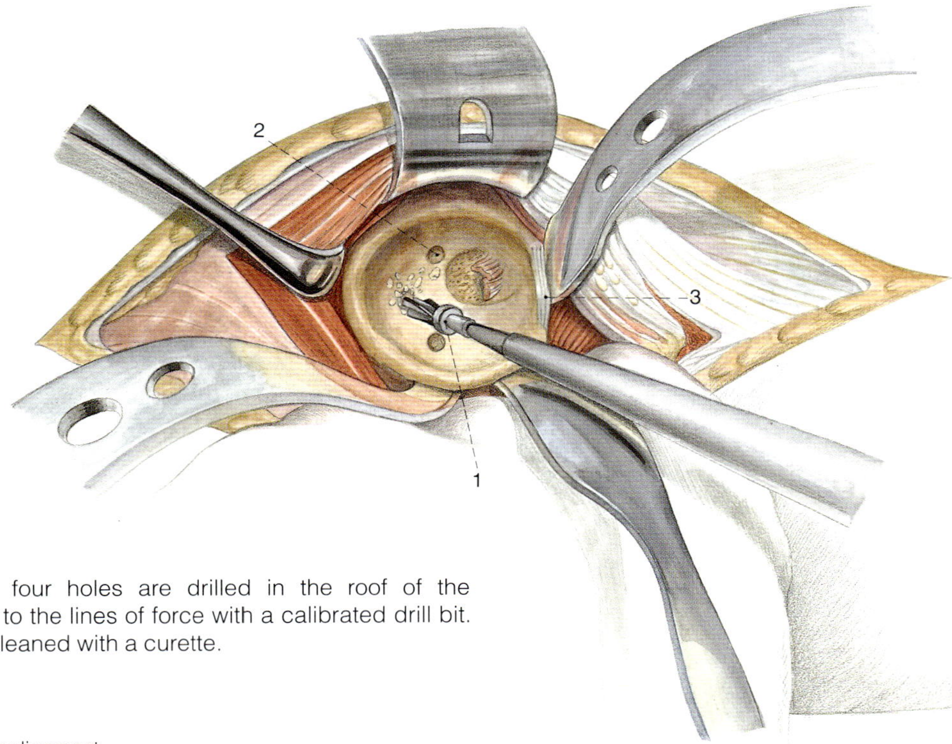

Fig. 3.**10** Three or four holes are drilled in the roof of the acetabulum parallel to the lines of force with a calibrated drill bit. The holes are then cleaned with a curette.

1 Calibrated drill
2 Hole in acetabulum
3 Transverse acetabular ligament

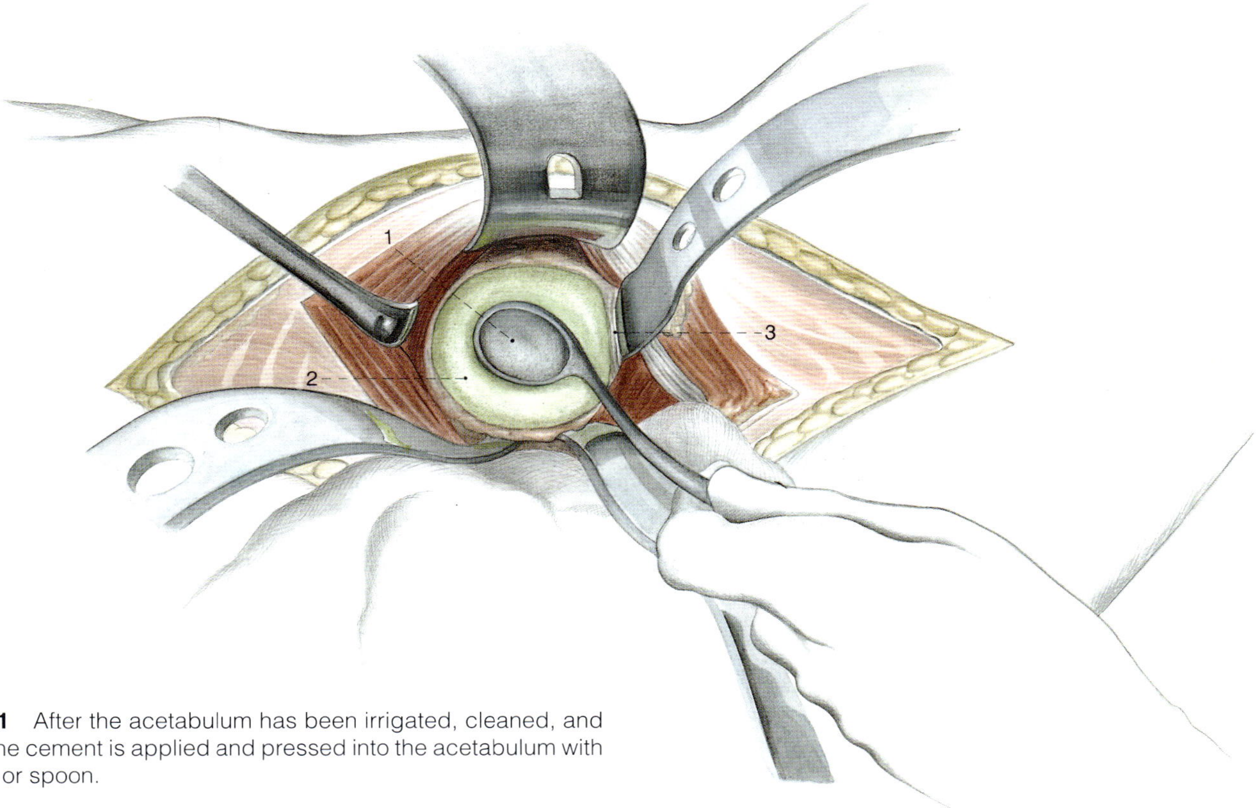

Fig. 3.**11** After the acetabulum has been irrigated, cleaned, and dried, the cement is applied and pressed into the acetabulum with a swab or spoon.

1 Cement
2 Spoon for pressing in cement
3 Transverse acetabular ligament

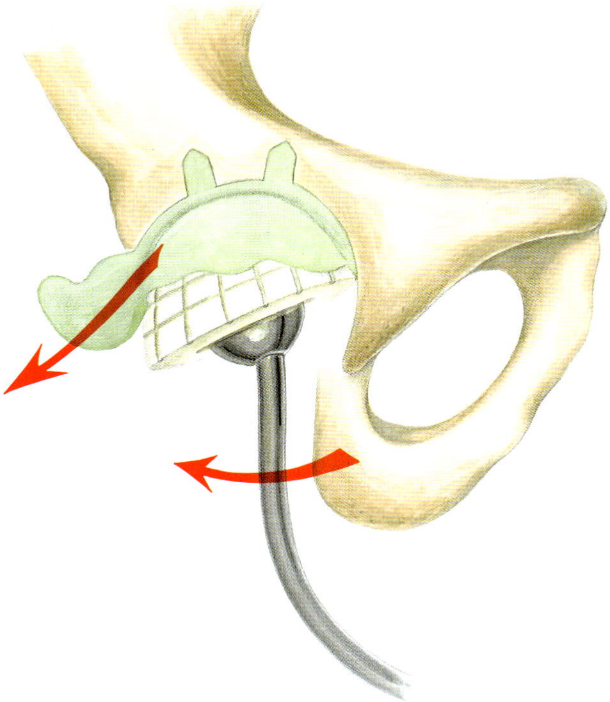

Fig. 3.**12a** The polyethylene acetabular cup is initially inserted into the acetabulum horizontally. Then the inserter is rotated so that it is parallel to the plane of the rim of the acetabulum. This permits deep insertion into the acetabulum while allowing excess cement to escape and avoiding lateral displacement.

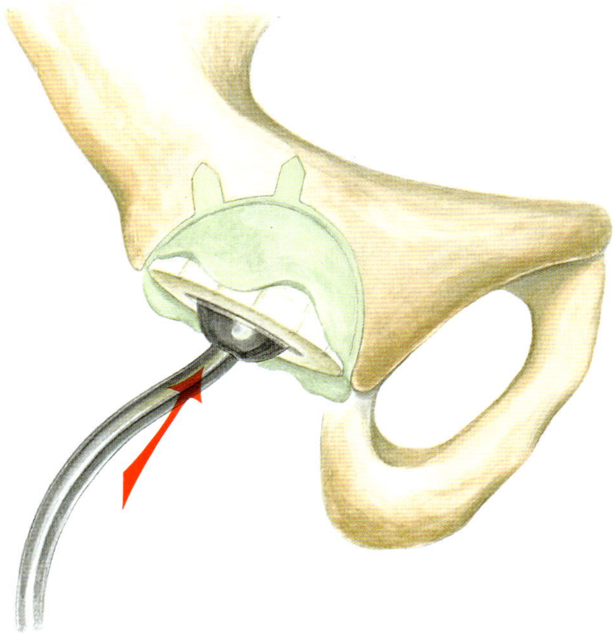

Fig. 3.**12b** Schematic diagram of the proper inclination with 10–20° anteversion. The inserter is held in this position, and light pressure is applied until the cement hardens.

While applying even pressure to the inserter, the surgeon cleans the excess cement from the circumference of the acetabulum with a curette (Fig. 3.**13**) to prevent any residual cement from breaking off and increasing polyethylene wear. The entire site is thoroughly irrigated during and after cement hardening.

Complications

Intraoperative and postoperative complications can occur if the circumference of the acetabulum is not sufficiently exposed. The acetabular labrum must be completely resected to expose the bony acetabular margin, particularly the superior rim. Often the surgeon will encounter bleeding from the medial femoral circumflex artery, which is easily overlooked if it is not located before implanting the stem. Drilling the holes in the roof of the acetabulum too deeply and penetrating the ilium can damage the superior gluteal artery, causing bleeding.

Using calibrated drill bits reduces the incidence of these complications. Careful reaming is necessary to avoid penetrating the floor of the acetabulum. Excessive traction on the elevator at the margin of the acetabulum can irritate the femoral nerve and cause paresis. Use of a curved Müller retractor has reduced the incidence of this complication. Paresis of the sciatic nerve is not generally the result of the acetabular dissection, but results from the nerve being stretched during the femoral dissection. The most common postoperative complication is dislocation of the hip in flexion, adduction, and internal rotation. This is generally the result of implanting the acetabular cup with insufficient anteversion; the surgeon should verify the stability of the implant components intraoperatively. Dislocation of the hip in extension and external rotation is generally the result of insufficient tension of the gluteal musculature or an acetabular cup that was implanted at too steep an angle or with too much anteversion.

Posterior dislocation can be corrected by adding a stabilizer (polyethylene spacer for the posterosuperior margin of the acetabulum), which is fastened to the polyethylene cup and the bone with two screws. If the hip dislocates in extension and external rotation, a longer femoral head component should be used.

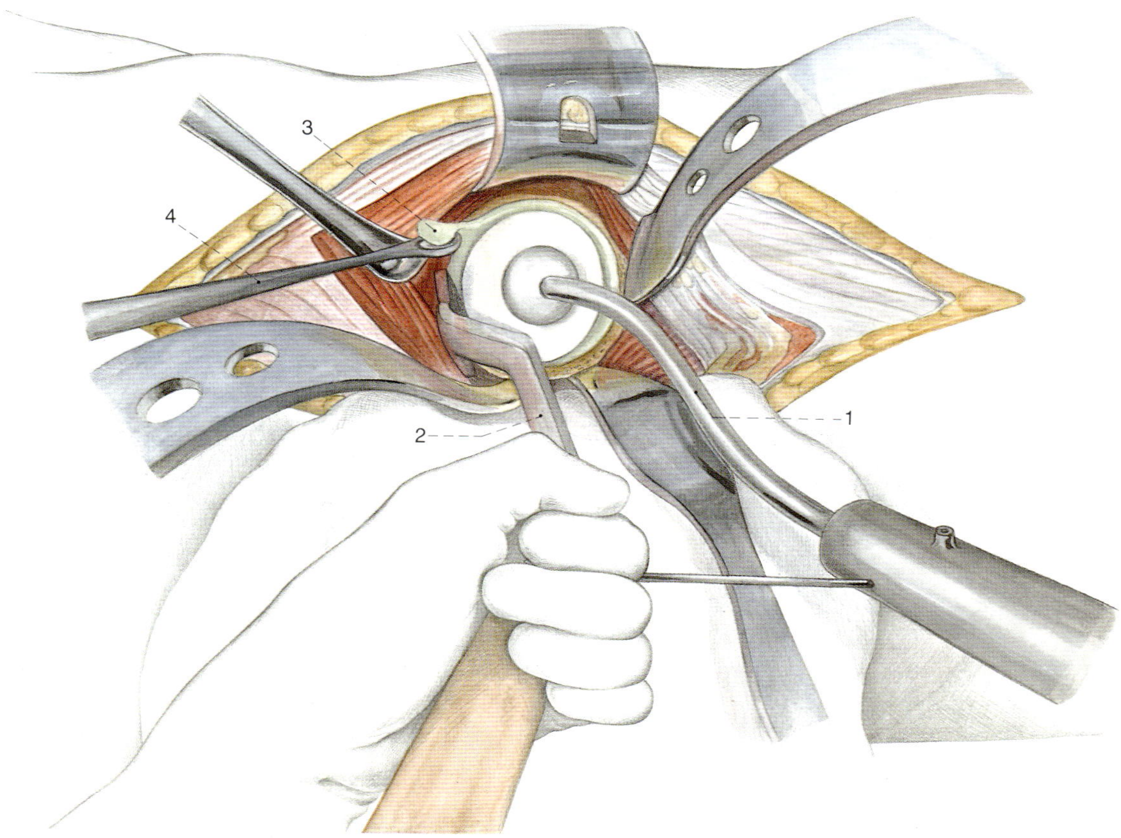

Fig. 3.**13** Excess cement is cleaned from the circumference of the acetabulum with a curette. Even pressure is applied to the inserter until the cement has hardened.

1 Cup positioner
2 Cement impactor
3 Cement
4 Curette

Zweymüller Cementless Acetabular Cup

Indications

Primary and secondary osteoarthritis of the hip, where the acetabular rim is intact.

Contraindications

- Severe osteoporosis
- Severe hip dysplasia with extensive acetabular defects

Principle

There are numerous cementless acetabular cups currently available. We will limit our discussion in this section, however, to the Zweymüller system, a conical self-threading titanium cup. These acetabular cups are anchored primarily around the circumference (and less on the floor) of the acetabulum. With this design, tilting is largely eliminated. Polyethylene liners in different shapes and thicknesses (for femoral heads of 28 or 32 mm diameter) with outer layers of titanium are inserted into the titanium cup.

This system generally provides high primary stability. We prefer not to use it in patients with severe osteoporosis, bony defects, or dysplastic acetabula.

Approach

Positioning, approach, and exposure of the acetabulum are identical to those described in the section "Cemented Acetabular Cups" (see Chapter 1: Approaches). Broad exposure of the acetabulum is the key to correct implantation. We recommend resecting the capsule and acetabular labrum completely to expose the bony margin of the acetabulum. The surgeon should retract the gluteal and rectus musculature sufficiently to prevent maceration when reaming the acetabulum and implanting the self-threading acetabular cup.

Surgical Technique

Residual cartilage is removed with a curved osteotome and an acetabular reamer (Fig. 3.**14**). Reaming is continued until bleeding subchondral bone is exposed. The soft tissue is completely resected from the floor of the acetabulum, and the osteophytes are removed to expose the plane of the acetabular rim (Fig. 3.**15**).

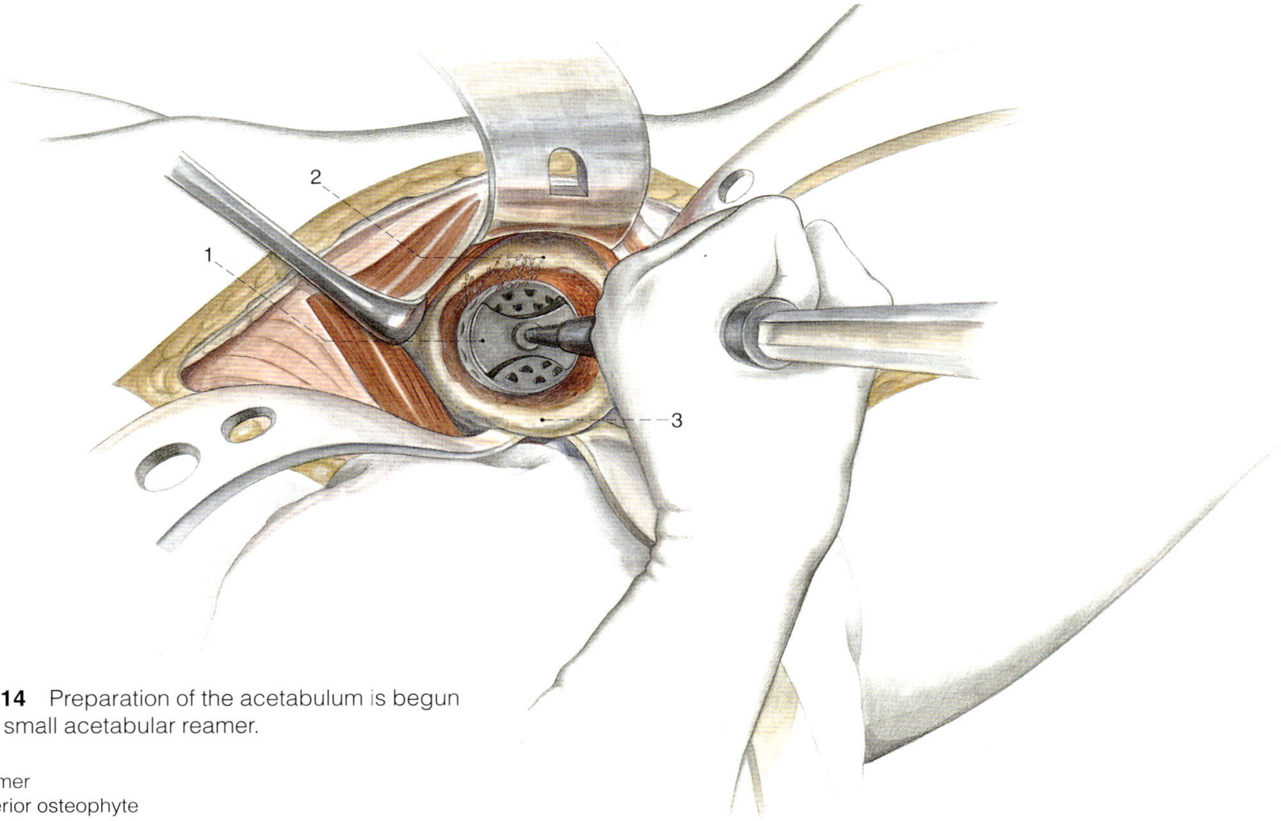

Fig. 3.**14** Preparation of the acetabulum is begun with a small acetabular reamer.

1 Reamer
2 Anterior osteophyte
3 Posterior osteophyte

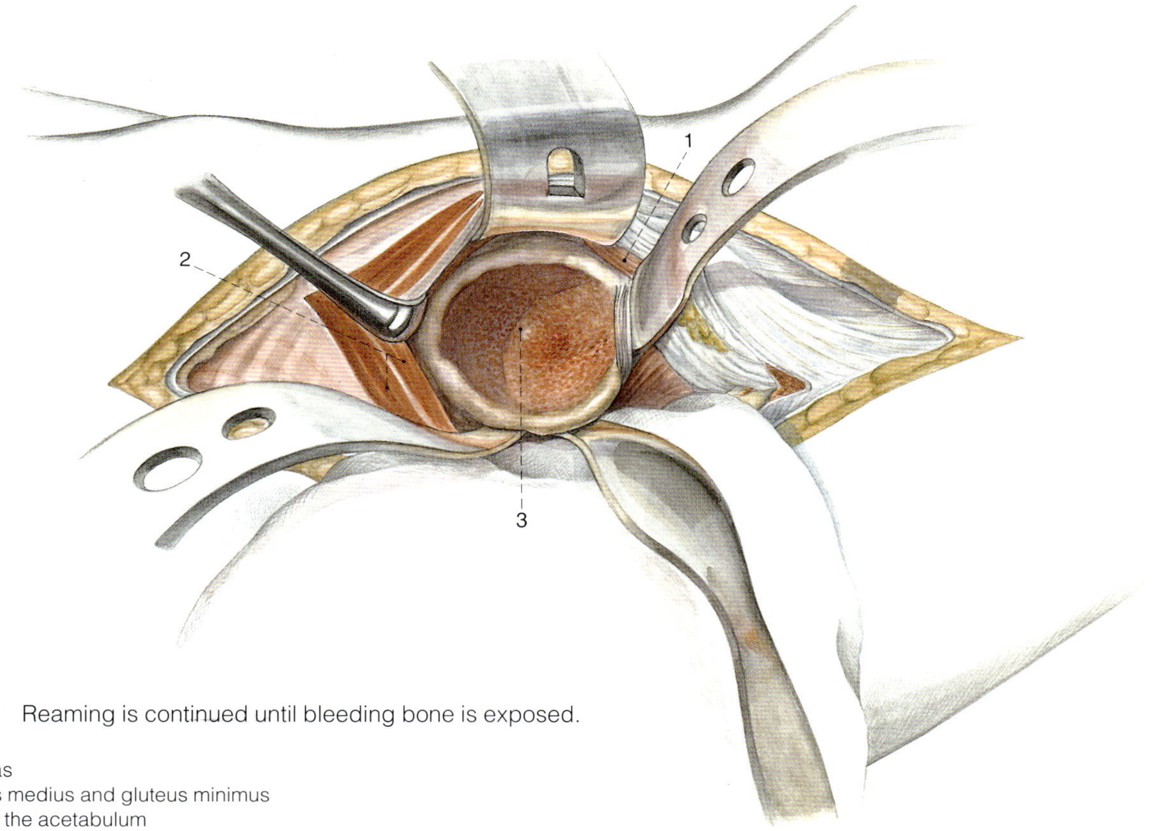

Fig. 3.**15** Reaming is continued until bleeding bone is exposed.

1 Iliopsoas
2 Gluteus medius and gluteus minimus
3 Floor of the acetabulum

Conical reamers are used to contour the initially hemispherical acetabulum to fit the titanium cup. We begin with the smallest reamer, inserting it at an angle of about 50° to horizontal with 10–20° anteversion (Fig. 3.**16**). We especially recommend this position for small and medium cups. For larger cups, we recommend a larger angle of inclination, i.e., the cup should be inserted at a steeper angle to avoid penetrating the floor of the acetabulum (Fig. 3.**17**). We continue reaming with successively larger cutting heads until the reamer engages the acetabular bone on all sides (Fig. 3.**18**). This is easy to judge because the surgeon can feel the reamer become slower as it encounters increasing resistance. Avoid removing too much bone, and ensure that the anterior and posterior rims of the acetabulum remain intact. Acetabula are not always ideally hemispherical, but are often oval or onion shaped; therefore, bony defects that are several millimeters deep often remain on the superior aspect. These defects are later filled with cancellous bone. In such an acetabulum, the surgeon should not use larger reamers in an attempt to seat the cup flush with the bone because this would compromise the stability of the anterior acetabular rim.

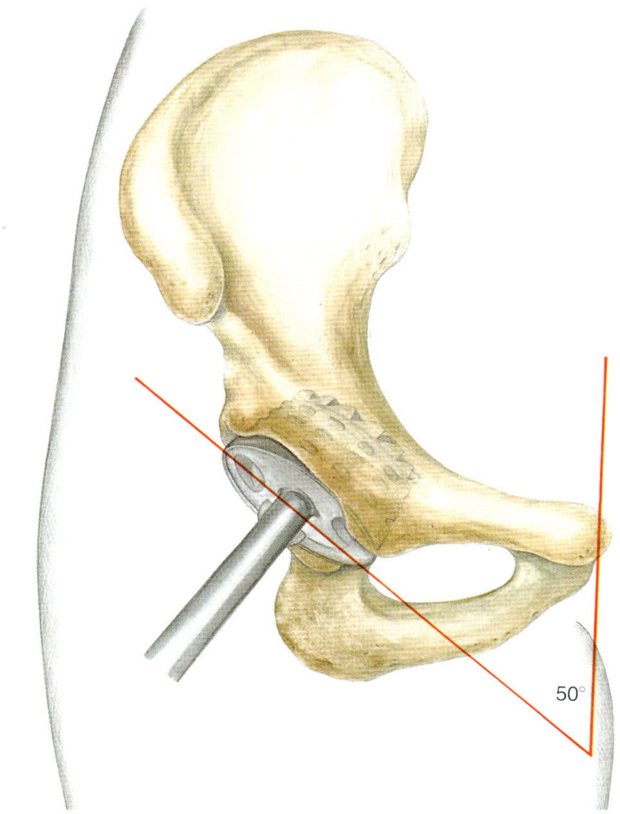

Fig. 3.**16** Schematic diagram of the position of a small conical acetabular reamer inclined 50°.

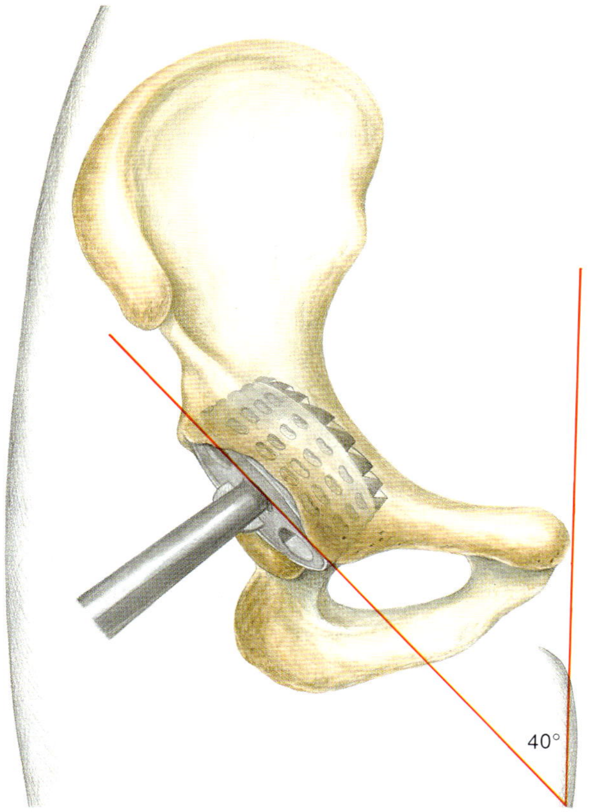

Fig. 3.**17** Schematik diagram of the conical acetabular reamer for larger implants inclined 40°.

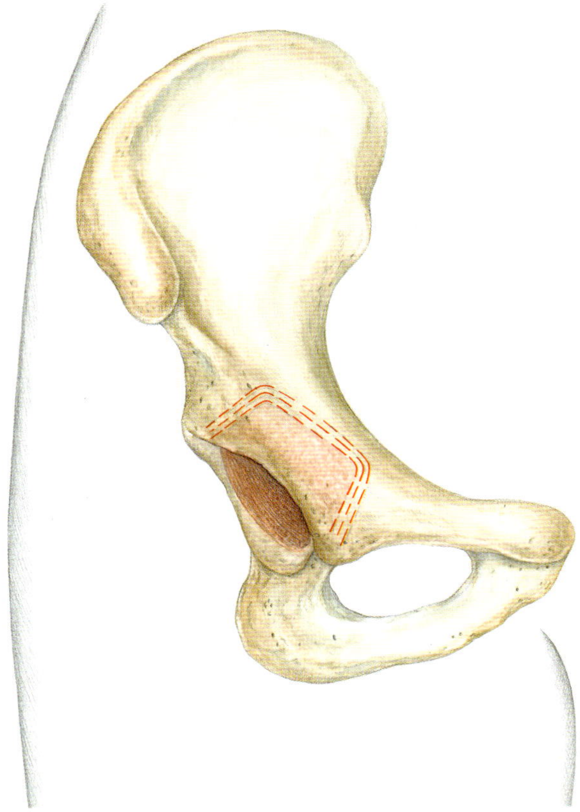

Fig. 3.**18** Schematic diagram of the prepared acetabulum. Conical reamers are used to contour the spherical acetabulum to accommodate the implant.

After the floor of the acetabulum has been irrigated and all reamings have been removed, the cup inserter is fitted with a self-threading titanium cup the same size as the last reamer. The cup inserter is centered in the same position as the reamer to ensure proper alignment, and the cup is impacted with two blows from a mallet to seat the cutting threads (Fig. 3.**19**). Since the cutting threads are still above the surface bone during this procedure, the surrounding soft tissue must be retracted to prevent maceration. Now the surgeon fits a ratchet handle onto the protruding shaft of the cup inserter (Fig. 3.**20**) and, having ensured proper alignment, turns the handle clockwise while applying slight pressure. The cup may be difficult to implant in male patients with sclerotic bone. The surgeon will notice this during the first few turns. If this is the case, a titanium cup that is 2 mm smaller can be used. However, the cup corresponding to the last reamer used can generally be screwed in as far as the floor of the acetabulum. Remove the cup inserter to check whether the cup has reached the floor of the acetabulum. In female patients with osteoporosis, the surgeon will encounter no resistance when screwing in the implant. Here, the surgeon should ascertain whether the implant has sufficient primary stability. If this is not the case, the cup should be removed and replaced with the next larger size.

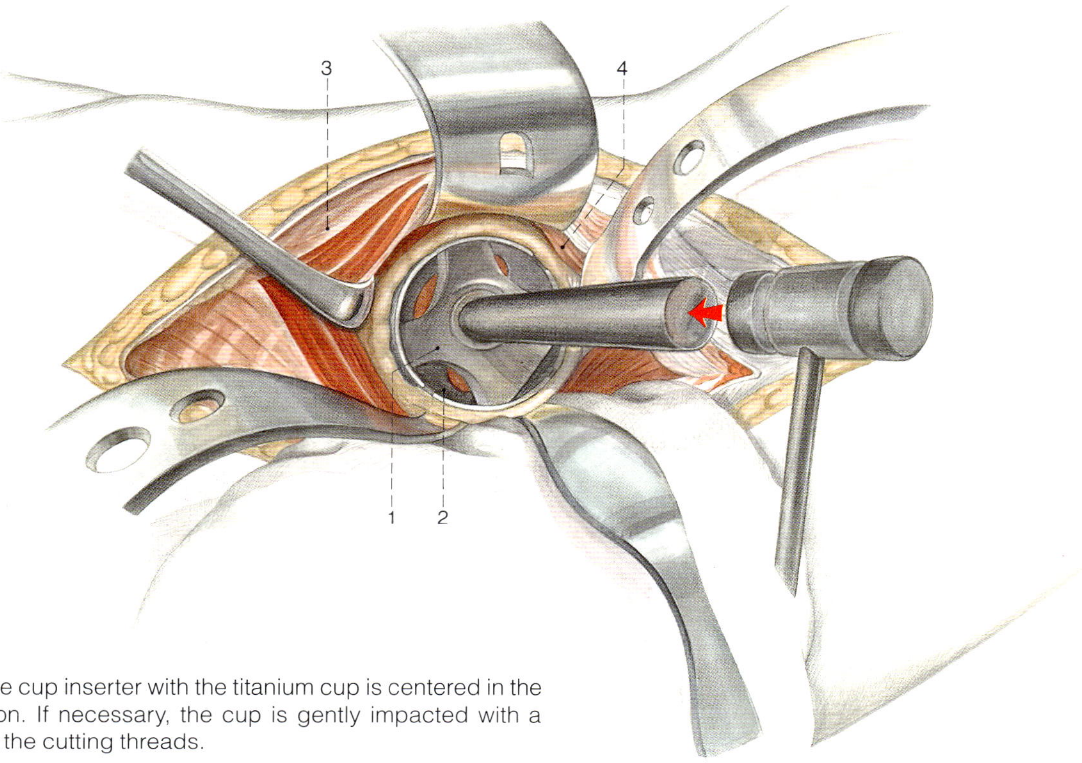

Fig. 3.**19** The cup inserter with the titanium cup is centered in the proper position. If necessary, the cup is gently impacted with a mallet to seat the cutting threads.

1 Cup inserter
2 Titanium cup with perforated floor
3 Gluteus medius
4 Iliopsoas

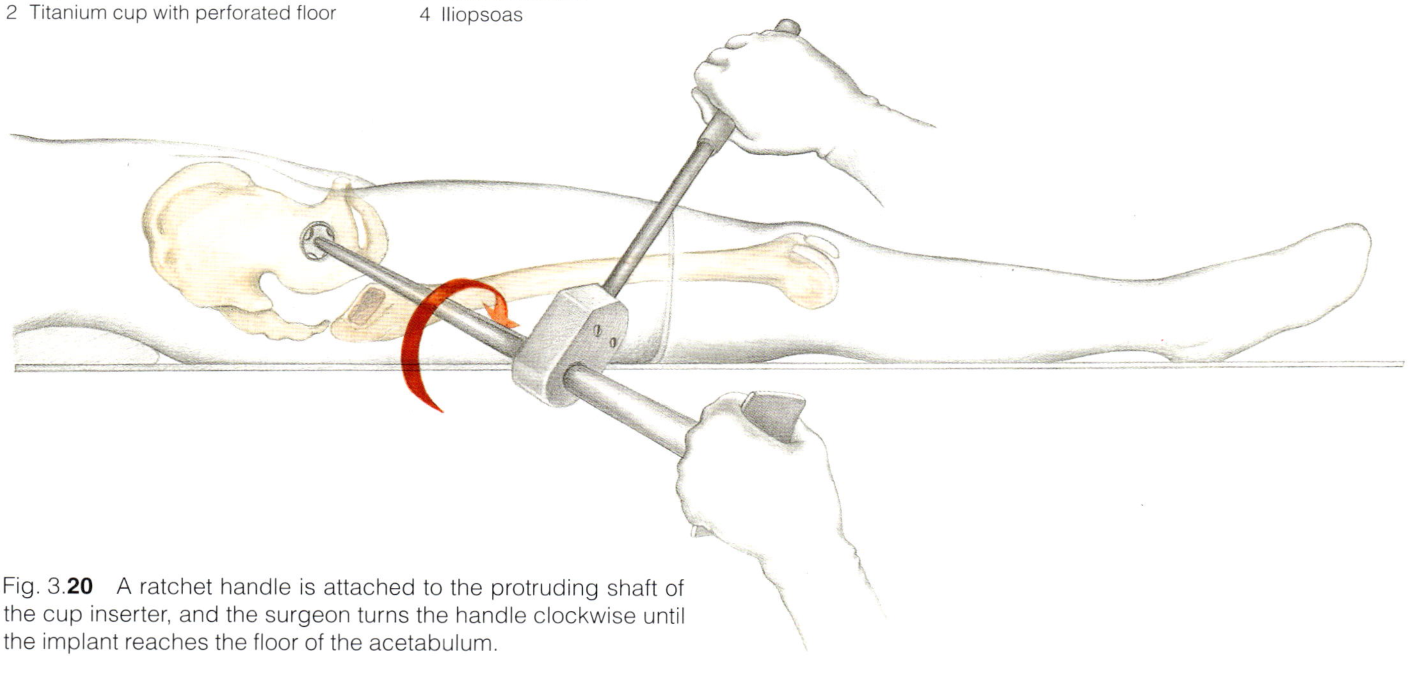

Fig. 3.**20** A ratchet handle is attached to the protruding shaft of the cup inserter, and the surgeon turns the handle clockwise until the implant reaches the floor of the acetabulum.

Bony defects in the floor or acetabular convexity (Fig. 3.**21**) can be filled with cancellous allograft or graft material from the resected femoral head. After cleaning the titanium cup, the surgeon inserts the polyethylene liner into the titanium cup. The four tabs snap into the notches on the rim (Fig. 3.**22**). A plastic impactor is used to seat the polyethylene liner in the titanium cup (Fig. 3.**23**).

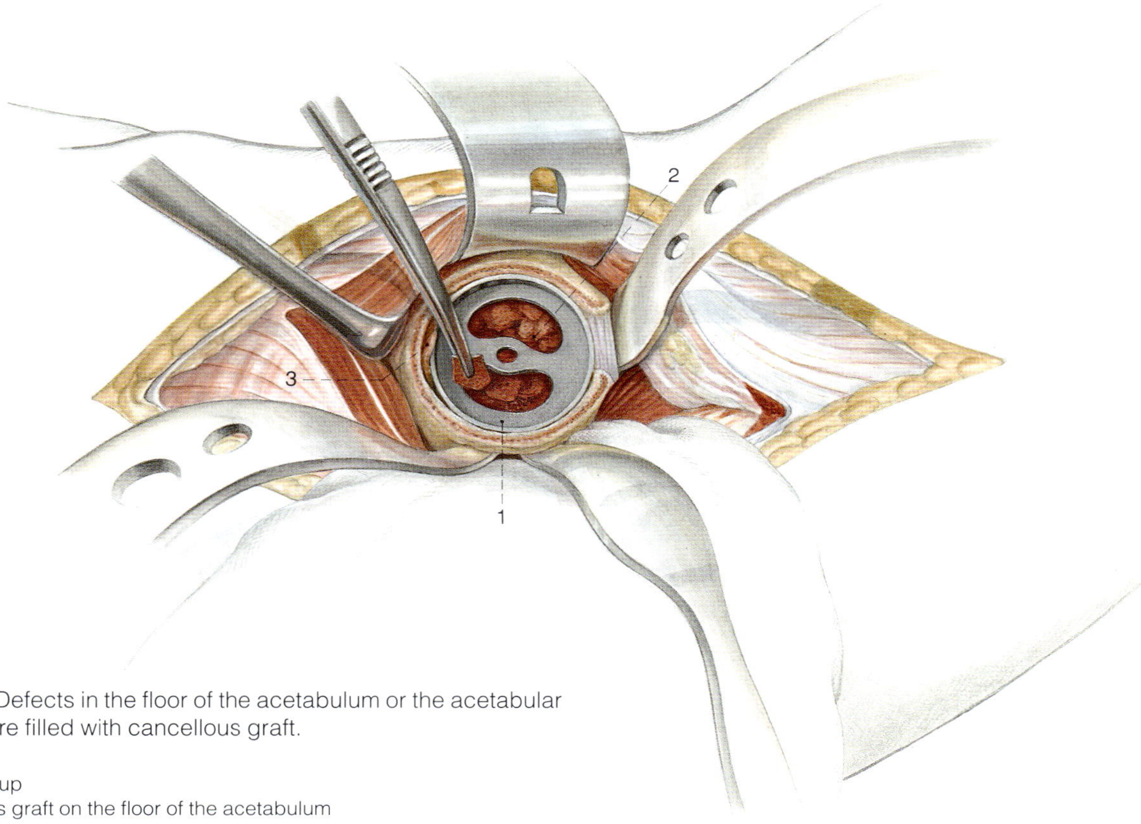

Fig. 3.**21** Defects in the floor of the acetabulum or the acetabular convexity are filled with cancellous graft.

1 Titanium cup
2 Cancellous graft on the floor of the acetabulum
3 Cancellous graft below the acetabular convexity

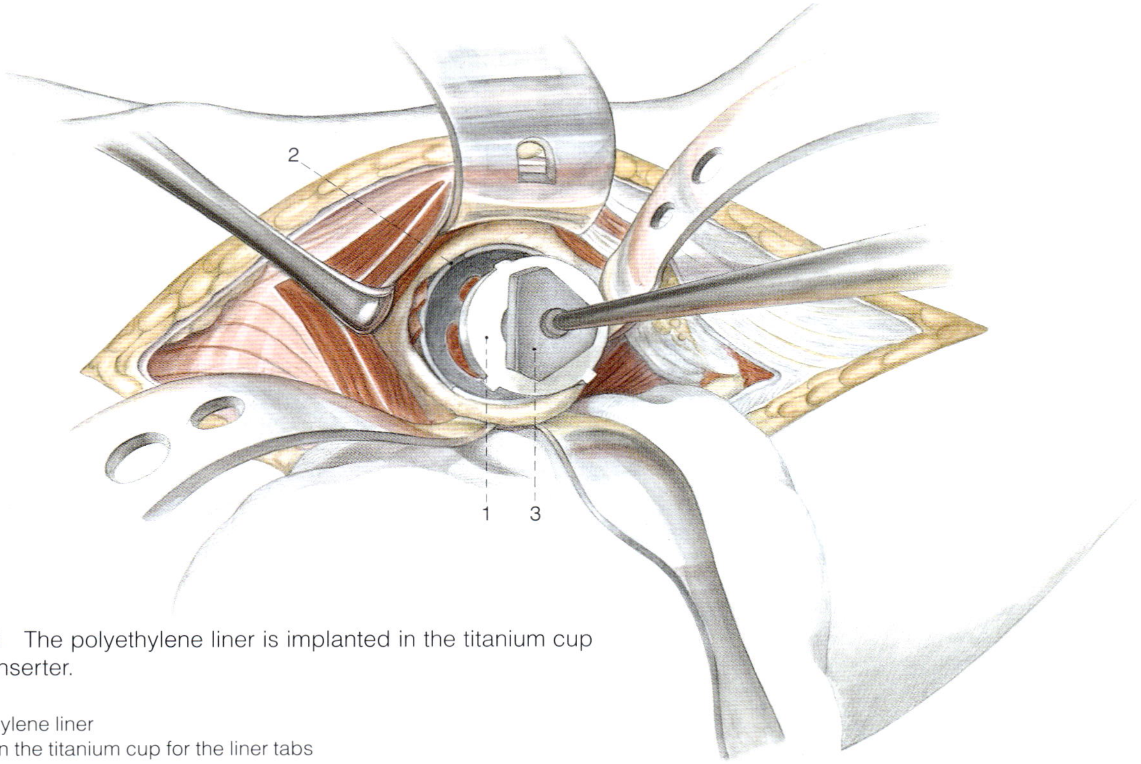

Fig. 3.**22** The polyethylene liner is implanted in the titanium cup with an inserter.

1 Polyethylene liner
2 Notch in the titanium cup for the liner tabs
3 Inserter for polyethylene liner

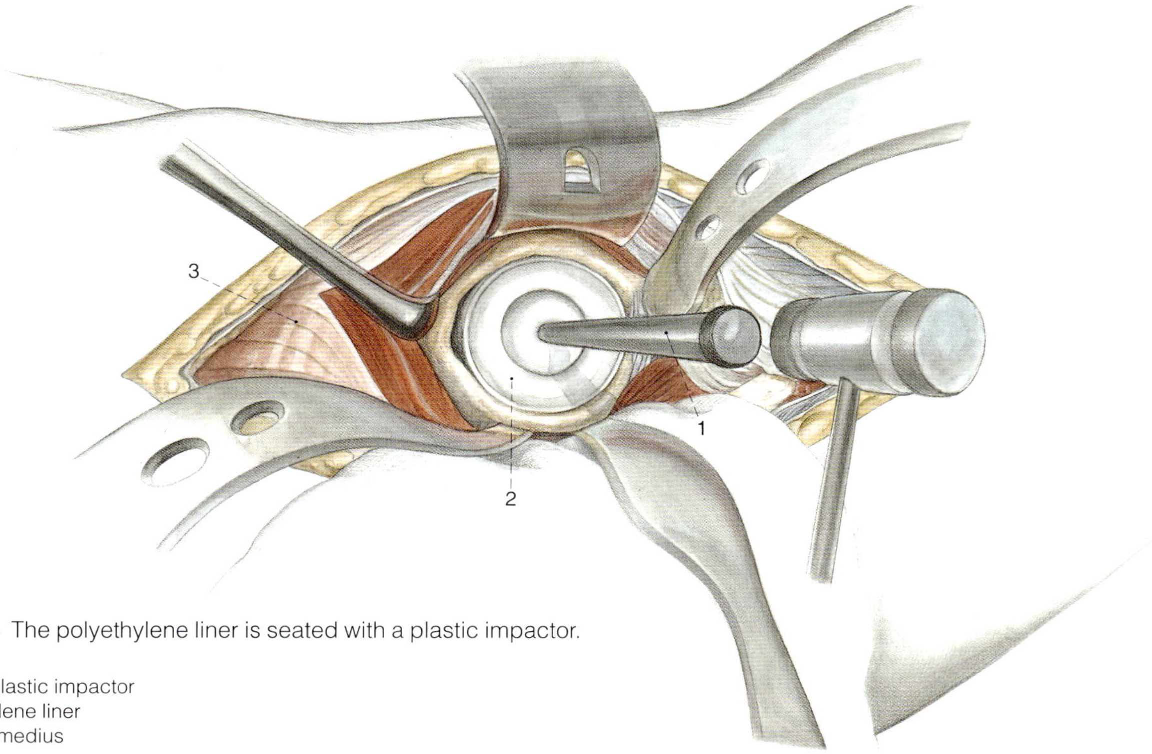

Fig. 3.**23** · The polyethylene liner is seated with a plastic impactor.

1 Grip of plastic impactor
2 Polyethylene liner
3 Gluteus medius

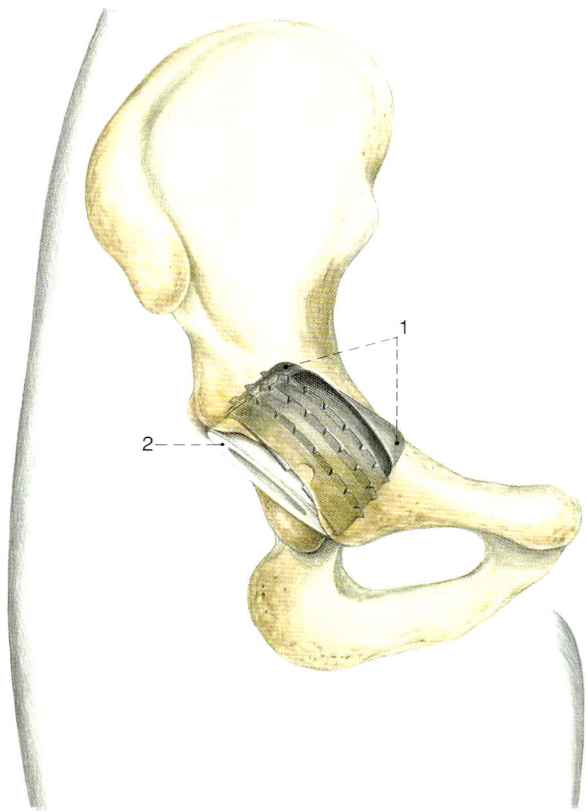

Fig. 3.**24** Schematic diagram of a steeply inclined implant after the floor of the acetabulum has been penetrated. The floor has been filled with cancellous graft.

1 Graft
2 Polyethylene liner with shoulder (for dysplastic acetabula)

If the cup has to be implanted at a steeper angle than originally planned and there is a tendency for the hip to dislocate when extended, we recommend using a polyethylene liner with a shoulder (Fig. 3.**24**).

Complications

The branches of the femoral artery may be damaged if soft tissue is not sufficiently retracted while the acetabulum is being reamed. This also applies to implanting the self-threading titanium cup. These complications can be avoided by adequately exposing the acetabulum. If the bleeding vessel cannot be located and ligated at the site, the femoral artery must be exposed through a curved inguinal incision and temporarily clamped until bleeding stops. Angiography of the femoral artery is indicated if postoperative bleeding occurs.

If the reamers are positioned incorrectly, they can penetrate the floor of the acetabulum. Minor perforations are not harmful, but where larger defects are encountered, the defects should be filled with cancellous graft; the inclination of the titanium cup should be reduced, and a polyethylene liner with an elevated rim should be used. The surgeon should ascertain whether the implant has sufficient primary stability. If this is not the case, we recommend using a cemented acetabular cup.

Special Cases

Protruding Acetabulum

A protruding acetabulum is seen in patients with inflammatory disorders and osteomalacia. In these patients, we recommend reinforcement of the acetabulum with a dysplastic acetabulum cup, reconstruction of the floor of the acetabulum, and lateral displacement of the acetabular component.

Surgical Technique

After the acetabulum has been exposed, degenerative changes can be seen, including bony defects that penetrate the center of the acetabular floor (Fig. 3.**25**). All cartilage is removed from the resected femoral head, and it is implanted in the floor of the acetabulum (Fig. 3.**26**). The graft that was wedged into the floor of the acetabulum is then reamed out to a concave shape (Fig. 3.**27**). Then a dysplastic acetabulum cup is impacted (Fig. 3.**28**). This dysplastic acetabulum cup is supported anteriorly, posteriorly, and along the superior rim of the acetabulum. Using a flexible drill, the surgeon drills three or four holes in the ilium (Fig. 3.**29**) and inserts cancellous screws, using an articulated screw driver. Now the polyethylene cup is cemented (Fig. 3.**30**). This method permits the surgeon to align the acetabular cup independently of the reinforcing cup. The polyethylene liner can also be fixed without cement using a hemispherical acetabular cup. Where there are large bony defects in the center of the floor of the acetabulum and insufficient anterior or posterior support for the reinforcing cup, we recommend implanting a reinforcing cup with a hook that engages the cotyloid notch after the acetabular defects have been filled (Fig. 3.**31**).

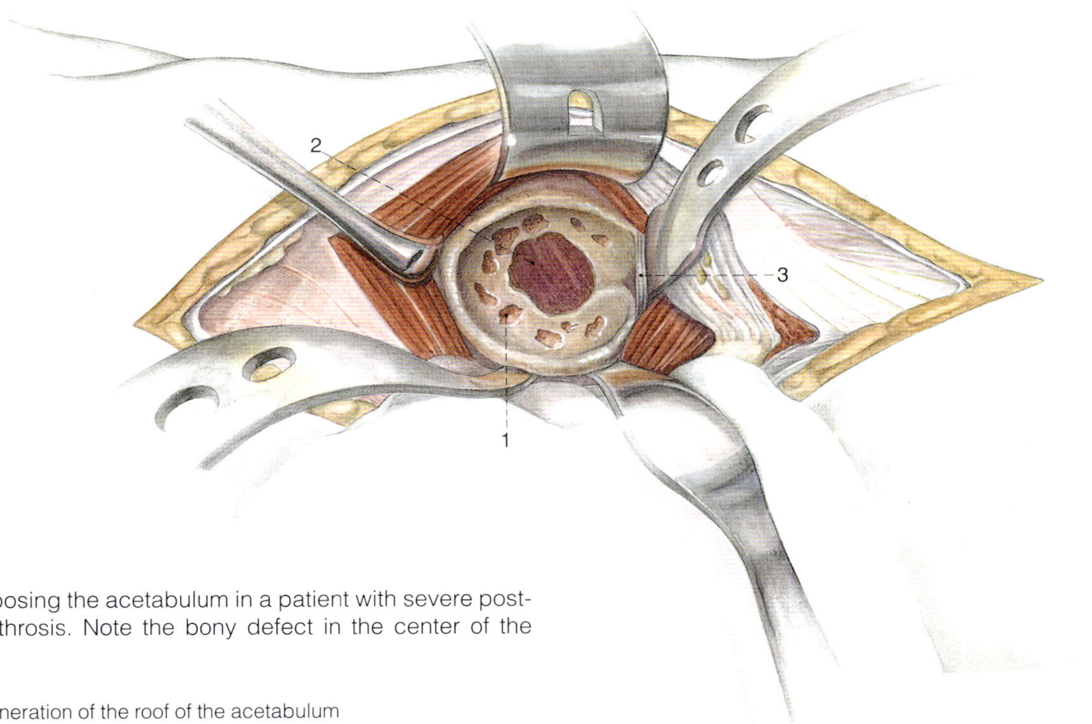

Fig. 3.**25** Exposing the acetabulum in a patient with severe post-arthritic coxarthrosis. Note the bony defect in the center of the acetabulum.

1 Arthritic degeneration of the roof of the acetabulum
2 Bony defect
3 Transverse acetabular ligament

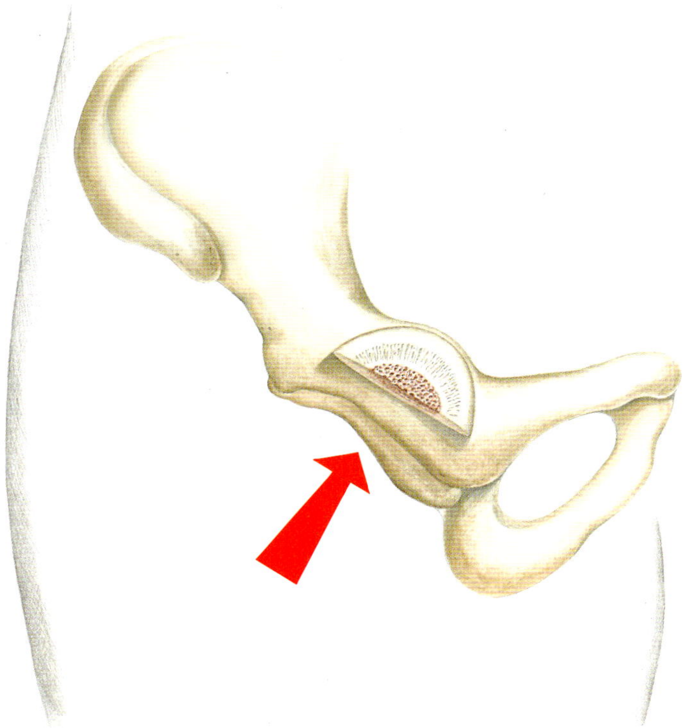

Fig. 3.**26** Reconstructing the bony defect in the center of the acetabulum. All cartilage is removed from the resected femoral head, which is then implanted in the floor of the acetabulum.

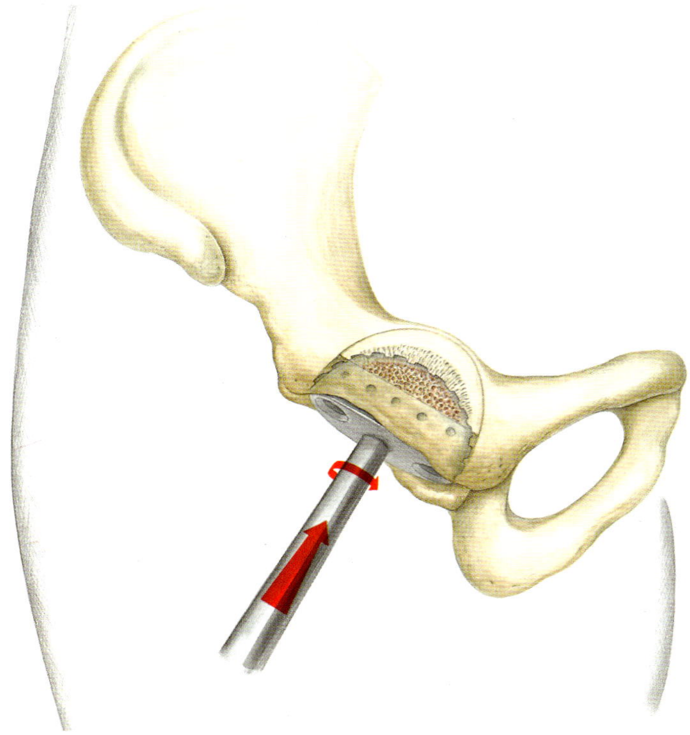

Fig. 3.**27** Preparing the acetabulum and the graft with an acetabular reamer.

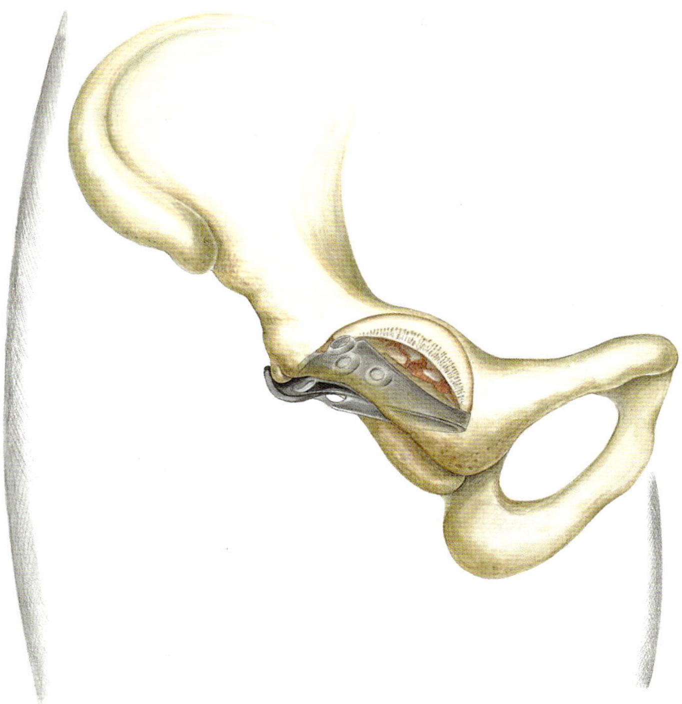

Fig. 3.**28** A Müller dysplastic acetabulum cup is impacted with a cup impactor.

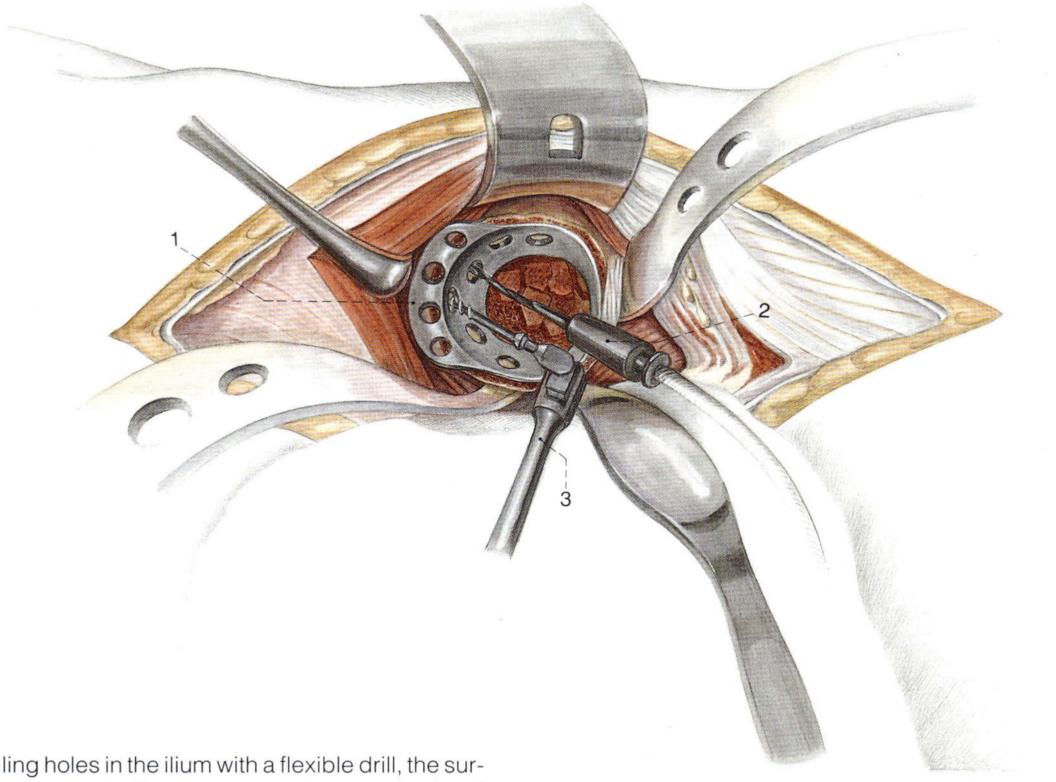

Fig. 3.**29** After drilling holes in the ilium with a flexible drill, the surgeon inserts three or four cancellous screws, using an articulated screw driver.

1 Müller dysplastic acetabulum cup
2 Flexible drill
3 Articulated screw driver

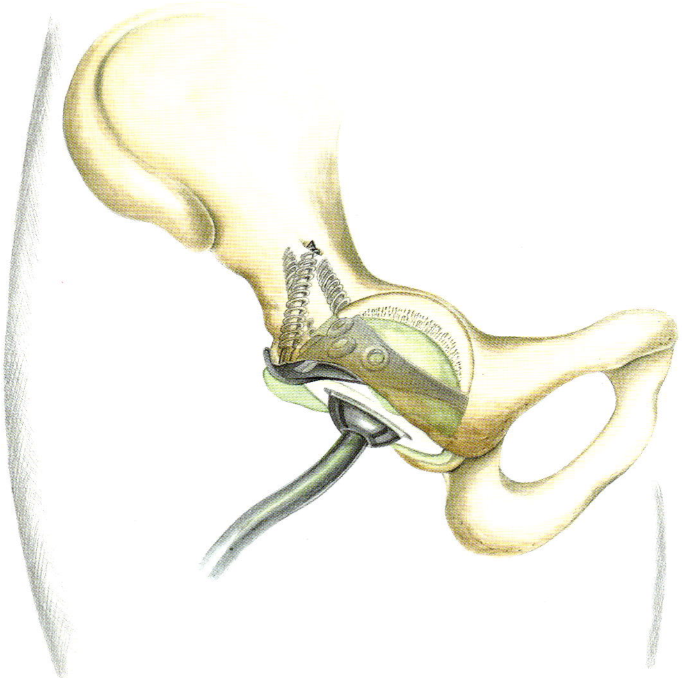

Fig. 3.**30** The polyethylene cup is cemented at an inclination of about 45° with 10–20° anteversion.

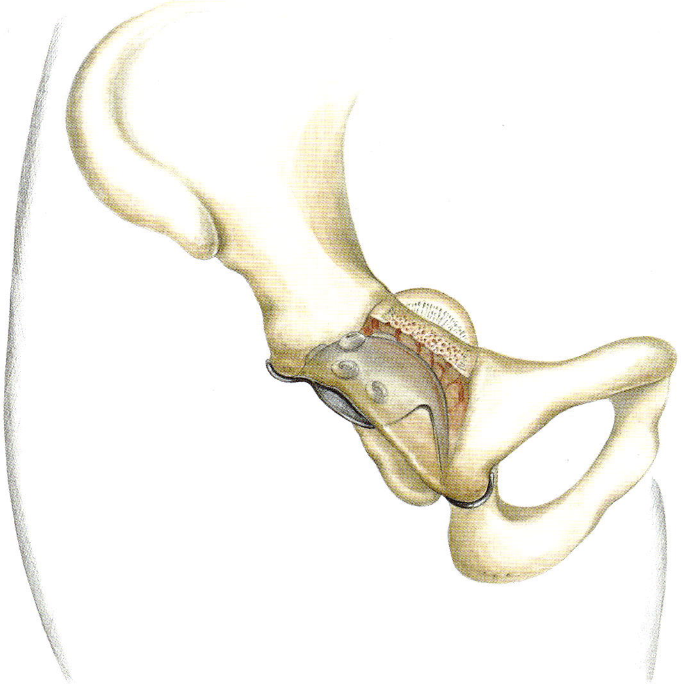

Fig. 3.**31** Where there are large bony defects in the center of the floor of the acetabulum or insufficient anterior or posterior support for the reinforcing cup, implanting a dysplastic acetabulum cup with a hook that engages the cotyloid notch is recommended after the acetabular defects have been filled (Ganz dysplastic acetabulum cup).

Dysplastic Acetabulum

We differentiate between the following stages of arthritic hip dysplasia according to the degree of deformity:

- Arthritic hip dysplasia with bony defects of the acetabular convexity (stage I)
- Arthritic hip dysplasia with subluxation (stage II, Fig. 3.**32**)
- Arthritic hip dysplasia with formation of a secondary acetabulum (stage III, Fig. 3.**33**)
- Superior (iliac) dislocation of the hip (stage IV, Fig. 3.**34**)

Principle

The surgical technique for reconstructing the acetabulum is similar for stages I and II; different procedures are used for reconstruction of arthritic dislocated hips (stages III and IV).

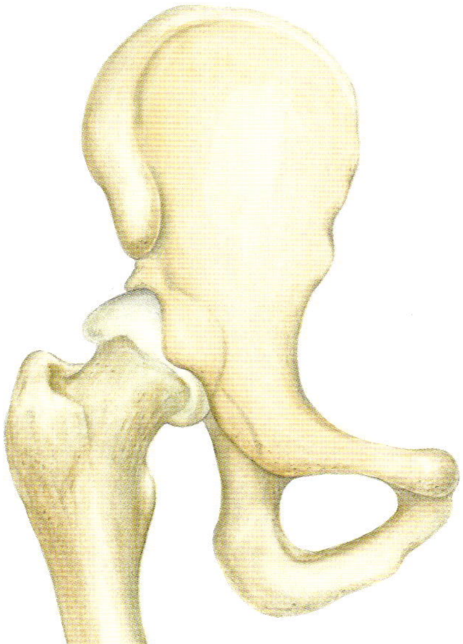

Fig. 3.**32**

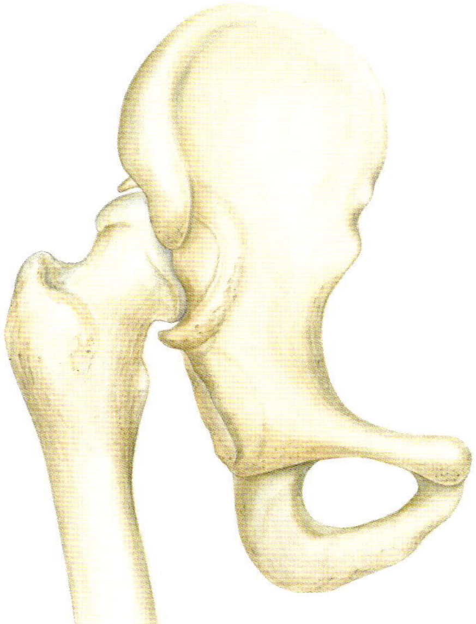

Fig. 3.**33**

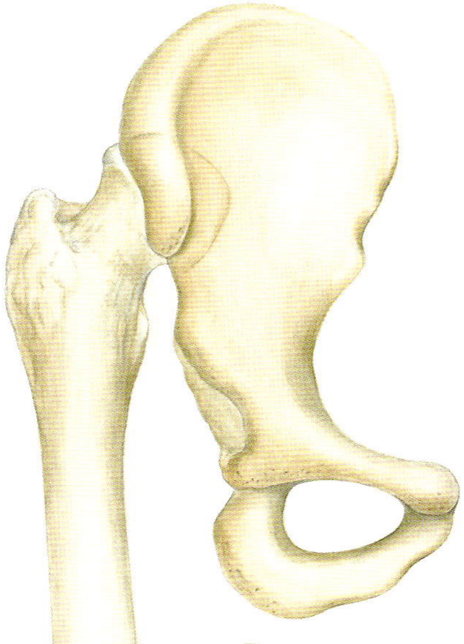

Fig. 3.**34**

Fig. 3.**32** Stage II arthritic hip dysplasia (subluxation).

Fig. 3.**33** Stage III arthritic hip dysplasia with a superior secondary acetabulum.

Fig. 3.**34** Superior (iliac) dislocation of the hip.

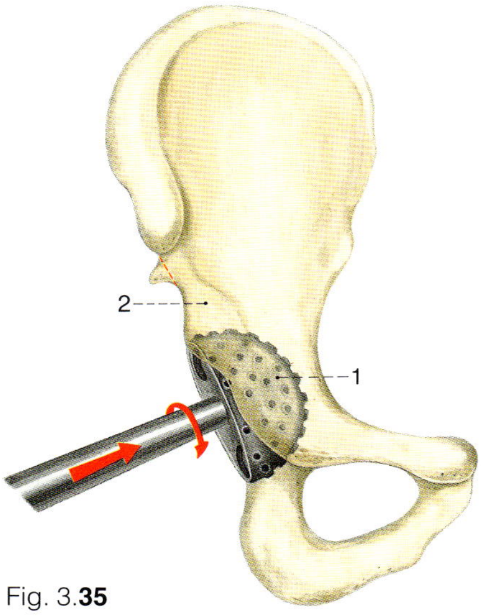

Fig. 3.**35**

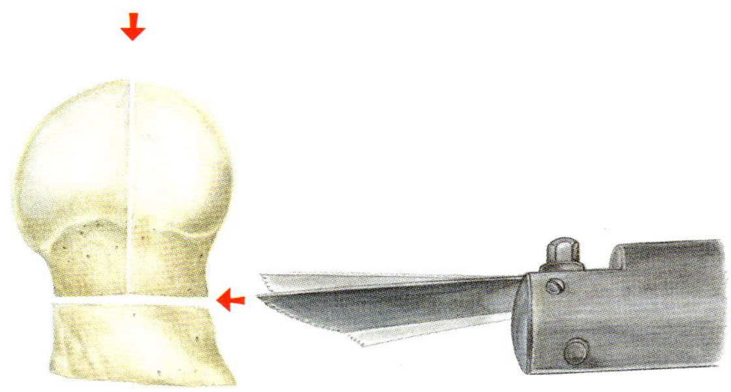

Fig. 3.**36**

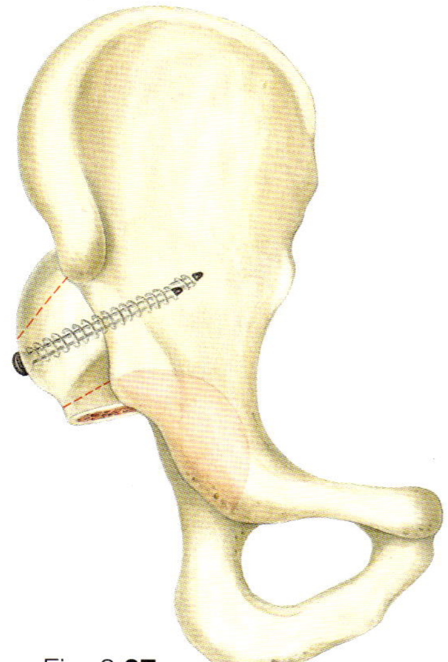

Fig. 3.**37**

Fig. 3.**35** Reaming the acetabulum down to the inner table.

1 Acetabular reamer
2 Defect in the acetabular convexity

Fig. 3.**36** Osteotomy of the resected femoral head for reconstructing the acetabulum.

Fig. 3.**37** Schematic diagram. Two screws are used to fix the segment of the femoral head to the ilium. The superior and inferior portions of the graft are resected.

Surgical Technique

In stage I or II arthritic hip dysplasia, the femoral head is resected, a complete capsulectomy is performed, and the acetabulum and bony defect are broadly exposed. The acetabulum is generally displaced laterally (the floor of the acetabulum is usually thickened), and must be reamed to achieve a more centered position (Fig. 3.**35**). The resected femoral head and neck are cut into three segments with an oscillating saw (Fig. 3.**36**). One head segment is placed in the secondary acetabulum and initially fixed with Kirschner wire and then fastened to the ilium with screws (Fig. 3.**37**). The superior portion of the graft is resected with an oscillating saw (Fig. 3.**38**). The inferior portion of the graft projecting above the roof of the acetabulum is ground off with an acetabular reamer (Fig. 3.**39**). After inserting a trial cup, the surgeon cements a polyethylene acetabular cup (Fig. 3.**40**). This procedure also permits cementless implantation. However, cementless cups with an outer diameter of less than 40 mm are only available as custom implants.

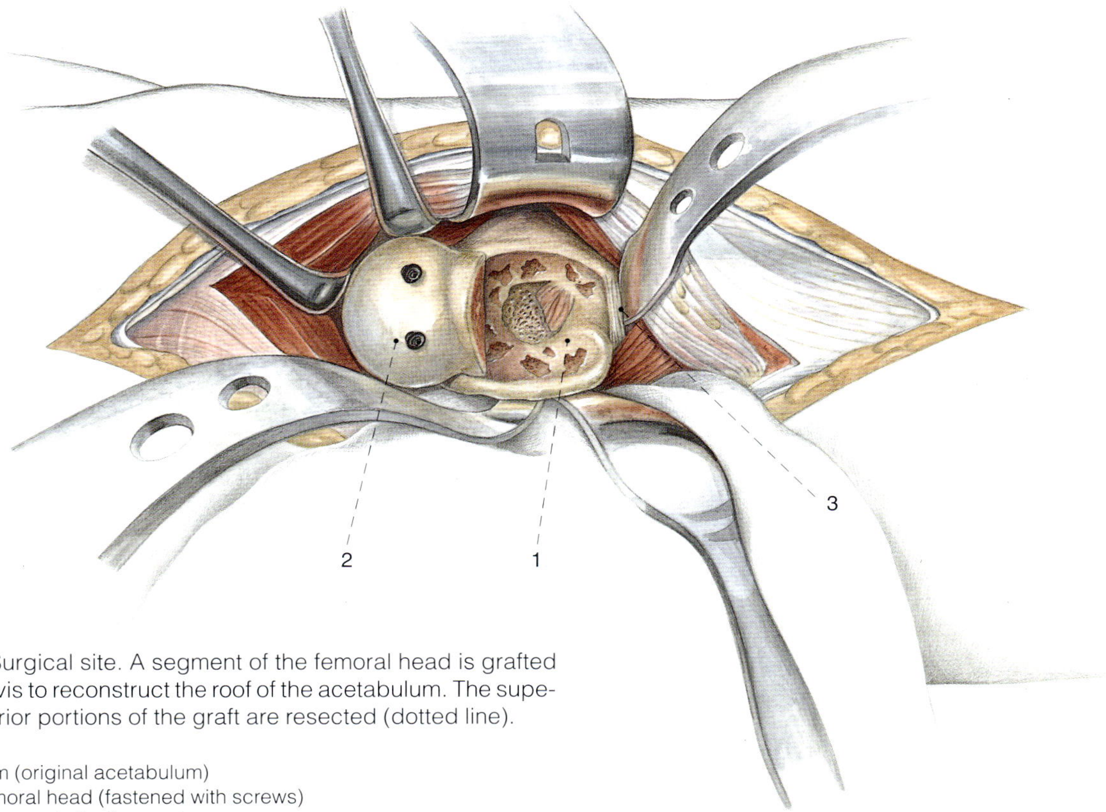

Fig. 3.**38** Surgical site. A segment of the femoral head is grafted onto the pelvis to reconstruct the roof of the acetabulum. The superior and inferior portions of the graft are resected (dotted line).

1 Acetabulum (original acetabulum)
2 Grafted femoral head (fastened with screws)
3 Transverse acetabular ligament

Fig. 3.**39** The inferior portion of the graft is ground off with an acetabular reamer to create a smooth transition between the original acetabulum and the grafted roof.

Fig. 3.**40** The surgeon may opt for cemented fixation (shown here) or cementless fixation of the acetabular component.

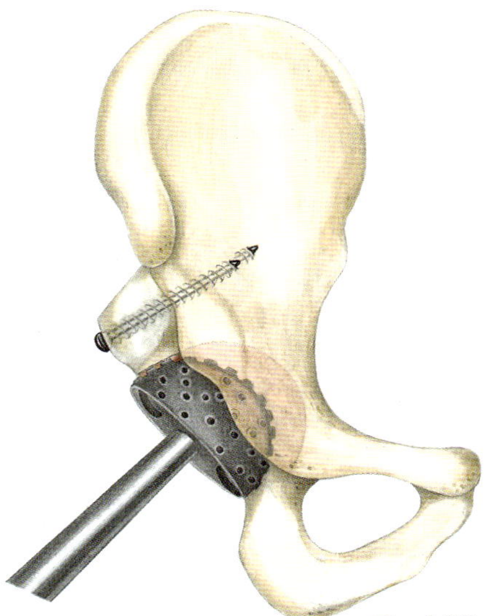

Fig. 3.**39**

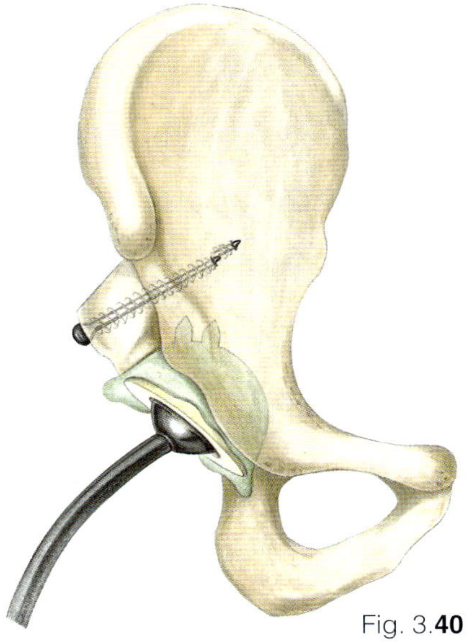

Fig. 3.**40**

Surgical Technique for Stage III and IV Arthritic Dislocated Hips

In a superior dislocation of the hip (Fig. 3.**41**), we prefer a lateral approach with a chevron osteotomy of the greater trochanter, a shortening osteotomy of the proximal femur corresponding to soft-tissue tension, and using the resected femoral head and neck segment to reconstruct the acetabulum (Fig. 3.**42**). In these patients, the capsule must be resected down to the original acetabulum. The rudimentary original acetabulum is small, shallow, and difficult to expose. We recommend using computerized 3-D models. The procedure requires smaller acetabular reamers from 36 to 42 mm (Fig. 3.**43**). The resected femoral head and neck segment is grafted so that it reconstructs the roof, the posterior wall, and

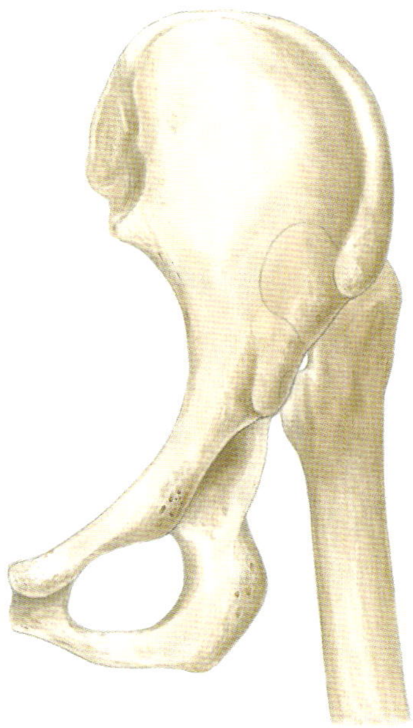

Fig. 3.**41** Superior (iliac) dislocation of the hip. Note the small, flat original acetabulum.

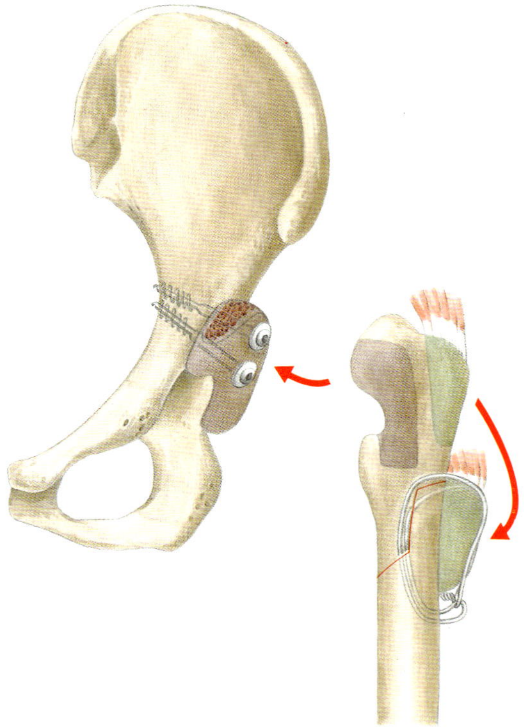

Fig. 3.**42** Schematic diagram of the trochanteric osteotomy, shortening osteotomy, and resection of the femoral head. The resected head is used to reconstruct the acetabulum.

part of the anterior wall of the acetabulum (see Figs. 3.**42** and 3.**43**). The surgeon reams the floor of the acetabulum down to the inner table, shaping the surrounding graft in the process. An acetabular cup of the proper size (22 mm femoral head) is cemented in place (Fig. 3.**44**). After preparing the proximal femur, the surgeon inserts the stem, performs a trial reduction, and resects additional bone if necessary. Cerclage wire, 1.2–1.5 mm in diameter, is then inserted into two holes drilled in the femur, and a dysplastic cylindrical straight-stem implant is cemented into the femur.

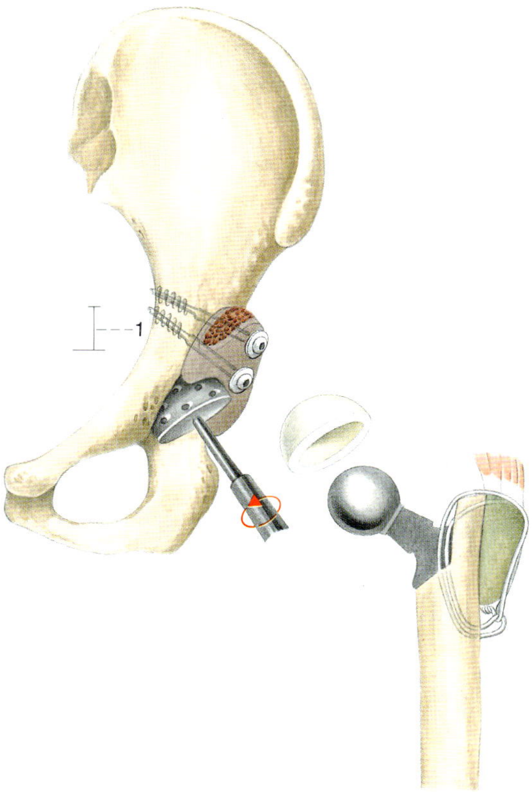

Fig. 3.**43** The original acetabulum is reamed out down to the inner table. The roof of the acetabulum is reconstructed from the head and neck fragment and then reamed to create a smooth transition to the original acetabulum. Then a dysplastic acetabular cup (22 mm femoral head) is cemented into the acetabulum. The femoral component consists of a dysplastic straight-stem cemented implant anchored in the femoral diaphysis.

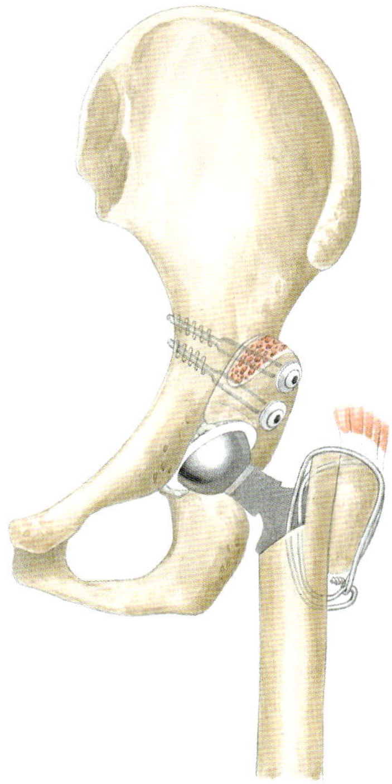

Fig. 3.**44** After reducing the dysplastic implants and fixing the greater trochanter.

Müller Cemented Stem

Indications

- Osteoporosis
- Cylindrical femoral shaft
- Altered femoral shaft after prior surgery

Surgical Technique

After the acetabular cup has been implanted, tenotomizing the piriformis and the short external rotators is recommended for better exposure of the proximal femur if the bone is osteoporotic (Fig. 3.**45a**). If the tenotomy is not performed, the subsequent flexion, adduction, and external rotation of the leg could cause an avulsion fracture of the apex of the greater trochanter. With the leg extended, a Hohmann retractor is inserted below the greater trochanter, and the proximal femur is lifted out over the fascia lata. The leg is flexed, adducted, and externally rotated. It is held in this position by the second assistant (Fig. 3.**45b**). This gives the surgeon good access to the femoral canal.

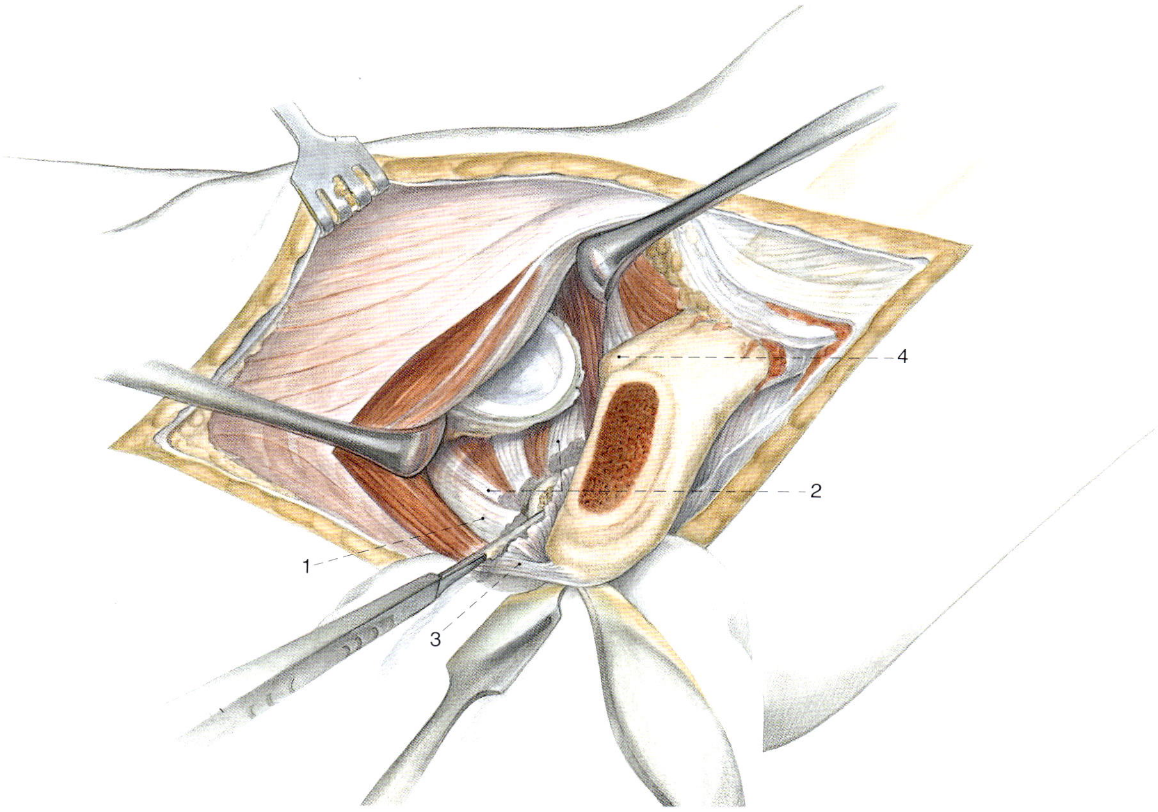

Fig. 3.**45 a** Tenotomizing the short external rotators and the piriformis tendon.

1 Piriformis
2 Gemellus and obturator internus
3 Tendons of the gluteus medius and gluteus minimus
4 Lesser trochanter

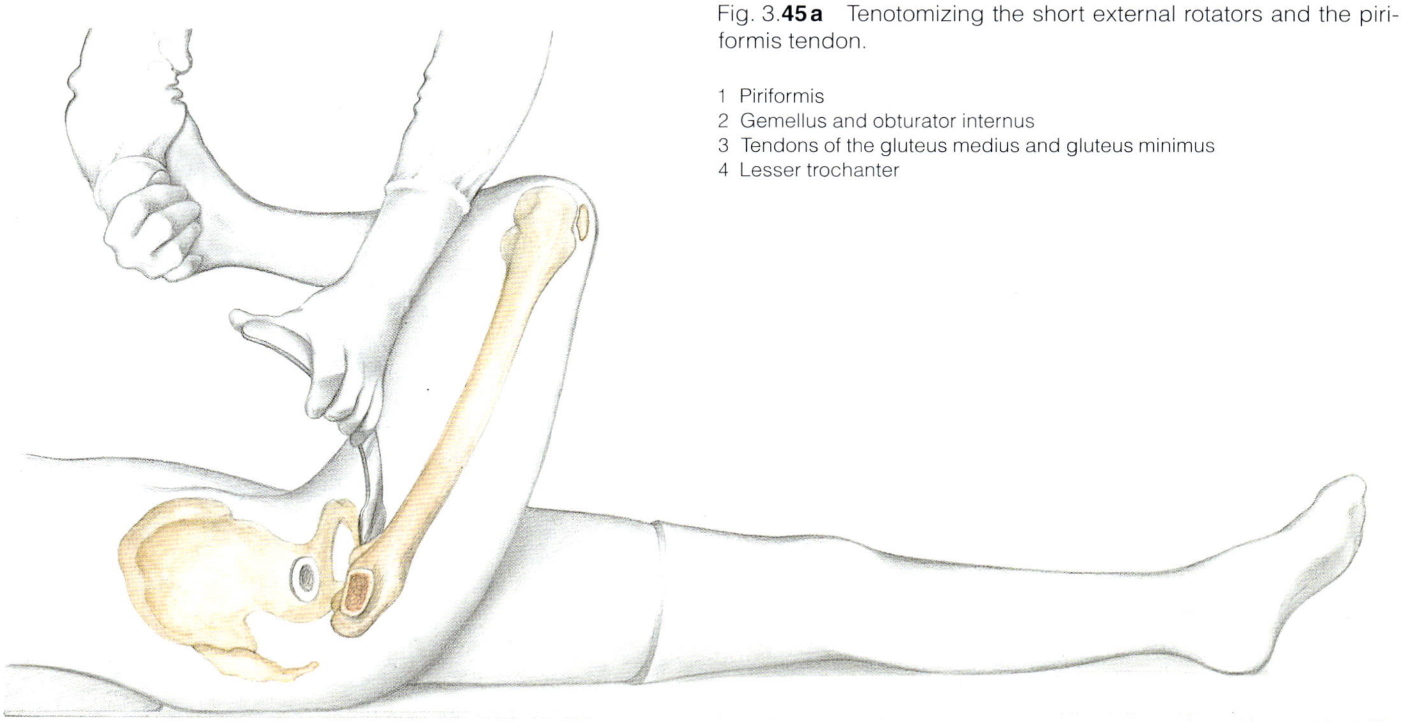

Fig. 3.**45 b** The leg is flexed, adducted, and externally rotated to expose the proximal femur.

Preparing the Femoral Canal

First the surgeon resects cancellous bone with a box osteotome (Fig. 3.**46a**).

When a straight-stem implant is to be used, the surgeon removes additional cortical bone from the superior and lateral end of the femoral neck osteotomy to allow him to center the implant when impacting it. Using an anatomic implant (right or left-handed stem with proper anteversion) eliminates the need for resecting bone at this site. The surgeon inserts a long medullary curette into the femoral medulla to cut a canal for the rasp and reduce the risk of fracturing the femoral cortex (Fig. 3.**46b**). Cancellous bone is then conservatively removed from the proximal femur. With a neck osteotomy guide, the surgeon uses the apex of the greater trochanter or that of the lesser trochanter as a landmark to verify the level of the osteotomy of the femoral neck.

If necessary, additional bone is resected from the femoral neck. If the original osteotomy has been performed correctly, the surgeon drives successively larger rasps into the femoral canal until the proximal portion of the final rasp lies flush with the osteotomy plane. When driving in the rasp, hold the handle in 10° of anteversion (Fig. 3.**47**). The handle has a quick-release coupling for use with different sizes of rasps (Fig. 3.**48**). After reaming the femoral canal with the largest possible rasp, the surgeon replaces it with a rasp one size smaller, which is fitted with a trial head with a medium-length neck (Fig. 3.**49**). The position of this trial implant is verified with a ruler. When we implant a cemented stem, we always ream the femoral canal to one rasp size larger than the final stem size to ensure uniform thickness of the cement mantle. For example, if the final rasp is size 12.5, we use a size 10 implant.

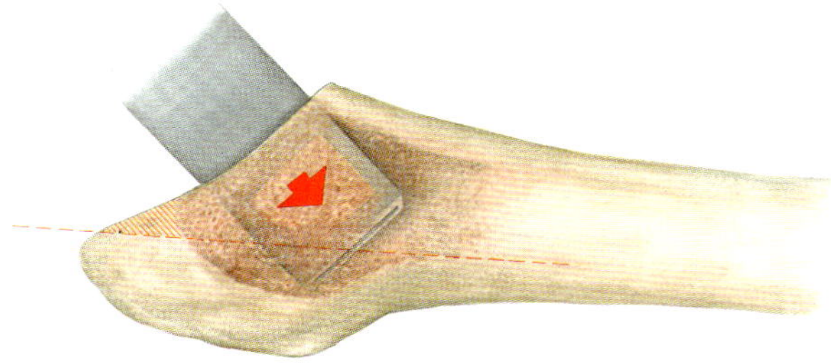

Fig. 3.**46a** Proximal cancellous bone is resected with a box osteotome. When a straight-stem implant is used, additional cortical bone is removed from the greater trochanter (dotted line).

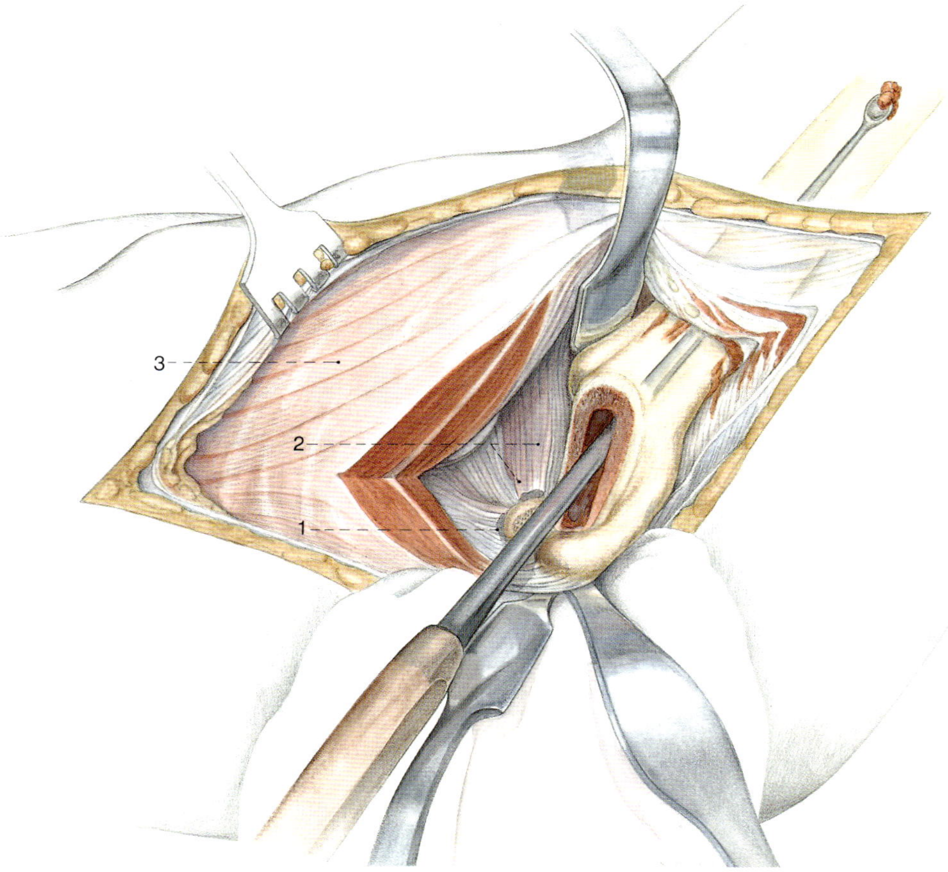

Fig. 3.**46b** A long medullary curette is used to cut a channel in the femoral medulla. To improve exposure, a Hohmann retractor is inserted below the greater trochanter, and the proximal femur lata is lifted out over the fascia lata.

1 Piriformis
2 Gemellus and obturator internus
3 Gluteus medius

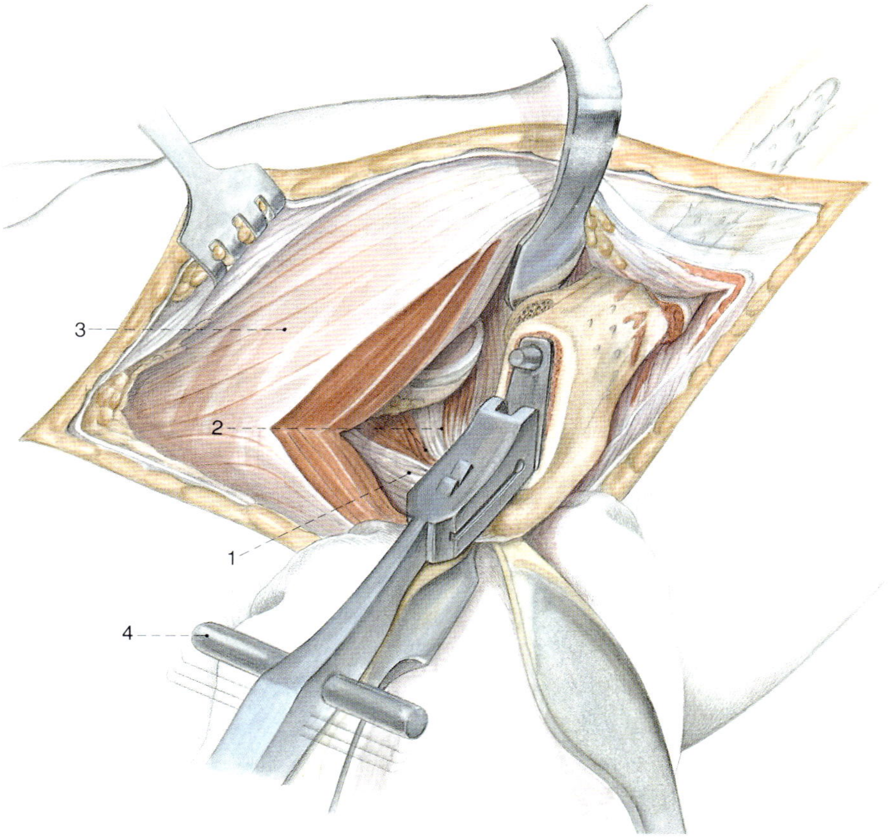

Fig. 3.**47** The femoral canal is widened with successively larger rasps. The alignment bar on the rasp handle should be held at about 10° of anteversion to the shaft of the femur.

1 Piriformis
2 Gemellus and obturator internus
3 Gluteus medius
4 Alignment bar for anteversion

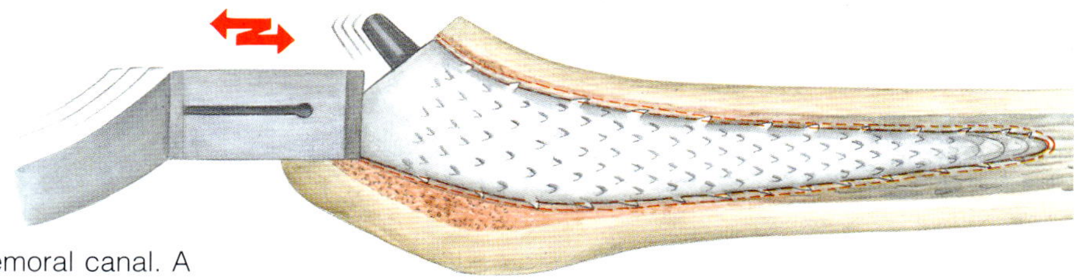

Fig. 3.**48** Schematic diagram of preparing the femoral canal. A handle with a quick-release coupling is used with successively larger rasps. A rasp one size smaller than the largest rasp is used as a trial implant.

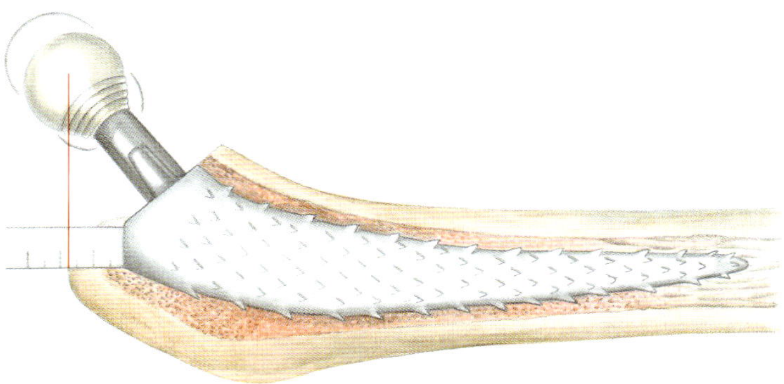

Fig. 3.**49** The proximal portion of the rasp must lie flush with the osteotomy plane of the femoral neck. The distance between the shoulder of the rasp and the greater trochanter corresponds to the preoperative drawing. Trial heads are available in three different neck lengths.

Trial Reduction

The hip is reduced with traction applied to the extended leg. The leg is abducted, adducted, and internally and externally rotated to assess the motion and stability of the artifical joint (Fig. 3.**50a**). Spontaneous dislocation in external rotation can be an indication of insufficient adductor tension. This can be resolved by using a head with a longer neck or a femoral implant with a longer stem. The hip should extend to 0° without excessive soft-tissue tension. If this is not the case, a head with a shorter neck or a femoral implant with a shorter stem should be used.

The points marked with asterisks (*) in Fig. 3.**50a** indicate osteophytes on the superior and inferior rim of the acetabulum that interfere with abduction and adduction and should be removed. Now the surgeon assesses leg length by comparing the distances between the iliac spines and the medial malleoli (Fig. 3.**50b**). Leg length differentials can be compensated for by selecting heads with longer necks or femoral implants with longer stems.

If the leg is too long, a smaller implant or a head with a shorter neck is used. Now the leg is placed in maximum flexion. The polyethylene acetabular cups currently available

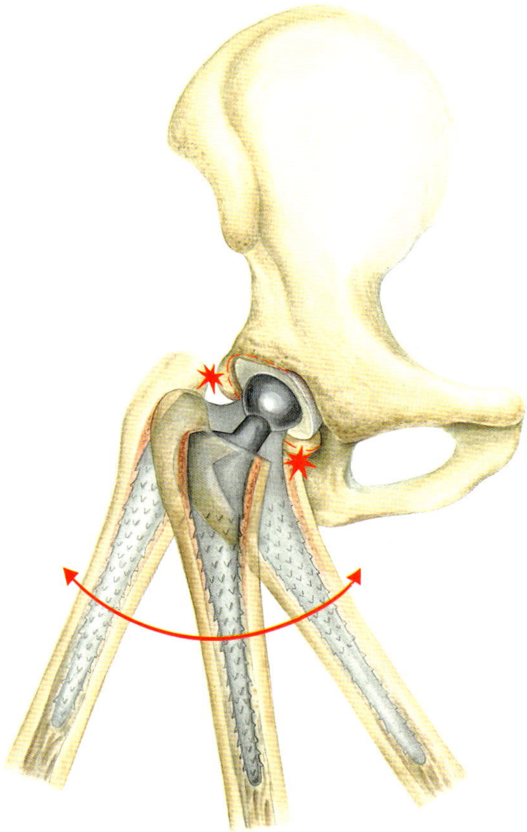

Fig. 3.**50a** The hip is reduced with the extended leg extended. The leg is then abducted, adducted, and internally and externally rotated to assess motion and stability. The asterisks (*) on the superior and inferior rim of the acetabulum indicate osteophytes that should be removed.

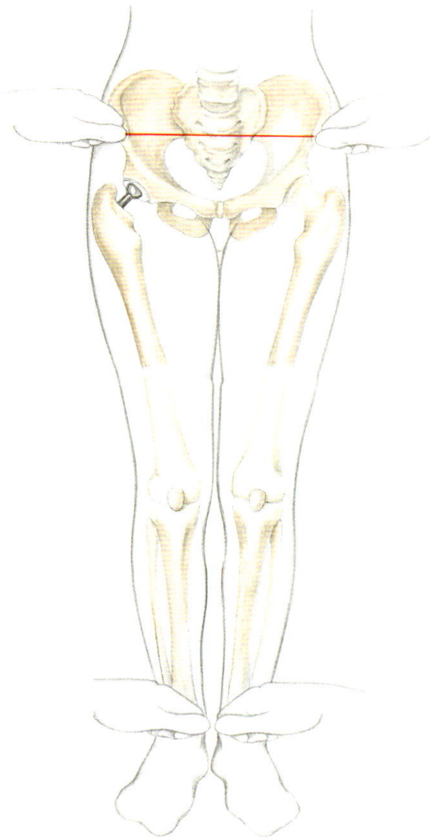

Fig. 3.**50b** Measuring leg length. The iliac spines and the medial malleoli are aligned parallel to each other.

should allow over 100° of flexion (Fig. 3.**50c**). Abduction and rotation are assessed at the same time. Instability in flexion, adduction, and internal rotation is usually an indication of insufficient anteversion of the implanted acetabular cup. If a cementless metal-backed acetabular cup is being used, the standard liner should be replaced with a liner with an elevated rim; if a cemented acetabular cup is being used, a polyethylene stabilizer with two posterosuperior screws can be fastened to the rim of the acetabulum (see chapter on revision total hip arthroplasty).

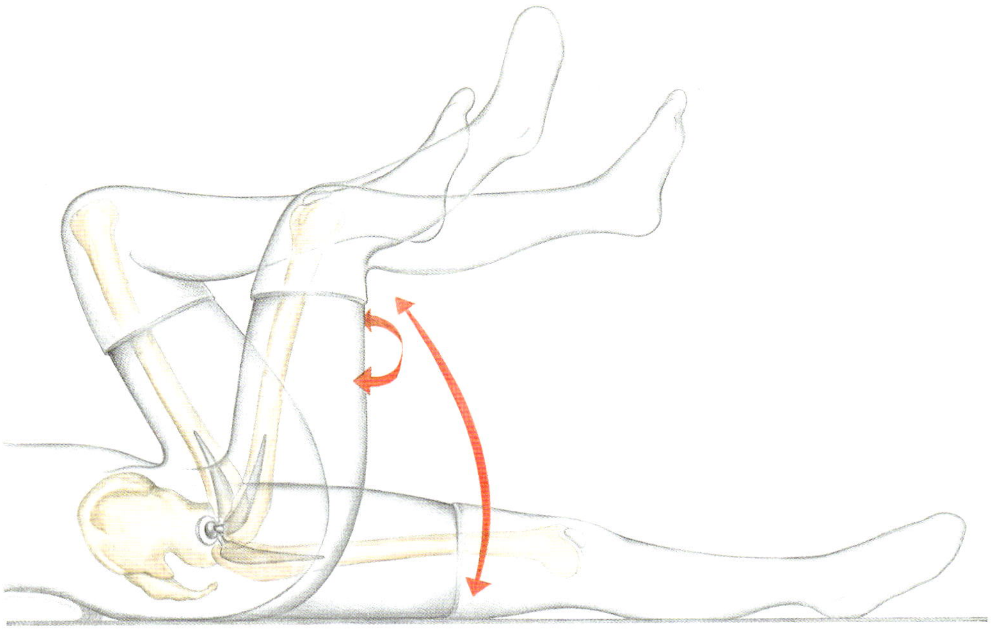

Fig. 3.**50c** Assessing flexion and stability of the hip with the leg in internal rotation, flexion, and adduction. Normal soft-tissue tension permits intraoperative flexion of 100°.

Preparing the Femoral Canal for Cement

We use a cylinder of autologous cancellous graft (taken from the resected femoral head) with a hollow reamer to seal the distal femoral canal (Fig. 3.**51 a** and **b**). After the marrow and residual cancellous bone have been removed, the femoral canal is irrigated (Fig. 3.**52**). Then the surgeon uses an impactor to drive in the cylinder of cancellous bone until it lies about 2 cm distal to the expected position of the distal tip of the stem (Fig. 3.**53**). A drain is inserted into the femoral canal, and the canal is packed with thrombin-impregnated compresses (Fig. 3.**54**).

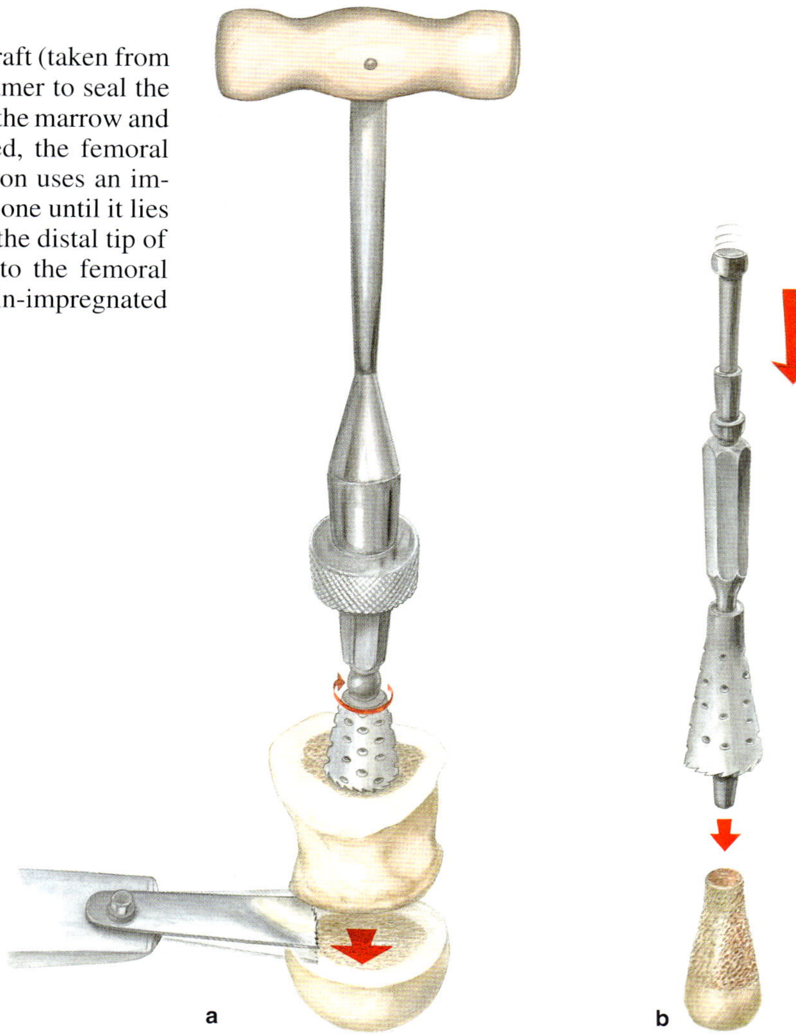

Fig. 3.**51 a** Sealing the distal femoral canal. A conical section of cancellous bone is removed from the resected femoral head with a hallow reamer.

Fig. 3.**51 b** Driving the cancellous section out of the conical reamer with an impactor.

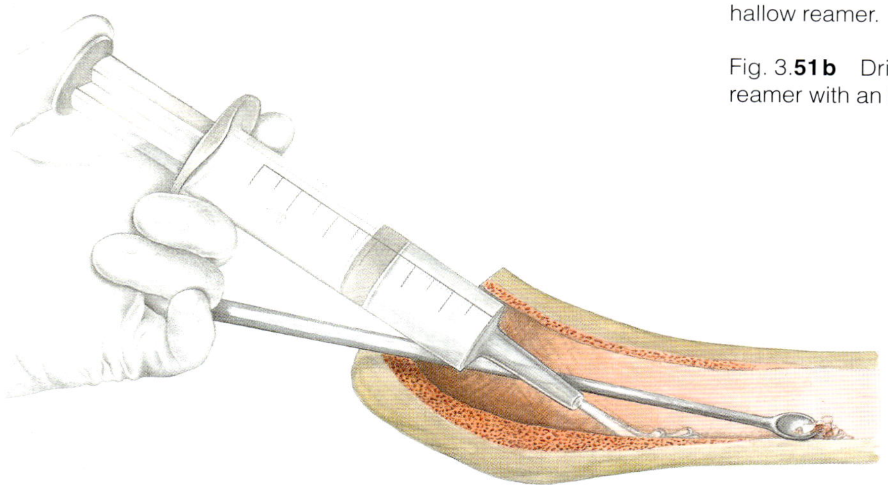

Fig. 3.**52** Curetting and irrigating the femoral canal.

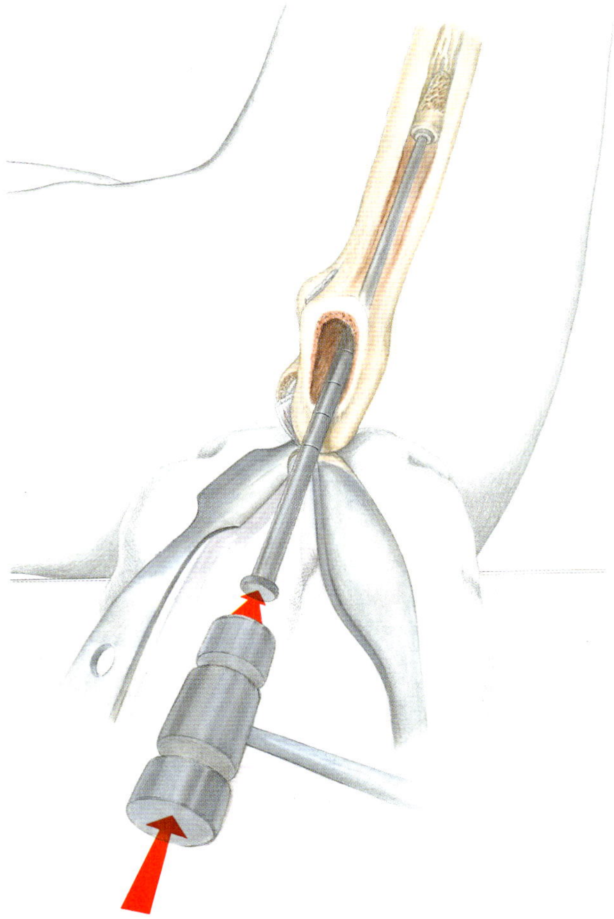

Fig. 3.**53** Driving in the cancellous cement restrictor with a graduated impactor. The cylinder of cancellous bone should lie about 2 cm distal to the distal tip of the stem. The length of the implant is indicated on the scale of the impactor.

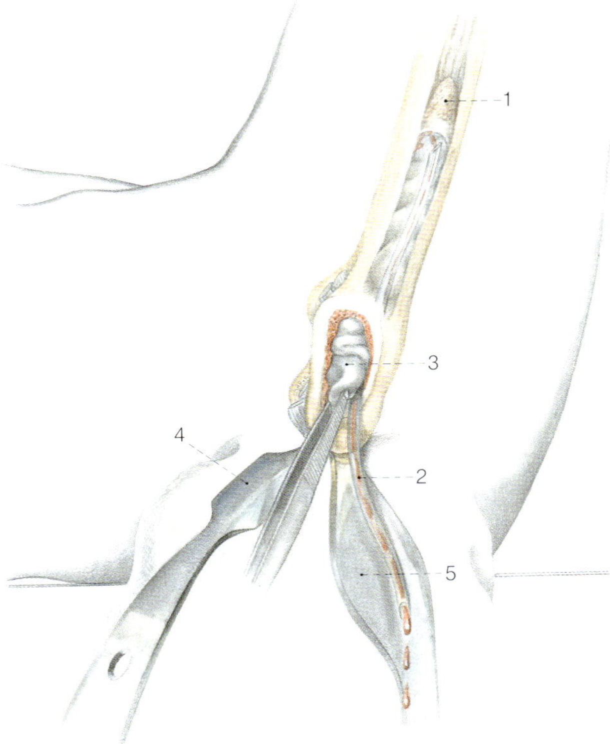

Fig. 3.**54** A drain is inserted as far as the cement restrictor, and the femoral canal is packed with thrombin-impregnated compresses.

1 Cement restrictor
2 Drain
3 Compresses
4 Gluteal reatractor
5 Fascia lata retractor

Cementing the Stem

We use precooled cement of normal viscosity, which we find easier to process and apply. The cement is precooled, vacuum mixed, and precompressed (Dränert system) to ensure a nonporous, homogeneous, bubble-free mixture.

After being mixed, the liquid cement is pressed into the cartridge from the mixing vessel (Fig. 3.**55**). The cartridge is attached to a compressed-air cement gun (Fig. 3.**56**) and is pressurized for 2 minutes. The gauze compresses are removed from the femoral canal, and the canal is checked to make sure it is dry. The cement is now injected into the femoral canal (Fig. 3.**57 a**). A "snorkel" can also be used (Fig. 3.**57 b**). It is our opinion that vacuum injection, using suction canulas and silicone seals is indispensable. The surgeon slowly inserts the stem while removing the drain (Fig. 3.**58**). After verifying the height and position of the implant, the surgeon applies slight compression while waiting for the cement to harden. Excess cement is cleaned off the shoulder of the stem. After cleaning and drying the taper, we attach a ceramic or metal head of the appropriate neck length (Fig. 3.**59**). Before reducing the hip, the surgeon should ensure that the articular surfaces are free of any interposed soft tissue. Finally, we assess motion and stability (Fig. 3.**60**).

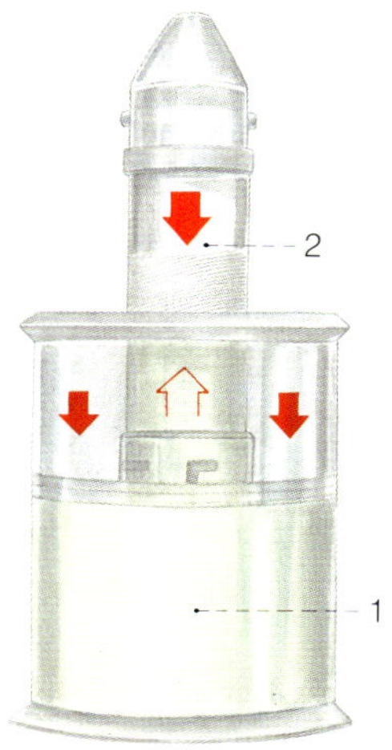

Fig. 3.**55** After being mixed, the precooled cement is pressed directly into the cartridge from the mixing vessel.

1 Mixing vessel with cement
2 Cartridge

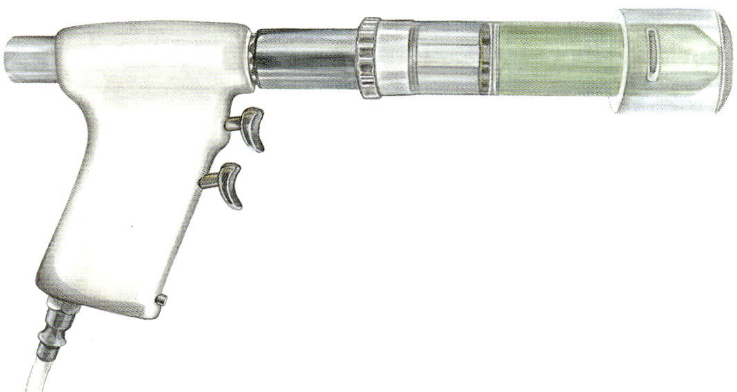

Fig. 3.**56** A Dränert cement gun is used to compress the cement (for 2 minutes) and inject it into the femoral canal.

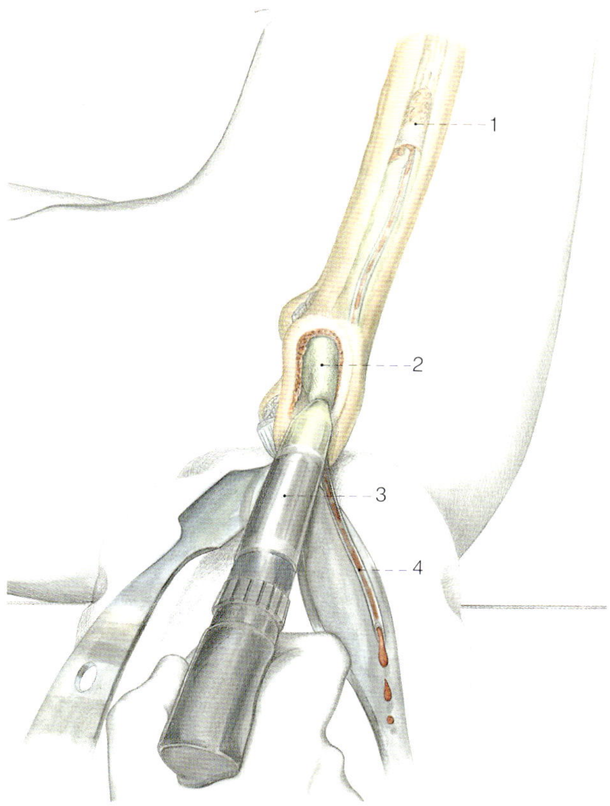

Fig. 3.**57 a** Filling the femoral canal with cement while relieving pressure with a drain.

1 Cement restrictor
2 Cement
3 Cement gun
4 Drain

Fig. 3.**57 b** An alternative method of cement injection utilizes a "snorkel" attachment. For clarity, this illustration shows a much thinner snorkel than the one used.

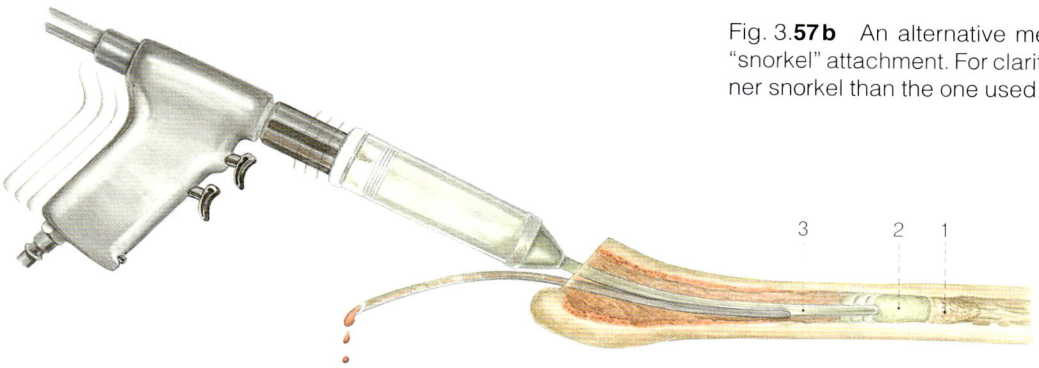

1 Cement restrictor
2 Cement
3 "Snorkel"

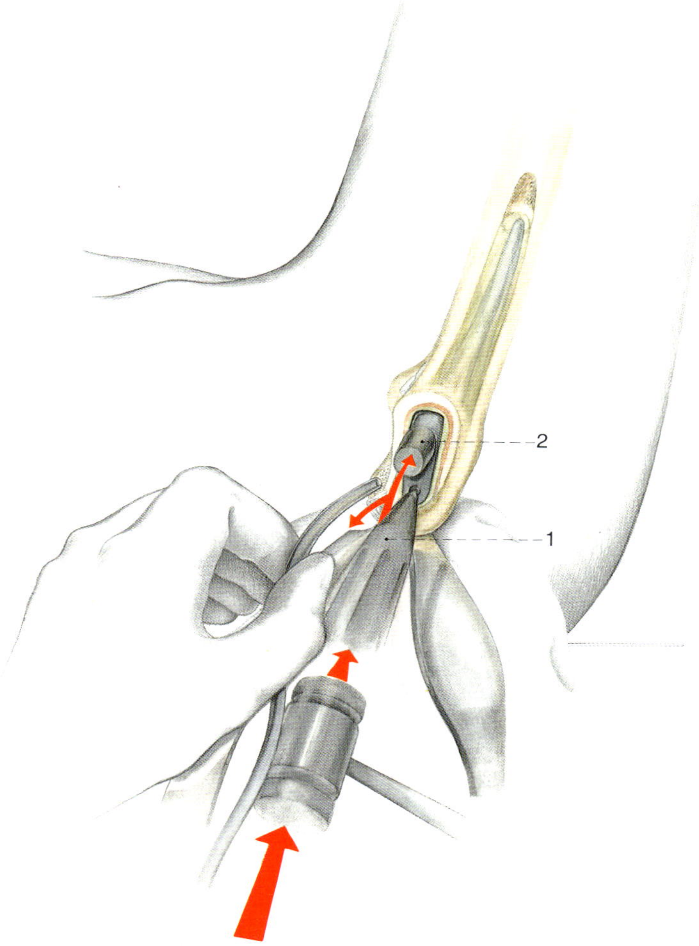

Fig. 3.**58** The stem is slowly pressed in while the drain is removed. When the implant has been fully seated, its position is verified with a ruler between the shoulder of the implant and the greater trochanter. If necessary, a mallet can be used to seat the implant deeper.

1 Impactor
2 Implant taper

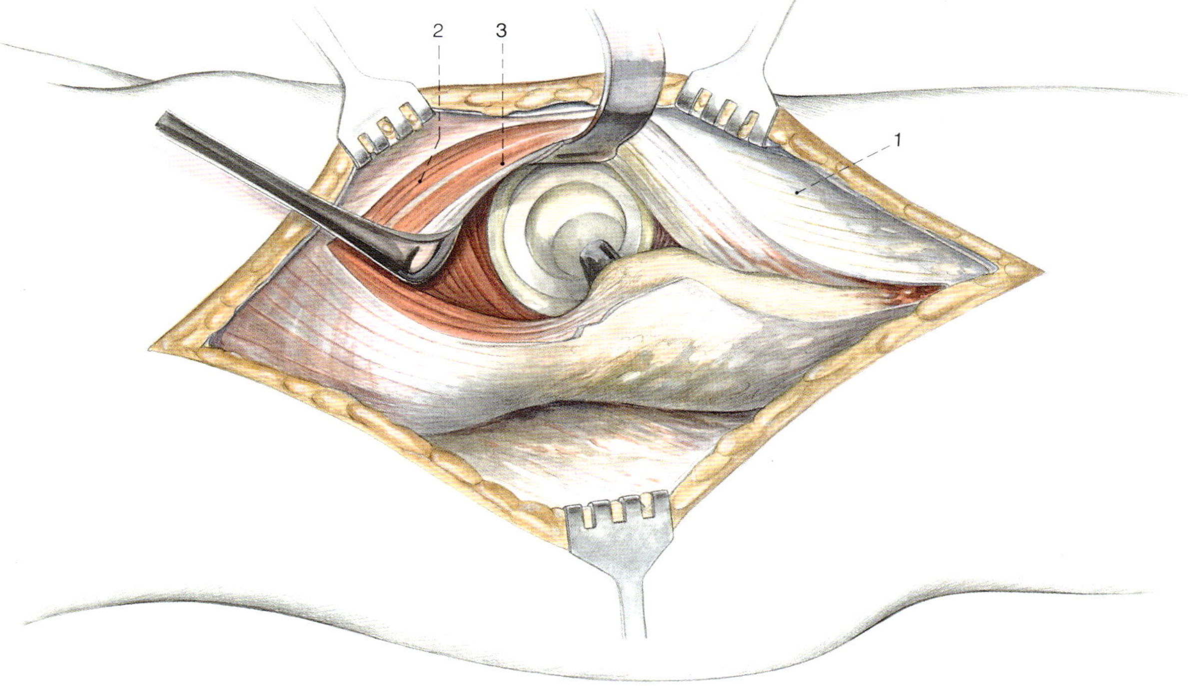

Fig. 3.**59** After the cement has hardened and any excess cement has been cleaned off the shoulder of the stem, the taper is cleaned and dried. Then a ceramic or metal head of the appropriate neck length is attached, and the hip is reduced.

1 Vastus lateralis
2 Gluteus medius
3 Gluteus minimus

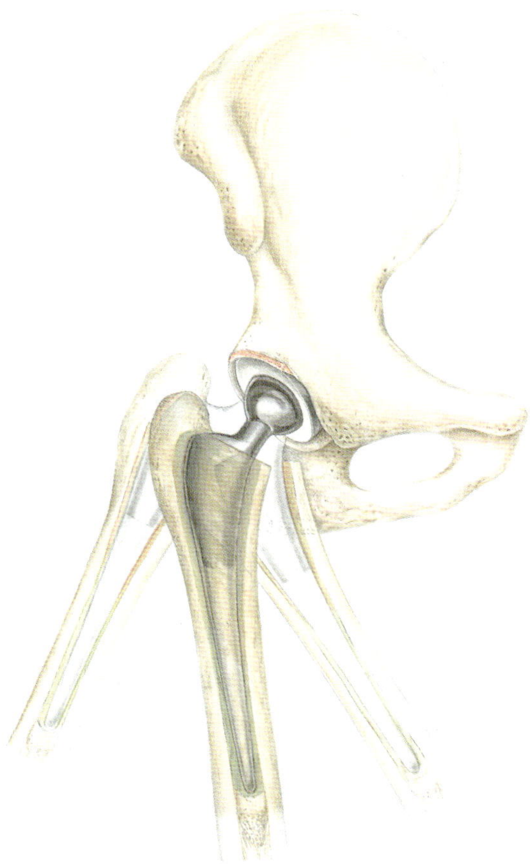

Fig. 3.**60** With the articular surfaces free of interposed soft tissue, the hip is reduced and motion and stability are assessed.

Closure

Placing the leg in flexion and internal rotation spontaneously closes the incision in the muscle fibers. The soft-tissue envelope formed by the vastus lateralis and gluteus medius is sutured in one or two layers; in either case, the suture includes the tendinous origins of the gluteus minimus. We use a vertical mattress stitch with nonabsorbable suture material to close the center of the incision over the greater trochanter (Fig. 3.**61**) after placing deep and subfascial drains. After closure, foam-rubber compression bandages are applied to both sides to compress the affected hip. A/P and lateral radiographs are prepared while the patient is still under anesthesia, and the leg is place in a foam-rubber splint.

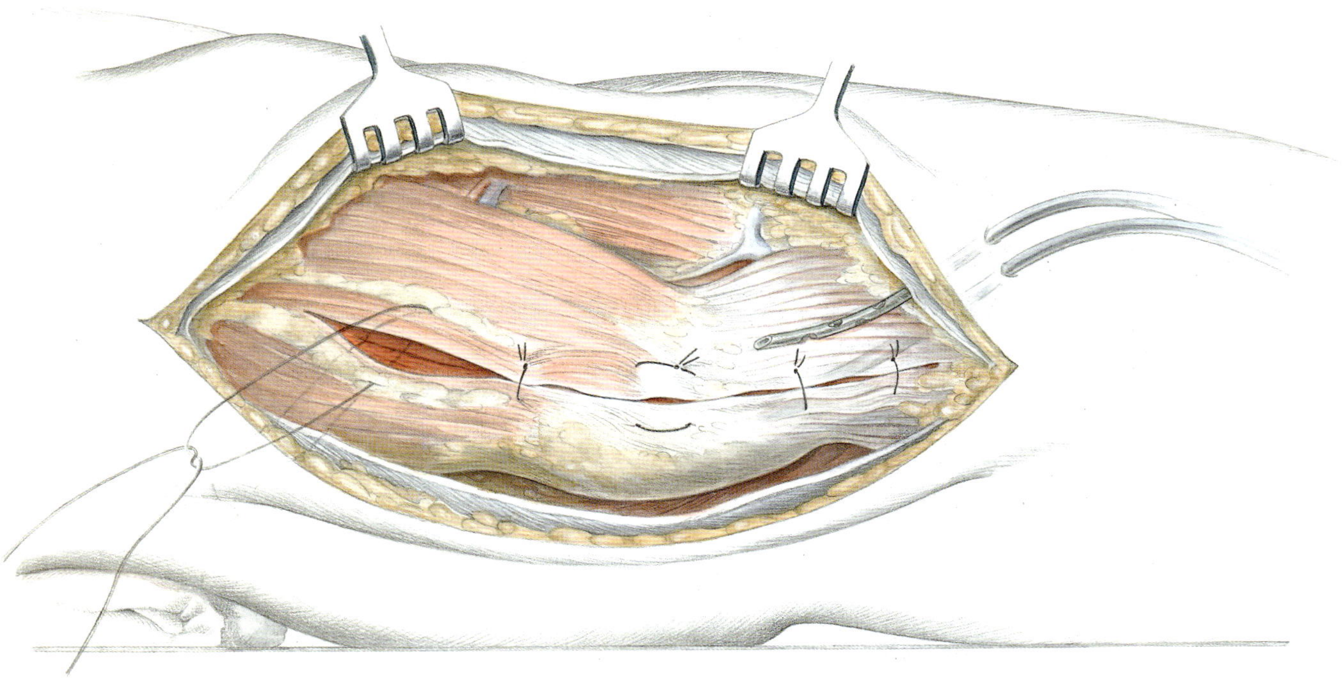

Fig. 3.**61** The soft-tissue envelope formed by the vastus lateralis and gluteus medius is sutured in one or two layers with the leg in internal rotation. Retention sutures are used where necessary, and deep and subfascial drains are placed.

Postoperative Treatment

Our patients receive perioperative prophylactic antibiotic therapy during surgery and within the first 24 hours postoperatively. We recommend compression bandages on the legs, mobilization on postoperative day one with gait training, and heparin therapy as deep-venous thrombosis prophylaxis. Partial weight bearing during the first 6 weeks postoperatively is recommended to protect soft tissue. After that, the patient may use a cane for an additional month.

Complications

Complications occurring in conjunction with cemented acetabular implants have been discussed. The most frequent stem complications are also attributable to insufficient exposure of the bone. This leads to a fracture of the posterolateral femoral cortex, particularly if the surgeon applies too much force and the bone is osteoporotic. Even in healthy bone, the surgeon should use the rasp carefully and avoid applying excessive force. If a fracture occurs, the incision should be extended distally and the vastus lateralis dissected to expose the fracture site. If it is a spiral fracture, the femur is reduced and stabilized with a plate. Bone fragments from spiral fractures can damage the perforating arteries. These arteries can bleed profusely and retract, making them difficult to locate. If this happens, we bluntly dissect the site between the vastus intermedius and the direct origin of the rectus femoris, palpate the deep femoral artery, and clamp it temporarily. Then we locate and ligate the bleeding stump of the artery. In muscular patients, it occasionally happens that the hip cannot be reduced with the final implant in place, although trial reduction did not present any problems. This can occur if the level of anesthesia is reduced prematurely. The duration of anesthesia should be discussed in advance with the anesthesiologist.

Spotorno Cementless Straight-Stem Implant

Indications

Primary and secondary osteoarthritis in younger patients.

Contraindications

- Severe osteoporosis
- Lack of primary stability due to other causes

Principle

The Spotorno cementless stem is a straight-stem press-fit implant. The prosthesis is conical in the coronal and sagittal planes, and has longitudinal ribs that provide a press fit in the metaphysis. If the metaphyseal anatomy does not provide suitable support (i.e., the shaft is cylindrical and osteoporotic), the stem is anchored proximally.

Preoperative Planning

Preoperative planning follows the criteria discussed in the introductory section on total hip arthroplasty. The requirements are a plain pelvic radiograph, acetabular and stem templates (provided by the manufacturer), and acetate sheets. The stem template is positioned so that under optimum shaft conditions (a funnel-shaped femoral shaft with bone stock of sufficient quality), there will be a layer of compacted cancellous bone about 1 mm thick between the implant and the cortex. In cylindrical or osteoporotic femurs, direct contact between the implant and the proximal diaphyseal cortex (i.e., the middle portion of the prosthetic stem) is desirable. The center of the implant femoral head should be at the apex of the greater trochanter. The osteotomy plane is also marked on the drawing, and the distance from it to the lesser trochanter is measured and recorded.

Surgical Technique

After the acetabular cup has been implanted, the proximal femur is exposed as described previously (see section on cemented stems). If the femoral neck is too long, a second osteotomy should be performed; ideally, the osteotomy level is about 1 cm proximal to the superior margin of the lesser trochanter. This is important for proper axial alignment of the straight-stem implant, which can only be achieved when the posterior segment of the osteotomized femoral neck is not longer than 1 cm.

Preparing the Greater Trochanter

Using an osteotome or a small oscillating saw, the surgeon removes a trapezoidal section of corticocancellous bone from the osteotomy plane, which includes part of the greater trochanter (Fig. 3.**62**). Particularly in a healthy femur, the surgeon will have to resect cortical bone from the apex of the greater trochanter to center the straight-stem implant. The femoral canal is broached with a long curette (Fig. 3.**63**), and then the medullary reamer is introduced into the femoral canal. The surgeon lateralizes the reamer as much as possible, rotating it while impacting it along the longitudinal axis of the femur. The canal can be widened laterally and posteriorly if required (Fig. 3.**64**). Now the reamer is replaced with successively larger rasps that are selected according to the preoperative plan (Fig. 3.**65a**). The rasps are held in 10° anteversion and impacted up to the mark (Fig. 3.**65b**).

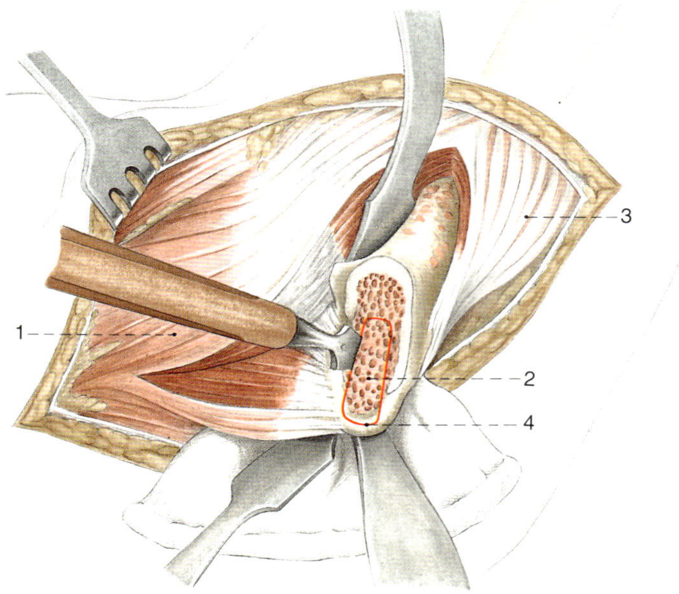

Fig. 3.**62** A trapezoidal section of corticocancellous bone is removed from the osteotomy plane with an osteotome or a small oscillating saw.

1 Gluteus medius
2 Trapezoidal section
3 Vastus lateralis
4 Greater trochanter

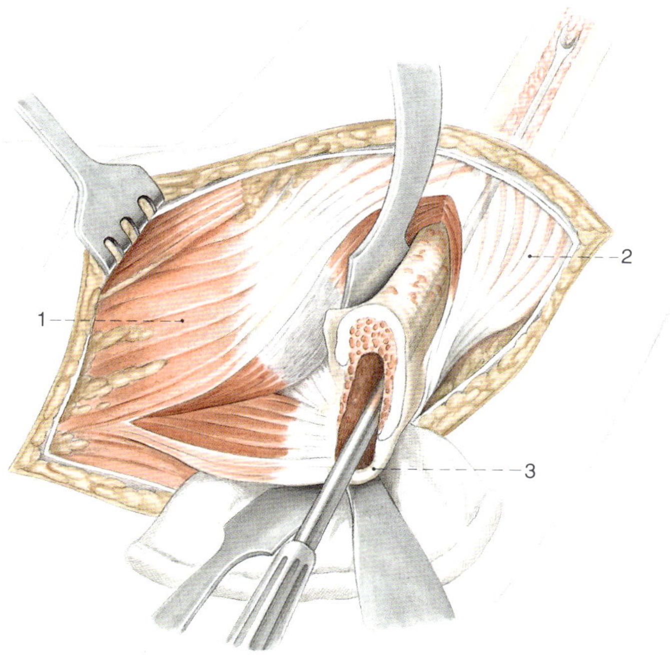

Fig. 3.**63** Broaching the femoral canal.

1 Gluteus medius
2 Vastus lateralis
3 Greater trochanter

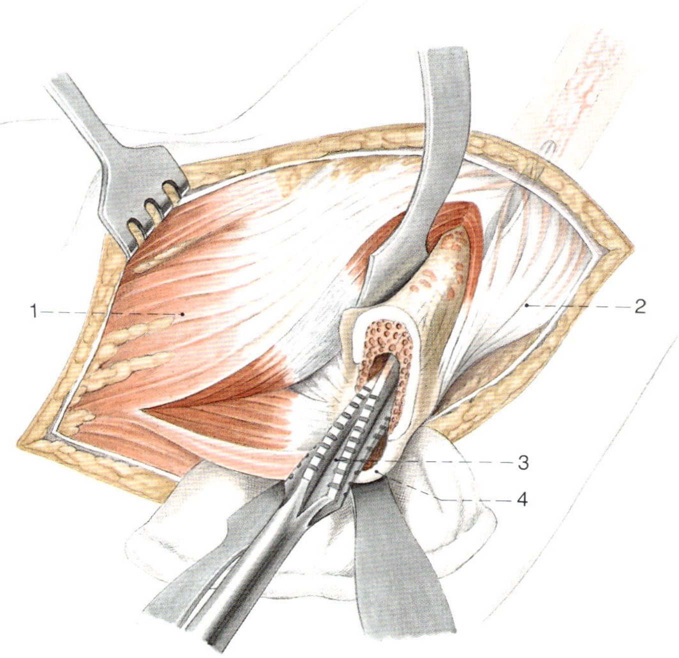

Fig. 3.**64** Preparing the femoral canal with a medullary reamer.

1 Gluteus medius
2 Vastus lateralis
3 Medullary reamer
4 Greater trochanter

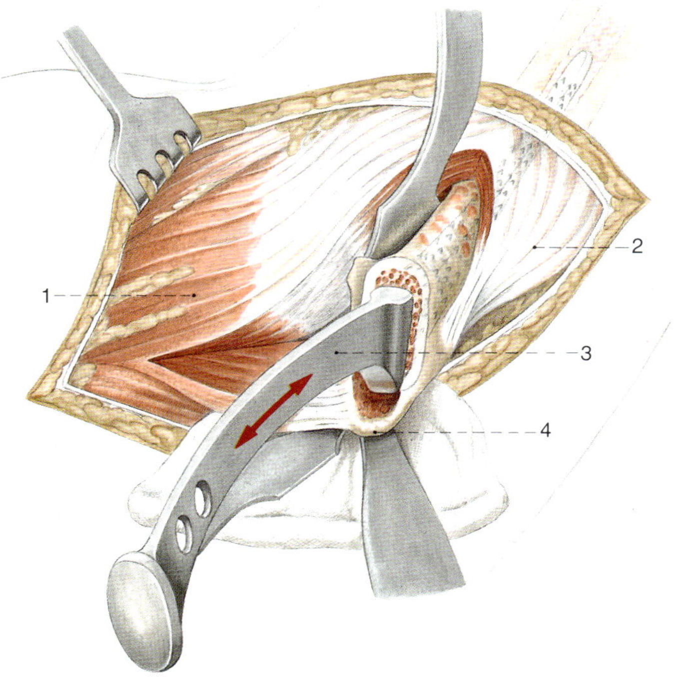

Fig. 3.**65a** Widening the femoral canal with successively larger raps.

1 Gluteus medius
2 Vastus lateralis
3 Rasp
4 Greater trochanter

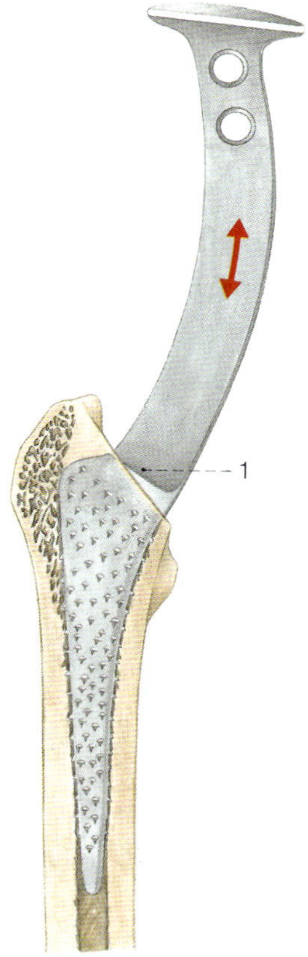

Fig. 3.**65b** Schematic diagram of the rasp partially impacted into the femoral canal. The rasp is driven in up to the mark.

1 Rasp mark

After the last rasp has been impacted, a 1-mm layer of cancellous bone should remain between the rasp and the medial cortex. The rasp is then removed, the femoral canal is irrigated and cleaned, and the implant is impacted with a mallet (Fig. 3.**66a**). The correct position of the implant is verified by measuring the distance between the apex of the greater trochanter and the shoulder of the implant with a ruler. Trial heads are attached and the optimum neck length is determined by reduction and evaluation of stability. The hip is reduced with the final ceramic head in place (Fig. 3.**66b**). Closure follows the procedure described in the section on cemented stems.

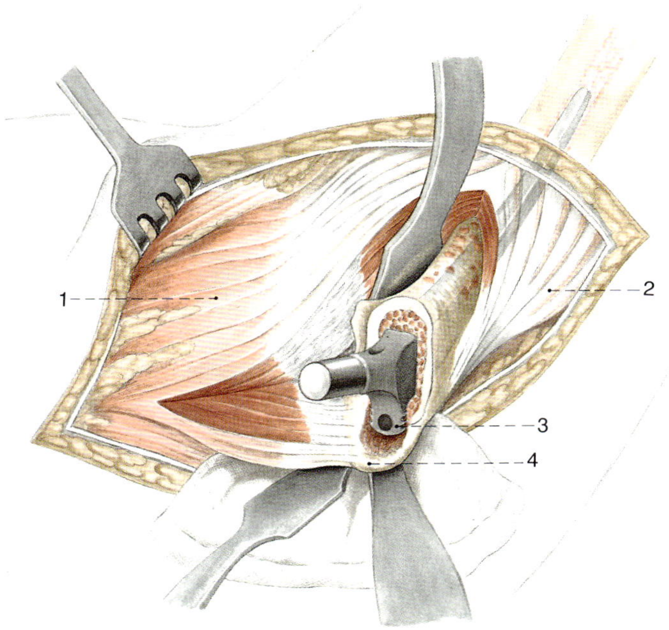

Fig. 3.**66a** After impacting the cementless stem.

1 Gluteus medius
2 Vastus lateralis
3 Shoulder of implant
4 Greater trochanter

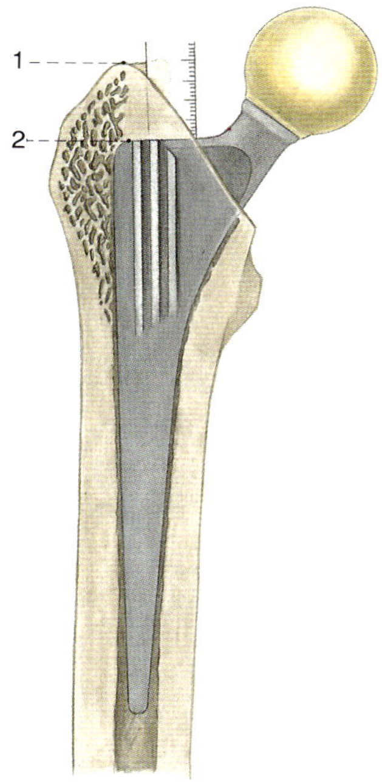

Fig. 3.**66b** Schematic diagram of the stem seated in the femur. The distance between the apex of the greater trochanter and the shoulder of the implant is measured and compared with the preoperative drawing.

1 Apex of the greater trochanter
2 Shoulder of implant

Postoperative Treatment

Immediate postoperative treatment is identical to that described in the section on cemented implants. We recommend partial weight bearing until the end of the sixth postoperative week.

Complications

Possible complications of implanting a straight-stem prosthesis include fractures of the proximal femur or greater trochanter. Proper preparation of the greater trochanter minimizes this risk but cannot eliminate it entirely. Avulsion fractures should be reduced with cerclage wire (1.2–1.4 mm). Postoperative management should include a longer period of partial weight bearing with forearm crutches, and rotation should be avoided.

Custom Implants

Aldinger Custom Cementless Stems Designed Using CT Scans

Indications

- Younger patients
- Arthritic hip dysplasia
- Osteoarthritis following slipped capital femoral epiphysis
- Osteoarthritis following osteotomy of the proximal femur

Principle

Custom implants designed using CT scans offer the following advantages:

1. Implant adapted to proximal femur ("fill and fit")
2. Increases leg length
3. Implant tailored to allow medial or lateral displacement of femur
4. Corrects anteversion

Preoperative Planning

In arthritic hip dysplasia, the superior aspect of the leg is shortened proportionately to the degree of subluxation. Total hip arthroplasty should strive to correct this.

First, the leg-length differential is assessed clinically. The difference in height between the two lesser trochanters in the standing anterior-posterior view pelvic radiograph is an indication of the superior displacement of the femur in the acetabulum. Clinical and radiographic measurements generally coincide, except in the presence of contractures with a functional reduction in leg length. The difference in height between the lesser trochanters is marked on the standing anterior-posterior view pelvic radiograph (Fig. 3.**67**). Then the surgeon traces the contours of the acetabular template level with the original acetabulum (Fig. 3.**68**), and marks the center of rotation of the acetabular cup (PM).

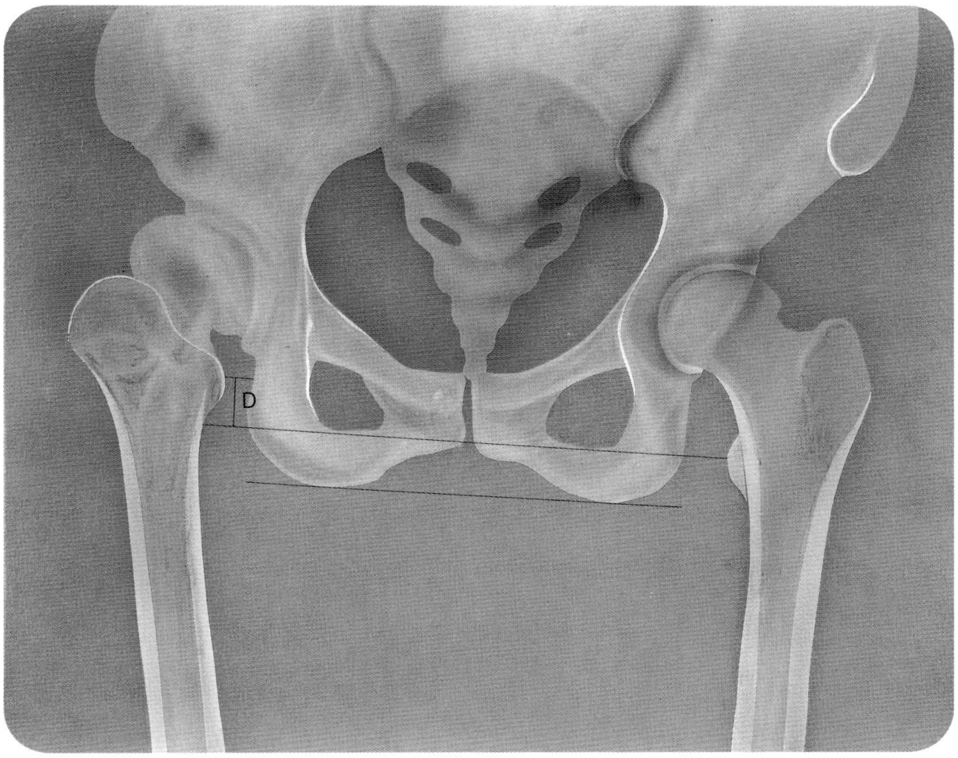

Fig. 3.**67** Measuring the leg-length differential on a standing anterior-posterior view pelvic radiograph. The superior displacement of the lesser trochanter in the affected hip (D) is corrected intraoperatively.

External rotation contractures can distort the appearance of the femoral neck in the radiograph. To achieve symmetrical femoral neck length, the surgeon superimposes an acetate sheet on the contralateral side and traces the contours and center of the contralateral femoral head (Fig. 3.**69**). This tracing is then reversed and superimposed on the affected hip so that the lesser trochanters align (Fig. 3.**70**). Now the surgeon marks the new center of rotation of the hip (KM).

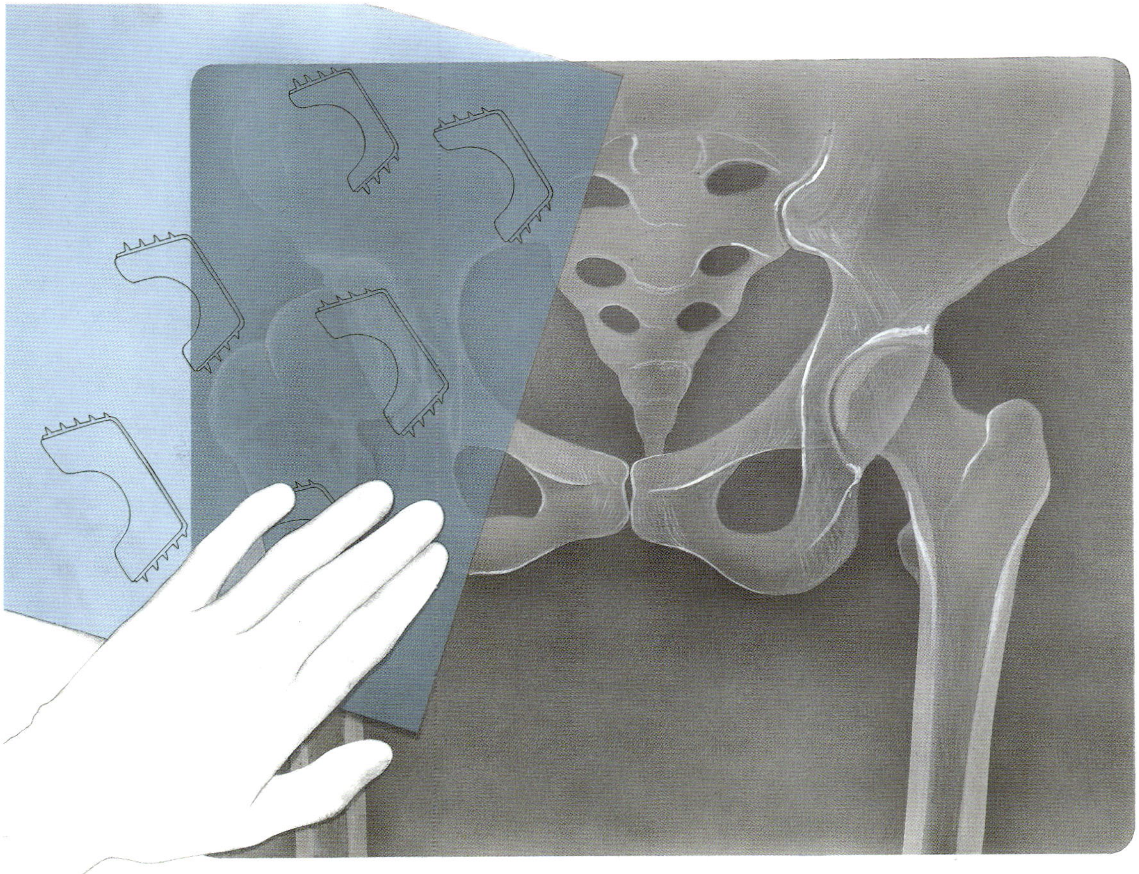

Fig. 3.**68** The contours of the acetabular template level and the center of rotation of the acetabular cup are marked on the radiograph.

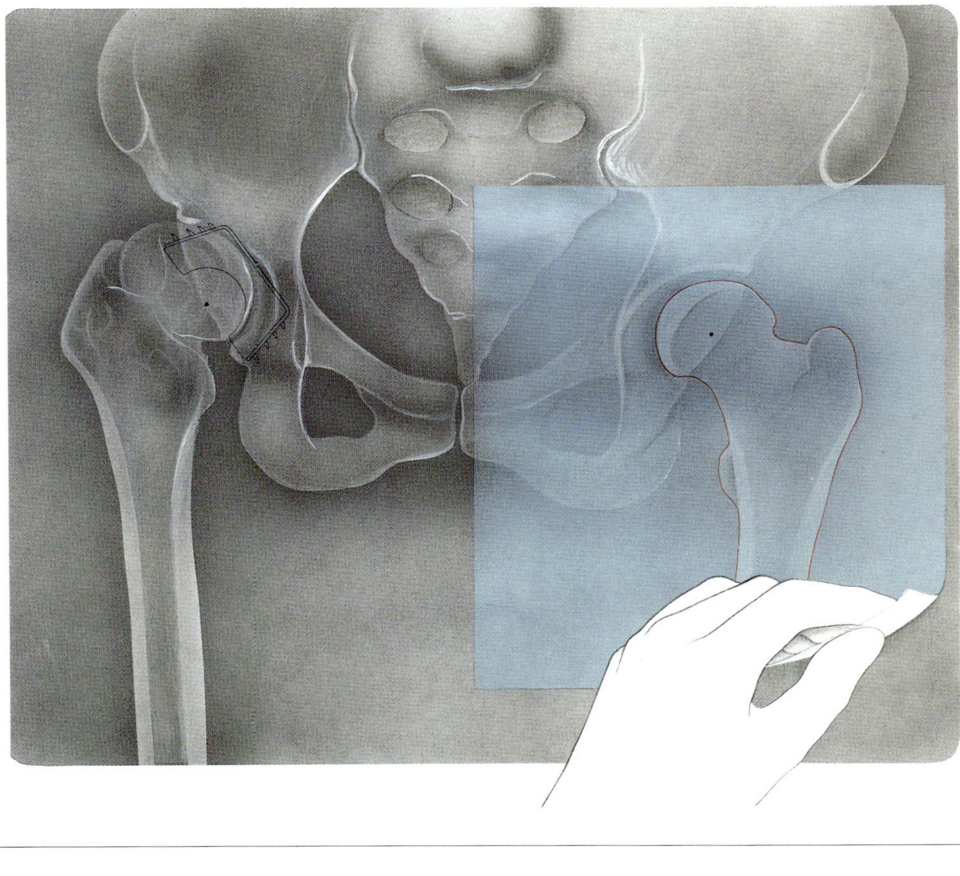

Fig. 3.**69** The contours and center of the contralateral femoral head are traced on a superimposed acetate sheet.

The horizontal and vertical distance between the points PM and KM define the increase in leg length and the lateral or medial displacement of the femur after reduction. Arthritic hip dysplasia frequently requires reconstruction of the roof of the acetabulum using bone from the resected femoral head. These corrections are recorded on the drawing as well (Fig. 3.**71**).

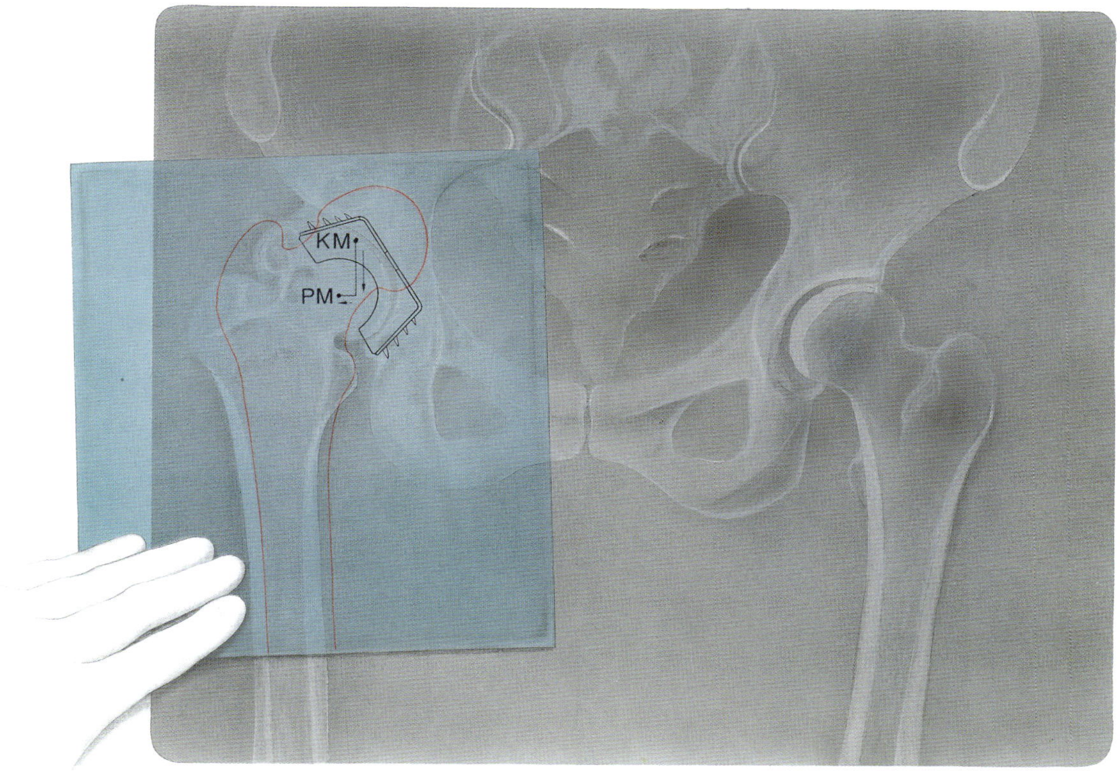

Fig. 3.**70** The tracing is reversed and superimposed on the affected hip so that the lesser trochanters align. The tracing shows the new center of rotation of the hip (KM). The horizontal and vertical distances between the points PM and KM define the increase in leg length and the lateral or medial displacement of the femur.

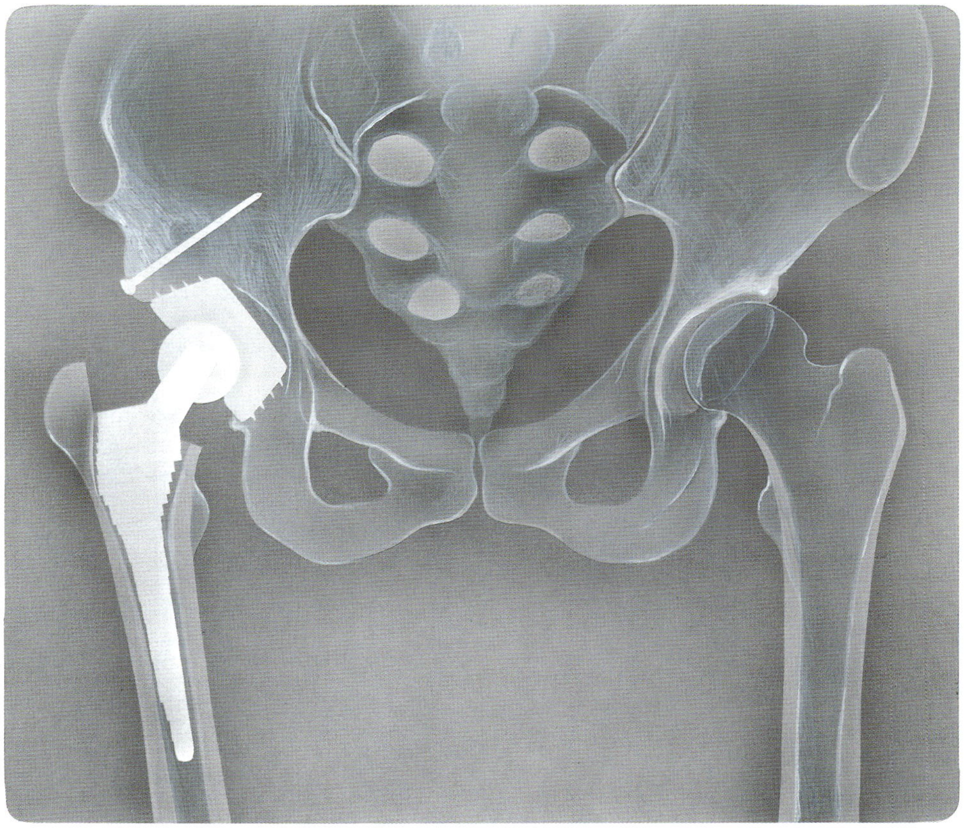

Fig. 3.**71** Any necessary reconstruction of the roof is recorded on the drawing as well. The manufacturer's templates (see Fig. 3.**74**) are traced on an acetate sheet and superimposed so that points PM and KM align.

Correcting anteversion may be indicated in the following situations:

1. Arthritic hip dysplasia with pathologic anteversion
2. Pathologic retroversion following slipped capital femoral epiphysis or osteotomy of the proximal femur

CT sections through the femoral neck and condyles reveal the version. If substantial deviation is detected, correcting the anteversion of the neck of the implant to a normal value of 10–15° may be indicated (Figs. 3.**72** and 3.**73**).

The manufacturer requires the following information to manufacture an implant based on CT scans:

- Plain pelvic radiograph and CT scan with the center of the implant head and center of the acetabular cup marked
- Desired increase in leg length
- Lateral or medial displacement of the femur
- Anteversion correction

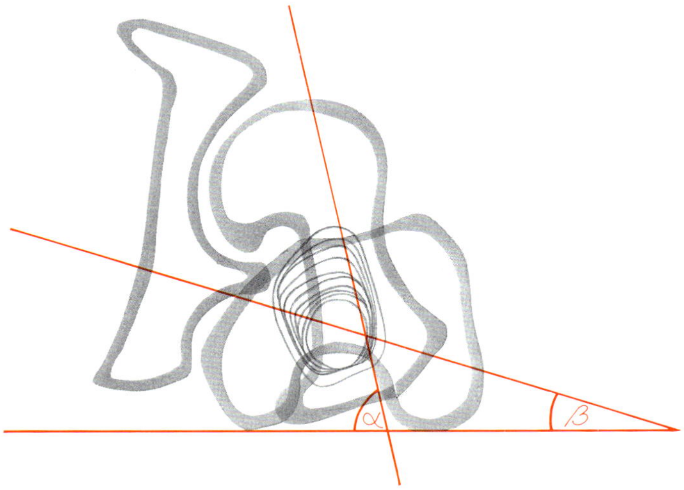

Fig. 3.**72** Pathologic anteversion (α) in arthritic hip dysplasia is revealed by two superimposing two CT scans (through the femoral neck and condyles). A 20° version correction (β) is required.

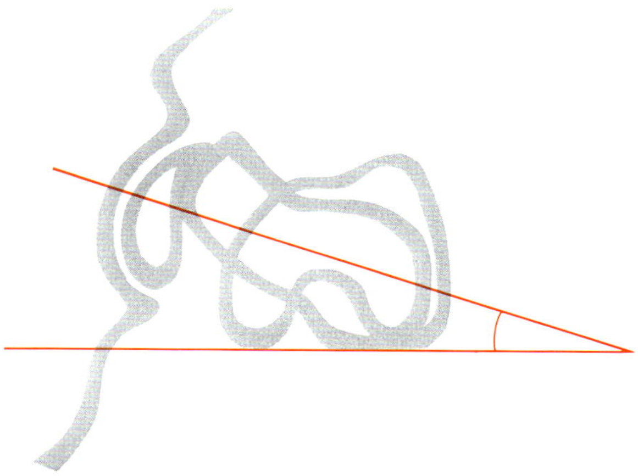

Fig. 3.**73** Following slipped capital femoral epiphysis, the anteversion may appear to be reduced. The prosthesis should be implanted in normal version.

Surgical Technique

The manufacturer supplies the implants with a planning drawing (Fig. 3.**74**), specifying the level of the osteotomy of the femoral neck and the implantation depth of the prosthesis. The manufacturer also provides the surgeon with important information, such as the details of a required osteotomy of the posterior femoral neck or required reaming in the femoral canal. This drawing provides the basis for definitive preoperative planning (see Fig. 3.**71**).

After the acetabular cup is implanted, the surgeon exposes the proximal femur as described in the section on cemented stems. Now the femoral neck osteotomy is performed at an angle of 60° to the axis of the femoral shaft (Figs. 3.**75** and 3.**76**).

The femoral canal is then broached with a long curette (Fig. 3.**77**).

Generally, the posterior portion of the femoral neck (trochanteric fossa) has to be removed with a Luer forceps (Fig. 3.**78**). Now the custom rasp is impacted into the femoral canal. The surgeon can impact the rasp manually or use a pneumatic impactor (Figs. 3.**79** and 3.**81**). While impacting the rasp, the surgeon shifts the pneumatic impactor posteriorly (Fig. 3.**80**). The rasp is impacted until the distance P between the rasp and the greater trochanter (20 mm in the illustration) corresponds to the distance determined in preoperative planning (Fig. 3.**82**). After the rasp is removed, the femoral canal is irrigated, and the stem is impacted to the planned depth (Fig. 3.**83**). With the stem in place, the surgeon attaches a trial head and reduces the hip to assess motion and stability. Then the final ceramic head is inserted and the hip is reduced. Closure follows the procedure described in the section on cemented stems.

Postoperative Treatment

We recommend 8 weeks of partial weight bearing with forearm crutches.

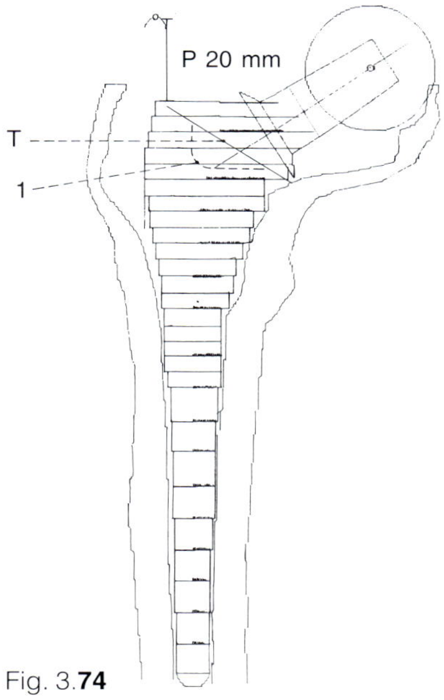

Fig. 3.**74**

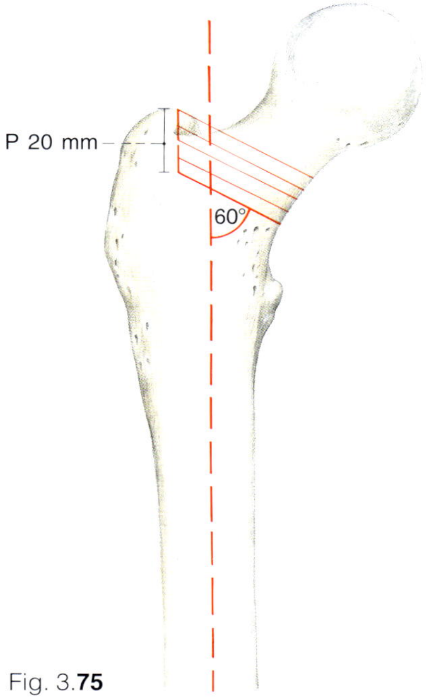

Fig. 3.**75**

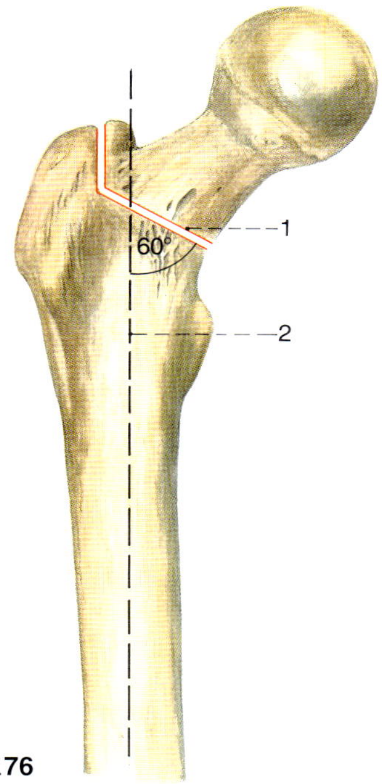

Fig. 3.**76**

Fig. 3.**74** Preoperative planning diagram provided by the manufactor.

P Distance between the greater trochanter and the shoulder of the implant
T Level of the osteotomy of the femoral nack
1 Posterior femoral neck osteotomy

Fig. 3.**75** Schematic diagram of the osteotomy of the femoral neck. In this example, a step-cut osteotomy is performed 2 cm inferior to the apex of the greater trochanter.

P Distance between the greater trochanter and the osteotomy plane

Fig. 3.**76** After the osteotomy of the femoral neck.

1 Level of the osteotomy of the femoral neck
2 Axis of the femoral shaft

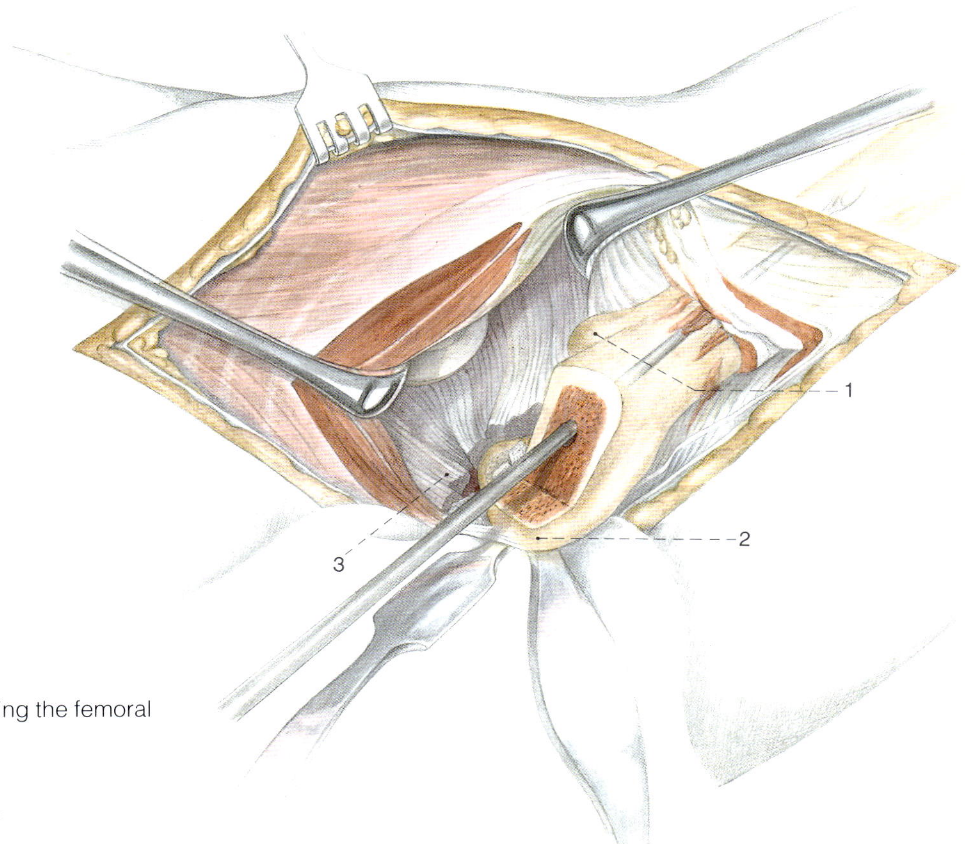

Fig. 3.**77** Broaching the femoral canal.

1 Lesser trochanter
2 Greater trochanter
3 Piriformis tendon

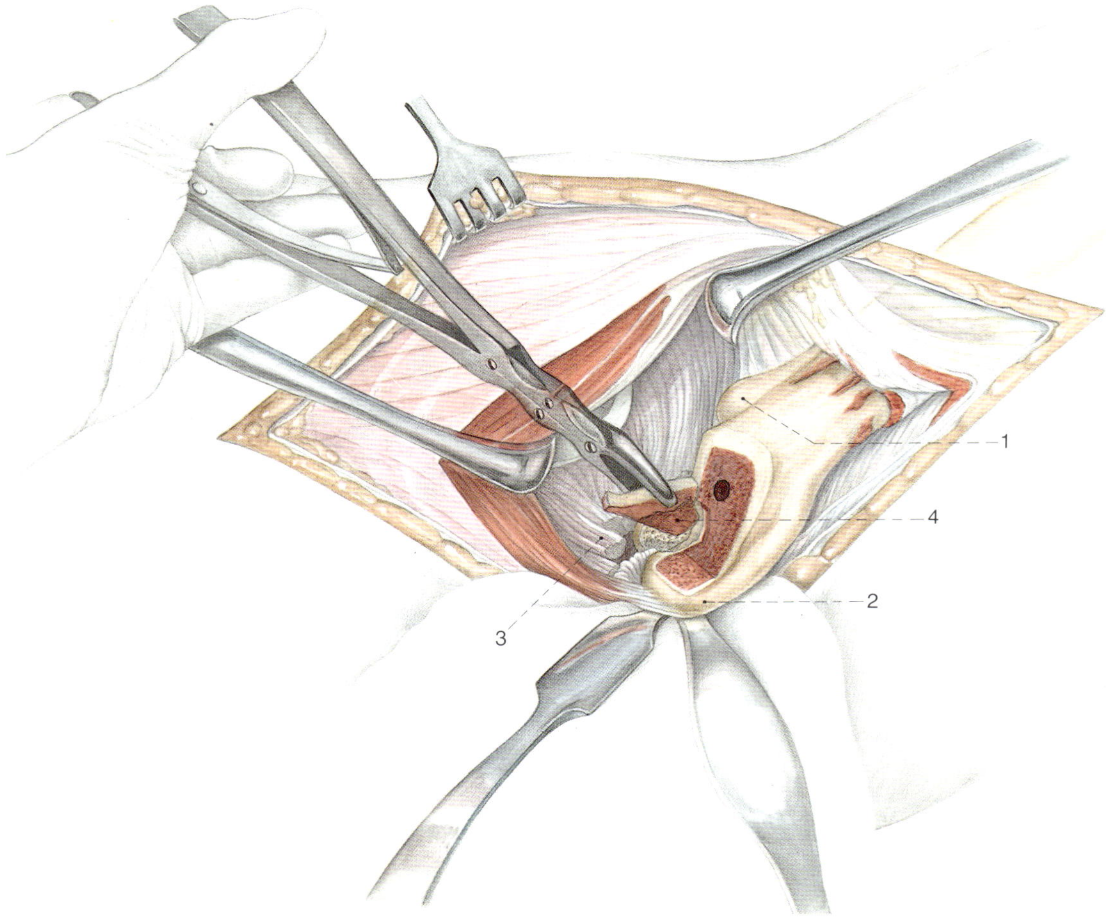

Fig. 3.**78** Removing cortical bone from the posterior femoral neck.

1 Lesser trochanter
2 Greater trochanter
3 Piriformis tendon
4 Cortical bone removed from the posterior femoral neck

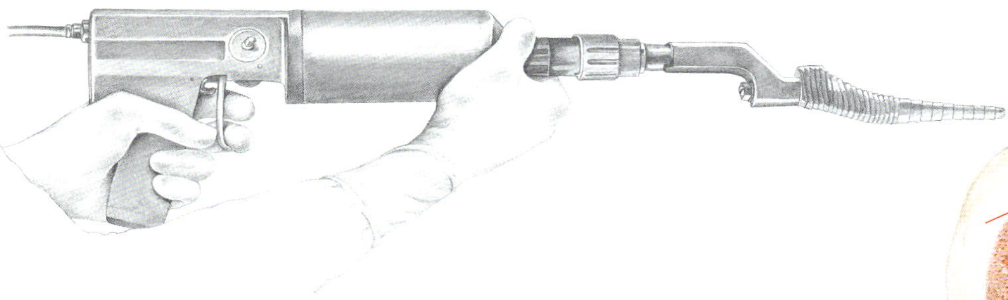

Fig. 3.**79** The custom rasp is attached to a pneumatic impactor.

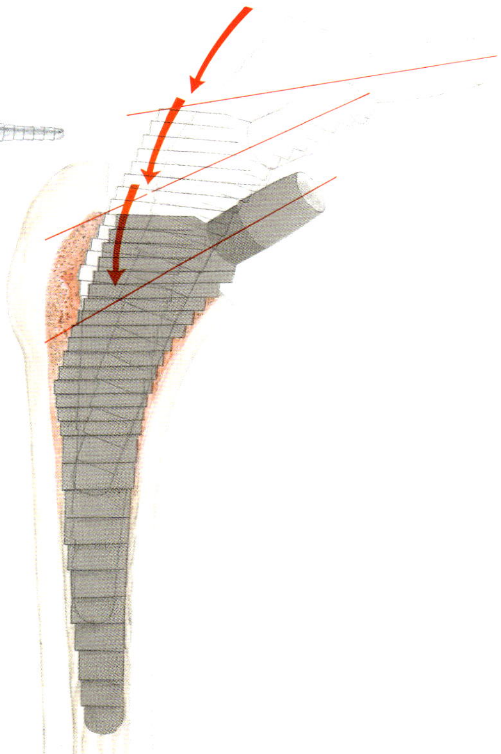

Fig. 3.**80** The rasp is shifted posteriorly as it is impacted. The ▶ position of the rasp is verified with fluoroscopy.

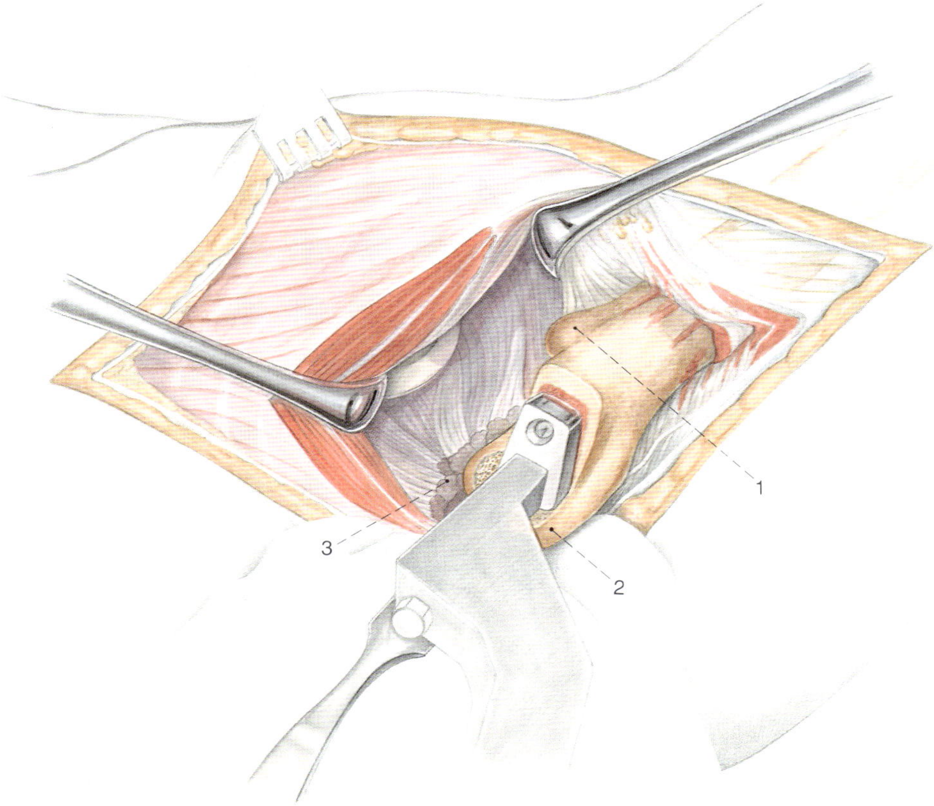

Fig. 3.**81** The rasp is impacted to the planned depth.

1 Lesser trochanter
2 Greater trochanter
3 Piriformis tendon

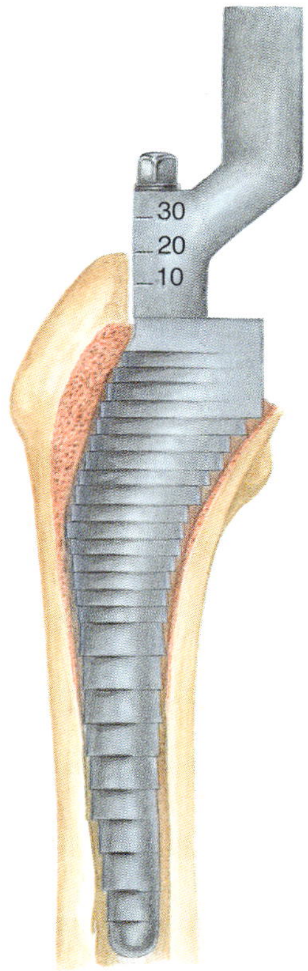

Fig. 3.**82** Schematic diagram of the rasp seated in the femur. The distance between the apex of the greater trochanter and the shoulder of the rasp is measured and compared with the preoperative drawing.

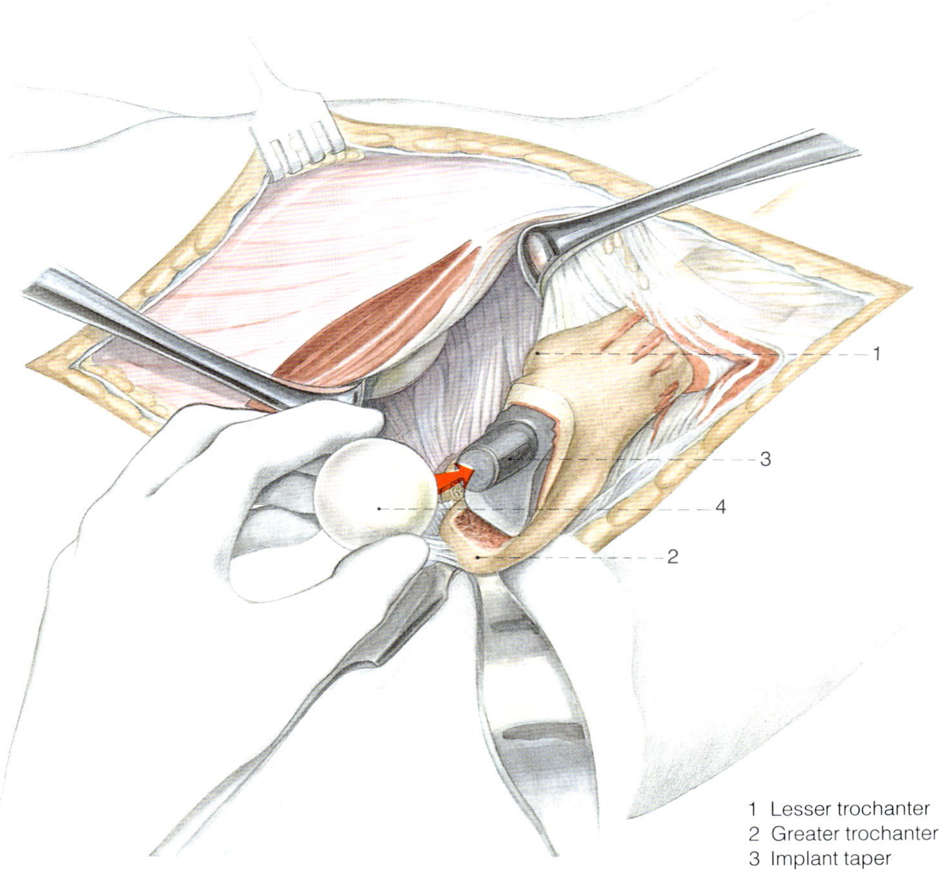

Fig. 3.**83** After the stem has been seated.

1 Lesser trochanter
2 Greater trochanter
3 Implant taper
4 Implant head

Egoform Custom Cementless Stems Designed Using Radiographic Measurements

Indications

- Osteoarthritis of the hip
- Younger patients without osteoporosis

Principle

Like the Aldinger prosthesis, the Egoform implant is a fill-and-fit system. Whereas the Aldinger system utilizes data from CT scans, the Egoform implant is designed on the basis of radiographic measurements. The shaft and the neck–shaft angle can be customized, but the version of the neck cannot be altered. This implant offers an optimum metaphyseal form fit and a collar for additional stress transfer, thus largely eliminating the need for diaphyseal fixation.

Preoperative Planning

Special anteroposterior and lateral radiographs are required for designing the implant and planning the procedure. A measuring band with a metal ring is applied to the patient's proximal thigh. The position of the ring should remain the same for both radiographs (Fig. 3.**84a** and **b**). The contours and center of the acetabular cup are traced on the anteroposterior radiograph as described in the section on the Aldinger implant. The surgeon then traces the contours of the proximal femur and the center of the contralateral femoral head on an acetate sheet, reverses this sheet, and superim-

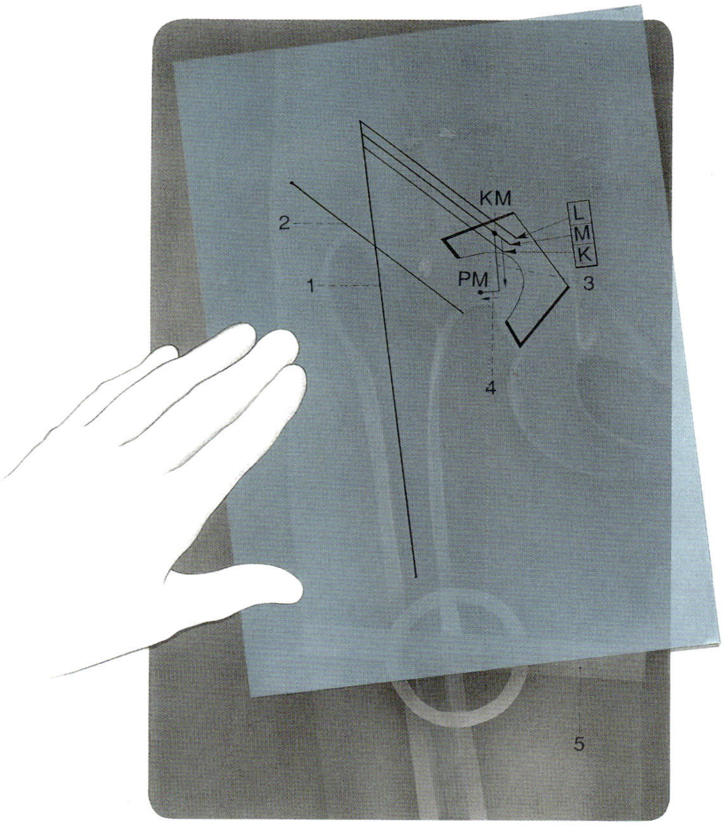

Fig. 3.**84a** The contours of the acetabular cup, the center of the cup (PM), and the center of the implant femoral head (KM) are traced on a special preoperative AP radiograph. Note the metal measuring band. The manufacturer's template is positioned so that the virtual axis of the stem is centered in the proximal femur. Line M should transect point KM.

1 Center axis of implant
2 Level of the osteotomy of the femoral neck
3 Increase in leg length
4 Lateral displacement (offset)
5 Measuring band
KM Center of prosthetic head
PM Center of acetabular cup

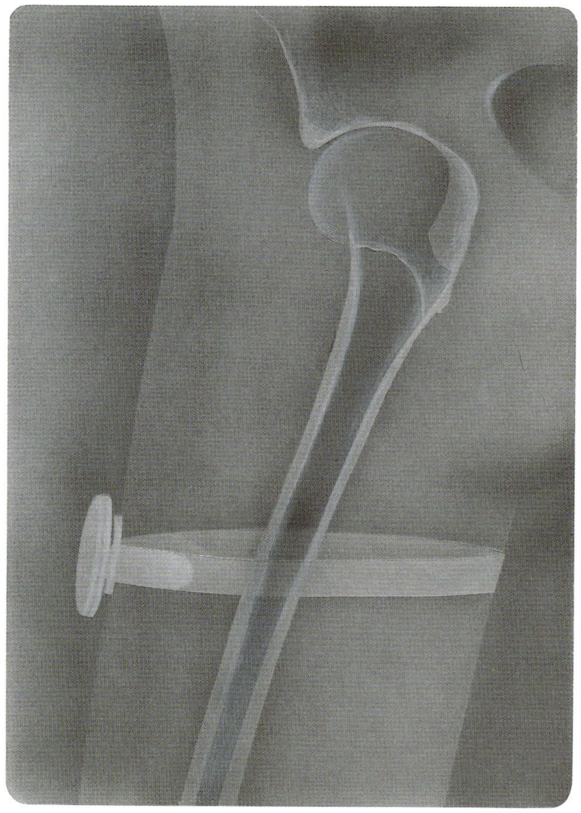

Fig. 3.**84b** Special lateral radiograph with measuring band for designing the Egoform prosthesis.

poses it on the affected hip. Next the surgeon superimposes an acetate sheet supplied by the manufacturer over the radiograph so that the axis of the prosthetic stem is centered in the proximal femur. This determines the plane of the femoral neck osteotomy. The middle line of the three parallel lines should transect point KM, the center of the head. These lines correspond to the three available head lengths (L = long, M = medium, K = short). The vertical and horizontal difference between points KM and PM correspond to the difference in leg length and the lateral or medial displacement. If no increase in leg length is desired, the femoral neck osteotomy can be performed further distally.

When the implant is finished, the manufacturer supplies drawings showing the contours of the implant. Acetate sheets showing the anteroposterior and lateral contours of the femur are superimposed on the manufacturer's respective drawings, and the surgeon traces the position of the implant in the proximal femur. Then the surgeon enters the distances from the apex of the greater trochanter to the shoulder of the implant and from the apex of the lesser trochanter to the collar of the implant in the planning drawing (Fig. 3.**85a** and **b**).

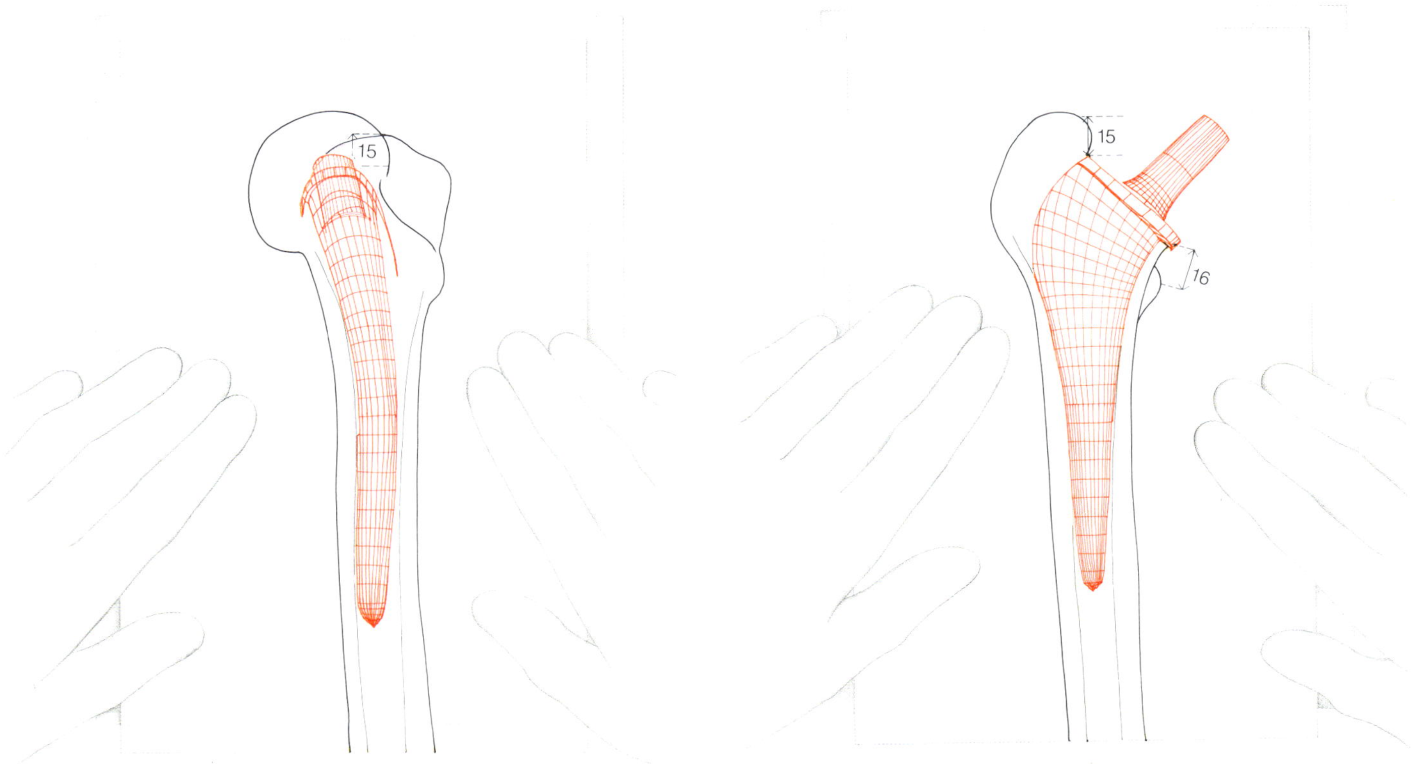

a b

Fig. 3.**85a** and **b** Acetate sheets showing the anteroposterior and lateral contours of the femur are superimposed on the manufacturer's respective contour drawings of the implant, and the position of the implant in the proximal femur is traced. The distances from the apex of the greater trochanter to the shoulder of the implant and from the apex of the lesser trochanter to the collar of the implant are entered in the planning drawing and verified intraoperatively.

Surgical Technique

After the acetabular cup is implanted, the surgeon exposes the proximal femur as described in the section on cemented stems. The medullary canal is first opened with a box osteotome and broached with a long curette, after which the surgeon impacts a custom rasp, which matches the exact size and shape of the implant. Impacting the rasp the last 2–3 cm is often difficult, particularly in male patients with hard bone. As the rasp is impacted, it automatically rotates according to the shape of the femur (Fig. 3.**86**). The surgeon should impact the rasp up to the collar; if this is not possible, its position is verified with fluoroscopy and any necessary corrections are made. When the rasp has been properly seated, the surgeon resects additional bone from the femoral neck if required (Fig. 3.**87 a** and **b**). With the rasp in place, the anterior cortex is osteotomized parallel to the collar. Then the rasp is removed and the posterior osteotomy is completed. The femoral canal is then irrigated and cleaned. The surgeon clamps the implant (whose proximal third is coated with hydroxylapatite) into the impactor and drives it into the femoral canal (Figs. 3.**88** and 3.**89**). Now the reference distances (from the apex of the greater trochanter to the shoulder of the implant and from the apex of the lesser trochanter to the collar of the implant) are checked to assess the position of the implant; the surgeon should verify that the collar rests on Bigelow's septum.

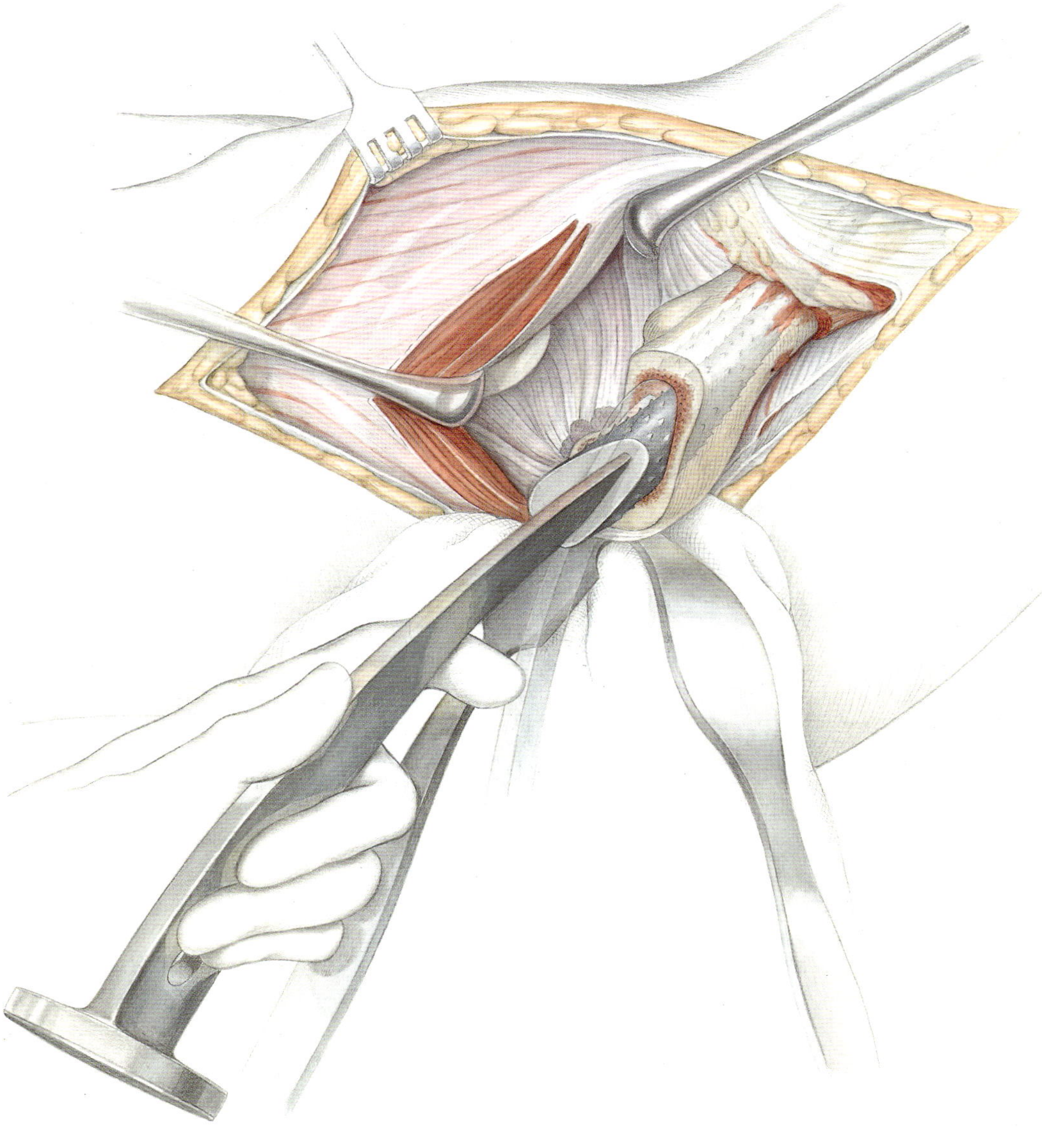

Fig. 3.**86** Impacting the custom rasp into the femoral canal. Impacting the rasp the last 2–3 cm is often difficult in osteosclerotic bone. As the rasp is impacted, it automatically rotates into proper version.

Fig. 3.**87a** Resecting additional bone from the femoral neck with the rasp in place.

Fig. 3.**87b** The edge of the rasp is parallel to the plane of osteotomy.

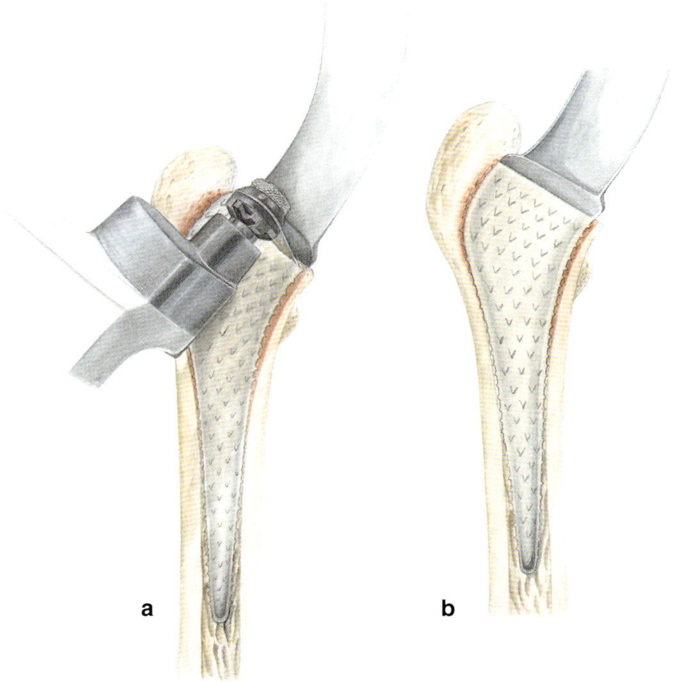

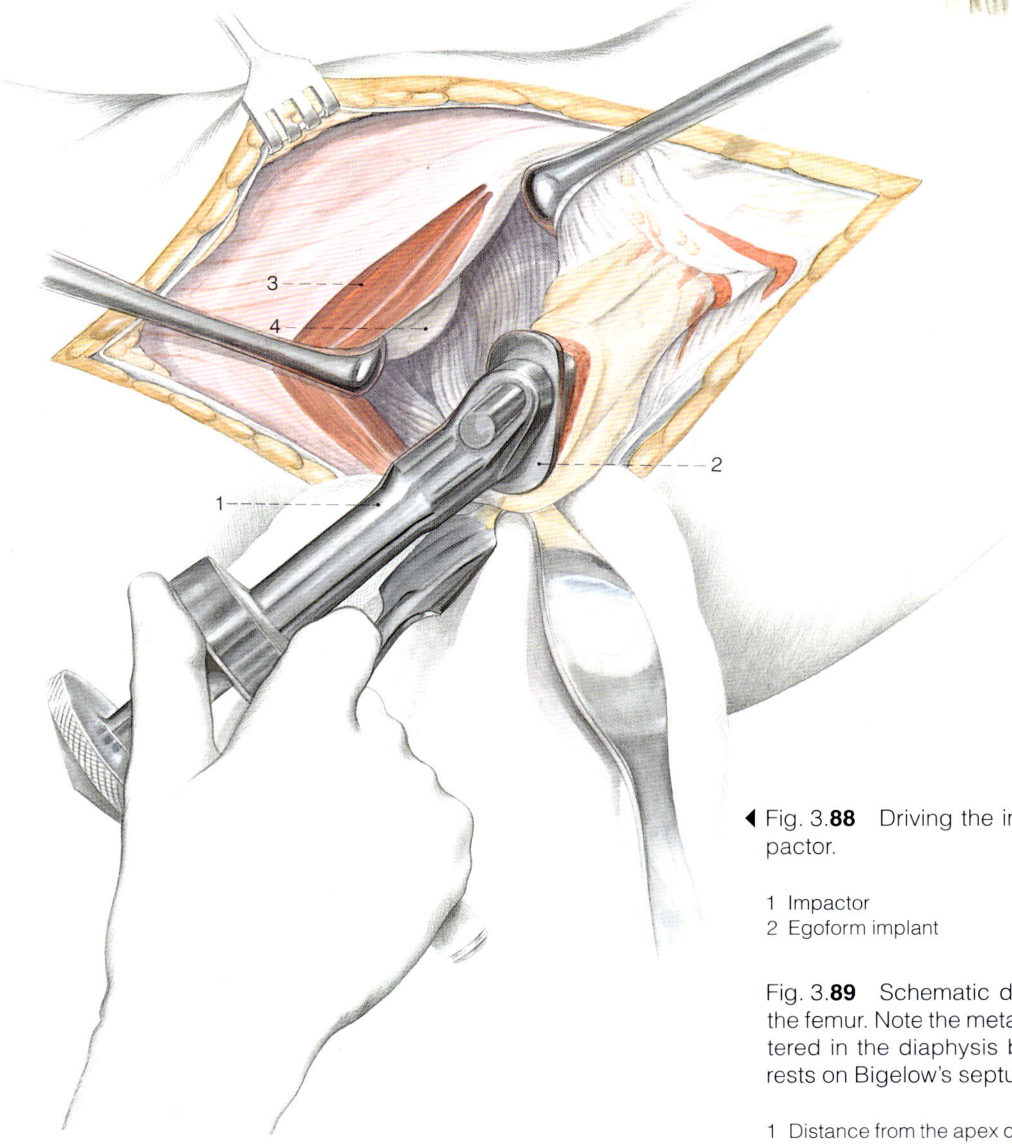

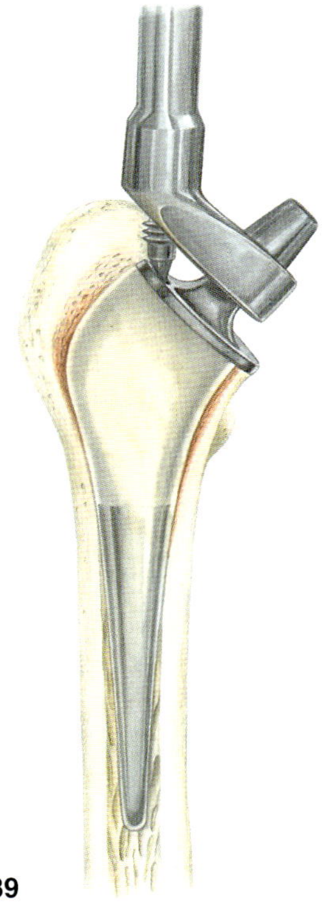

Fig. 3.**89**

◀ Fig. 3.**88** Driving the implant into the femoral canal with the impactor.

1 Impactor
2 Egoform implant
3 Gluteus medius
4 Acetabular cup

Fig. 3.**89** Schematic diagram of the implant correctly seated in the femur. Note the metaphyseal support; the distal implant is centered in the diaphysis but not fixed. The collar of the prosthesis rests on Bigelow's septum.

1 Distance from the apex of the lesser trochanter to the collar of the implant

References

Aldinger G, Fischer A, Kurtz B. Computer-assisted manufacturing of individual endoprostheses. Arch Orthop Traumatol Surg. 1983; 102:31.

Charnley J. Low Friction Arthroplasty of the Hip. Heidelberg: Springer; 1979.

Draenert K. Beobachtungen zur Zementierung von Implantkomponenten. Med Orth Technik 1986; 6.

Moretton JC, Claudon B, Cravoisy JC, Magnien P. Conception et fabrication assistee par ordinateur d'une prothese femoral de haunch. Rev Chir orthop. 1986; 72:89.

Müller ME. Total hip prostheses. Clin Orthop. 1970; 72:46.

Spotorno L, et al. Unsere Erfahrungen mit nicht zementierten Prothesen. Orthopädie. 1987; 16.

Starker M, Heipertz W. Frühergebnisse bei individuell gefertigten Endoprothesen. Praktische Orthop. 1991; 22:431.

4 Revision Total Hip Arthroplasty

E. Nieder

The chapter on revision total hip arthroplasty presents the procedures used to replace implants after aseptic failure. The procedures are divided into preoperative, intraoperative and postoperative phases and are described in sequence. The phases include preoperative planning, surgical approach, implant removal, reimplantation, soft-tissue reconstruction, closure and postoperative management.

Regardless of the type of fixation used with the primary implant, we favor using cement with the revision implant for the following reasons:

- Reliable pain relief and immediate full weight bearing
- Long-term studies show results to be reliable
- Easy clinical and radiological assessment postoperatively
- It allows bone-conserving removal techniques even in the absence of loosening
- Antibiotics can be eluted from the cement for prophylaxis against periprosthetic infection and for treatment of this most serious complication following replacement.

Cement itself is nontoxic. However, its wear particles (like those of many implant materials) may induce progressive osteolysis. Therefore, cemented implants should be checked regularly and revised early before this occurs, even in the absence of loosening. If it occurs, defects must be grafted in aseptic cases and the new implant should again be fixed with cement. If these rules are observed, cemented implants remain a viable surgical option.

The implants and tools described here (except those which are referred to other authors) were designed and are used by the group of surgeons at the Endo-Klinik in Hamburg. They are therefore called ENDO-Modells.

Preoperative Planning

Differential Diagnosis

When a patient complains of pain following total hip arthroplasty, physical examination to isolate the possible causes of the pain is the first step in preoperative planning. Pain can be caused by the implant and bone, or have its origin in the soft tissue surrounding the joint, or is due to neurological alterations. It may also be referred from a pathologic condition in a different region or it may be a sign of periprosthetic infection.

Pain caused by the implant and bone is generally a sign of loosening of one or both components. In cementless implants, this is either due to a failure to achieve biologic fixation or to loosening after biologic fixation has been achieved. Patients with cementless stems may also experience persistent pain in spite of biologic fixation. Asymptomatic loosening is rare, but it can occur in both cemented and cementless implantation. Loosening of the acetabular component generally causes pain in the groin or buttocks, while thigh or knee pain is often due to stem problems. Trochanteric nonunion causes localized pain, which often radiates into the iliotibial tract. Recurring dislocations and fractures are further (albeit obvious) causes of pain.

Pain associated with soft-tissue changes may be the result of heterotopic ossification, scarred adhesions, trochanteric bursitis, fascial defects, irritation of the psoas tendon due to anteroinferior protrusion of the acetabular component, myotendinitis, or tendinitis of muscular insertions (for example where there is improper weight bearing due to increase or decrease in leg length or other implantation errors, or abductor insufficiency).

Pain due to neurological alterations occurs when a nerve has been damaged in previous surgery or is irritated by postoperative scars. Depending on the sensory or motor functions of the nerves in question, the result can be neuralgia, altered sensation, or paresis in the affected regions (namely those supplied by the femoral, sciatic, anterior and lateral femoral cutaneous nerves, and, occasionally by the obturator nerve).

Many of these sources of pain originating in the hip must be isolated from pain projected from a different region, for example the lumbar spine or the sacroiliac joint. Their pain characteristics can be very similar, particularly when there are no radicular symptoms.

Periprosthetic infection is the obvious diagnosis when pain, erythema, warmth, soft-tissue swelling or fistulas are present. However, other infections are only distinguished by uncharacteristic pain or discomfort, increased erythrocyte sedimentation rate and C-reactive protein (CRP) value, or they remain free of symptoms.

The physician must decide whether revision surgery should include implant replacement. The main indications for replacement of the prosthesis are:

- Loosening of one or both components
- Thigh pain in a cementless stem where biologic fixation has been achieved
- Fracture jeopardizing the fixation of the implant
- Material failure
- Malposition of one or both components resulting in recurring dislocation or improper weight bearing
- Periprosthetic infection (if a one-stage revision operation is planned).

All other causes of pain may be indications for revision surgery without implant replacement.

Following physical examination and aside from the standard preoperative tests, certain microbiological, transfusion-related and radiographic procedures are required.

Microbiological Evaluation

Microbiological examination of infected joints is required before any revision surgery (with or without implant replacement) is performed, because, besides clinically detectable infections, there is always the possibility of an occult periprosthetic infection without significant symptoms.

Antibiotics should be discontinued at least three days prior to any microbiological examination involving aspiration of the hip, specimen from a sinus, and pre- or intraoperative biopsy (quinolones should be discontinued seven days prior to examination). If the patient absolutely requires antibiotic therapy, then the specimens should be treated with an ion exchanger raisins to absorb the antibiotics prior to analysis. However, results obtained in this manner will remain tentative because such a specimen may falsely fail to reveal any vital pathogens.

Arthrocentesis

Arthrocentesis is the simplest, most cost-effective and most reliable method of detecting infection preoperatively. Aspirated specimens permit correct assessment in over 90% of cases (depending on laboratory and clinical conditions). Indirect methods are less reliable and more expensive.

Aspirating the hip under fluoroscopy requires sterile conditions. Arthrocentesis should not be performed on the ward or in the cast room. When skilled personnel perform the procedure with a long, thin needle, local anesthesia is unnecessary. This eliminates variables due to the anesthetic's slight antimicrobic effect. The surgeon targets the neck of the implant and can feel the needle stop at the metal or be deflected off it. If no fluid can be aspirated, the surgeon moves the joint slightly. This pumps in synovial fluid and thus often prevents a "dry aspiration". Heterotopic ossification or deep protrusion can prevent arthrocentesis. If only a small quantity of fluid is aspirated, no crystalloid solution should be added to the specimen to prevent it from drying out. This could dilute the bacteria to below the biological detection limit, and the oxygen content of the diluting fluid could inhibit anaerobes. When aspirating, as much fluid as possible should be collected. The minimum sample size is greater than one milliliter.

If the hospital has appropriate laboratory facilities, the specimen should be delivered directly to the lab without further processing. A larger quantity of aspirated fluid acts as a natural transportation medium. If delayed delivery by courier or mail is required, specimens must be sealed to prevent desiccation, and anaerobes must be protected against exposure to oxygen. An anaerobic jar or transportation medium may be used for this purpose. An anaerobic jar is an airtight container with a chemically produced anaerobic environment. A transportation medium is an agar that maintains the quantity and vitality of the bacteria including anaerobes for a certain period of time without permitting them to reproduce in significant numbers. If the specimen has to be stored overnight, it should be stored in an anaerobic jar or transportation medium at +4°C and not in an incubator. Storing the specimen in an incubator at +35°C can inhibit certain bacteria while others will continue to reproduce; thus, the stored sample no longer corresponds to actual conditions.

Sinus Specimen

In obvious infections accompanied by drainage and sinus formation, a smear will not be sufficient. Smears are often contaminated with skin flora and dry quickly. To obtain a representative specimen, the surgeon must thoroughly clean the opening of the sinus and then curette material from the sinus tract. Since the specimens are often small enough to dry out in an anaerobe container or become lost in a transportation medium, the specimen is generally placed directly in a suitable culture medium (such as anaerobic blood-culture flask) and brought in this medium to the laboratory as quickly as possible. If the specimen cannot be forwarded immediately, it is incubated at +35°C; a temperature of +35°C is chosen in this case because a culture medium is used instead of a transportation medium.

Arthrocentesis should be performed in addition to obtaining a specimen from a sinus because the results are more reliable and contamination with germs or skin flora is less likely.

Biopsy

The impact of correct microbiological diagnosis on the therapeutic procedure is so great that the surgeon should not hesitate to perform a preoperative biopsy when in doubt. In most cases, however, biopsies are performed intraoperatively. This is done either to permit the surgeon to alter his surgical strategy on the basis of immediate microscopic examination, or to obtain a culture for postoperative monitoring. The transportation and storage conditions for aspirates also apply to biopsies.

Processing and Assessing the Specimens

Macroscopic assessment of the quantity, consistency, and color of the specimen by the surgeon and by laboratory personnel indicate whether the aspirate is a representative specimen and not aspirated tissue fluid or blood. A cloudy specimen may indicate an infection. Some anaerobes have a distinct odor.

Gram's stain and microscopic assessment provides further information. Before staining, aspirates and specimens from a sinus are centrifuged to concentrate the cellular components. Biopsies are homogenized prior to centrifuging because many pathogens have an affinity to collagen fibers. Homogenization yields better culture results.

If microscopic examination reveals that there is a large quantity of erythrocytes in aspirated fluid, one may reasonably assume that blood has been aspirated. Protein structures, such as those found in synovial fluid are an indication of a representative specimen. A large quantity of leukocytes in aspirated fluid is a sign that infection may be present. Bacteria found outside of leukocytes may be attributable to contamination, whereas phagocytized bacteria found within leukocytes are evidence of infection. Some species of bacteria can be tentatively identified on the basis of their shape, configuration, and their Gram's stain properties. Use of special stains or phase-contrast microscopy may also be required.

For culture assessment, aspirated fluid, specimens from a sinus, and biopsies have to be incubated under aerobic and anaerobic conditions in a nutrient medium that is also suitable for fungus. Since the pathogens responsible for periprosthetic infection are often only present in small quantities and/or grow slowly, particularly if the patient was previously treated with antibiotics, the microbiologist should select methods that are suitable for long-term observation and not susceptible to contamination. The specimens should be handled similarly to blood cultures; cultures should be observed over a period of 18 to 21 days. The material should be examined for mycobacteria if there is reason to suspect their presence (e.g. medical history or unexpected negative microbiological findings).

Identification and sensitivity testing follow the procedures used with other materials.

Since a large proportion of the pathogens responsible for periprosthetic infection are skin flora germs, validation of the culture results is not always easy, especially when clinical suspicion of infection is borderline. Obtaining another specimen and excluding possible sources of contamination is often indicated to substantiate inconclusive results.

The most frequent causes of false negative results are failure to suspend antibiotic therapy prior to microbiological diagnostics, improper technique in obtaining the specimen, failure to observe transportation and storage requirements, improper culture conditions, insufficient observation periods, and neglecting or underestimating skin flora as a cause of periprosthetic infection.

The surgeon and the microbiologist should cooperate very closely and both should consider the spectrum and the biological characteristics of the pathogens causing periprosthetic infection, which is the most serious complication following implantation of an artificial joint into bone. It is a complex problem, because it represents an infection of the bone in the presence of a large foreign body.

Blood Product Management

Large quantities of blood are required in total joint arthroplasty, especially in revision surgery. Since most operations can be planned, it is best to develop a program of autologous transfusion to minimize or even eliminate the need for donor blood. This reduces the problems associated with allogenic blood, i.e., infections (AIDS, hepatitis), immunomodulating or immunosuppressive effects; incompatibility, hemolytic reactions, and dysfunction of cellular blood components due to damage during storage.

Autologous transfusion techniques include:

- Preoperative plasmapheresis (PPH)
- Preoperative autologous blood donation (PABD)
- Acute normovolemic hemodilution (ANH)
- Mechanically processed autologous transfusion (MAT)

These four procedures are combined into an autologous transfusion program (acc. to Schleinzer and Mehrkens; Fig. 4.**1**). Depending on the patient and on the quantity of blood required, the blood product management will include some or all of these procedures. Blood salvage and retransfusion should not be performed in the presence of infection or a tumor; hemodilution should be restricted to patients without cardiac or renal dysfunction and with normal hemoglobin values.

Preoperative Plasmapheresis

Autologous plasma can be obtained as early as 2 years before surgery. Whole blood is taken from the patient. The cellular components are separated by centrifugation or filtration and immediately returned to the patient; the plasma (900 ml per session) is quick frozen and stored at –40 °C. The volume deficit is compensated for by infusing colloids and having the patient drink fluids. After intraoperative hemostasis is obtained and in the postoperative period, the plasma is reinfused. This promotes coagulation, stabilizes the volume better than colloids, and improves the coagulatory function.

Preoperative Autologous Blood Donation

Autologous blood donation can begin 7 weeks preoperatively. Generally, a volume of 500 ml per session is taken. A "three-bag system" is used in separating the blood into plasma, erythrocytes, and "buffy coat" (leukocytes and platelets). The "buffy coat" is discarded because the leukocytes and platelets deteriorate within several hours, negatively influence the quality of the erythrocytes and acidify the milieu. The plasma is stored at –40 °C; the erythrocytes are suspended in an additive solution and stored at +4 °C. Here too, the volume deficit is compensated for by infusing colloids and having the patient drink fluids. Both plasma and erythrocytes are returned to the patient during and after surgery. The plasma has the functions described previously, and the erythrocytes provide oxygen-carrying capacity.

Acute Normovolemic Hemodilution

After anesthetic induction and before surgery, 10–20 ml of blood per kilogram of body weight are withdrawn and replaced with a colloid. As a result, the viscosity of the whole blood decreases, thus improving tissue perfusion and oxygen delivery. This autologous blood, which is of high quality, is stored at room temperature and is retransfused in inverse order at the end of the operative procedure.

Mechanically Processed Autologous Transfusion

The patient's blood lost during surgery and postoperatively is collected and then mechanically processed by a centrifugation and washing device ("cell-saver"). This results in autologous packed red blood cells which reveal in-vivo normal physiological function and survival time. The erythrocytes' yield can be as high as 75%. The erythrocyte concentrate is immediately returned to the patient. Volume deficits are managed intraoperatively with colloids and postoperatively with autologous plasma.

Fig. 4.**1** Autologous blood product management (acc. to Schleinzer and Mehrkens). ▸

PPH	Preoperative plasmapheresis
PABD	Preoperative autologous blood donation
ANH	Acute normovolemic hemodilution
MAT	Mechanically processed autologous transfusion
Yellow	Plasma
Red	Erythrocytes
Green	Colloidal solution
Blue	Storage at –40 °
1	Centrifugation and washing device ("cell saver")
2	Centrifuge and optoelectric separator
3	Roller pump and centrifugation device or filter respectively

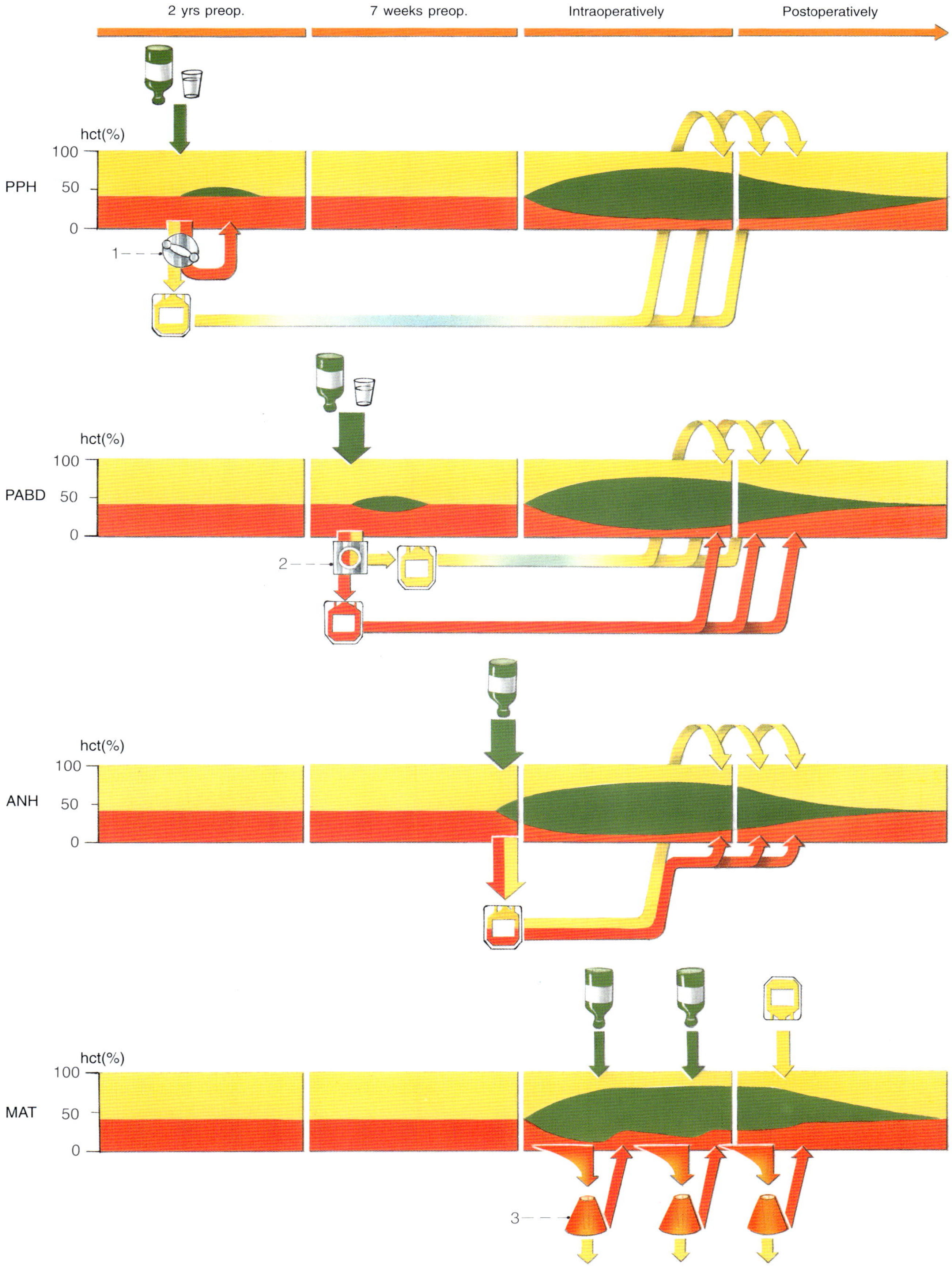
2 yrs preop.
7 weeks preop.
Intraoperatively
Postoperatively
hct(%)
100
50
0
PPH
1
hct(%)
100
50
0
PABD
2
hct(%)
100
50
0
ANH
hct(%)
100
50
0
MAT
3

Radiographic Evaluation

Follow-up radiographs in two planes are sufficient to detect most evidence of change. Loosening will almost invariably show up on the plain pelvic radiograph, significantly more distinctly in cemented implants than in cementless ones. Aseptic loosening can often be radiologically distinguished from periprosthetic infection. The most definite radiological sign of periprosthetic infection is the lack of a sclerotic line separating the bone from the band-shaped or cystic lucency seen in aseptic cases. In typical cases the radiograph is generally cloudy; ill-defined areas of cancellous bone and sclerotic bone can be seen, and indistinct periosteal deposits may also be visible.

Three-phase radionuclide bone scans and radionuclide-labeled leukocyte scans can help to reveal an infection in uncertain cases. However, aspirating the joint is the simplest, least expensive, and most direct method and takes priority over other methods. If a sinus is present in a periprosthetic infection, injecting the sinus with contrast medium may be indicated to determine its size and orientation. If the sinus lies in the groin or within the pelvis, a combination of sinus injection, angiography, and computed tomography can help the surgeon to determine the size and orientation.

In addition to becoming increasingly important in the design of custom implants (generally cementless) for primary total hip arthroplasty, CT can also be used in revision arthroplasty, provided that metallic artifacts can be suppressed. This technique is used to help design custom implants beyond the scope of modular systems and to provide the surgeon with a more detailed picture of the pathoanatomy (particularly that of the pelvis).

Conventional radiographs are generally sufficient to determine the length, diameter, and curvature of cemented custom implants. Determining implant dimensions on the basis of radiographic values requires radiographs of known magnification; either the radiograph includes a scale or the focal length and the distance between the film and the object (bone or implant) must be known.

The radiopaque scale is fixed on a stand level with the bone (Fig. 4.**2**). Like the bone or implant, the magnification of its image in the radiograph depends on the focal length and the distance between the film and the object. Any value x (length or width of an implant or bone) will be in the same proportion to its dimension in the radiograph x' as l is to l', where l is the actual length of the scale, and l' is the length of the image.

$$\frac{x}{x'} = \frac{l}{l'} \quad \text{thus } x = \frac{l \cdot x'}{l'}$$

If the bone is not parallel to the imaging plane (for example in a flexion contracture), then the scale must be inclined with the bone to permit the surgeon to determine the specific dimensions at any one point because in this case there are varying proximal and distal magnifications.

An alternative procedure is to affix two spheres with known diameters to the skin in the same plane as the bone, one proximal and one distal. The dimensions can be determined on the basis of the respective magnifications of the spheres.

If the focal length and the distance between the object and the film are known (Fig. 4.**3**), then the following equation applies:

$$\frac{x}{x'} = \frac{f-h}{f} \quad \text{thus } x = \frac{(f-h)\,x'}{f}$$

The value x again stands for any dimension that is to be determined; x' is the scale of its image; f is the focal length; and h is the distance between the object and the imaging plane. If the object does not lie parallel to the imaging plane, then that must also be compensated for in this method. This is done by determining the varying distances to the imaging plane.

Regardless of the method, the longer the focal length is, the lower the magnification and thus the smaller the possible error will be.

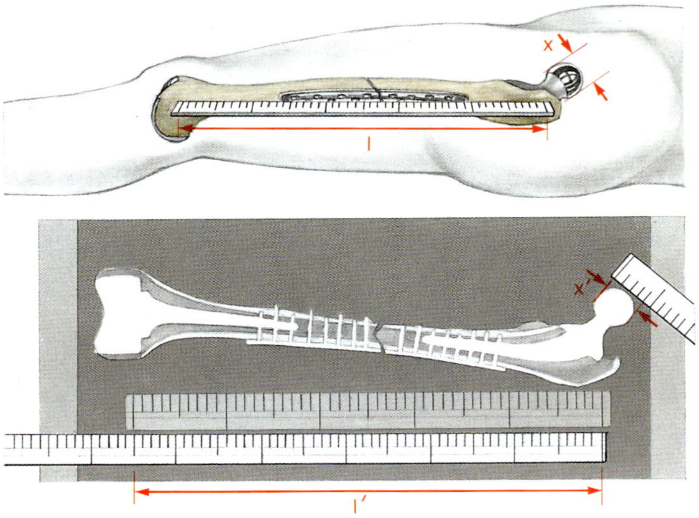

Fig. 4.**2** Determining the actual dimensions of bones and implants by including a scale in the radiograph.

l = Actual length of scale in radiograph
l′ = Length of its image
x = Actual dimension of a length to be determined (in the example diameter of prosthetic head)
x′ = Dimension of its image

$$x = \frac{l \cdot x'}{l'}$$

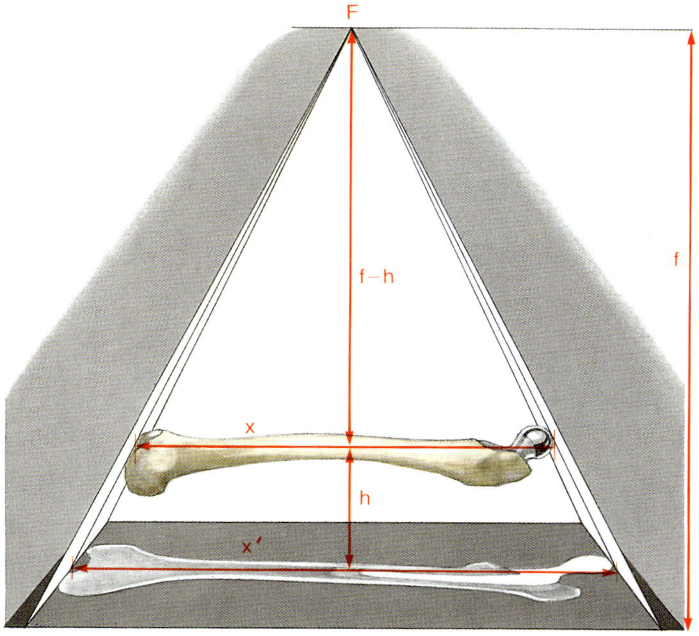

Fig. 4.**3** Determining the actual dimensions of bone and implants from focal length and distance between the object and the film.

F = Focus
f = Focal length
h = Distance between object and film
x = Actual dimension of a length to be determined (in the example length of femur)
x′ = Dimension of its image

$$x = \frac{(f - h)\, x'}{f}$$

Approaches to the Hip

Depending on specific requirements, the following approaches are recommended for revision total hip arthroplasty (Fig. 4.**4**):

- Posterior approach
- Transtrochanteric approach
- Transgluteal approach

Anterolateral and anterior approaches are less suitable. Please refer also to the chapter on the approaches.

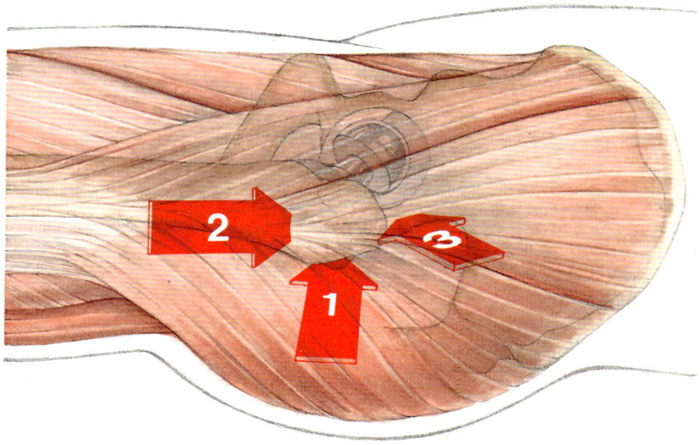

Fig. 4.**4** Approaches to the hip in revision total hip arthroplasty.

1 Posterior approach
2 Transtrochanteric approach
3 Transgluteal approach

Positioning

The patient is positioned laterally for the posterior approach. A hollow cushion is used to provide better access to the surgical sites. The patient's thorax and abdomen are supported anteriorly and posteriorly; the posterior support leaves the sacrum exposed so that it can be palpated intraoperatively to determine the position of the pelvis. The surgeon stands (or occasionally sits) posterior to the patient. When the left hip is operated on, the first assistant generally stands on the surgeon's right side (sometimes on the surgeon's left side), and the second assistant always stands on the opposite side of the operating table. The table is adjusted to medium height (Fig. 4.**5a**).

For a transtrochanteric or transgluteal approach, the patient is supine. The part of the operating table under the patient's legs is turned slightly to the involved side. The surgeon sits (or occasionally stands). When the left hip is operated on, the first assistant generally stands to the surgeon's right (sometimes to the surgeon's left), and the second assistant always stands on the opposite side of the operating table. The table is adjusted to maximum height (Fig. 4.**5b**).

If the patient is positioned on an evacuable "bean bag," the surgical staff can change the patient's position intraoperatively from lateral to supine by tilting the table and reshaping the cushion (Fig. 4.**5c**).

Where difficult acetabular procedures are planned that involve a danger of damaging intrapelvic structures, the entire abdomen should also be prepared and draped to permit a laparotomy.

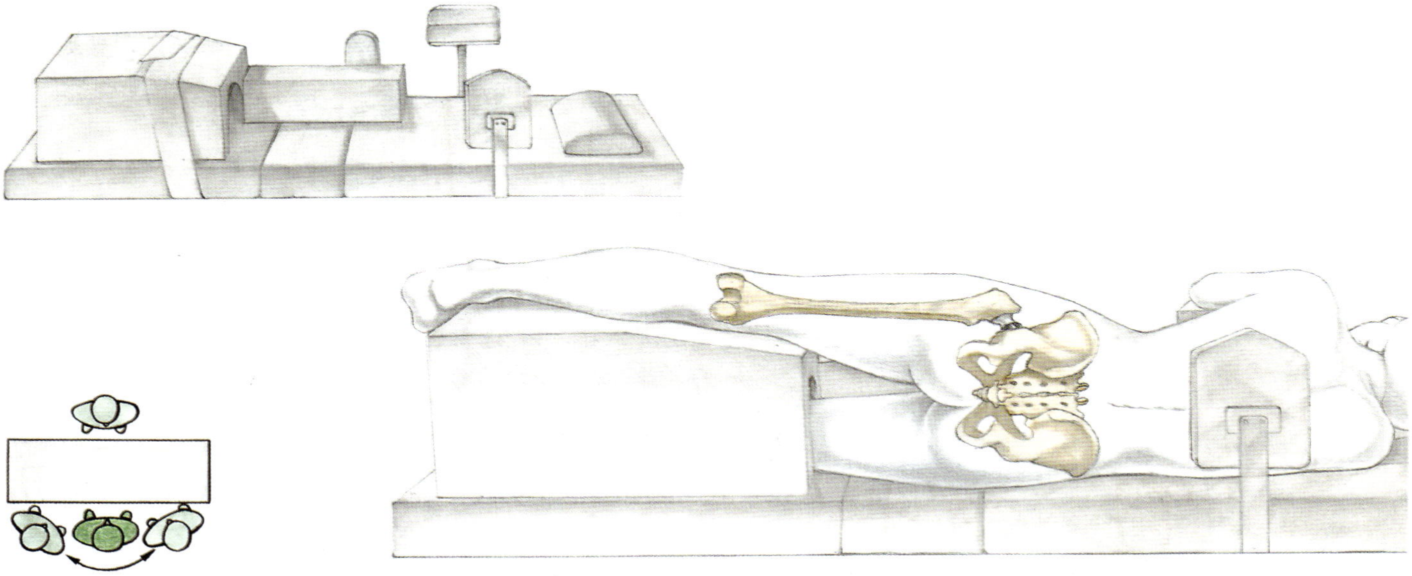

a

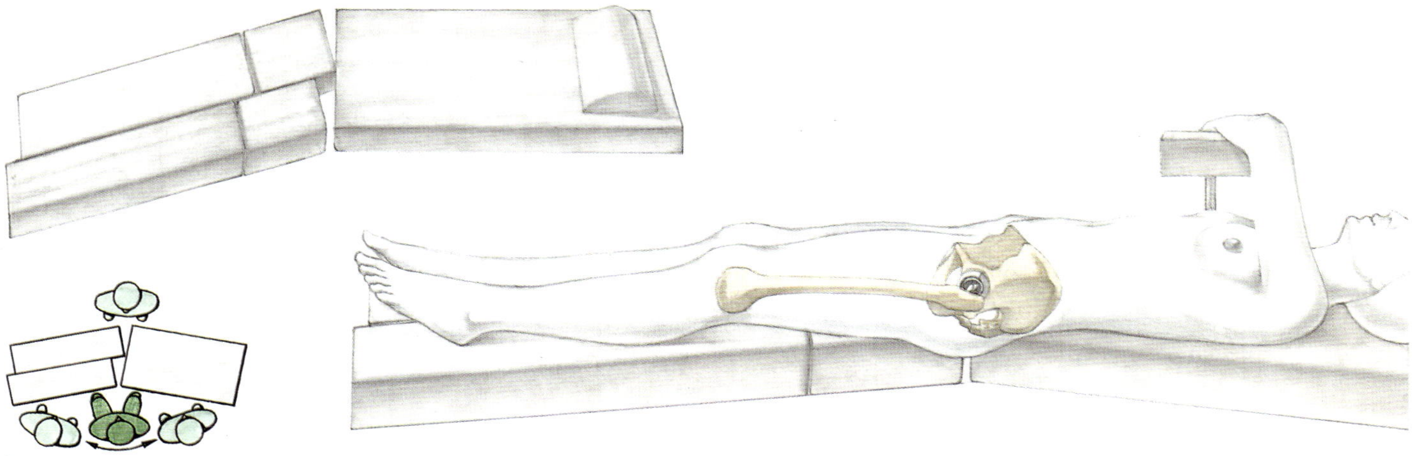

b

Fig. 4.**5a–c** Positioning the patient for the three approaches.

a Lateral position for posterior approach using hollow cushion. Note positions of surgical staff.

b Supine for transtrochanteric or transgluteal approach. The part of the operating table under the patient's legs is turned slightly to the involved side. Note positions of surgical staff.

c Universal positioning on a "bean bag".

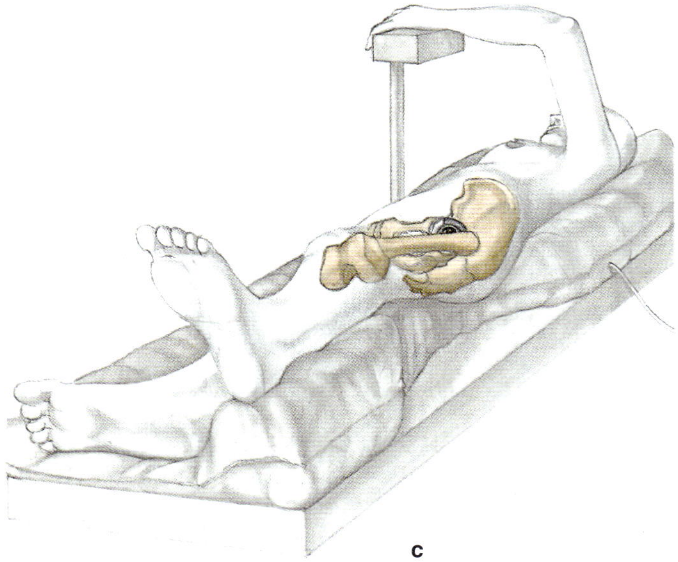

c

Skin and Fascial Incision

The skin and fascial incision is identical in all three approaches. A lateral skin incision begins proximal to the greater trochanter and is carried distally. The proximal third of the incision lies proximal to the greater trochanter and the remaining two-thirds lie distal to it (Fig. 4.**6a**).

Distal to the greater trochanter, the incision follows the iliotibial tract (along the axis of the femur). The surgeon should avoid damaging the tensor fasciae latae anteriorly. Posteriorly the insertion of the gluteus maximus into the femur should also be handled with care.

The proximal third of the incision courses over the anterior fibers of the gluteus maximus and follows their posterior curvature (Fig. 4.**6a**). When extending the incision proximally to improve exposure, there should be only slight posterior curvature. Increasing the posterior curvature brings the incision into an area of thicker gluteal fat and more profuse bleeding. Irritation of the gluteus maximus is increased, and the patient will lie on part of the wound postoperatively.

Old scars should be excised. If the prior incision cannot be used for the approach, the surgeon should maintain sufficient distance between it and the new incision. Crossing the old scar or deviating from it at an acute angle endangers healing (Fig. 4.**6b**).

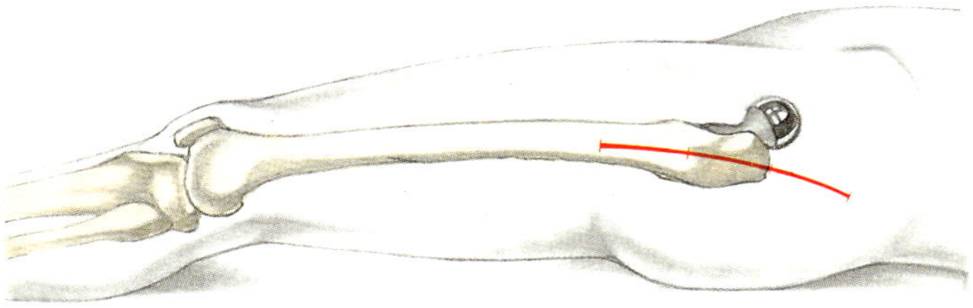

a

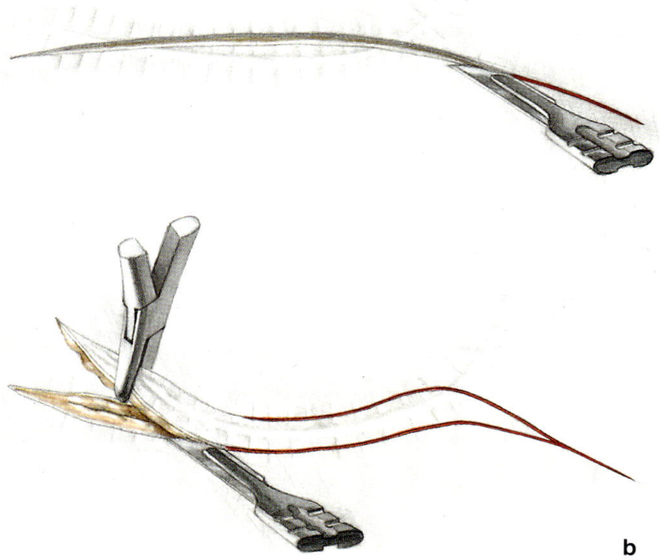

b

Fig. 4.**6a–c** Making the skin incision, excising the scar, and opening the fascia lata.
a Skin incision for the posterior, transtrochanteric, and transgluteal approach.
b Managing scars from previous surgery. *Above:* wrong. *Below:* correct.

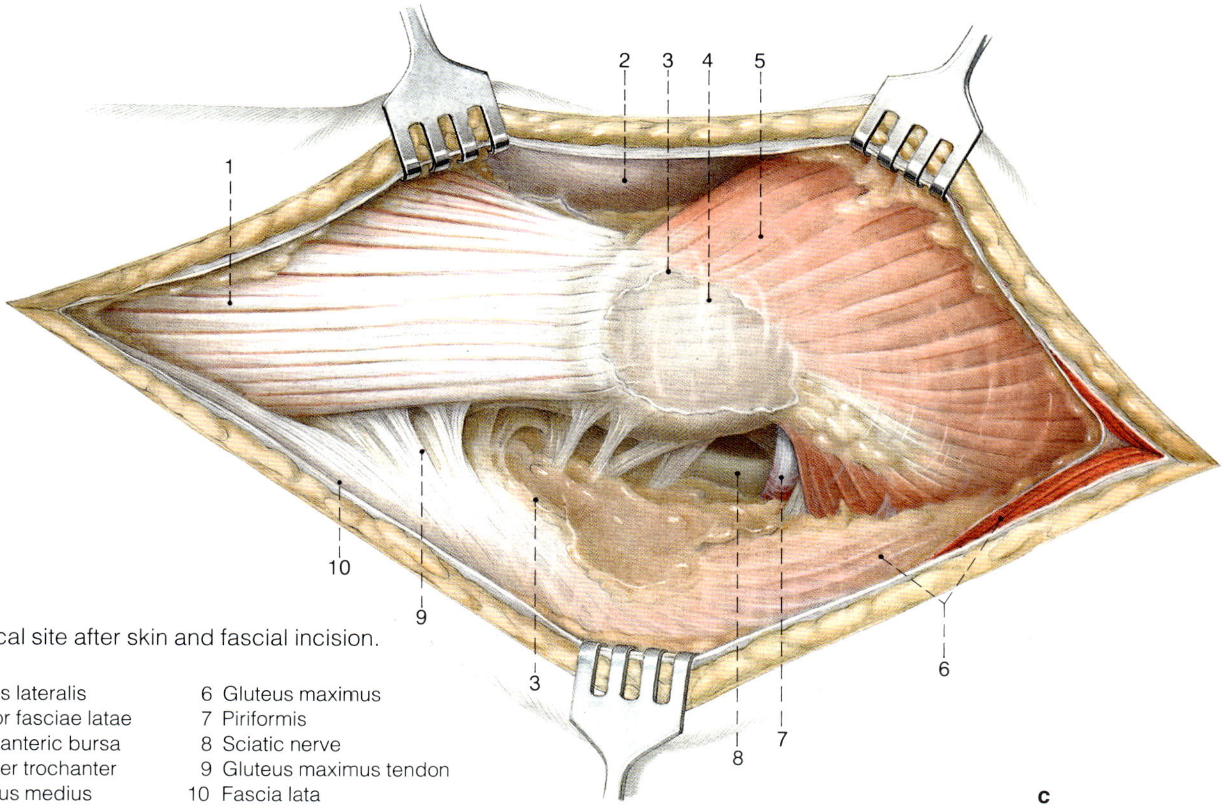

c

c Surgical site after skin and fascial incision.

1 Vastus lateralis
2 Tensor fasciae latae
3 Trochanteric bursa
4 Greater trochanter
5 Gluteus medius
6 Gluteus maximus
7 Piriformis
8 Sciatic nerve
9 Gluteus maximus tendon
10 Fascia lata

If severe scarring is present between the fascia lata and the muscles, the surgeon can best locate the boundary between them distally in an area unaffected by previous surgery. When the skin and fascia lata have been opened, the anterior fibers of the gluteus maximus are bluntly dissected. All three approaches will expose the same surgical site (Fig. 4.**6c**).

Moistened cloths are sutured to the fascia lata to protect the subcutaneous tissue (Fig. 4.**7**).

Next the surgeon locates the sciatic nerve. The sciatic nerve is surrounded by fatty tissue, and in revision surgery, it is often obscured by scarring. First the surgeon should try to locate it by palpation. The open hand is inserted into the wound with the fingertips pressed against the ischium. The nerve is located by sliding the fingertips toward anterior (Fig. 4.**8**). If the surgeon suspects that scarring has shifted the nerve towards the posterior margin of the acetabulum, then the nerve should be exposed. The easiest way to do this is to begin distally (where there is generally less scarring) at the point where the nerve disappears into the deep layer medial to the gluteus maximus tendon.

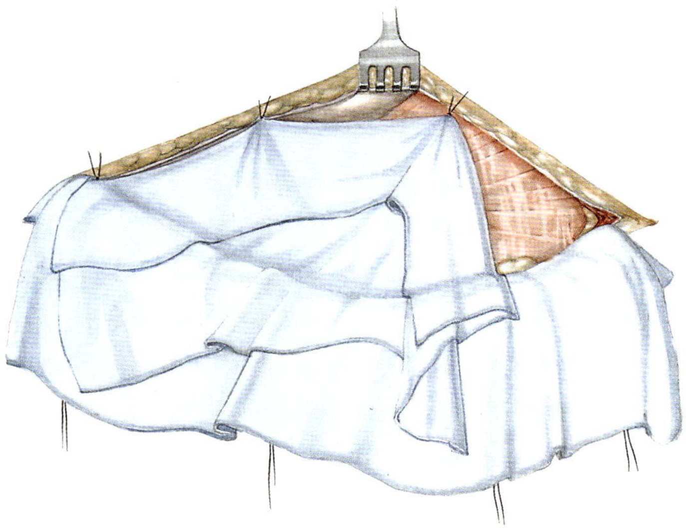

Fig. 4.**7** Moistened cloths are sutured to the fascia lata (not shown in the following illustrations).

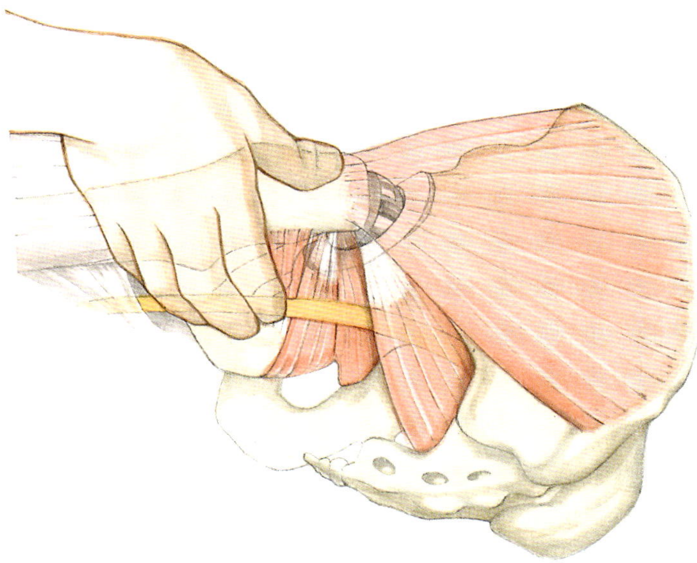

Fig. 4.**8** Palpating the sciatic nerve.

Posterior Approach to the Hip

With the patient in a lateral position, the surgeon uses the flexed calf as a lever to place the hip in maximum internal rotation. This extends the external rotators, making them easier to differentiate, and it moves their femoral insertions away from the sciatic nerve. The external rotators are (from proximal to distal): the posterior fibers of the gluteus minimus (covered by the gluteus medius), the piriformis, the superior gemellus, the obturator internus, the inferior gemellus, the obturator externus (covered by the quadratus femoris), the quadratus femoris, and the part of the gluteus maximus that inserts into the femur (Fig. 4.**9**). The gluteus maximus tendon is only incised if the posterior fascia is to be released (see Fig. 4.**10**).

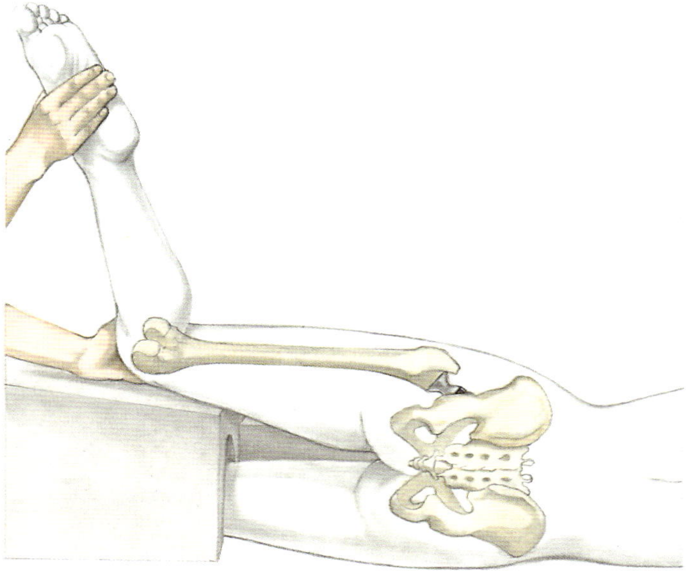

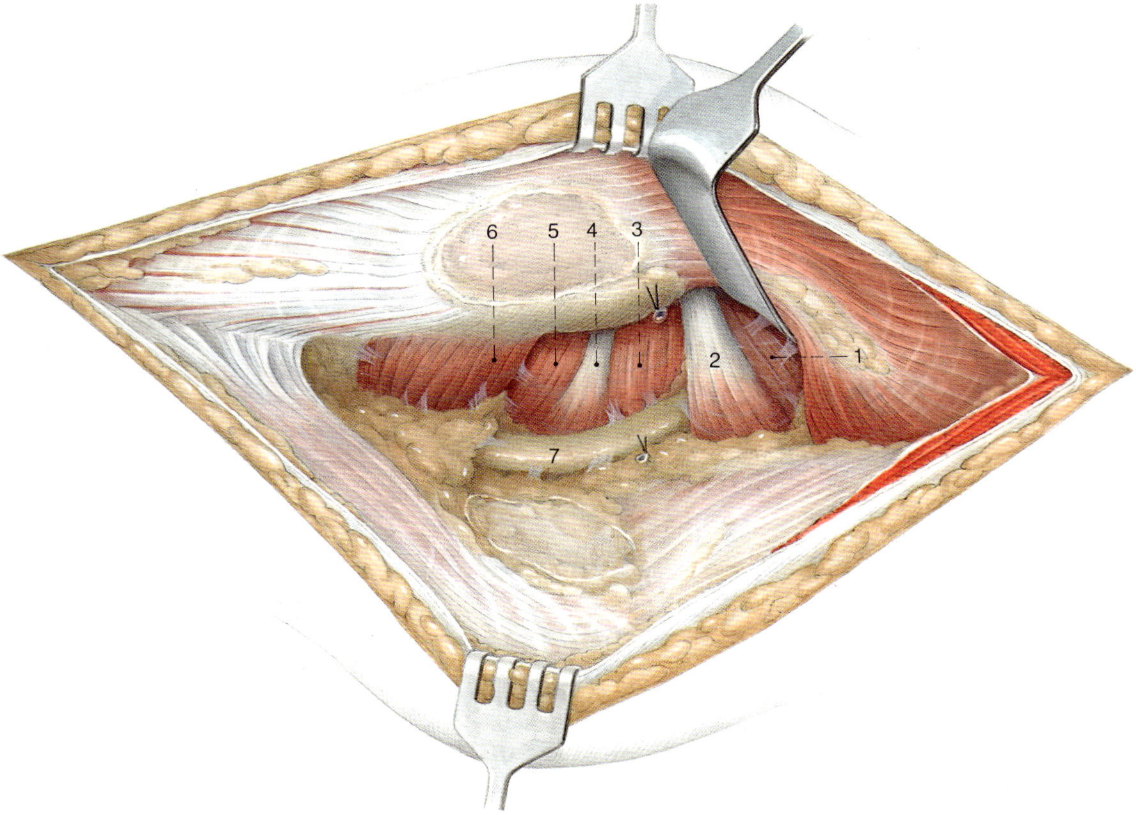

Fig. 4.**9** Posterior approach. With the leg in maximum internal rotation and extension the external rotators are maximally extended.

1 Gluteus minimus
2 Piriformis
3 Superior gemellus
4 Obturator internus
5 Inferior gemellus
6 Quadratus femoris
7 Sciatic nerve

We recommend releasing the external rotators from the femur in the following order to expose the hip.

First, the surgeon dissects the posterior margin of the gluteus medius and lifts the muscle. If excessive scarring or fatty tissue is present, the posterior margin can be located by palpating the round tendon of the piriformis. The coarse fibers of the gluteus minimus are now visible proximal to the piriformis tendon. After the quadratus femoris is dissected directly from the femur, the lesser trochanter becomes visible. The tendinous and muscular insertions of the muscles between the gluteus minimus and the lesser trochanter are incised as close to the bony insertion on the trochanteric fossa as possible. The surgeon should preserve as much of the piriformis and obturator internus tendons as possible for subsequent reattachment (see Fig. 4.**170**). In revision total hip arthroplasty, the external rotators are often scarred to the capsule so that dissecting the muscles generally opens the capsule as well. Next, the surgeon performs a capsulotomy parallel to the posteroinferior margin of the gluteus minimus. The capsulotomy extends as far as the acetabulum (Fig. 4.**10a**).

Opening the incised capsule exposes the implant. Next, the posterior fibers of the gluteus minimus are retracted from the superior capsule, and the surgeon incises the capsule close to the femur, or the muscle fibers are incised along with the capsule if they are fused with it (Fig. 4.**10b**).

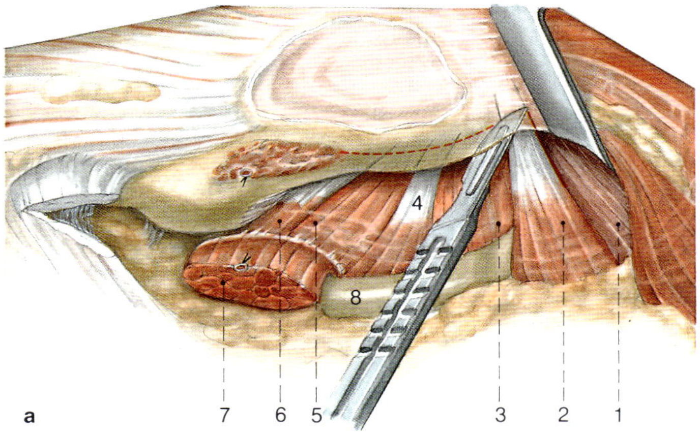

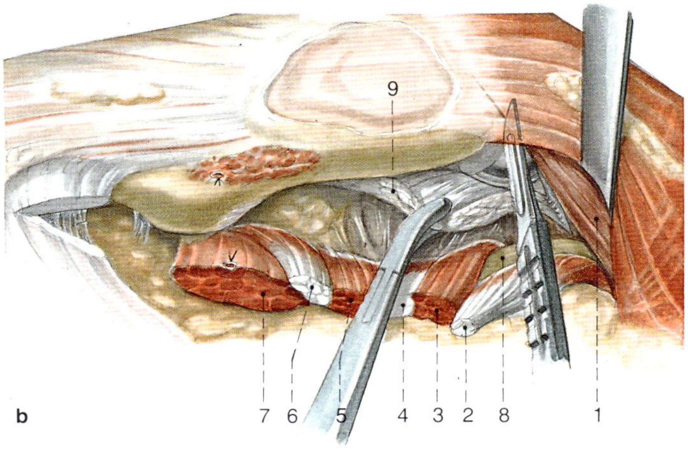

Fig. 4.**10a** and **b** Exposing the joint.

a Dissecting the external rotators and performing a posterior capsulotomy.

1 Gluteus minimus
2 Piriformis
3 Superior gemellus
4 Obturator internus
5 Inferior gemellus
6 Obturator externus
7 Quadratus femoris
8 Sciatic nerve

b Superior capsulotomy.

1 Gluteus minimus
2 Piriformis
3 Superior gemellus
4 Obturator internus
5 Inferior gemellus
6 Obturator externus
7 Quadratus femoris
8 Sciatic nerve
9 Joint capsule

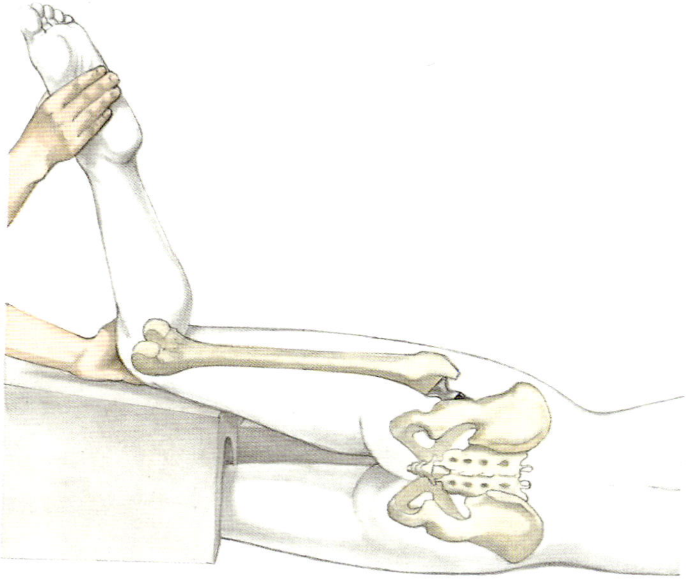

With the leg in the same position, all accessible parts of the capsule are excised. The surgeon should avoid damaging the abductors superior to the site and the psoas tendon inferior to it. This is sometimes difficult in the presence of heterotopic ossification. Note that the sciatic nerve can lie very close to the site, particularly when previous surgery has removed the layer of external rotators protecting the nerve, and the formation of scar tissue has moved it closer (Fig. 4.**11**).

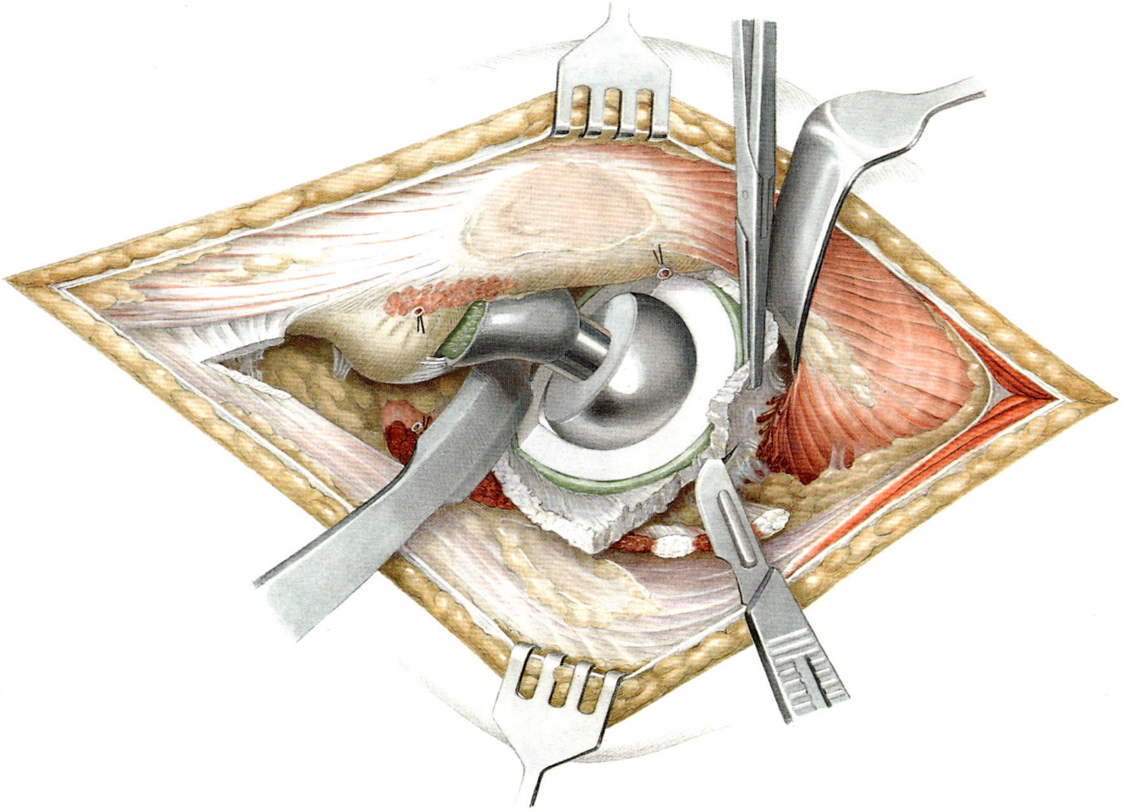

Fig. 4.**11** Excision of the superior, posterior, and inferior capsule with the leg in maximum internal rotation and extension.

The posterior approach provides easy access to the roof of the acetabulum and the posterior and superior periacetabular bone. The attachments (origins) of the abductors can be dissected from the iliac bone superiorly and posteriorly as far as the sciatic notch with a periosteal elevator (Fig. 4.**12**).

The surgeon dislocates the hip using a bone hook inserted around the prosthetic femoral neck (Fig. 4.**13**). Applying excessive force to the calf can lead to femoral fracture. Anterior scarring can hinder dislocation. In this case the surgeon pulls on the bone hook to tighten the scars, palpates them, and incises them close to the femur. After dislocating the joint and removing the femoral component, the surgeon resects the anterior scars.

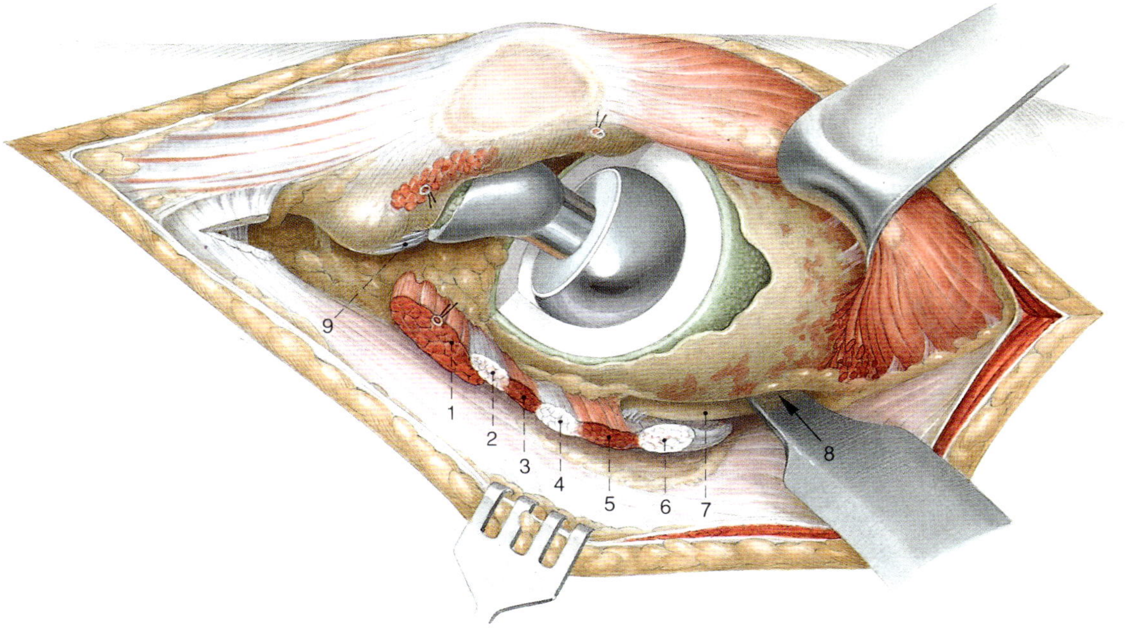

Fig. 4.**12** Exposing the roof of the acetabulum and the posterior and superior periacetabular bone.

1 Quadratus femoris
2 Obturator externus
3 Inferior gemellus
4 Obturator internus
5 Superior gemellus
6 Piriformis
7 Sciatic nerve
8 Greater sciatic notch
9 Psoas tendon

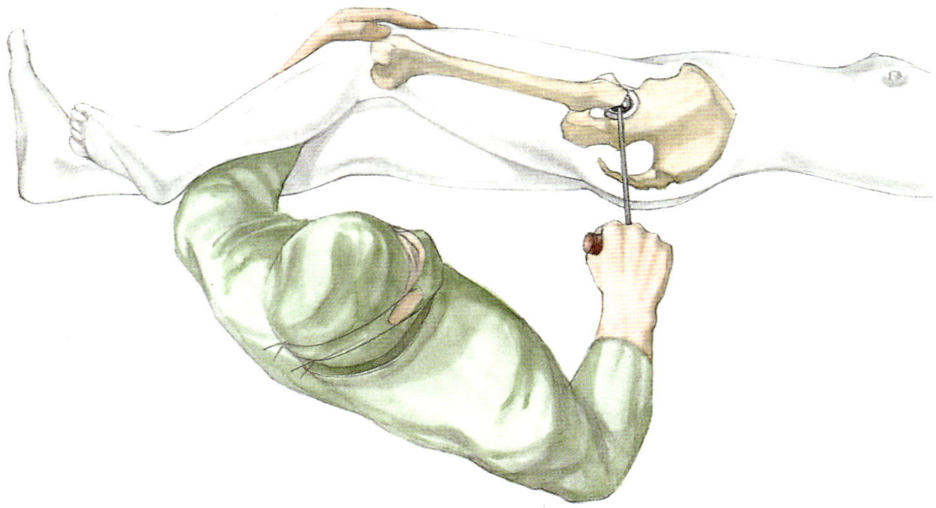

Fig. 4.**13** Posterior dislocation of the hip. With the leg slightly internally rotated, flexed, and adducted, traction is applied with a bone hook inserted around the prosthetic femoral neck.

Limited anterolateral exposure of the hip with the leg externally rotated and extended is helpful where excessive anterior scarring or heterotopic ossification prevents dislocation, and the obstructions cannot be removed from posteriorly. The surgeon should avoid damaging the superior gluteal nerve, which supplies the tensor fasciae latae (Fig. 4.**14**). If dislocation still cannot be safely carried out, then a trochanteric osteotomy (see Fig. 4.**19**) provides better exposure.

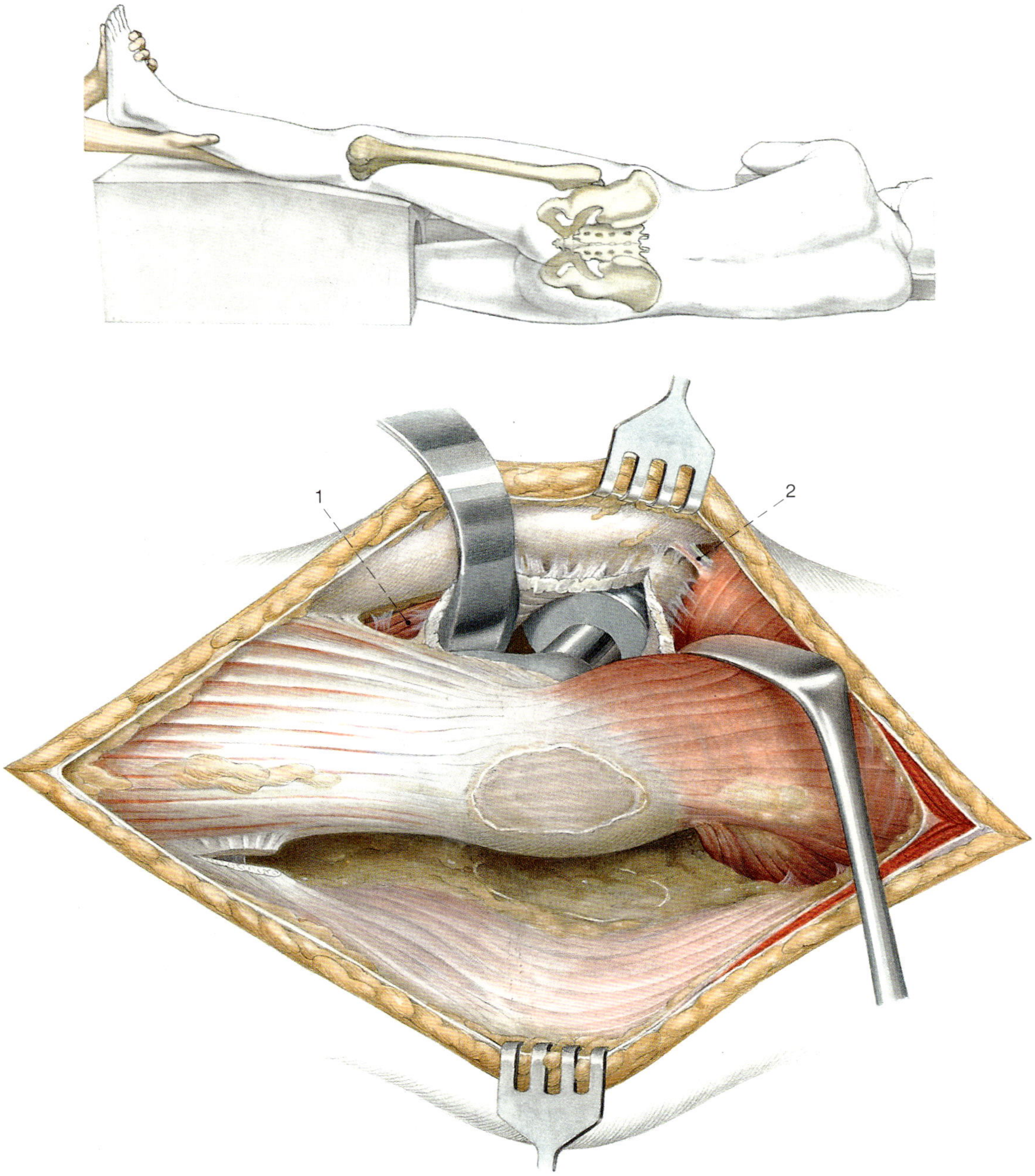

Fig. 4.**14** Limited anterolateral exposure of the hip with the leg externally rotated and extended.

1 Iliacus
2 Superior gluteal nerve

To remove the femoral component, the leg is maximally internally rotated, partially flexed, and slightly adducted. Two retractors are inserted to expose the femoral canal (Fig. 4.**15**). The surgeon is seated for this procedure, and the operating table at maximum height, inclined slightly away from the surgeon.

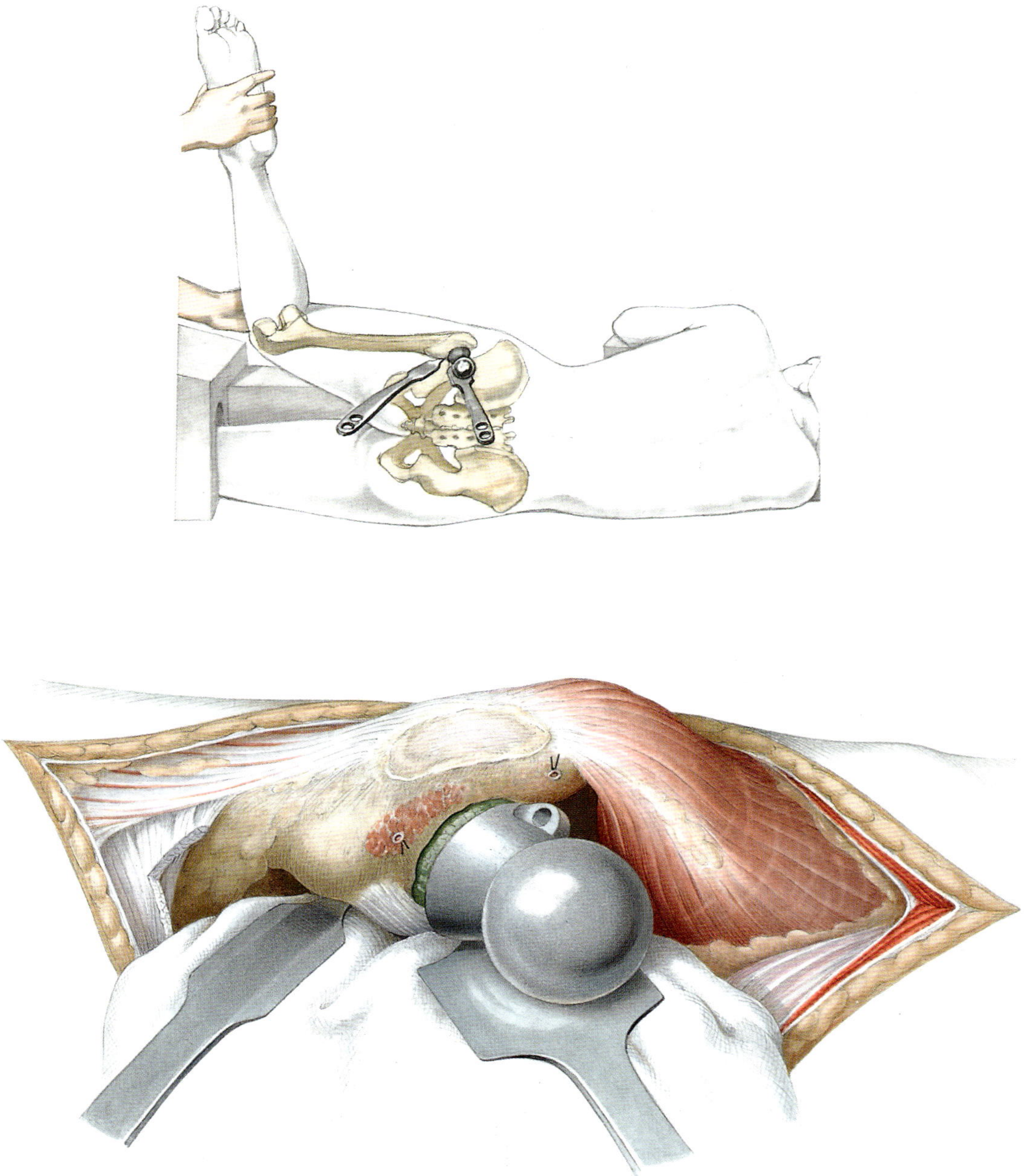

Fig. 4.**15** Removing the femoral component. The leg is maximally internally rotated, partially flexed, and slightly adducted.

To expose the acetabular component, the leg is in a neutral position, and the surgeon pulls the femur anteriorly with a broad bone hook while pressing the iliac crest posteriorly. The external rotators can be retracted by impacting a curved plate into the ischium posteroinferior to the acetabulum. This eliminates the need for an assistant. Damage to the sciatic nerve can be avoided by impacting the pin of the plate anterior to the external rotators (Fig. 4.**16**).

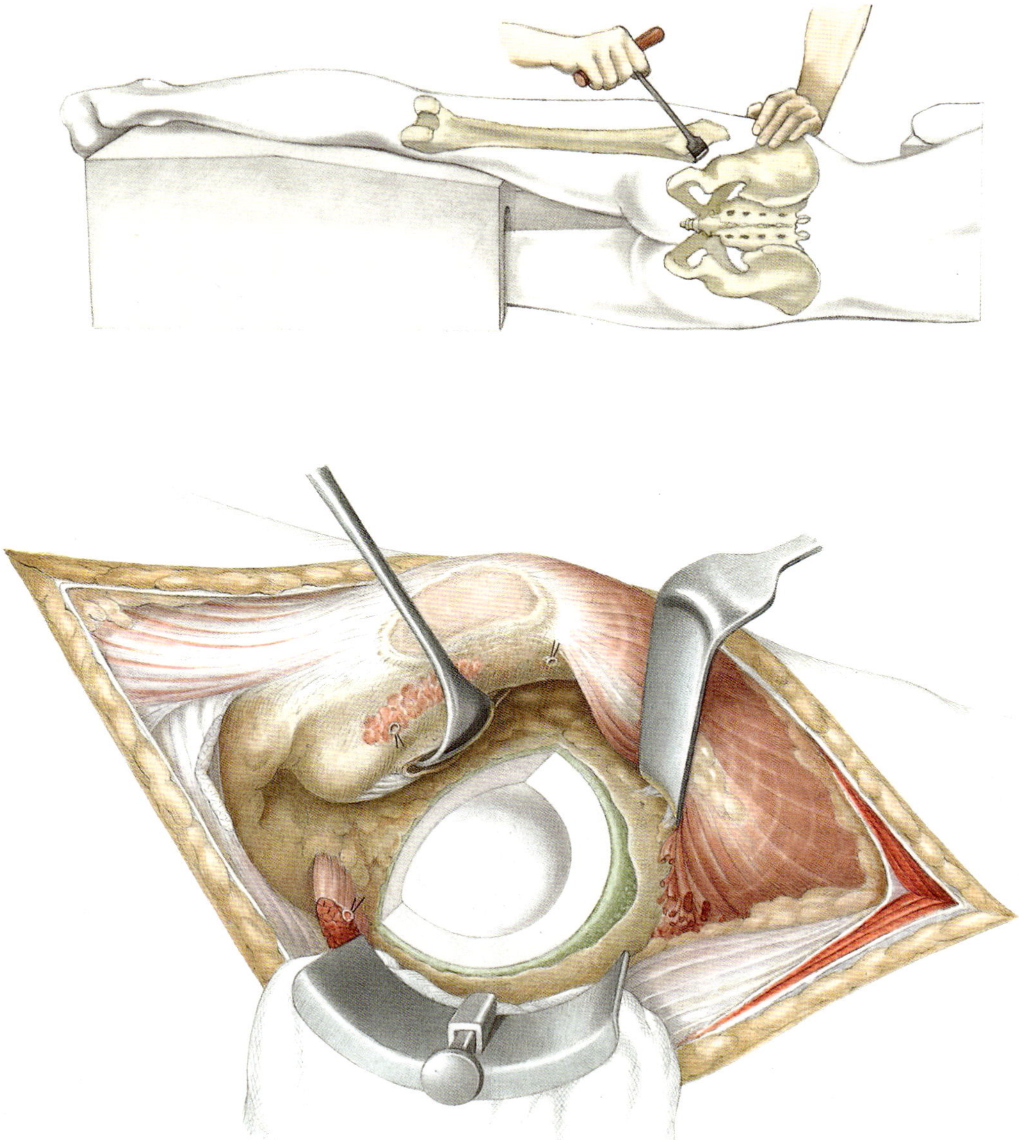

Fig. 4.**16** Exposing the acetabular component with the leg in a neutral position. The surgeon pulls on the bone hook while pressing on the anterior superior iliac spine. A curved plate fastened to the ischium with a pin retracts the external rotators posteriorly.

To replace only the acetabular component, the surgeon must perform very thorough excision of scarred adhesions (particularly anteriorly) to prevent the head or taper of the femoral component from interfering with the procedure. A retractor is inserted directly against the pelvic bone to push the superiorly displaced femur anteriorly (Fig. 4.**17**). Here also, the surgeon may obtain increased exposure by performing a trochanteric osteotomy (see Fig. 4.**19**).

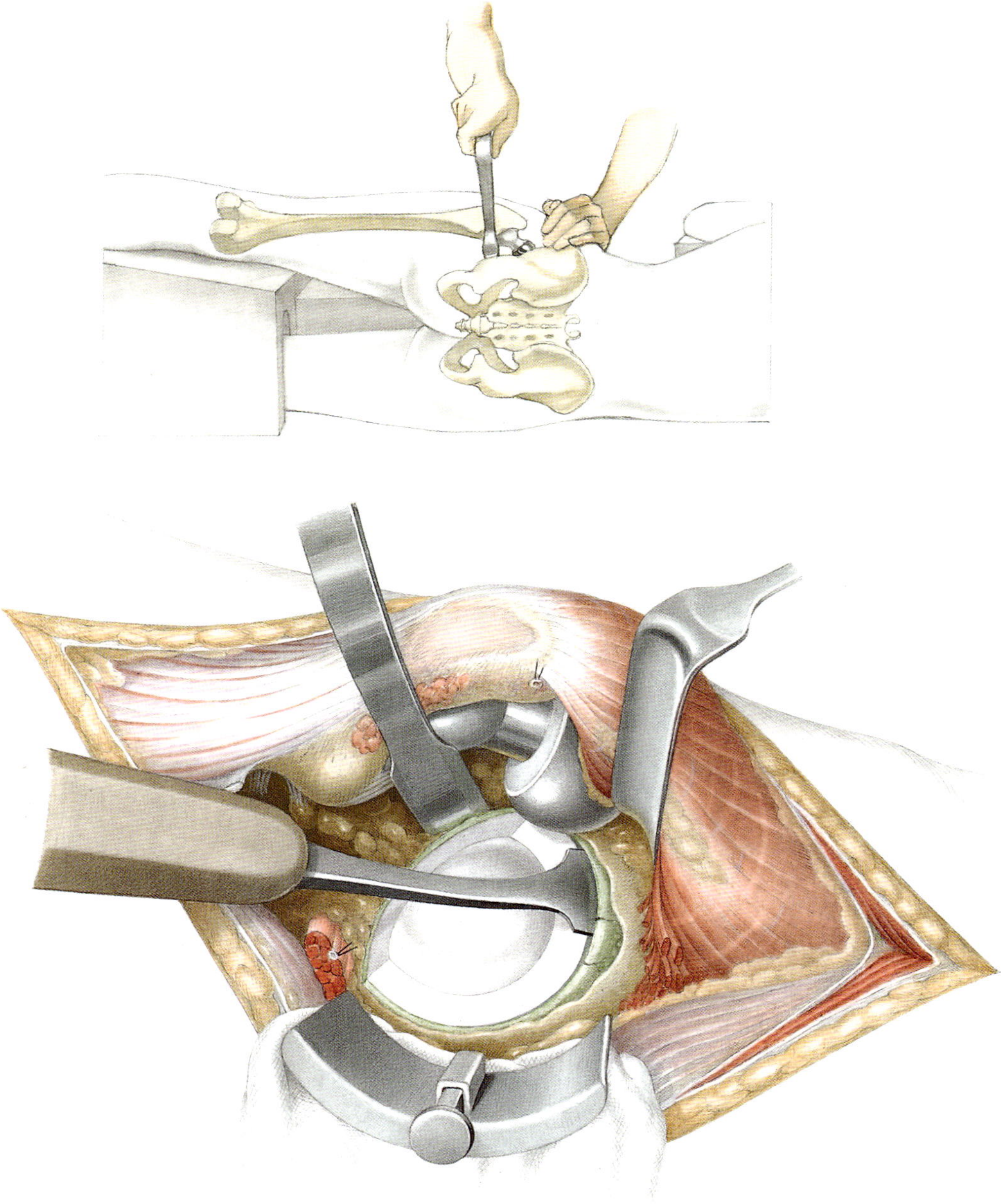

Fig. 4.**17** Exposing and removing the acetabular component while leaving the femoral component in place.

Transtrochanteric Approach to the Hip

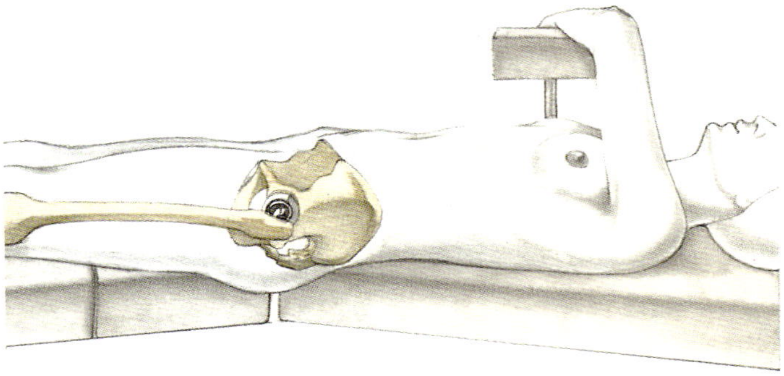

With the patient supine and the leg in a neutral position, the tendinous insertion of the vastus lateralis at the greater trochanter is incised transversely to permit osteotomy of the greater trochanter (Fig. 4.**18**).

We recommend lifting the abductors with a curved retractor or probe inserted anteriorly and performing a chevron osteotomy (Müller's technique) with a saw or osteotome (Fig. 4.**19**).

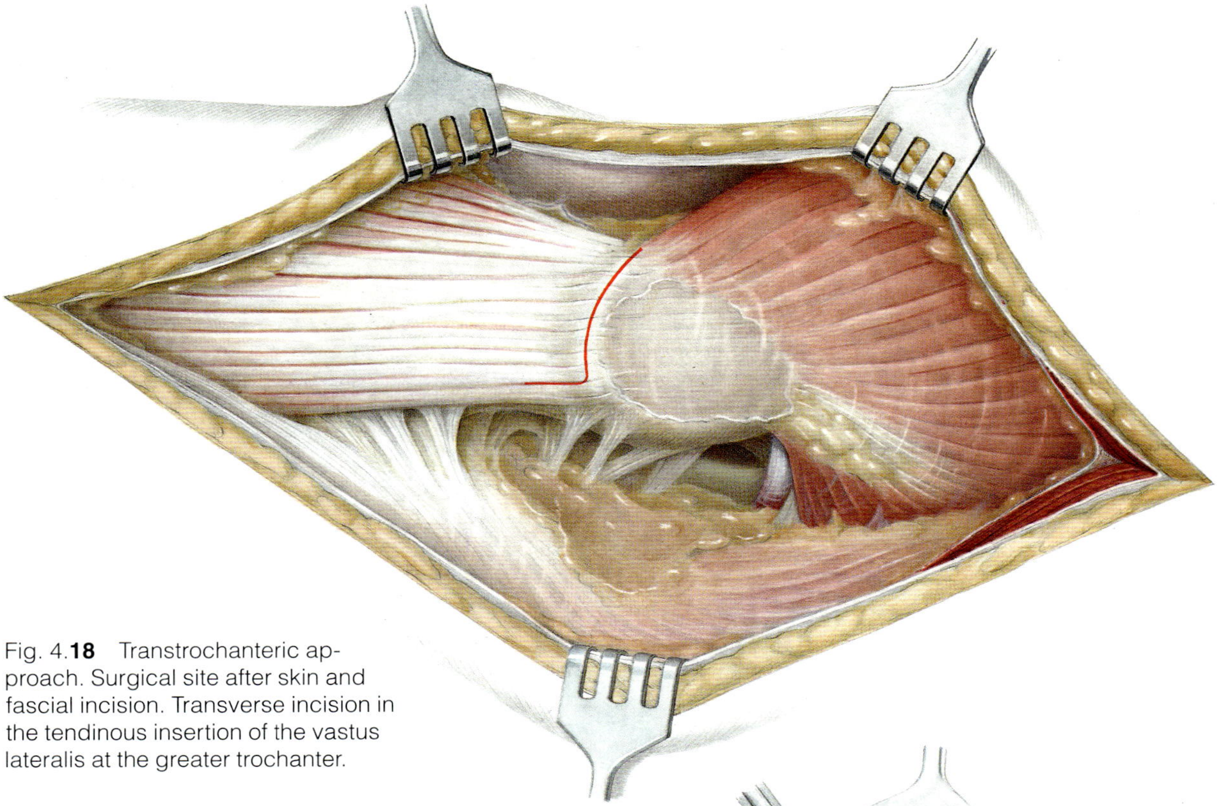

Fig. 4.**18** Transtrochanteric approach. Surgical site after skin and fascial incision. Transverse incision in the tendinous insertion of the vastus lateralis at the greater trochanter.

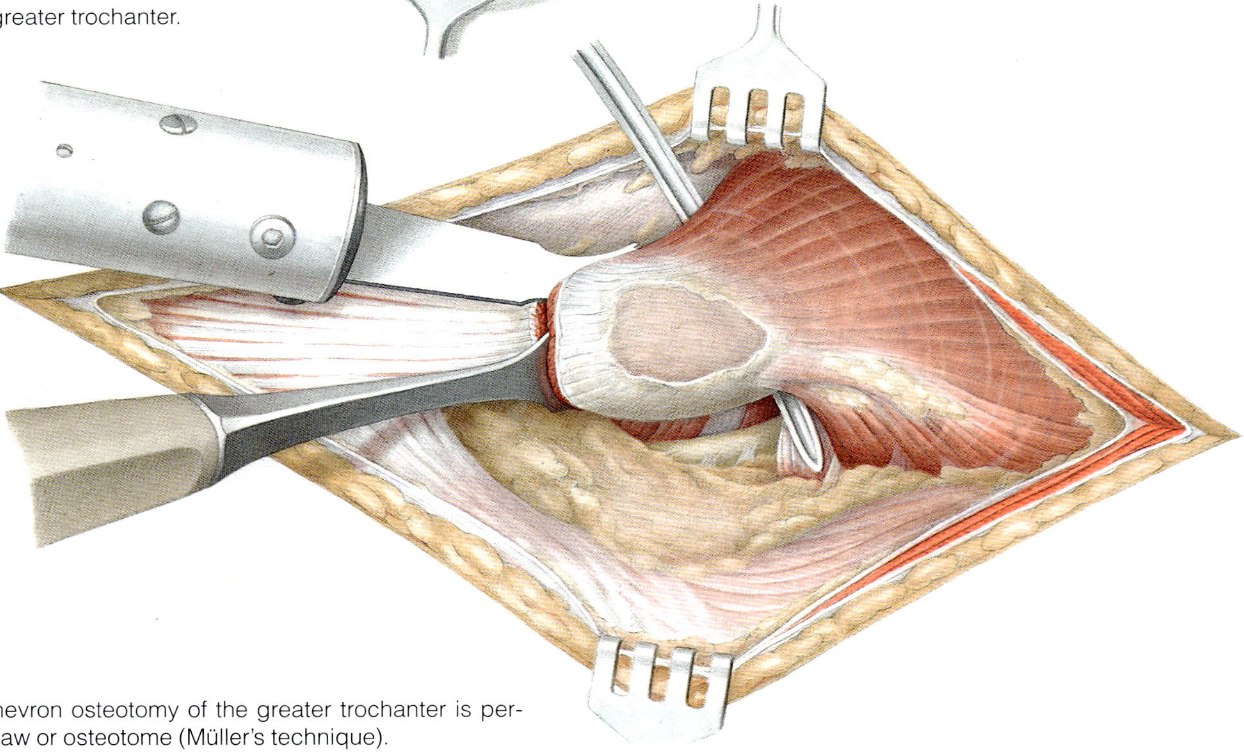

Fig. 4.**19** A chevron osteotomy of the greater trochanter is performed with a saw or osteotome (Müller's technique).

The angle and shape of the osteotomy determines how stable subsequent fixation of the trochanter fragment will be (see Fig. 4.**171**).

A flat osteotomy performed at a greater angle to the sagittal plane than the angle of the force vector of the abductors is more likely to fail than a steep osteotomy at an angle less than that of the force vector. The greater angle decreases the friction forces that relieve stress on the wire suture after refixation of the trochanter fragment (see Fig. 4.**171**), and, in addition, it decreases the area of contact between the osteotomy surfaces.

When the trochanter fragment is reduced, an osteotomy with an even surface is less able to resist the flexion and internal rotation forces of the anterior fibers of the abductors than a Müller chevron osteotomy (Fig. 4.**20**).

An alternative to this osteotomy is to mobilize the proximal origin of the vastus lateralis without dissecting its insertion off the distal aspect of the greater trochanter. An osteotome is inserted beneath the muscle to remove the trochanter fragment. The fragment retains its soft-tissue attachments and more vascular supply despite the osteotomy, and the additional distal tension of the vastus lateralis stabilizes subsequent internal fixation. A curved osteotome is the instrument of choice for this procedure (Fig. 4.**21**).

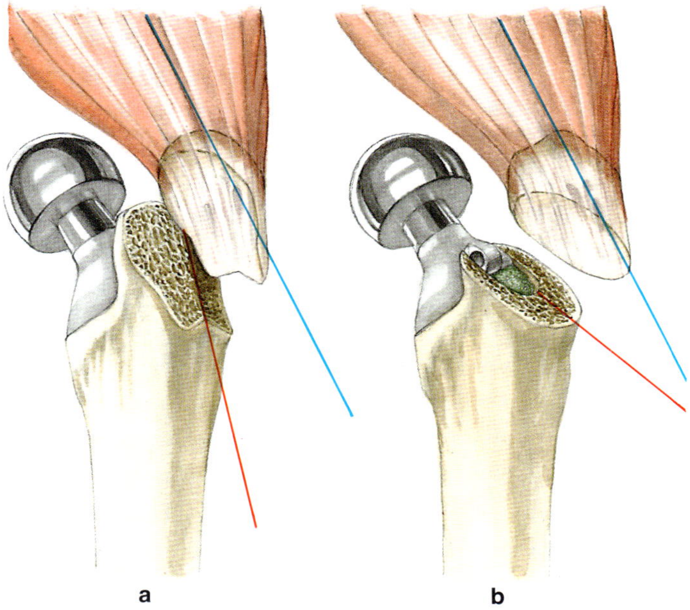

Fig. 4.**20** Correct (**a**) and incorrect (**b**) trochanteric osteotomy technique.

Red Angle of osteotomy
Blue Line of action of abductor force vector

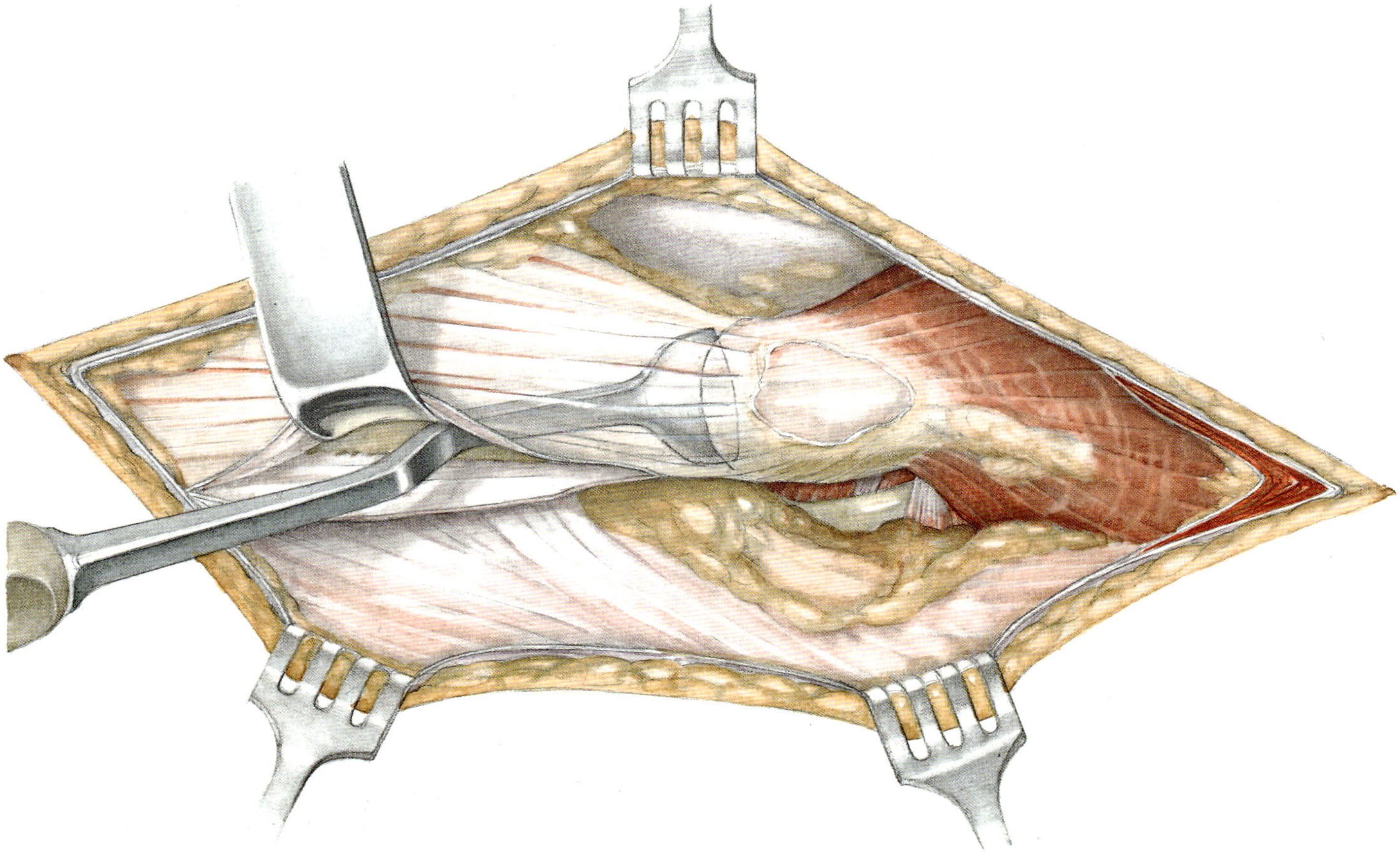

Fig. 4.**21** An alternative trochanteric osteotomy preserves the soft-tissue attachments between the greater trochanter and the vastus lateralis. The osteotomy is performed with a curved osteotome.

If the insertion of the piriformis tendon has been dissected with the trochanter fragment and the tension of the piriformis prevents exposure of the posterior superior periacetabular bone or places excessive strain on the region of the superior gluteal nerve, the surgeon should dissect the tendon from the trochanter fragment. The surgeon then resects the anterior, superior, and inferior portions of the capsule and any heterotopic ossification with the leg slightly adducted, flexed, and externally rotated (Fig. 4.**22**).

The leg is slightly abducted, extended, and internally rotated to resect the posterior portion of the capsule and posterior heterotopic ossification. Dissecting the insertions of the external rotators greatly improves exposure, but is not essential. A pin is impacted into the ilium superior to the acetabulum to retract the trochanter fragment (Fig. 4.**23**).

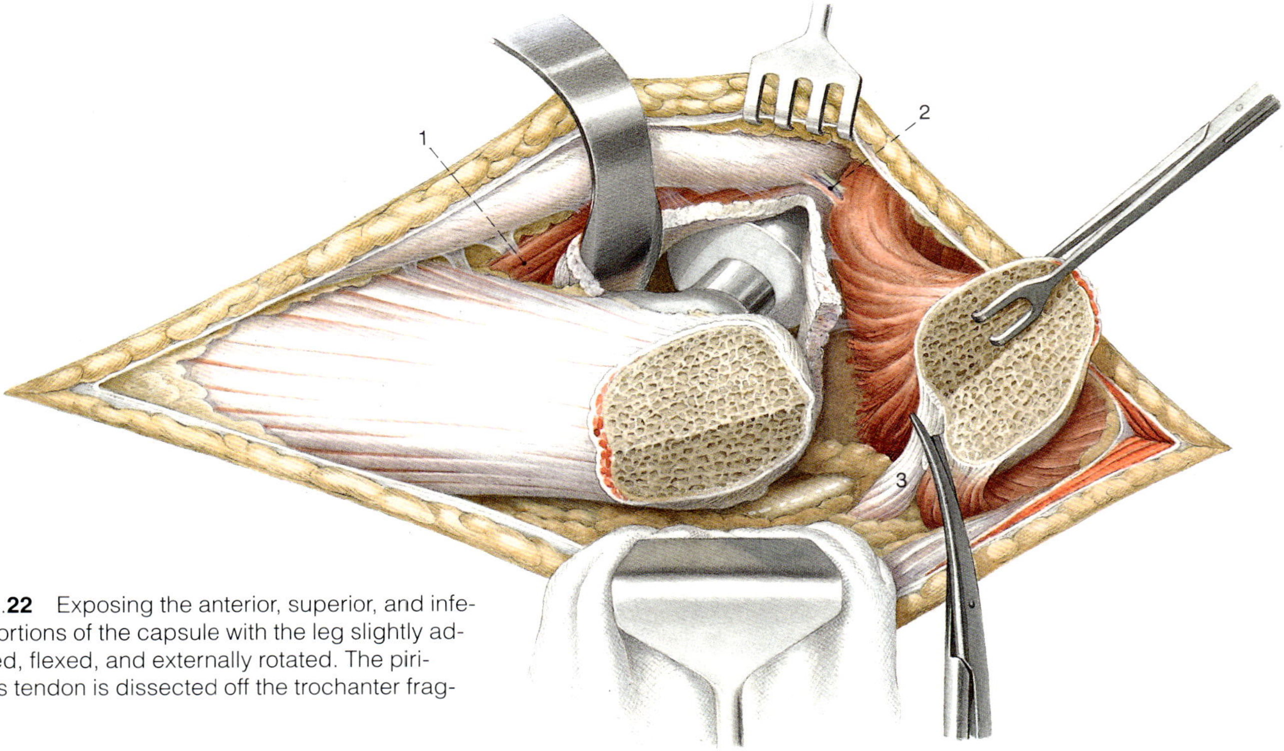

Fig. 4.**22** Exposing the anterior, superior, and inferior portions of the capsule with the leg slightly adducted, flexed, and externally rotated. The piriformis tendon is dissected off the trochanter fragment.

1 Iliacus
2 Superior gluteal nerve
3 Piriformis

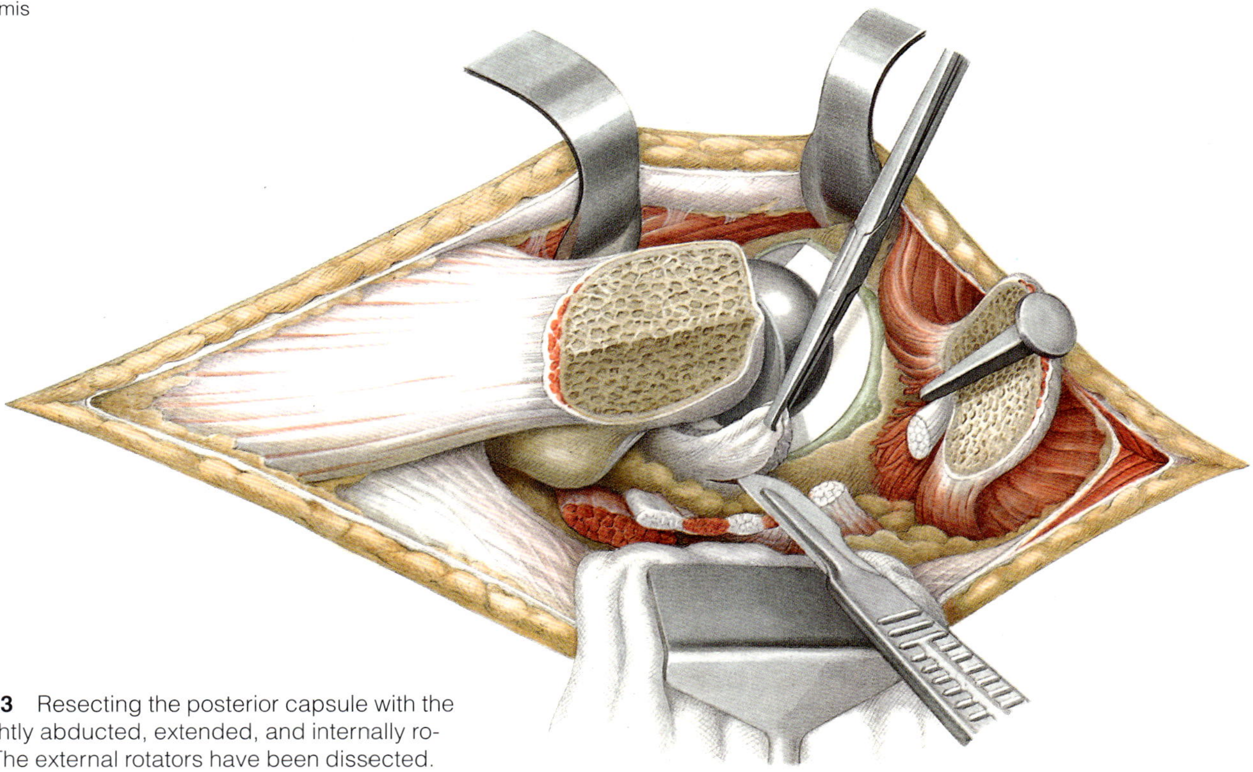

Fig. 4.**23** Resecting the posterior capsule with the leg slightly abducted, extended, and internally rotated. The external rotators have been dissected.

The surgeon dislocates the hip with the leg slightly flexed, adducted, and externally rotated, while pulling on a bone hook inserted around the prosthetic femoral neck (see Fig. 4.**13**). After dislocating the joint, the surgeon resects the anterior scars.

To extract the femoral component and expose the femoral canal, the affected leg is placed over the opposite leg. The proximal femur is raised by pressing on the knee of the affected leg, using the opposite leg as a fulcrum (Fig. 4.**24**).

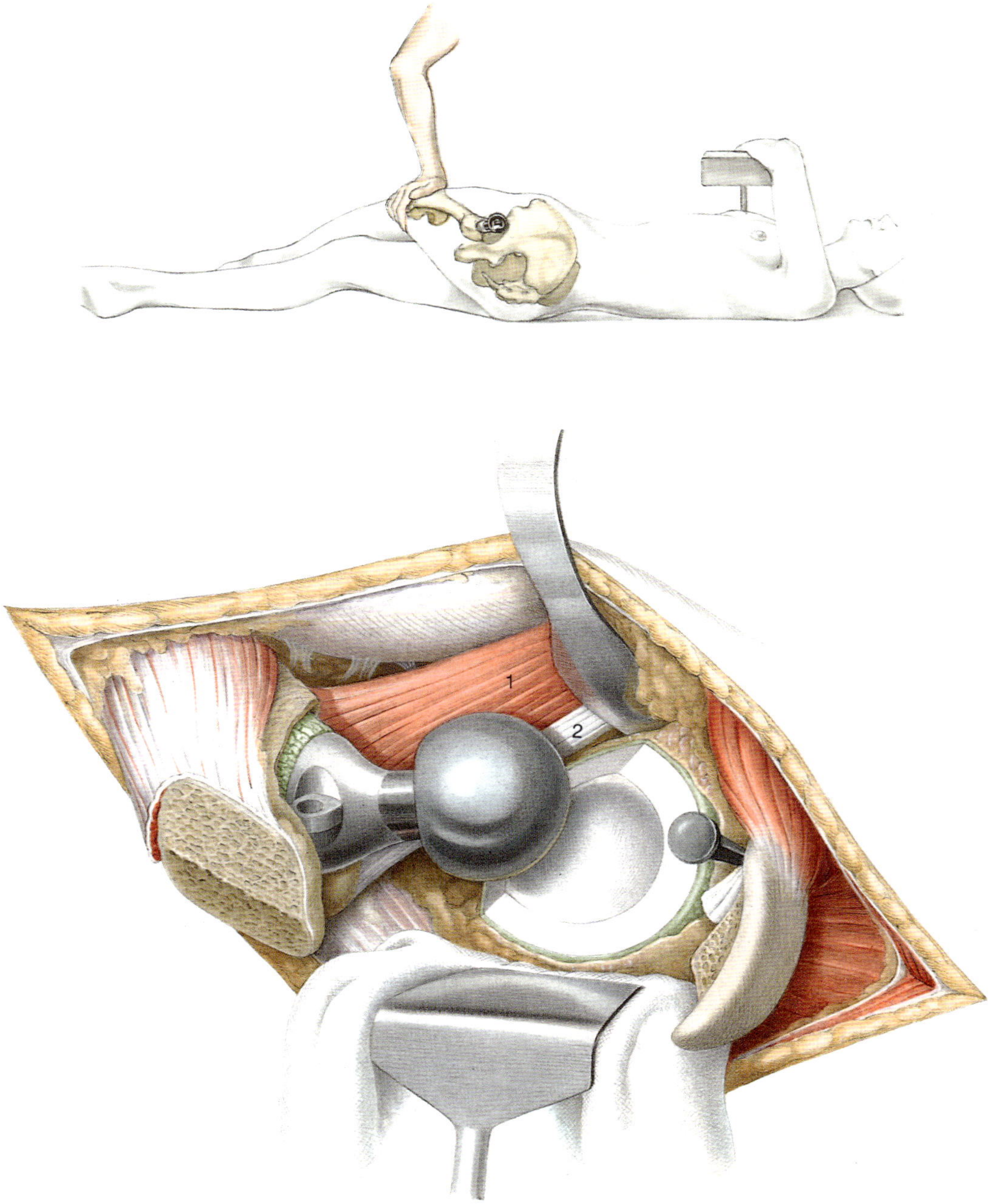

Fig. 4.**24** Exposing the femoral component. The affected leg is placed over the opposite leg, and pressure is applied to the knee.

1 Iliacus
2 Psoas tendon

To expose the acetabular component, flexion is increased and the proximal femur is shifted posteriorly by placing a roll between the legs and pulling on the prosthetic femoral neck with a bone hook. This provides good exposure of the acetabulum even when the stem is left in place (Fig. 4.**25**).

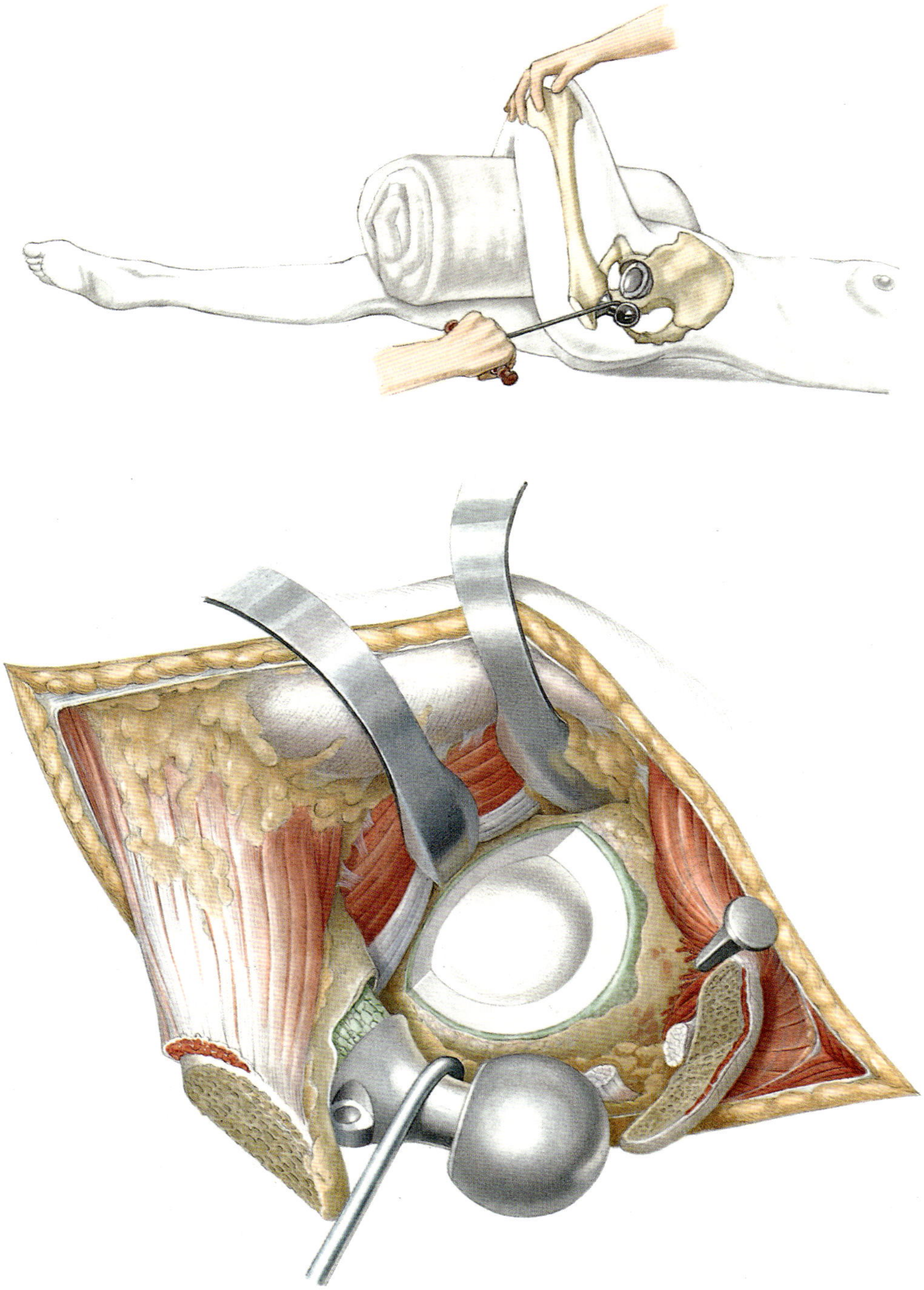

Fig. 4.**25** Exposing the acetabular component. With a roll in place between the legs, traction is applied on the prosthetic femoral neck with a bone hook.

If exposure of the iliac wing is required (see Fig. 4.**125**), the proximal skin and fascial incision deviates anteriorly from the greater trochanter and is carried toward the anterior superior iliac spine. The incision then courses parallel to the iliac crest. The surgeon dissects the abductors off the iliac crest, leaving a small portion of the tendinous origin to facilitate subsequent reattachment. The superior gluteal nerve is sacrified. Dissection can extend as far as the greater sciatic notch if necessary (Fig. 4.**26**).

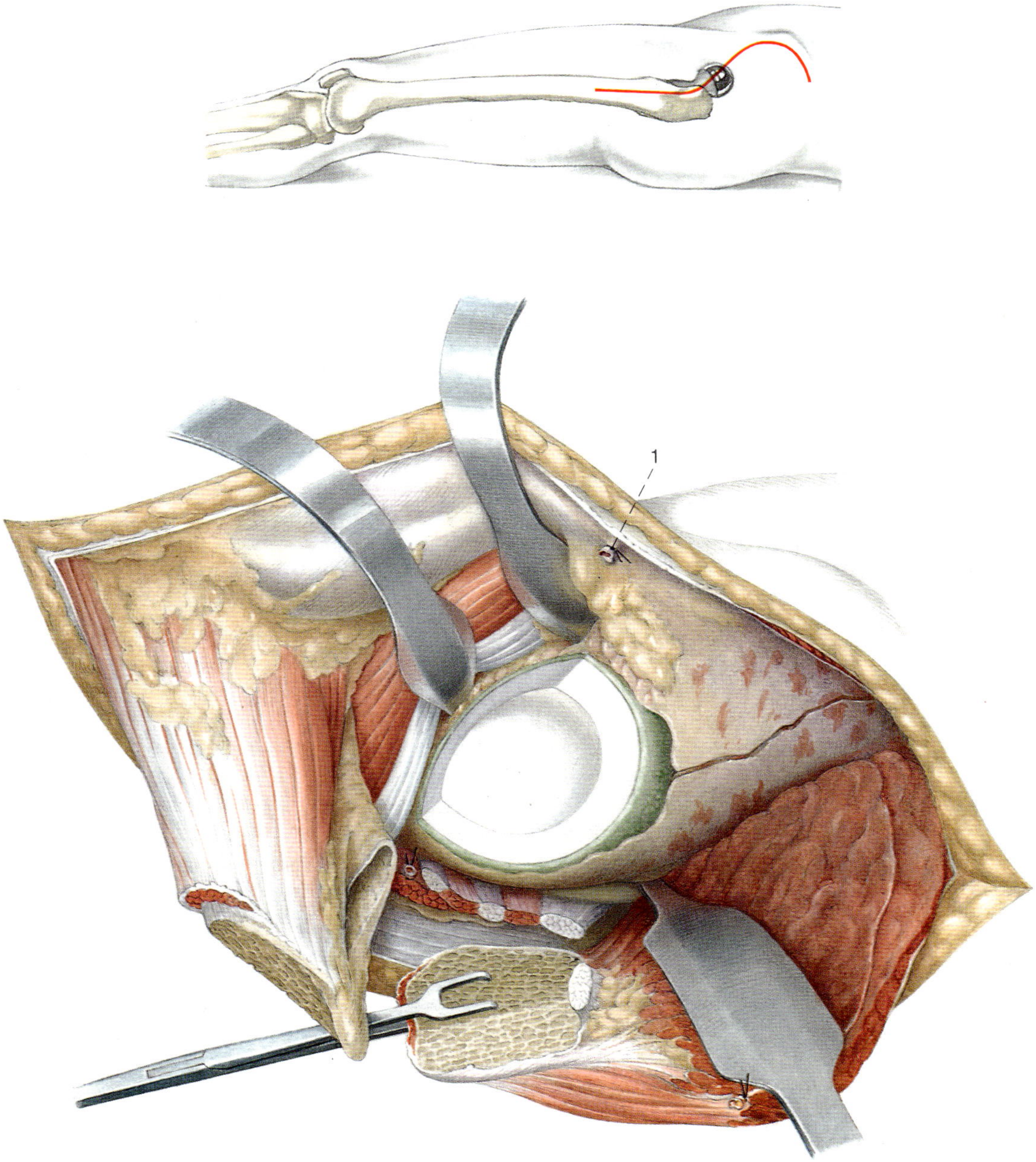

Fig. 4.**26** Exposing the iliac wing through a different incision.

1 Superior gluteal nerve, superior gluteal vessels

Transgluteal Approach to the Hip

With the patient supine and the leg in a neutral position, the surgeon splits the fascia of the gluteus medius along the boundary between the anterior and lateral thirds of the muscle. If only the hip is to be exposed, the incision is carried distally over the greater trochanter into the tendinous tissue and fascia of the vastus lateralis. If the procedure also requires exposure of the proximal femur, the incision curves posteriorly along the distal aspect of the greater trochanter and then continues distally along the linea aspera to permit dissection of the vastus lateralis (Fig. 4.**27**).

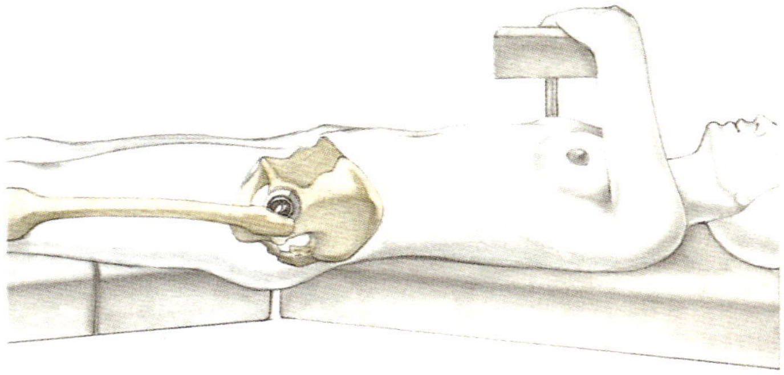

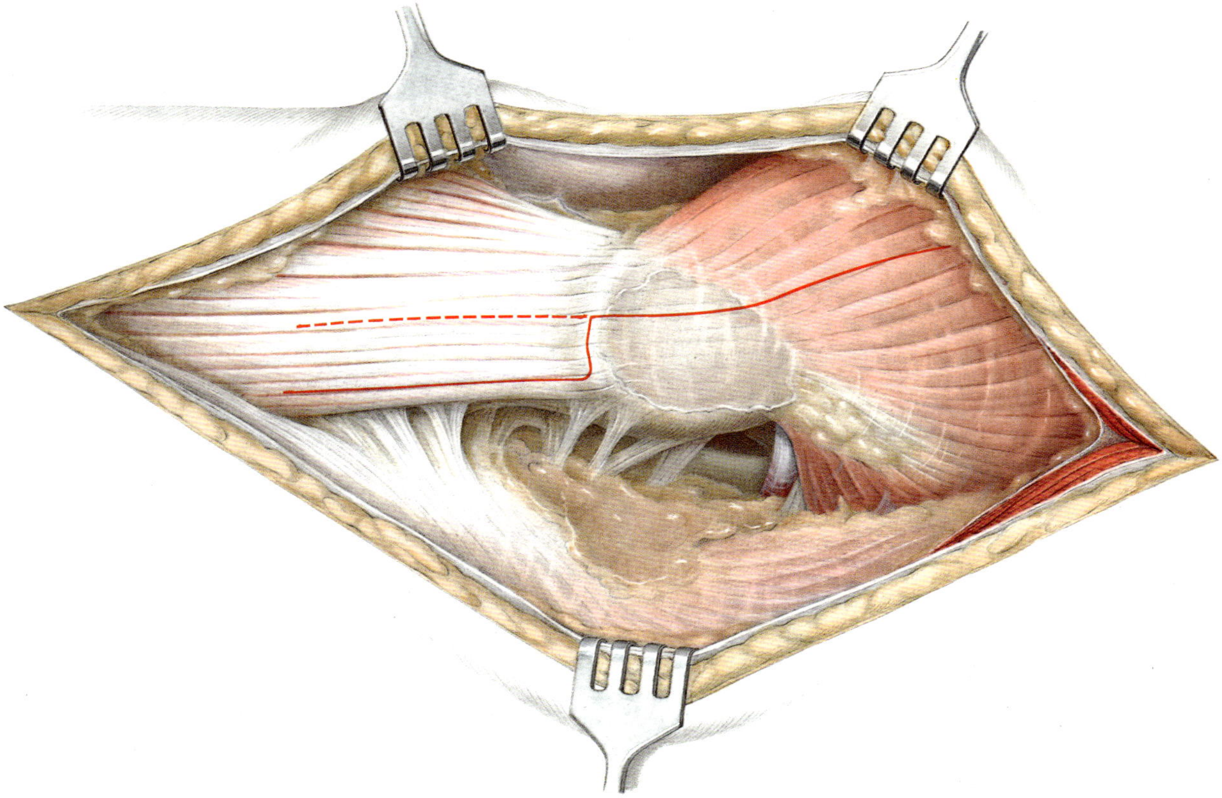

Fig. 4.**27** Transgluteal approach. Surgical site after skin and fascial incision. A transgluteal incision has been made proximal to the greater trochanter. Distal to the greater trochanter, the incision either splits the vastus lateralis parallel to its fibers (dotted line) or the vastus lateralis is dissected off the proximal femur (solid line).

The gluteus medius and the gluteus minimus beneath it are split parallel to their fibers. The tendinous soft tissue attached to the anterior greater trochanter and connected with the tendinous insertion of the vastus lateralis is then sharply dissected off the greater trochanter. This soft tissue should be subperiosteally dissected off the bone in a single layer. The vastus lateralis is split parallel to the direction of its fibers if only the hip joint is to be exposed; or its proximal origin is dissected off the femur as shown in the illustration. Avoid stretching and avulsing the dissected tendinous tissue when retracting it anteriorly.

The lateral and posterior thirds of the gluteus medius remain attached to the greater trochanter, since their fibers insert directly without any distal tendinous tissue connected with the vastus lateralis. The superior gluteal nerve between the gluteus medius and the gluteus minimus is protected if the abductors are not split too far superiorly. With the leg in external rotation, the surgeon exposes the capsule and performs an anterior capsulectomy (Fig. 4.**28**).

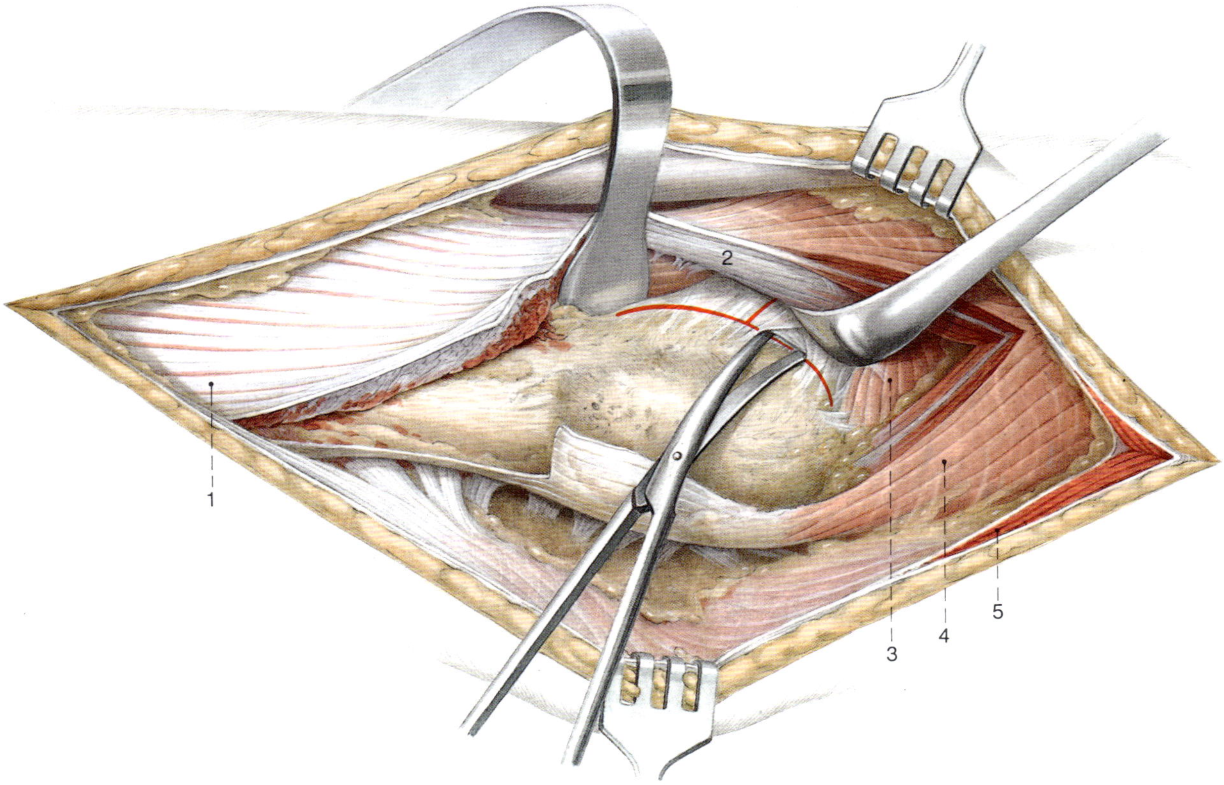

Fig. 4.**28** Dissecting the vastus and gluteal tendinous insertion and soft tissue off the anterior capsule. The red line indicates the capsulotomy.

1 Vastus lateralis
2 Anterior Vastus and gluteal tendinous insertion
3 Gluteus minimus
4 Gluteus medius
5 Gluteus maximus

After performing an anterior, superior, and inferior capsulectomy and removing any heterotopic ossification, the surgeon dislocates the hip transgluteally with a bone hook (see Fig. 4.**13**). With the joint dislocated, the posterior capsule is resected. Incising the insertions of the external rotators improves exposure (Fig. 4.**29**).

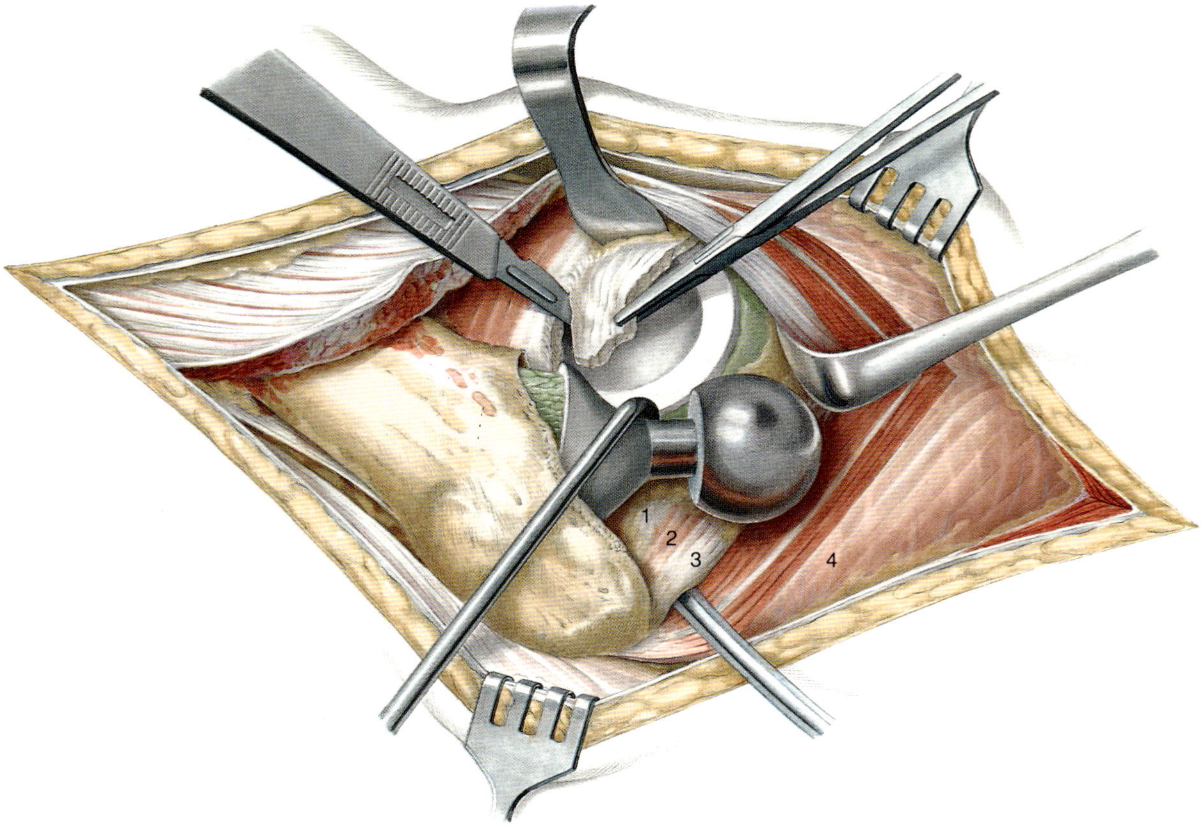

Fig. 4.**29** Capsulectomy. A probe can be inserted beneath the external rotators to improve exposure before their femoral insertions are transected.

1 Obturator internus
2 Superior gemellus
3 Piriformis
4 Gluteus medius

To extract the femoral component and expose the femoral canal, the affected leg is placed over the opposite leg and the surgeon presses on the knee of the affected leg as in the transtrochanteric approach. A roll and bone hook are used to increase flexion and adduction for exposure of the acetabular component. Exposure is not as good as in the transtrochanteric approach because the lateral and posterior abductors attached to the greater trochanter limit mobility of the proximal femur, and the superior gluteal nerve limits the superior splitting in the abductors (Fig. 4.**30**). Revising the acetabular component with the femoral component left in place is more difficult using this approach, but it is also possible if the posterior capsule is carefully excised and the insertions of the external rotators are incised.

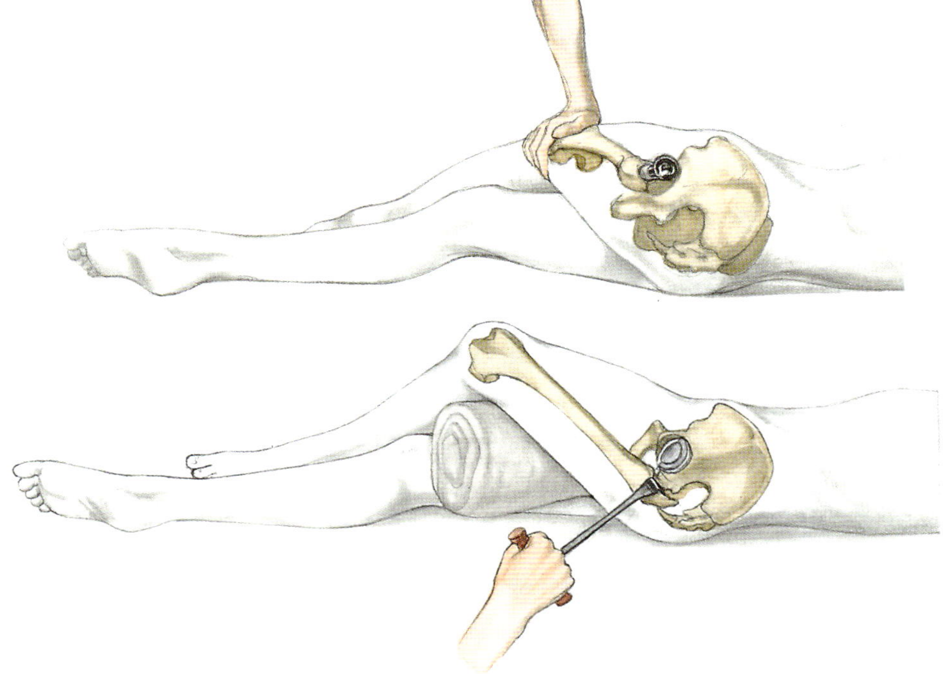

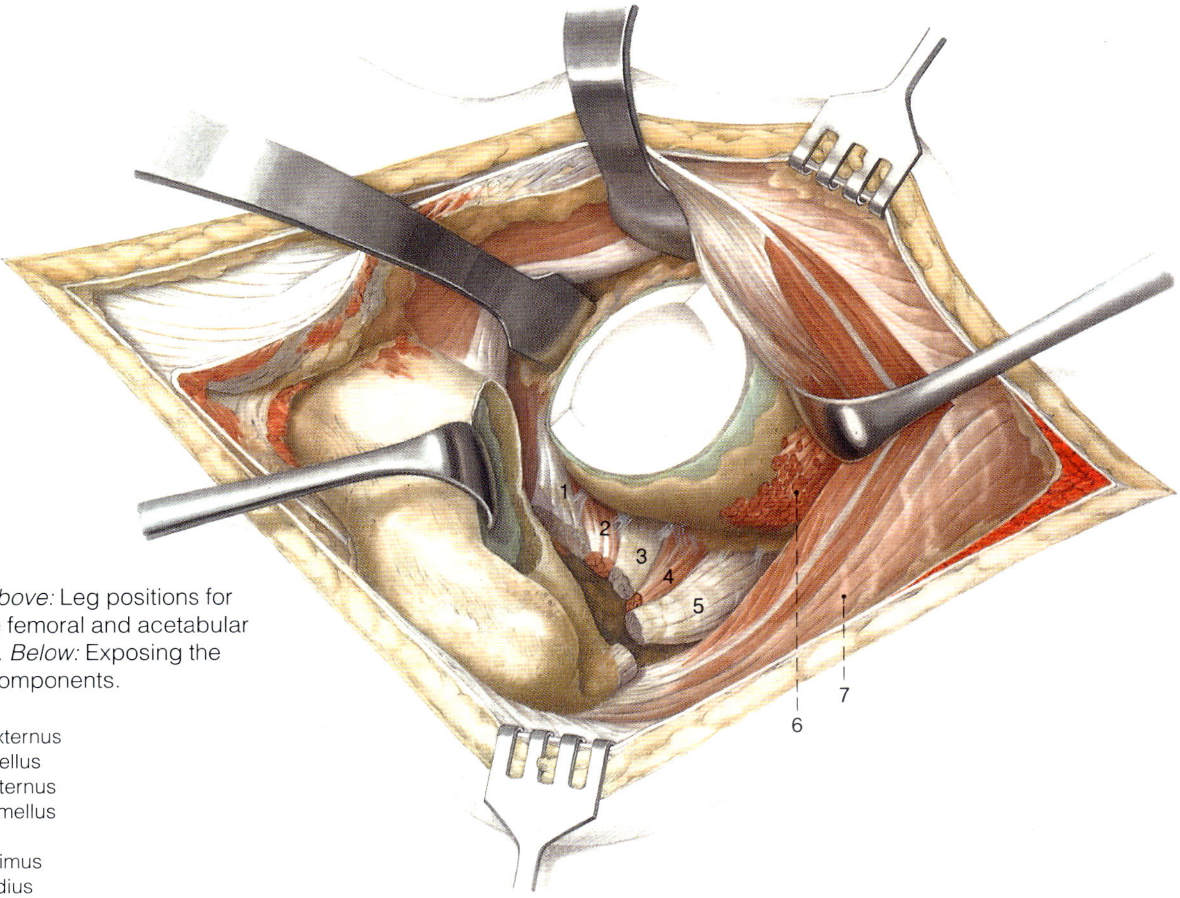

Fig. 4.**30** *Above:* Leg positions for exposing the femoral and acetabular components. *Below:* Exposing the acetabular components.

1 Obturator externus
2 Inferior gemellus
3 Obturator internus
4 Superior gemellus
5 Piriformis
6 Gluteus minimus
7 Gluteus medius

Extending the Approaches Distally

Lateral Approach to the Femur

If the proximal femur is to be exposed, the skin and fascial incision is extended distally. With the hip in internal rotation, the surgeon incises the fascia and the tendinous attachments of the vastus lateralis near the linea aspera and dissects the vastus lateralis from its origins, ligating its blood vessels.

Combining the lateral approach to the femur with a transgluteal (Fig. 4.**31**) and transtrochanteric approach (Fig. 4.**32**) to the hip makes it easy to change the position of the leg when exposing either the proximal femur or the femoral canal (e. g. while removing the cement through a window in the femur and from proximal). The affected leg is extended or placed over the opposite leg, depending on the exposure required.

When, alternatively, a posterior approach to the hip (Fig. 4.**33**) is used, exposing the femur with the patient in a lateral position requires maximum external rotation and extension (see Fig. 4.**14**), and exposing the femoral canal requires maximum internal rotation, partial flexion, and slight adduction (see Fig. 4.**15**) so that exposure of these two regions makes difficult re-positioning of the patient necessary. In addition the height and inclination of the operating table must be adjusted accordingly, and the surgeon may stand or sit, depending on the particular phase of the procedure.

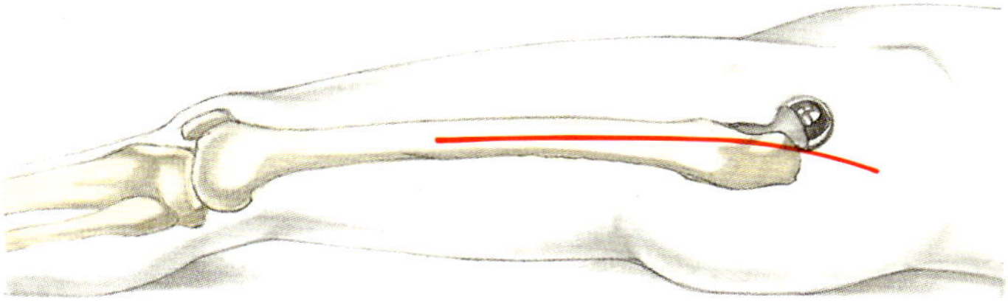

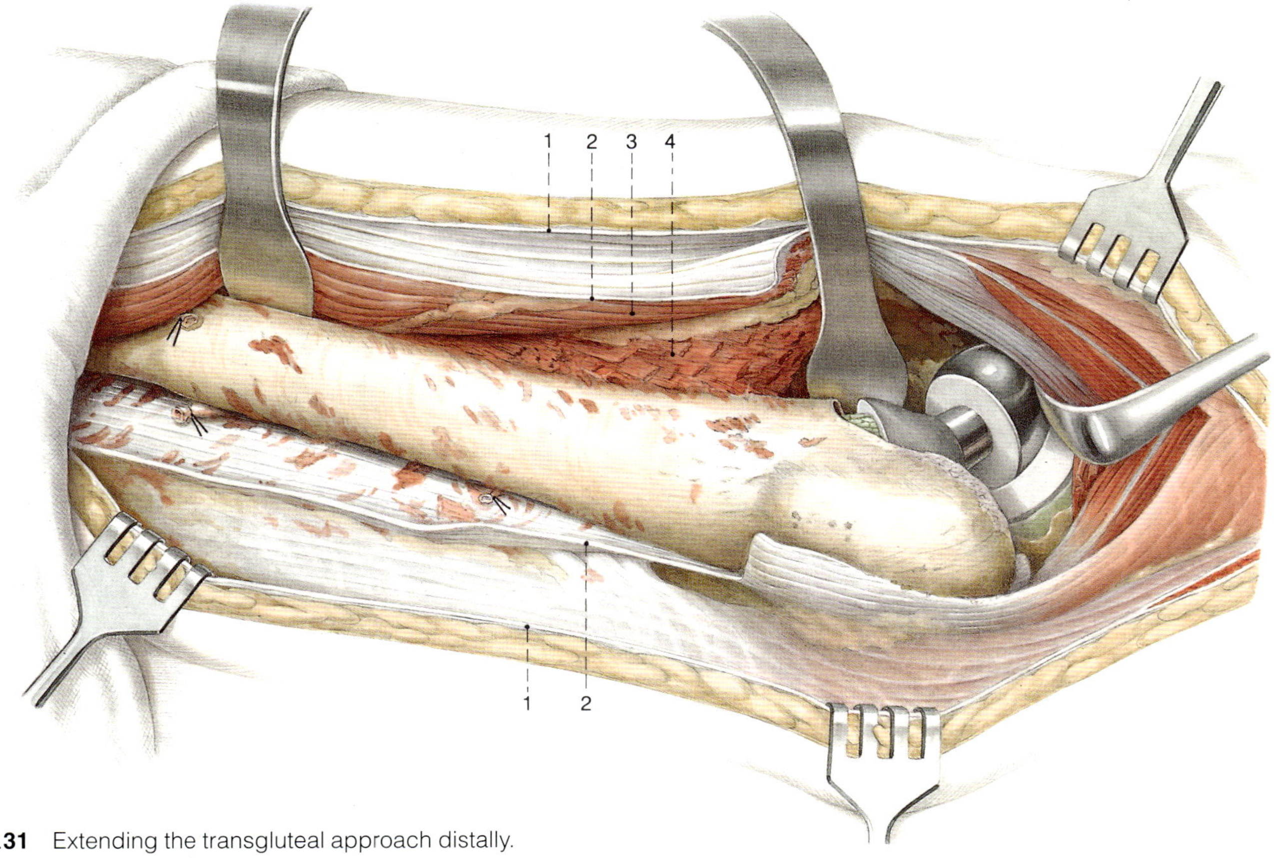

Fig. 4.**31** Extending the transgluteal approach distally. Lateral approach to the femur.

1 Fascia lata
2 Vastus lateralis tendon
3 Vastus lateralis
4 Vastus intermedius

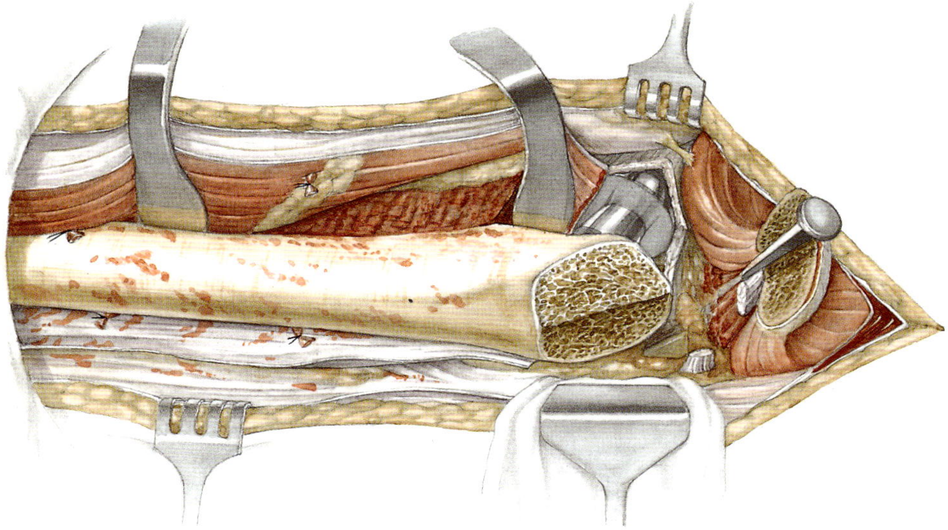

Fig. 4.**32** Extending the transtrochanteric approach distally. Lateral approach to the proximal femur.

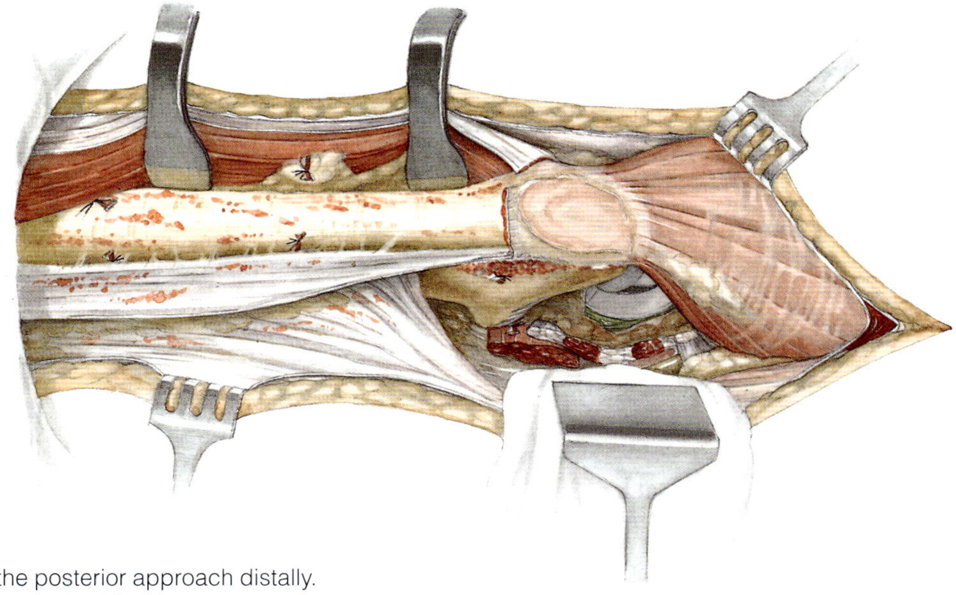

Fig. 4.**33** Extending the posterior approach distally. Lateral approach to the proximal femur.

Lateral Approach to the Knee

If the knee is also to be exposed, the skin and fascial incision is extended to the knee joint past the patella, ending lateral to the tibial tuberosity. After dissecting the vastus lateralis completely off the femur, the surgeon incises the capsule of the knee joint to a point lateral to the tibial tuberosity and opens the joint space. After dissecting the retropatellar fat body, the surgeon dislocates the patella medially with the knee flexed. Medial dislocation of the patella is difficult in a lateral approach to the knee joint alone, but it is easily performed in combination with a lateral approach to the femur, since the vastus lateralis has been dissected from its origin, relieving the tension on the extensors.

If a total femoral prosthesis (see Fig. 4.**153**) is indicated, then the popliteus tendon, lateral collateral ligament (Fig. 4.**34**), cruciate ligaments (Fig. 4.**35**), and medial collateral ligament (Fig. 4.**36**) are successively dissected off the femur.

This results in the exposure of the entire femur (Fig. 4.**37**) and permits the femoral and reimplantation of all implants in total hip revision surgery.

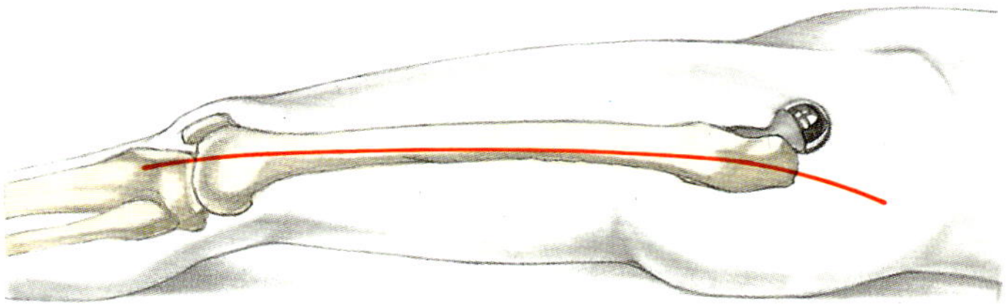

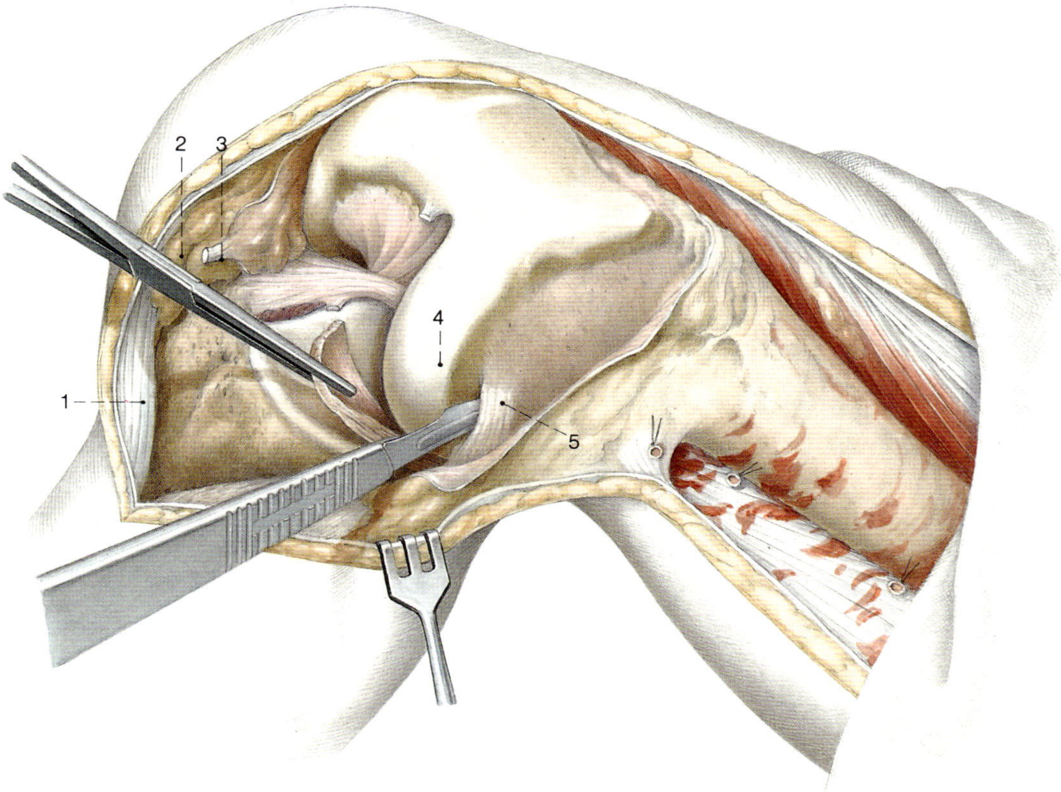

Fig. 4.**34** Extending the lateral approach to the proximal femur distally to the knee. Medial dislocation of the patella, dissection of the lateral collateral ligament and the popliteus tendon at the femoral insertion, and meniscectomy.

1 Patellar ligament
2 Retropatellar fat body
3 Retropatellar synovial fold
4 Lateral condyle
5 Lateral collateral ligament

Evaluating the Approaches to the Hip

Posterior Approach

This approach avoids damage to the abductors. Periacetabular dissection prior to dislocation sometimes requires an additional anterolateral approach if there is pronounced anterior scarring or heterotopic ossification. This technique is generally sufficient. If not, the surgeon may always perform a secondary trochanteric osteotomy, but this requires a greater trochanter that is suitable for osteotomy.

Maximum internal rotation is required for removing and reimplanting the femoral component, and can endanger a weakened femur. The torque created by internal rotation also interferes with the reduction of preoperative and intraoperative fractures. Exposing the femoral canal from proximal and then the femur from lateral (e.g. when removing cement from proximal and through a window in the femur) requires repeated and time-consuming re-positioning of the leg and the table.

The posterior approach provides good exposure of the superior and posterosuperior periacetabular region, which is the most frequent site of deficient bone stock. Exposure permits extensive reconstruction, but this may be difficult if the femoral component is left in place. Thorough release of all periarticular scars is required in these cases; if this proves insufficient, a secondary trochanteric osteotomy may be performed.

This approach rarely damages anterior neurovascular structures. The sciatic nerve is easily exposed and protected with the patient in the lateral position.

The lateral position is advantageous for intraoperative blood salvage because blood does not flow out of the wound and can be almost completely recovered by suction.

After a posterior approach, the patient can be rapidly mobilized with minimal pain and without a postoperative period of partial weight bearing, unless contraindicated by other considerations. The risk of postoperative dislocation is always somewhat higher where there is extensive dissection of the external rotators.

Indications for the Posterior Approach

The approach is indicated for replacement of the complete hip implant or only the femoral or acetabular component and is suitable for the majority of all revision cases. Almost any degree of acetabular reconstruction is permitted.

Extensive heterotopic ossification and scarring (primarily anterior), weakening of the proximal femur, and a femoral component left in place may limit the application of this approach.

Transtrochanteric Approach

If the greater trochanter is suitable for osteotomy (i.e., it contains enough cancellous bone) and the osteotomy and fixation of the trochanter fragment are performed properly, the risk of non-union at the osteotomy site and hip instability will be slight. This risk increases significantly where these conditions are not met. Periarticular dissection and debridement is easily performed prior to dislocation, even in patients with extensive heterotopic ossification and deep protrusion with scarred adhesions.

Exposing the femoral canal does not result in any appreciable stresses that may fracture a weakened femur because there is no torque created by internal rotation as with the posterior approach. The transtrochanteric approach is therefore especially suitable for the reduction of fractures or when the proximal femoral bone is weak. The femoral canal and the femur can be exposed from proximal respectively lateral by simply changing the position of the leg.

The approach provides optimal exposure of the periacetabular region, even when the femoral component is left in place.

The risk to major neurovascular structures is slight due to the good exposure. Posteriorly mobilizing the abductors after the osteotomy protects the superior gluteal nerve.

A period of limited weight bearing is advisable in postoperative management because of the trochanteric osteotomy. The risk of postoperative dislocation increases when the external rotators have been dissected or if fixation of the trochanter fragment fails.

Indications for the Transtrochanteric Approach

The approach is indicated when optimal exposure is necessary and no torque should be applied to the femur, for instance in cases with extensive heterotopic ossification, deep protrusion with scarred adhesions, extensive acetabular reconstruction and a weakened femur or femoral fracture.

Deficient trochanteric bone stock limits the range of indications.

Transgluteal Approach

The damage to the abductors remains tolerable. The lateral and posterior abductor fibers left attached to the greater tochanter interfere with excising posterior periarticular scars and ossifications prior to dislocation.

Exposing the femoral canal places only slight stresses on a weakened femur and the position of the leg is easily changed if the femoral canal and the femur have to be exposed alternately as in the transtrochanteric approach.

Exposure of the periacetabular region is limited especially when the femoral component is left in place because the lateral and posterior abductor fibers retain their attachments to the greater trochanter, limiting the mobility of the proximal femur. A secondary posterior trochanteric osteotomy is possible, but refixation of this trochanter fragment is doubtful.

Splitting the abductors too far superiorly can damage the superior gluteal nerve. The risk of damage to other major neurovascular structures is slight, but higher when scars and ossifications obstruct exposure.

Risk of postoperative dislocation increases when the insertions of the external rotators are dissected to improve exposure, or when fixation of the anterior tendinous insertion of the vastus lateralis and abductors fails. Partial weight bearing promotes healing of these structures.

Indications for the Transgluteal Approach

The approach is indicated in a weakened femur in which the greater trochanter is not suitable for osteotomy.

Heterotopic ossification and scarring (primarily posterior) and a femoral component left in place limit the range of indications.

Anterior and Anterolateral Approach

The anterior and anterolateral approaches are not recommended for revision total hip arthroplasty because they do not provide sufficient exposure. An anterior approach requires dissecting the origins of the abductors from the iliac wing, while the anterolateral approach may entail damage to or anteriorly incising the insertions of the abductors on the greater trochanter. Both procedures weaken the hip muscles.

Posterior scars or heterotopic ossification is difficult to remove. Periacetabular exposure within the posterosuperior region is limited and nearly impossible when the femoral component is left in place.

With these approaches in revision surgery there is a greater danger of damaging the femoral nerve, major anterior blood vessels and the lateral femoral cutaneous nerve. The superior gluteal nerve is transected in an anterolateral approach.

After both these approaches, revision is problematic if the operation is followed by an infection, particularly with anterior fistulas.

Removing Total Hip Implants

In the absence of implant loosening, removing a femoral component is generally more complicated than removing an acetabular component, and cementless stems often require a more invasive procedure than cemented ones. There are several reasons for this:

Design elements that impair removal have been largely eliminated from cemented implants without sacrificing implant longevity.

Cemented femoral components with a conical shape, regular curvature and an even surface lacking any complex structures are easily extracted from the cement. Generally, the design has a hole or other feature that permits use of an extraction instrument. These stems can usually be removed even from an intact cement mantle without loosening once the cement between the implant shoulder and the greater trochanter has been chiselled out. Remaining loose cement can be easily removed because the connective tissue that forms in areas of bone resorption adheres poorly to bone and cement and is not as strong as that encountered when cementless implants are loose. Even cement which is not loose can in most cases be removed without opening the femur, provided the surgeon is equipped with appropriate instruments. Problem areas are easily located in the preoperative radiographic evaluation. Thus, if the surgeon must resort to cutting a window in the cortex to remove the implant or residual cement, this can be done precisely at the site of the problem and therefore in the majority of cases the window need only be a small one (Fig. 4.**38a**). Opening the entire femur initially to simplify the procedure by performing a transfemoral removal is recommended only in severe cases of chronic stem loosening where a weakened femur is likely to fracture during the approach, during removal or in later phases of the procedure. Before doing so, every effort should be made to preserve even very thin femoral bone so that bone grafting is possible.

Cemented acetabular components rarely cause major problems, unless protrusions of cement in the pelvis that are larger than the bone defects through which they have been pressed require removal (e. g. when the acetabulum is to be reconstructed with graft or in the presence of periprosthetic infection).

Design features that impair removal are often crucial to the fixation of cementless implants.

Cementless femoral components of older designs have holes or undercuts while newer designs often employ complex surface treatments (such as coarse or fine texturing, or coarse or fine-porous coatings covering all or part of the stem). The stems rarely have longitudinal structures that are conducive to removal. Often there is no feature that permits use of an extraction instrument. A non-removable collar can prevent access to the bone-implant interface, and thus eliminate the surgeon's only non-invasive option for removing a fixed stem. Where the bone-implant interface is accessible, coarse surface structures often interfere with the instruments. Bony

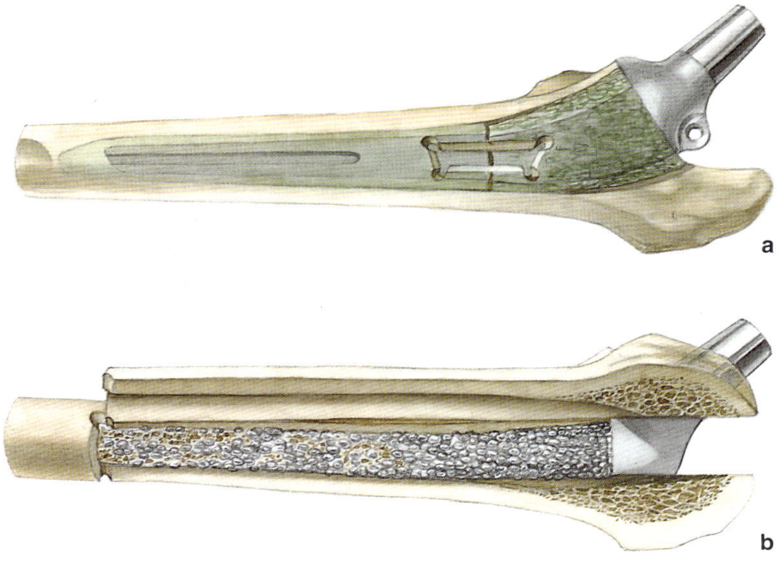

Fig. 4.**38a** and **b** Invasive procedures for removal of cemented and cementless stems.
a Small, precisely localized window at the site of the problems for removing firmly fixed or partially loosened cemented stems (e.g. stem fractures).
b If a firmly fixed or even loosened cementless stem is to be removed (e.g. thigh pain where biologic fixation has been achieved) often an initial longitudinal osteotomy is performed or a window covering the entire length of the implant is opened.

and connective tissue attachments adhere far better to cementless implants than to cemented ones. Areas of strong biologic fixation are often difficult to locate precisely in the preoperative radiographic evaluation. While these sites depend in part on the respective implant design and surface structure, they may occur in different areas, even when the same implant system is used. Even a small area of biologic fixation can prevent extraction. But also in cases of severe loosening the connective tissue may interfere with removal. Thus, in difficult cases a small window is insufficient, and the surgeon must split the femur longitudinally or open a window covering the entire length of the implant (Fig. 4.**38b**).

Cementless acetabular components are less problematic than stems. However, bone and connective tissue can cause problems when a threaded acetabular cup with undercuts transverse to the threads is to be removed even in the presence of severe loosening.

When both components require replacement, the surgeon first removes the stem and then the acetabular component. To minimize blood loss when removing a cemented stem, it is recommended that the surgeon remove the stem but leave the cement intact initially. Then the acetabular component is removed, the acetabulum is reconstructed if necessary, and the new cup is implanted, before the surgeon continues work on the femur.

Removing Cemented Stems

The surgeon removes the stem first. This is followed by removal of the cement in the proximal cancellous and distal cortical bone of the femur, the residual plug of cement in the femoral diaphysis, and (if present and a longer stem is indicated) a shelf of cortical bone separating the femoral medullary canal.

Removing the Stem from the Cement Mantle

Before extracting the stem, the surgeon removes the cement between the implant shoulder and the greater trochanter. This sometimes involves hollowing out the greater trochanter. A narrow Lambotte osteotome is best for splitting the cement (Figs. 4.**39** and 4.**40**).

After this, stems designed for easy removal can generally be extracted from an intact cement mantle that adheres to the walls of the femoral canal. If a system-specific extraction instrument can be attached to the stem, then the extraction force can be applied along the axis of the stem (Fig. 4.**41**).

If an extraction instrument is not provided or available but the implant has a collar, then the surgeon can use a mallet and an impactor to extract the implant by applying force obliquely instead of axially. Traction applied to a bone hook around the prosthetic femoral neck prevents the transverse component of this force from damaging the femur (Fig. 4.**42**).

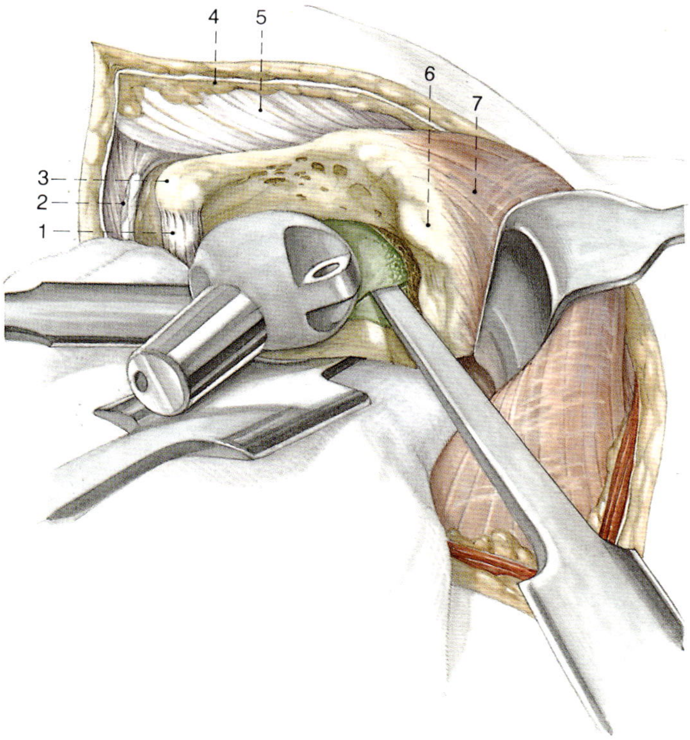

Fig. 4.**39** Exposing the proximal femur through a posterior approach to remove a cemented stem. Splitting the cement between the implant shoulder and the greater trochanter.

1 Psoas tendon
2 Incised gluteus maximus tendon
3 Lesser trochanter
4 Fascia lata
5 Vastus lateralis
6 Greater trochanter, hollowed out
7 Gluteus medius

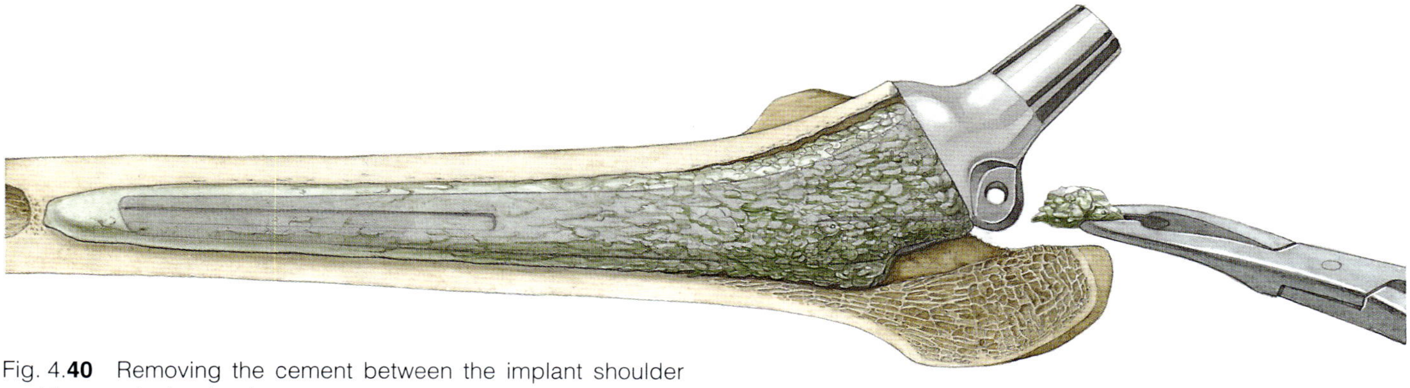

Fig. 4.**40** Removing the cement between the implant shoulder and the greater trochanter.

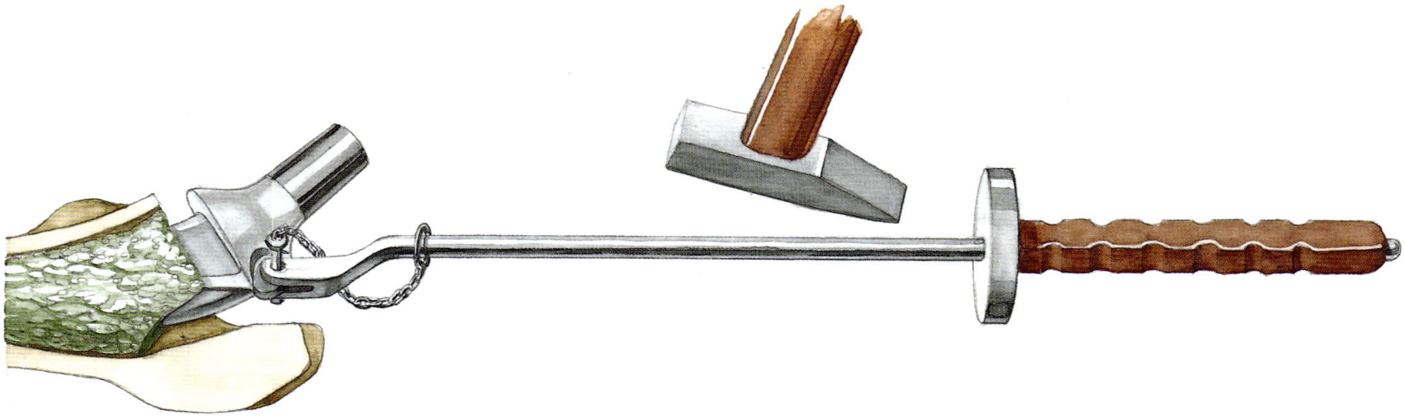

Fig. 4.**41** Attaching a system-specific extraction instrument. The extraction force is applied along the axis of the stem.

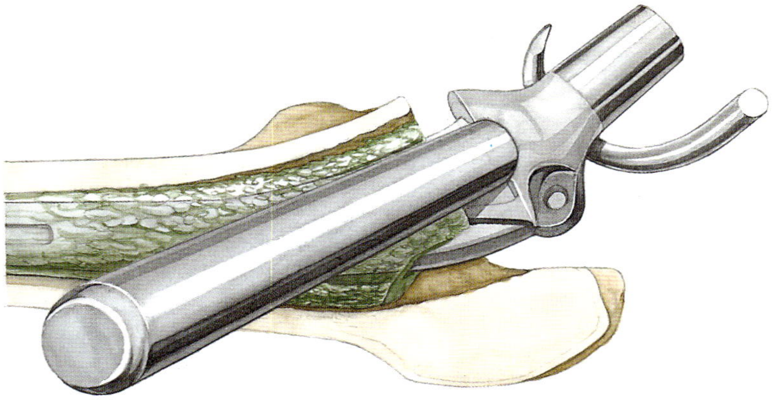

Fig. 4.**42** Using an impactor to extract a collared stem. Traction applied to a bone hook compensates for the transverse component of the obliquely applied force.

A universal extraction instrument may be used on nonmodular stems with fixed heads. The socket of the instrument engages the prosthetic femoral head; a slap hammer screwed onto a corner of the socket opposite the slot for the femoral neck is used to apply extraction force axially. Since the slap hammer can be attached on both corners opposite the slot, the instrument permits right and left-handed use and anterior or posterior application to the femoral head (Fig. 4.**43**).

Implants without a fixed head or collar can cause significant problems if they do not permit attaching an extraction instrument or have a proximal groove or undercut that an impactor or center punch can engage. If a diamond saw is available, then the surgeon can cut a groove in the taper, and a screw clamp can be attached to provide a surface for the impactor to engage. Traction applied with a bone hook compensates for the transverse force (Fig. 4.**44**).

Another improvised solution when removing an implant without a fixed head or collar is to expose a flat part of the stem either proximally or through a window. Using a carbide-tipped bit, the surgeon drills a hole and attempts to extract it with center punch (Fig. 4.**45**). Carbide-tipped bits will have increasing difficulty penetrating steel, cobalt-chrome, or titanium. Low speed drilling and constant pressure without changing the direction of drilling are necessary to avoid separating the cutting edge or hardening the metal of the implant. The site must be irrigated.

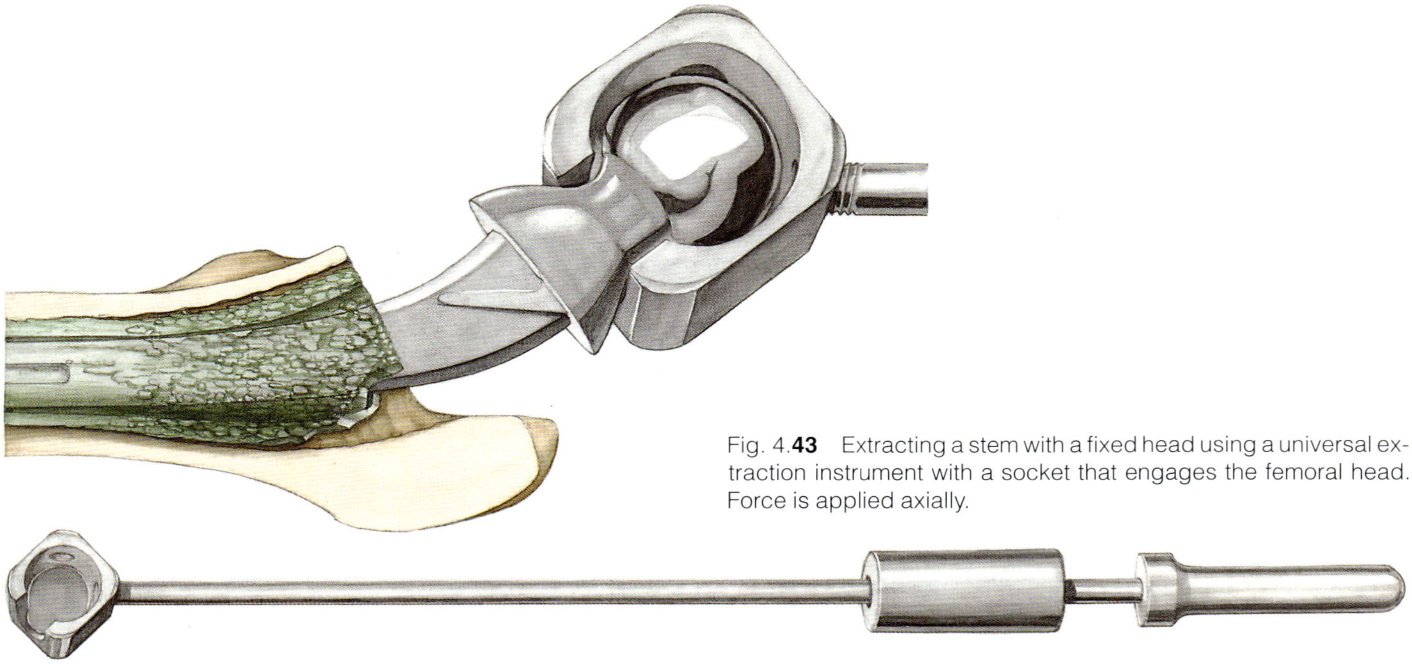

Fig. 4.**43** Extracting a stem with a fixed head using a universal extraction instrument with a socket that engages the femoral head. Force is applied axially.

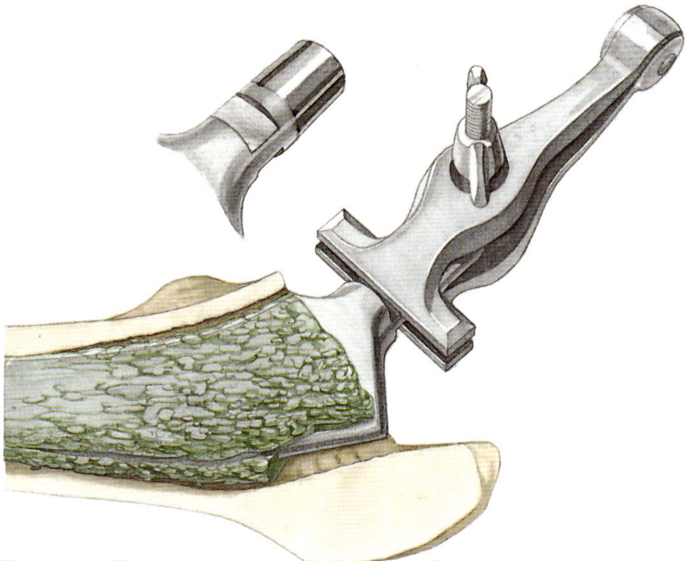

Fig. 4.**44** Extracting a stem without a fixed head or collar. A groove is cut in the taper, and a screw clamp is attached to provide a surface for the impactor to engage.

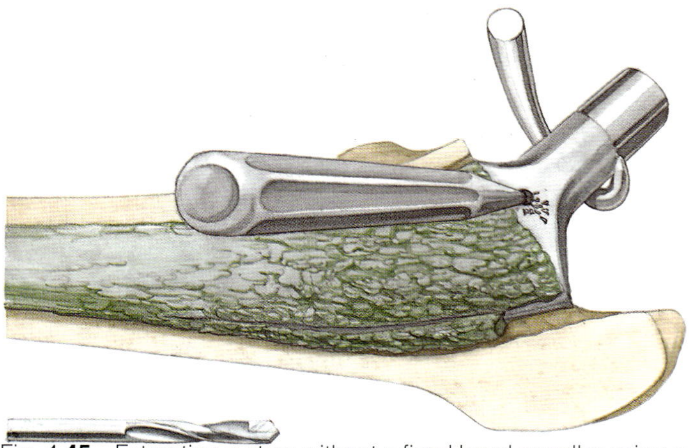

Fig. 4.**45** Extracting a stem without a fixed head or collar using a center punch inserted in a hole drilled in the flat surface of the proximal part of the implant. Traction applied with a bone hook compensates for the transverse component of the applied force.

In such cases, an extraction instrument that attaches directly to the taper and permits application of axial force is helpful. An instrument with an axial impacting plate and a shaft with an angled collar matching the taper and equipped with threaded holes is impacted onto the taper so that the shaft of the instrument is lies within the axis of the stem. A drill guide is successively screwed into two or three of the holes in the collar, and the surgeon drills through the guide about 2 mm into the taper using a carbide-tipped bit (Fig. 4.**46a**). After removing the drill guide, the surgeon inserts set screws into the threaded holes of the collar. Their tapered tips engage the drillholes in the taper. The farther distal the screws are, the better they transfer force to the taper. The most important screw is the one opposite the base of the instrument shaft. When extracting the implant (Fig. 4.**46b**), the surgeon should repeatedly retighten the screws after every few blows with the mallet to avoid loosening of the collar due to deformation of the tips of the set screws.

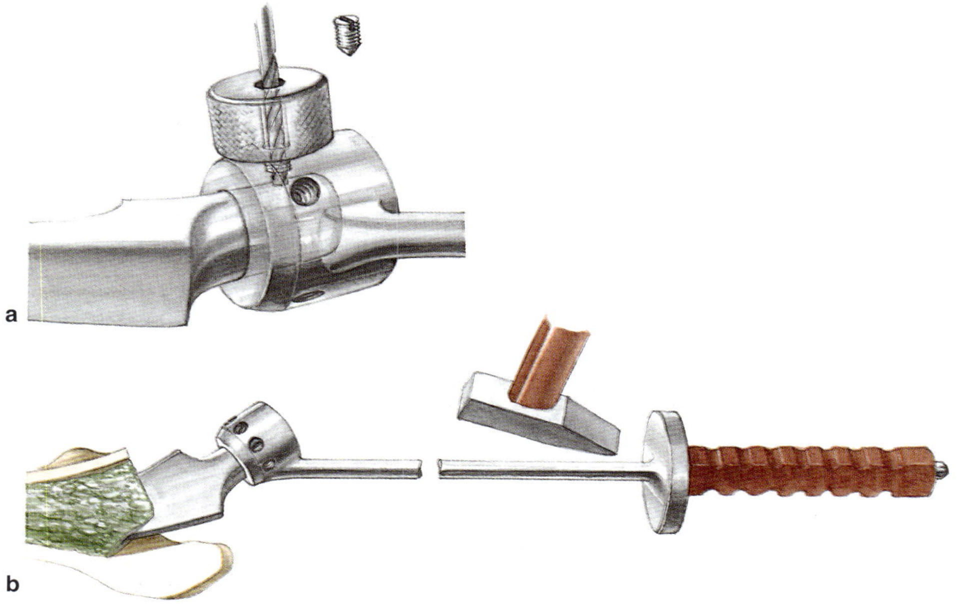

Fig. 4.**46a** and **b** Extraction instrument with an angled collar for engaging the implant taper. Force is applied axially.
a Drilling a hole in the taper with a drill guide.
b Inserting set screws into the holes (on the distal side of the collar whenever possible).

Removing Cement from the Proximal Cancellous Bone

Narrow osteotomes, chisels and gouges are the surgeon's most important instruments for removing the remains of the cement after the stem has been extracted. Using proper instrumentation conserves bone. Different widths, blade shapes (straight, curved, sharpened symmetrically or either on the inside or the outer edges), and shaft lengths and shapes are used for specific tasks. All are honed at an extremely steep angle suitable for cutting the brittle cement without causing damage to the bone. They are designed either as full-metal models like the Lambotte osteotome or composites with a metal blade enclosed in an outer handle so that the full force of the mallet is transmitted directly to the cement.

In the proximal cancellous area, the cement mantle is split radially with such instruments with straight symmetrically honed blades (Fig. 4.**47a**). The lug chisel has a blade with a lug that prevents the chisel from deviating from the femoral canal into the bone (Fig. 4.**47b**).

The flakes of cement are broken off into the lumen. Gouges sharpened on the inside penetrate well between the bone and cement, but they only pry the flakes of cement off the bone slightly and can easily penetrate the bone (Fig. 4.**48a**). Gouges sharpened on the outside do not penetrate well and are only suitable for proximal use where the surgeon can tilt the shaft of the gouge into the lumen. Once driven into the interface they provide better leverage and do not much endanger the bone (Fig. 4.**48b**). The attempt to break flakes of cement off by tilting the gouge outwards may result in a cortical fracture (Fig. 4.**48c**).

Flakes of cement can be broken off by impacting a narrow osteotome with a straight, symmetrically sharpened blade into the interface and rotating the chisel around its longitudinal axis. If the bone is strong, it can be used as a fulcrum for turning the blade (Fig. 4.**49a**). If the bone is weakened, it can be perforated, and the surgeon should use the adjacent cement as a fulcrum to relieve the load on the bone (Fig. 4.**49b**).

Another method of distributing the load is to impact a wide gouge with a curved blade, sharpened on the inside into the bone–cement interface and a second narrower chisel with a straight or curved blade between it and the flake of cement. The flake usually breaks off when the inner chisel is carefully tapped with a mallet, while the outer gouge protects the bone behind it (Fig. 4.**50**).

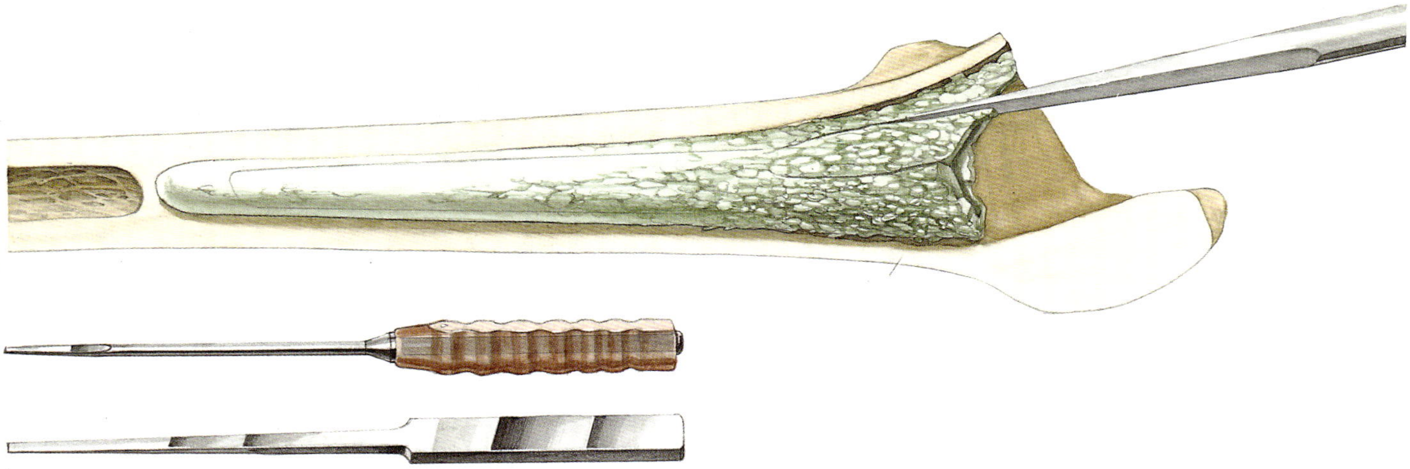

a

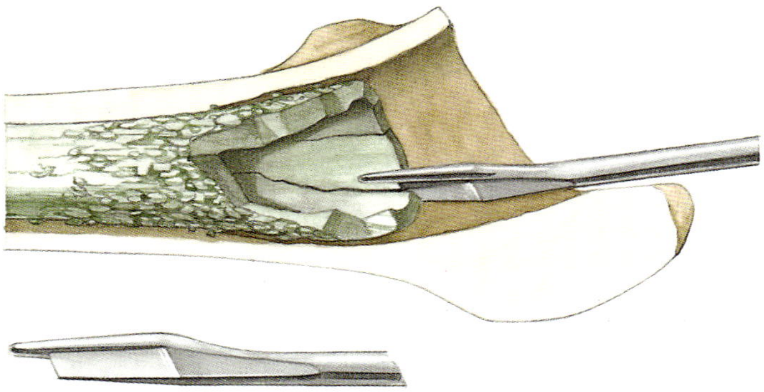

b

Fig. 4.**47a** and **b** After the stem has been removed, the cement mantle remaining in the cancellous bone is split radially with cement chisels with straight, symmetrically honed blades.
a Full-metal Lambotte osteotome.
b Lug chisel. The lug prevents the chisel from deviating from the femoral canal into the bone.

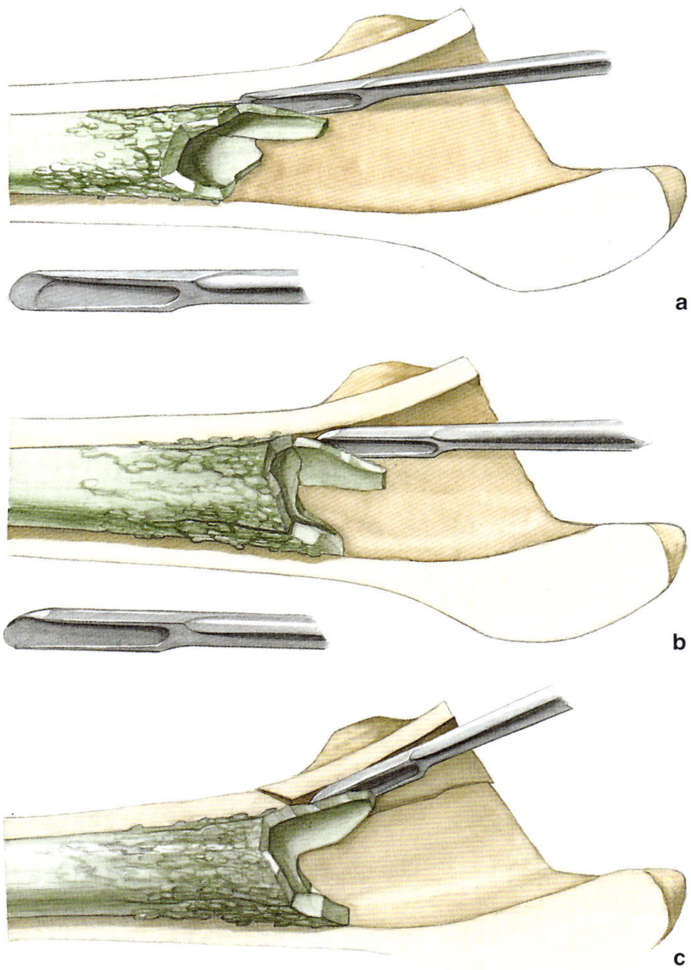

Fig. 4.**48a–c** Breaking off cement flakes with gouges.
a Gouges sharpened on the inside penetrate well between the bone and cement, but provide poor leverage and can easily penetrate the bone.
b Gouges sharpened on the outside do not penetrate well, but provide better leverage and do not endanger the bone.
c Cortical fracture resulting from the attempt to break flakes of cement off by tilting the gouge outwards.

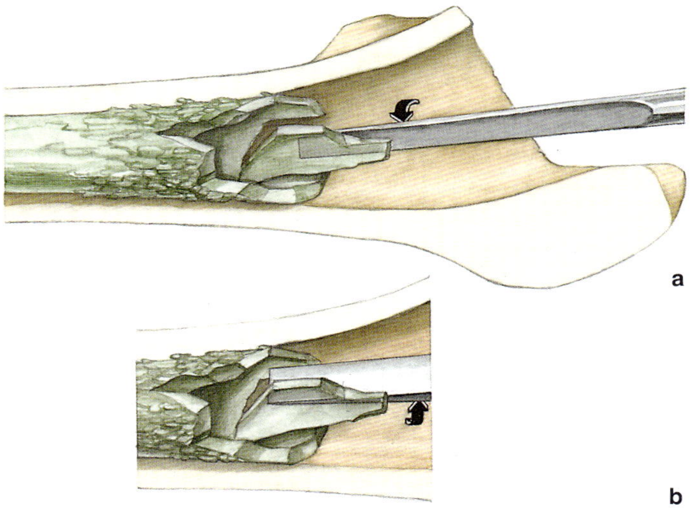

Fig. 4.**49a** and **b** A narrow osteotome with a straight, symmetrically sharpened blade is driven into the interface and rotated around its longitudinal axis.
a Using bone as fulcrum.
b Using cement as fulcrum.

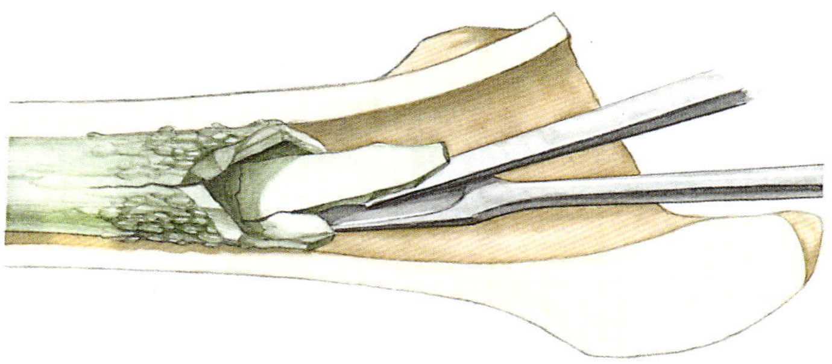

Fig. 4.**50** Distributing the load with two instruments. The outer gouge protects the bone, the inner one breaks off the cement.

If the bone in that region cannot be subjected to any stress at all, then the surgeon should try hammering transversely against the shaft of a gouge inserted between the cement and the bone. This method is very effective in the proximal femoral canal, but is less effective in removing cement further distally because the resulting ratio of work arm to power arm is less favorable (Fig. 4.**51**).

Often, a chisel will glance off a thin sliver of cement that adheres to the wall of the femoral canal. The surgeon can toy to break off the tip of the sliver by impacting a gouge (sharpened on the inside with an angled distal shaft) along the bone–cement interface immediately proximal to the sliver (Fig. 4.**52 a**) or through the cement distal to the sliver (Fig. 4.**52 b**). The surgeon has to be careful, because this can easily produce a perforation in a weakened femur. Breaking off the sliver forms a ledge that a gouge can engage. Slivers that stubbornly adhere to the wall of the femoral canal can be broken off by drilling a hole through the cortex and driving a narrow impactor through the hole (Fig. 4.**52 c**).

Longer gouges with shafts with a proximal offset are useful for removing cement from the distal portion of the femoral canal. They provide a better view of the distal femoral canal because the surgeon's hand and the instrument's grip are not in the surgeon's line of sight. Using a head lamp is recommended (Fig. 4.**53**).

Where extreme femoral anteversion or the medial greater trochanter impairs the surgeon's view into the femoral canal, a distal window is opened over the affected region. Gouges with a shaft having a distal offset are useful here (Fig. 4.**54**).

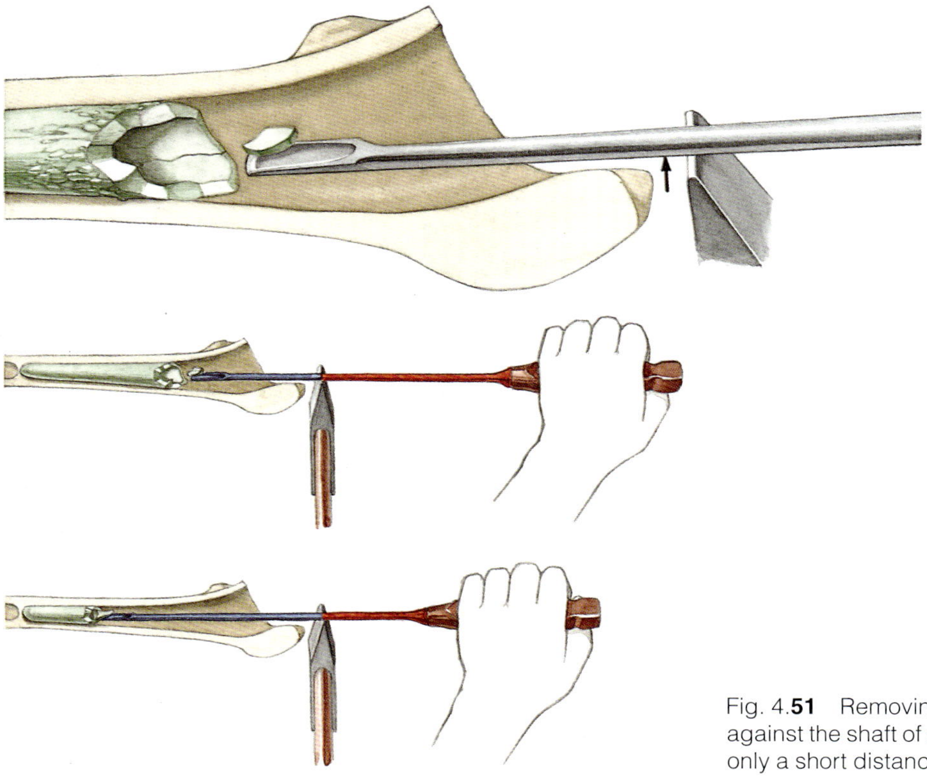

Fig. 4.**51** Removing a flake of cement by hammering transversely against the shaft of a gouge. This method is effective when there is only a short distance between the blade and the hammer.

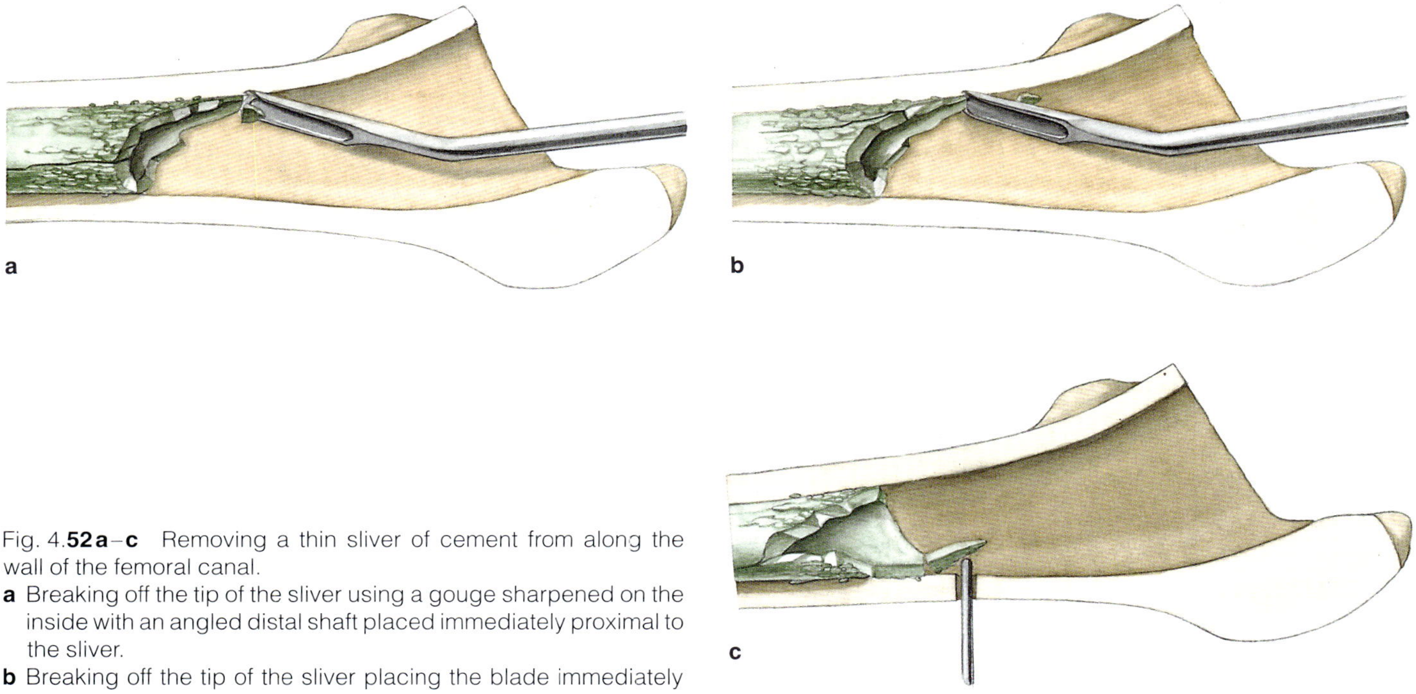

Fig. 4.**52a–c** Removing a thin sliver of cement from along the wall of the femoral canal.

a Breaking off the tip of the sliver using a gouge sharpened on the inside with an angled distal shaft placed immediately proximal to the sliver.

b Breaking off the tip of the sliver placing the blade immediately distal to the sliver.

c Breaking off cement splinters with a narrow impactor through a hole drilled in the cortex.

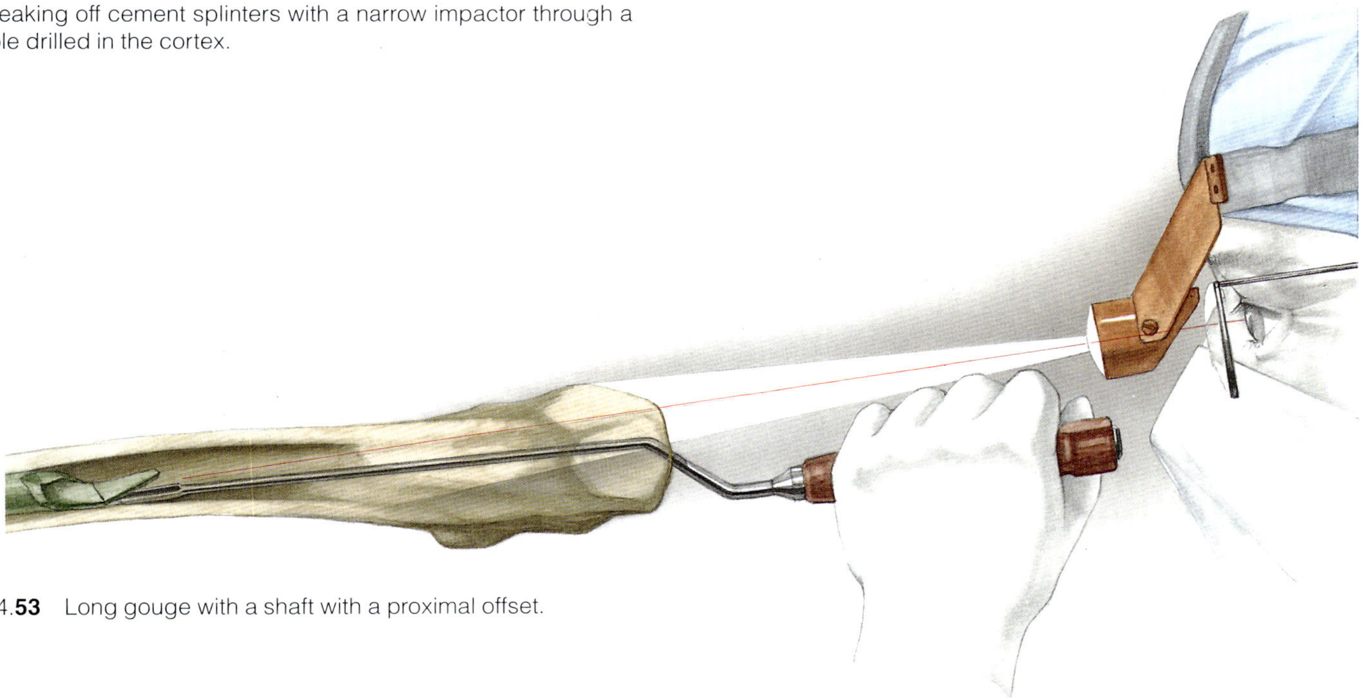

Fig. 4.**53** Long gouge with a shaft with a proximal offset.

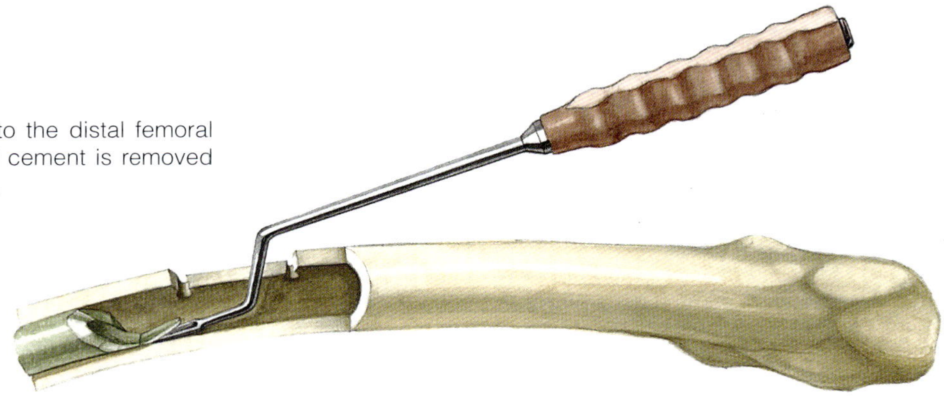

Fig. 4.**54** Where the view from proximal into the distal femoral canal is impaired, a window is opened and cement is removed using a gouge with a shaft with a distal offset.

Removing Cement from the Distal Cortical Bone

Taps of various sizes are the most important instruments to remove cement from the distal cortical bone of the femoral canal. The tap cuts threads in the cement mantle as it is advanced. The surgeon then uses a mallet to extract the instrument, which pulls a segment of the cement mantle with it. Use the largest tap that the cement mantle will accommodate, and break off only short segments; only three or four threads should engage the cement. The surgeon should extract the instrument upon feeling resistance and hearing an audible grinding sound; advancing the tap any further could fracture the cement mantle and the femoral cortex. After a few blows with the mallet, the surgeon advances the tap slightly because the mallet blows can loosen the tap within the cement (Fig. 4.**55a**). If the surgeon uses a smaller tap in order to extract longer segments, it will not engage the cement mantle deeply enough to overcome the friction of the femoral canal and will strip the threads it cuts in the cement (Fig. 4.**55b**). The method becomes risky if the cement mantle is open on one side. The tap then migrates into the softer bone. This generally happens laterally in the far distal femoral canal when the stem was implanted in varus (Fig. 4.**55c**).

When working with the tap, the surgeon checks from the preoperative radiographs in two planes to see whether cement from previous surgery has penetrated into cavities in femoral

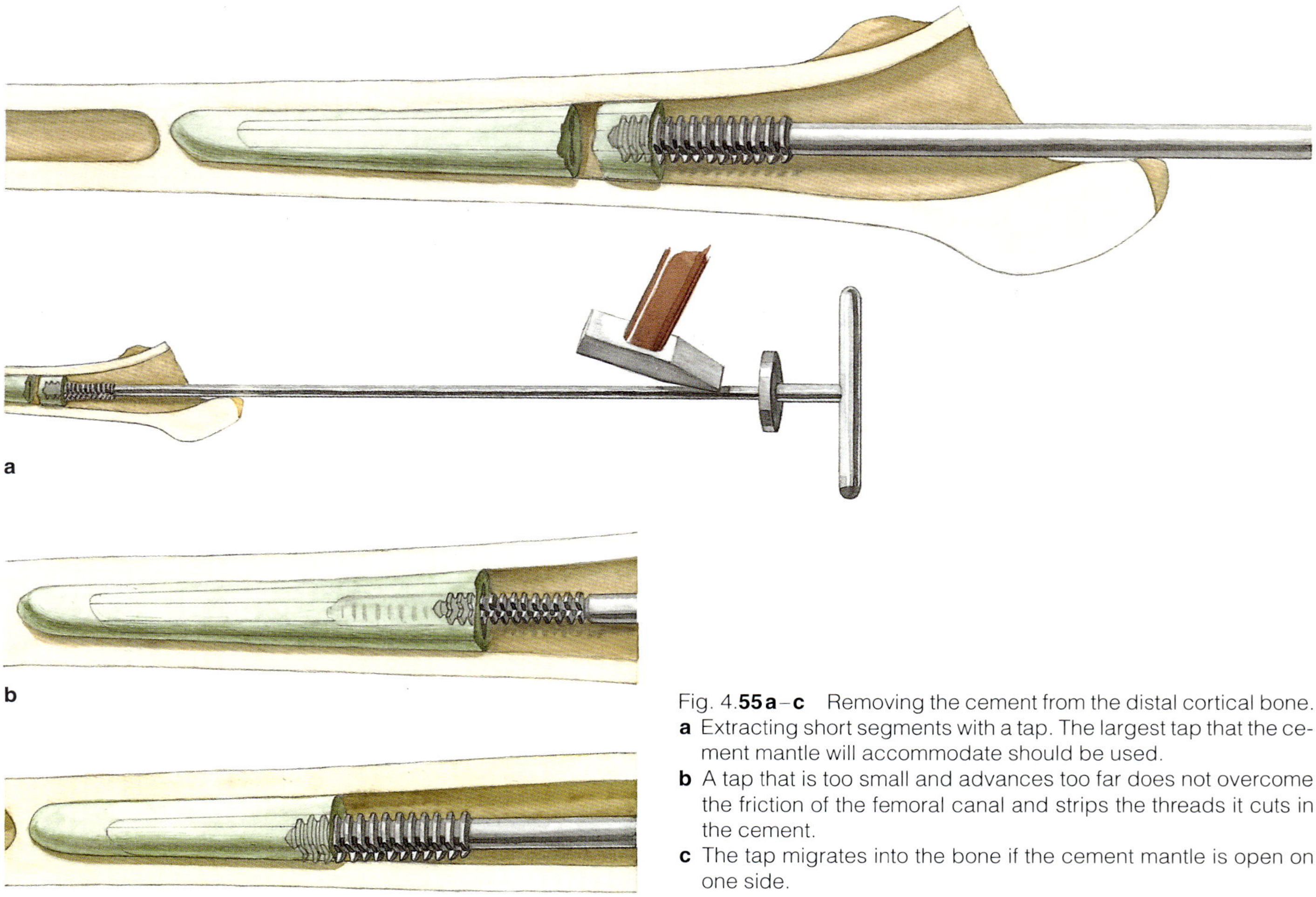

a

b

c

Fig. 4.**55a–c** Removing the cement from the distal cortical bone.
a Extracting short segments with a tap. The largest tap that the cement mantle will accommodate should be used.
b A tap that is too small and advances too far does not overcome the friction of the femoral canal and strips the threads it cuts in the cement.
c The tap migrates into the bone if the cement mantle is open on one side.

cortex or into an old window. If this is the case the tap may not be used. To avoid fracturing the femoral cortex, the surgeon should also verify the absence of any stenosis proximal to the cement segment being removed.

If the femoral cortex is thick enough, a stenosis proximal to the cement segment can be widened with a reamer (Fig. 4.**56a**). The reamer should have a rigid shaft; articulated reamers are difficult to control because they will take the path of least resistance and migrate into the bone. If the cortex is not thick enough to permit reaming the stenosis, then a cortical window is opened at the stenosis or distal to it. The surgeon uses the tap to draw the segments into the window, where they are broken up (Fig. 4.**56b**).

If the tap cannot extract any more segments, a reamer can be used to remove the residual cement. The surgeon starts with a small reamer, widens the hole in the cement with a larger reamer, and then uses a smaller reamer again to deepen the hole. To avoid damaging the femoral cortex, this should only be done when the femoral canal can be directly inspected. The surgeon repeats this procedure until the cement has been removed or the region is no longer visible, checking the reamings frequently. To prevent the reamer from migrating into the softer cortex, the surgeon discontinues this procedure as soon as bone is found in the reamings (Fig. 4.**57**).

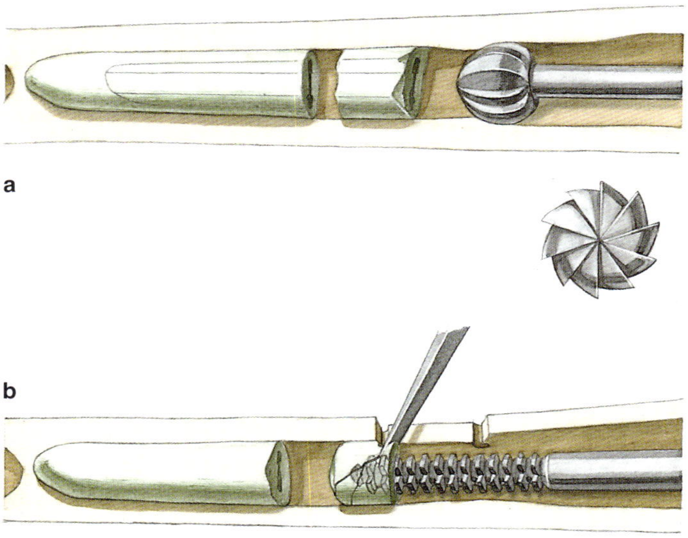

Fig. 4.**56a–c** Removing cement from the distal femoral canal in the presence of a stenosis.
a Eliminating a stenosis proximal to the cement using a reamer with a rigid shaft.
b Pulling a segment from the region distal to a stenosis into a cortical window.

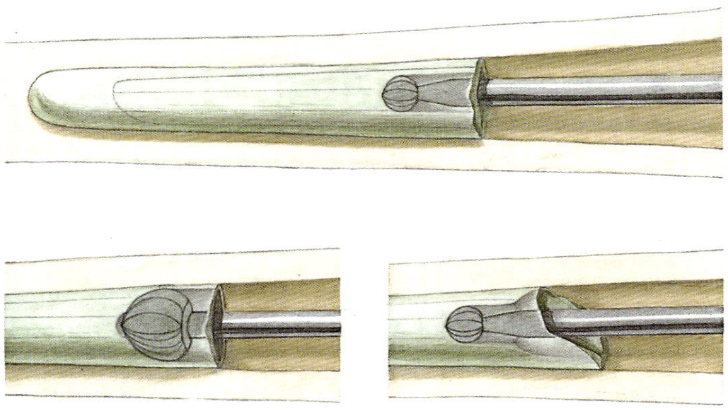

Fig. 4.**57** Reaming out a cement mantle with a reamer (femoral canal must be directly visible).

Removing a Residual Plug of Cement and a Diaphyseal Cortical Bone Bridge

After the cement mantle has been removed, a residual plug of cement will often remain behind in the distal femoral canal. If this plug must be removed to accommodate a longer revision stem, the surgeon can drill through it and, if present, an underlying diaphyseal cortical bone bridge in one step. The plug must be visible with a level face, and there may be no significant femoral anteversion (Fig. 4.**58a**). If the plug contains an impression of the implant tip that lies in the center of the plug, it can be used to guide the drill bit (Fig. 4.**58b**). If the face of the plug is oblique, the drill bit can be deflected and penetrate the cortex. A drill sleeve is recommended in such cases to center the bit (Fig. 4.**58c**). If the surgeon is successful in drilling a hole in the plug, a suitable tap is used to extract it (Fig. 4.**58d**). Blindly relying on a drill sleeve inserted deeply in the femoral canal to center the bit can lead to cortical perforation, especially in the presence of pronounced femoral anteversion (Fig. 4.**58e**) or if the sleeve becomes dislodged in the femoral canal. Where there is a risk of damaging the bone, the surgeon should remove the plug through a cortical window (see Fig. 4.**65b**).

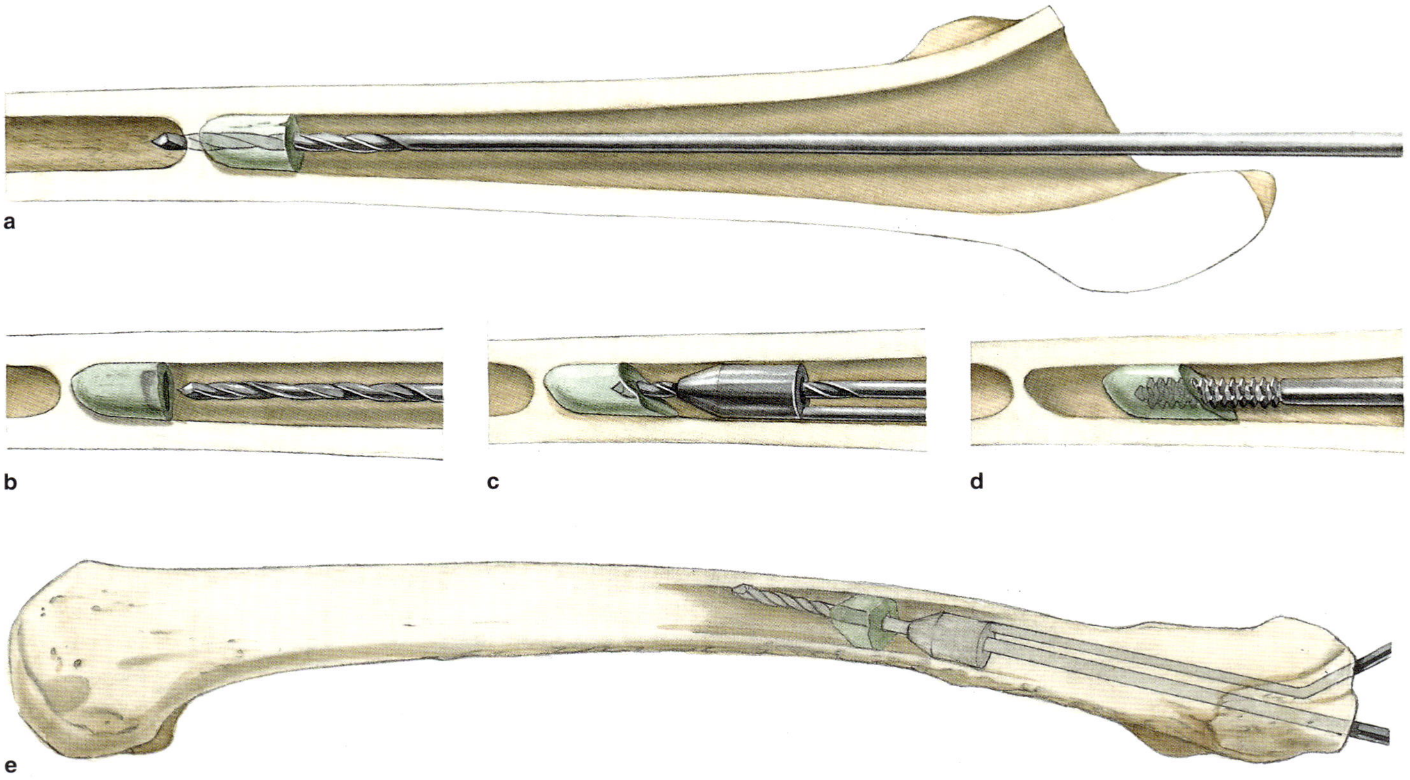

Fig. 4.**58a–e** Removing a residual plug of cement from the femoral diaphysis.
a Drilling through a level-face plug and diaphyseal cortical bone bridge.
b Using the impression left by the implant tip to guide the drill bit.
c Using a drill sleeve to drill through a plug with an oblique face.
d Extracting the drilled plug with a tap.
e Using a drill sleeve fails to prevent cortical penetration in the presence of pronounced femoral anteversion.

A hook-shaped chisel (with the blade sharpened on the inside) can be used to remove a fragment of a residual cement plug that cannot be drilled. This method can also be used to remove remaining slivers of cement that adhere to the wall of the femoral canal. The surgeon should exercise care to prevent damaging the cortex with the blade (Fig. 4.**59**).

In the absence of infection, a plug can also be left in place if a long-stem revision implant is not indicated. It will act as a cement restrictor for the new cement. In aseptic cases where a long-stem revision implant is required (to bridge a defect, or due to deficient proximal bone stock), a plug that cannot be removed can be impacted distally unless a diaphyseal cortical bone bridge prevents this (Fig. 4.**60**).

A diaphyseal cortical bone bridge must be removed when a long-stem implant is indicated. If one is not indicated, the bridge is left in place as a cement restrictor. If the most distal point of a bridge requiring removal lies in the center of the femoral canal, then the bridge may easily be perforated with a drill and removed with a reamer. If the previous stem migrated laterally or was implanted in varus, the most distal point may be eccentric and the drill or reamer could penetrate the cortex. Such bridges are removed with a gouge that is sharpened on the inside (Fig. 4.**61**). This should only be done when the femoral canal can be directly inspected; if the distal femoral canal is not visible from proximal, the surgeon must open a small distal window immediately proximal to the bridge.

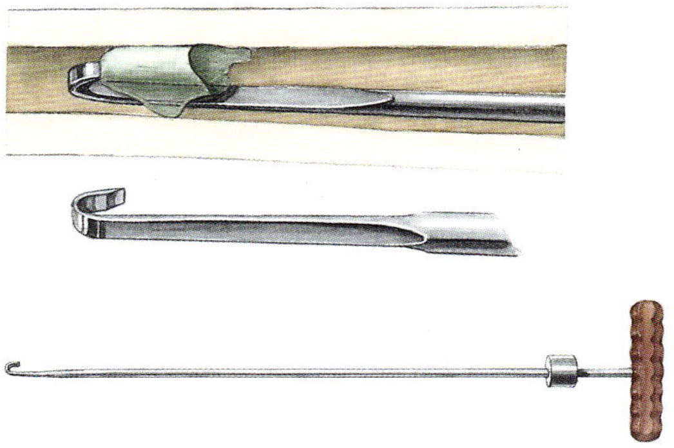

Fig. 4.**59** Using a hook-shaped chisel to remove a fragment of a residual cement plug or sliver of cement adhering to the wall of the femoral canal.

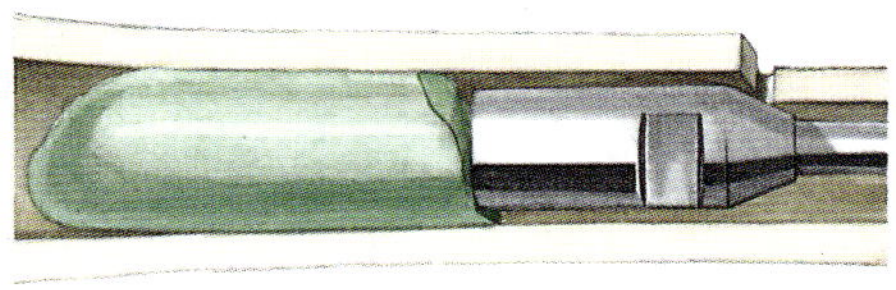

Fig. 4.**60** Impacting a residual plug distally in aseptic cases.

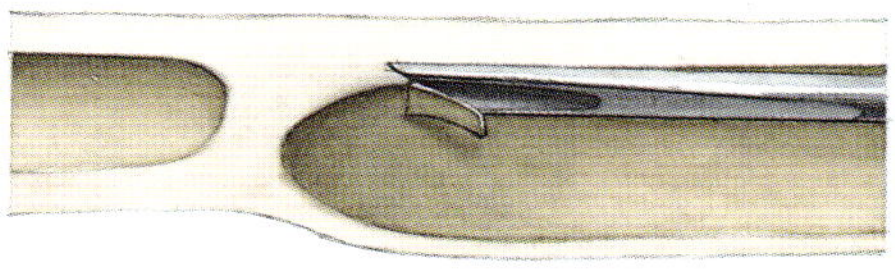

Fig. 4.**61** Removing an asymmetrical diaphyseal cortical bone bridge by chiseling. Drilling and reaming can easily penetrate the femoral cortex.

Checking for Perforations

If there is the slightest suspicion that the femoral cortex has been penetrated, the femoral canal should be inspected with a flexible sound, the distal end of which is slightly curved. If the sound passes through a perforation into the surrounding soft tissue, this will be palpable through the grip; in slender patients it will be palpable through the skin as well. The sound of the instrument scraping on bone will also stop. Most perforations are anterior, lateral, or anterolateral, depending on the direction of anteversion or the position of a migrated stem tip. The distance between the perforation and the plane of osteotomy is measured on the scale on the sound (Fig. 4.**62**), and the femur is exposed at that site.

A direct approach through the quadriceps is sufficient to inspect small perforations and where there is little musculature. A lateral approach to the femur should be used for larger lesions or perforations that lie further medial.

Exposing an intraoperative penetration is imperative for several reasons. The extent of the defect must be assessed. When implanting the revision stem, the surgeon must ensure that the stem passes and bridges the defect instead of migrating through it. Excess cement must be removed when the stem is cemented, and cancellous graft should be inserted before closure. Sometimes the perforation can be used as a window through which the problem can be eliminated.

Finally, the femoral canal is cleaned. Patches of cement adhering to the walls are removed with a reamer with a rigid shaft, and the connective tissue in the region of bone resorption is removed with a curette (Fig. 4.**63**).

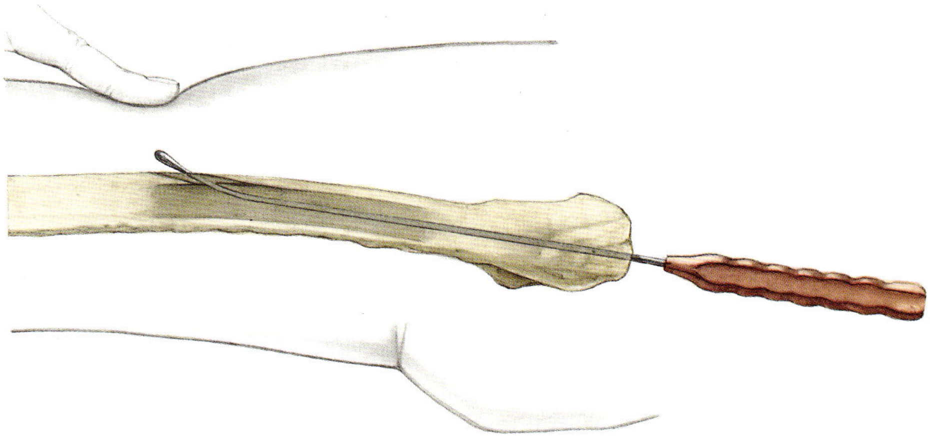

Fig. 4.**62** Checking for perforations on the femoral cortex. Localizing the perforation using the scale on the sound.

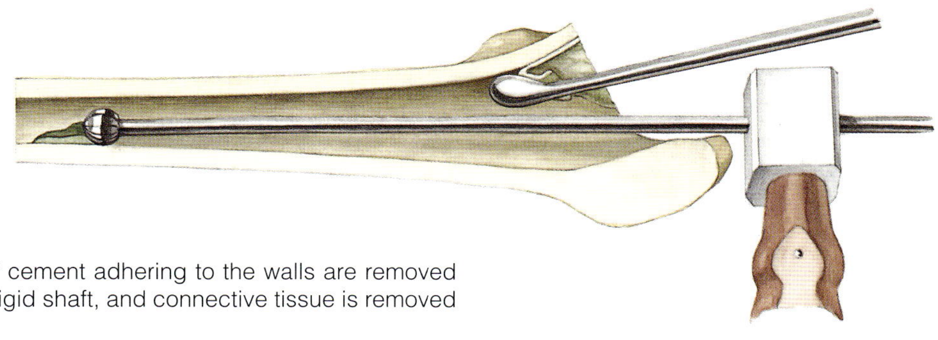

Fig. 4.**63** Patches of cement adhering to the walls are removed with a reamer with a rigid shaft, and connective tissue is removed with a curette.

Cortical Windows for Removing Cemented Stems

Except for transfemoral implant removal, cutting a cortical window is the most invasive procedure used in removing cemented stems and cement. A window can be opened as required in any phase of implant extraction.

Anterior windows weaken the femur least because the fibers they interrupt do not belong to major load-bearing structures. The anterior femur is easily accessible through a small incision in the quadriceps, or through a lateral approach to the femur. A posterior window (an option in a posterior approach with the hip in internal rotation) weakens the linea aspera, a major load-bearing structure, and also requires dissecting important muscle insertions in an area with good vascular supply. Both are disadvantages. Lateral windows should be avoided because they interrupt tensile fibers that protect against fracture. The exception is when a lateral perforation is extended to form a window. Medial windows are unsuitable because the region is difficult to gain access to, and the compressive fibers should not be interrupted.

The anterior femur is the optimum location for a window (Fig. 4.**64a**). It should only be as large as necessary. The recommended shape is a trapezoid; this ensures a gradual transition in rigidity from the bone weakened by the window to the intact femur. First the four corners of the window are marked with a drill. This prevents the bone from splitting past the intended window when the osteotomy is performed. Next, the surgeon saws the long side, irrigating to prevent thermal necrosis, and then uses an osteotome to cut the short sides (Fig. 4.**64b**). The osteotomized surfaces are beveled outward (if the cortex is thick enough) to provide a sufficient area of contact between the window and the femur so that the window nests in the opening when it is replaced. The "lid" will sink into the bone somewhat, since the osteotomy creates a slight gap (Fig. 4.**64c**). The gap is smallest when an extremely fine flexible osteotome is used instead of a saw or a standard osteotome. A blade guide placed on the bone prevents the chisel blade bending when the cut is made (Fig. 4.**64d**).

A window should always lie as far proximal as possible, either at or immediately proximal to the site of the problem, never distal to it if possible (Fig. 4.**65**). Every window must be bridged by a longer revision stem extending a few centimeters distal to it. If the tip of the revision stem lies level with a window, subsequent femoral fracture might result, especially if the window lies laterally.

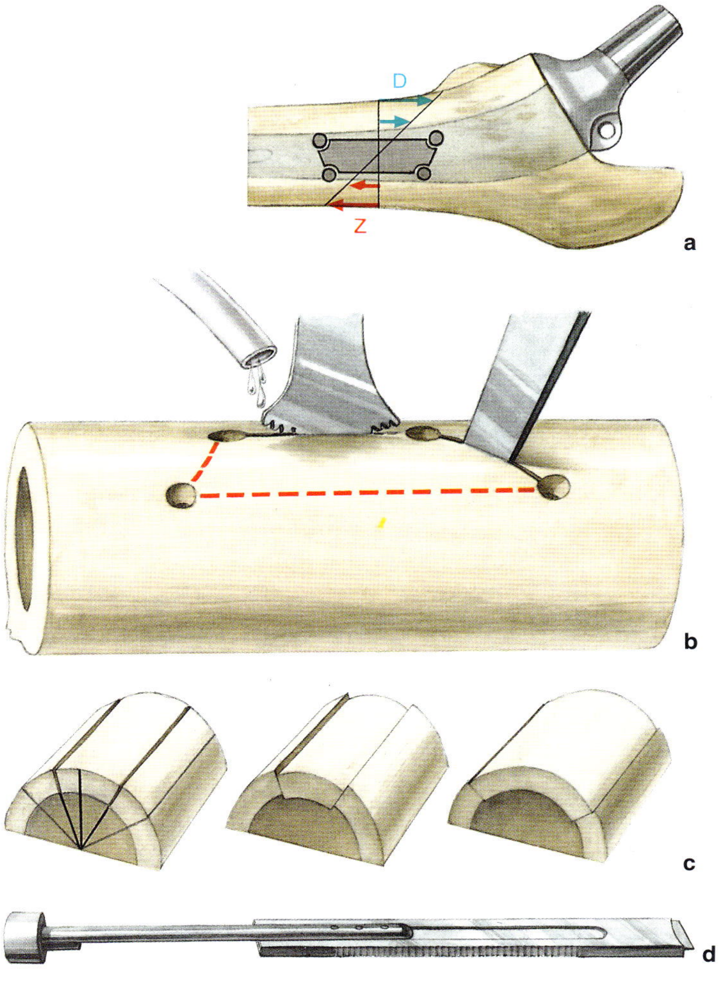

Fig. 4.**64a–d** Windowing technique for cemented stems.

a Anterior windows interrupt fibers that do not belong to major load-bearing structures. Trapezoidal shape.
b The corners of the window are marked with a drill. The long sides are cut with a saw while the site is irrigated; the shorter sides are cut with an osteotome.
c The "lid" sinks into the window when it is replaced. The osteotomy surfaces are beveled outward.
d Flexible osteotome with blade guide leaves a narrow osteotomy gap.

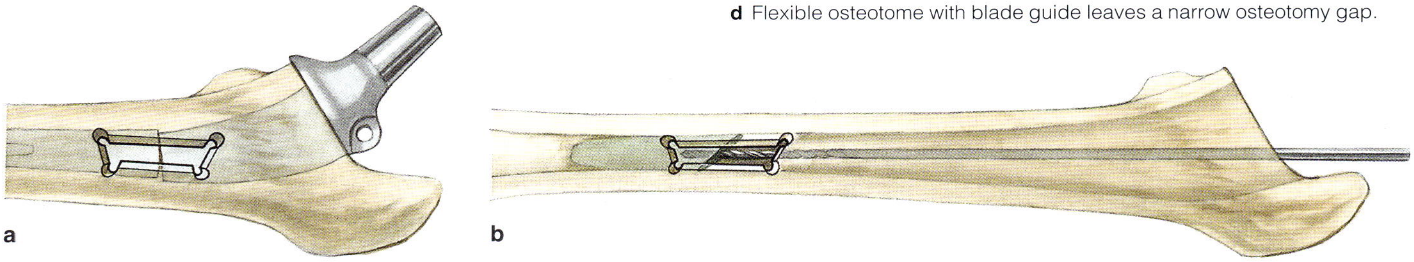

Fig. 4.**65a** and **b** Examples of windows.
a Window over the shaft fracture, not distal to the distal fragment (see also Fig. 4.**68** and 4.**69**).
b Window over a residual cement plug with an oblique face.

Transfemoral Removal of Cemented Stems

Transfemoral removal of the stem and cement (Wagner's method) is indicated where advanced bone resorption, fractures, or other defects have weakened the proximal femur so that a fracture is expected during the approach, implant removal, or a later phase of the procedure. The surgeon dissects the vastus lateralis off the femur near the linea aspera in a strip 1 cm wide and ligates the transected blood vessels. Half of the circumference of the femur is exposed over the distal end of the stem, and two holes are drilled, which are then connected with a transverse osteotomy. One hole is drilled near the linea aspera and the other anterior or anterolateral. A longitudinal osteotomy is performed from the hole near the linea aspera to the apex of the greater trochanter. This is best done with a flexible osteotome. Beginning at the anterior or anterolateral hole, the surgeon then osteotomizes the femur longitudinally in short intervals using a Lambotte osteotome to create a cortical window. This is done through the muscle without dissecting the vastus lateralis off the femur (Fig. 4.**66**).

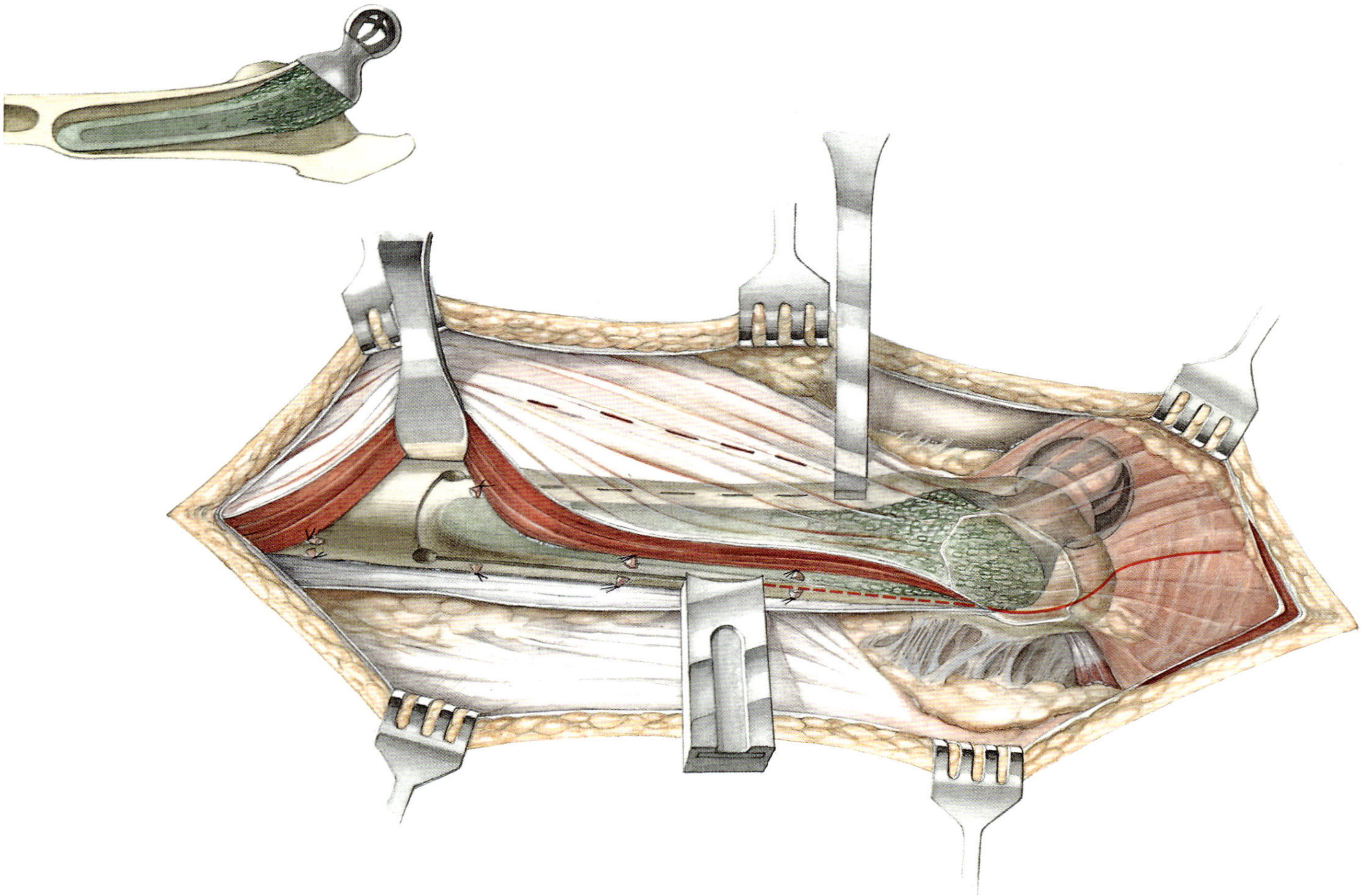

Fig. 4.**66** Transfemoral removal of a cemented stem (Wagner's method). A semicircular transverse osteotomy is performed between holes drilled over the distal tip of the implant. A longitudinal osteotomy is performed along the linea aspera through the middle of the greater trochanter. The gluteus medius and gluteus minimus are split parallel to their fibers. A series of partial longitudinal osteotomies performed through the muscle with a Lambotte osteotome provide a "hinge" for the femoral window. The vastus lateralis is only dissected off the femur next to the linea aspera and at the site of the distal semicircular transverse osteotomy.

The gluteus medius and gluteus minimus are split parallel to their fibers from the apex of the greater trochanter proximally as in a transgluteal approach. Then the surgeon opens the anterolateral window with wide osteotomes. This permits transfemoral and transgluteal removal of the implant and cement (Fig. 4.**67**). The revision implant must be significantly longer than the implant removed because the osteotomized proximal femur can no longer provide sufficient support for fixation (see Fig. 4.**148**).

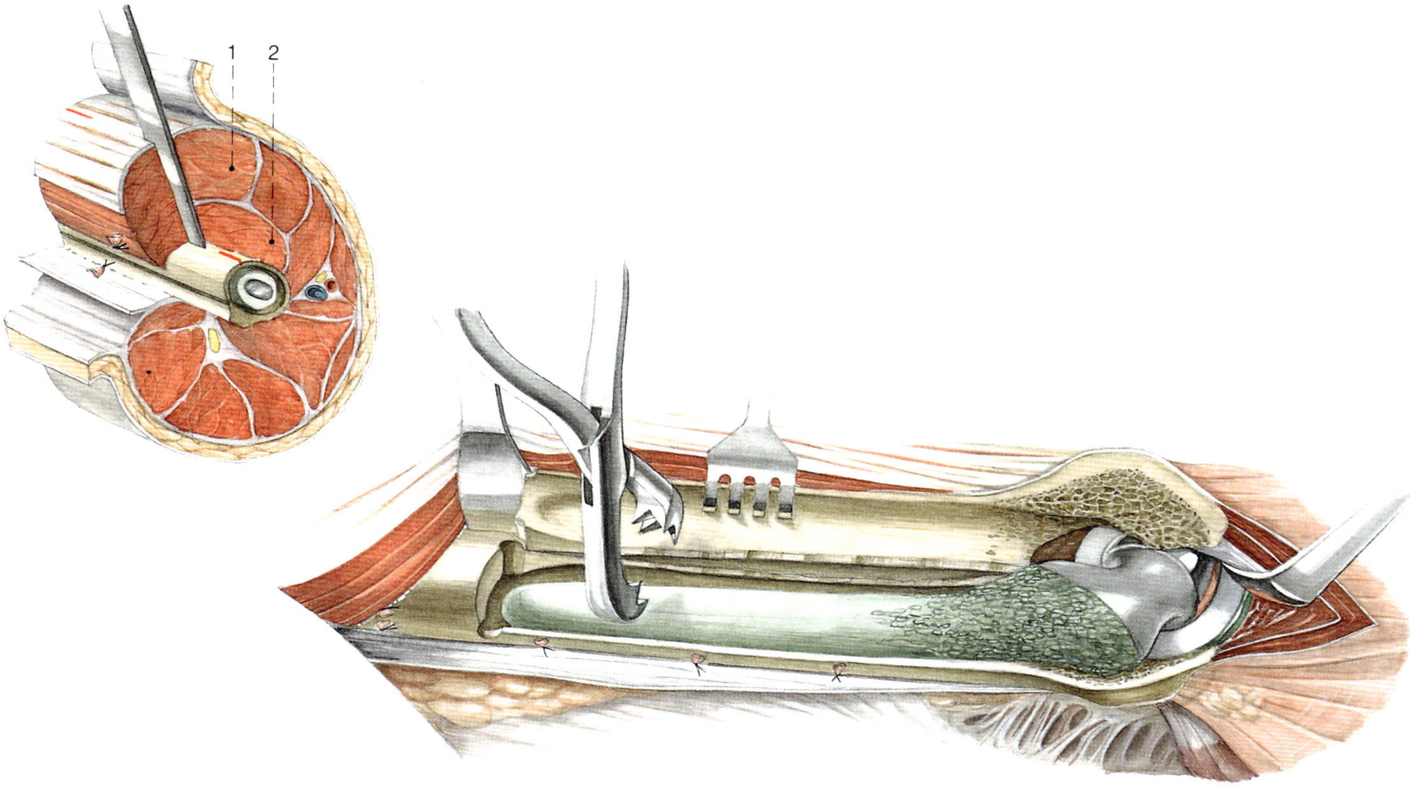

Fig. 4.**67** Opening the anterolateral window. The "lid" retains its soft-tissue attachments with the vastus lateralis. A transgluteal approach is made to the hip, permitting transfemoral and transgluteal removal of the implant and cement.

1 Vastus lateralis
2 Vastus intermedius

Removing Fractured Cemented Stems

Stems can fracture due to material quality, stem geometry, surface quality, or excessive load cycles, if the proximal stem has loosened while the distal stem is still rigidly fixed in sturdy bone. Fatigue fractures generally occur between the proximal and middle thirds of the implant. The proximal fragment can almost always be easily removed (Fig. 4.**68a**). The distal fragment poses the most problems because it is generally rigidly fixed. While fractured cementless stems with fixed distal fragments almost always require a window extending the length of the distal fragment (see Fig. 4.**98**), cemented distal fragments can generally be removed with less invasive procedures.

Drilling a Hole in the Implant through a Proximal Window and Extracting it with a Center Punch

A universal method, which is nearly always successful and requires no special instruments, involves cutting a small window over the fracture site after the proximal fragment has been removed. The cement is cleaned off the part of the distal fragment visible in the window. A hole is then drilled into the implant with a carbide-tipped bit (Fig. 4.**68b**), and the surgeon pushes the fragment out using a center punch that engages the hole. The technique of opening a distal window to push the fragment out proximally with an offset impactor (Fig. 4.**68c**) is not recommended because a longer revision stem must be implanted to bridge the defect.

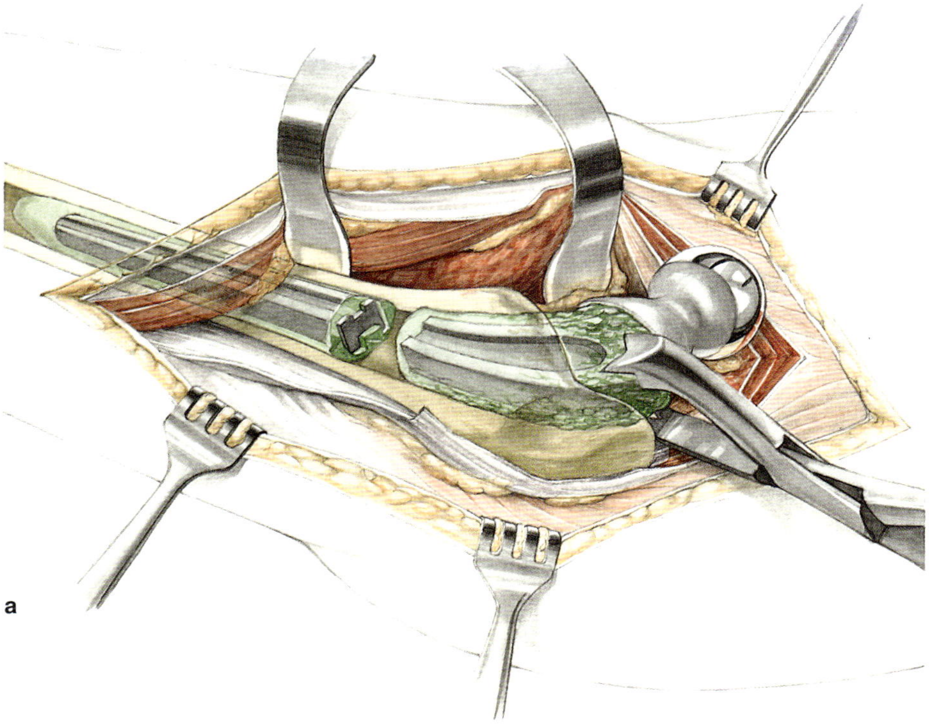
a

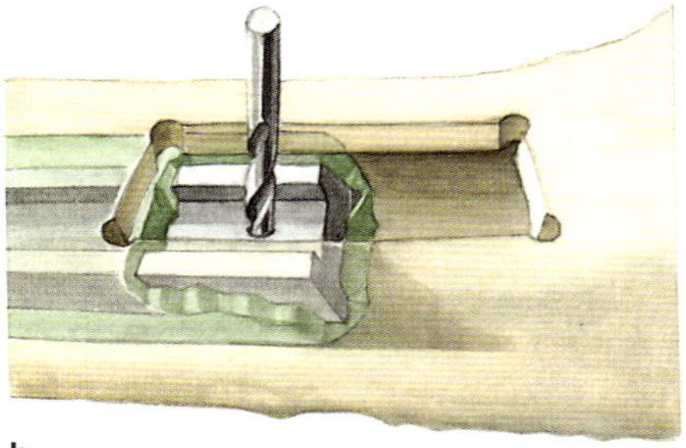
b

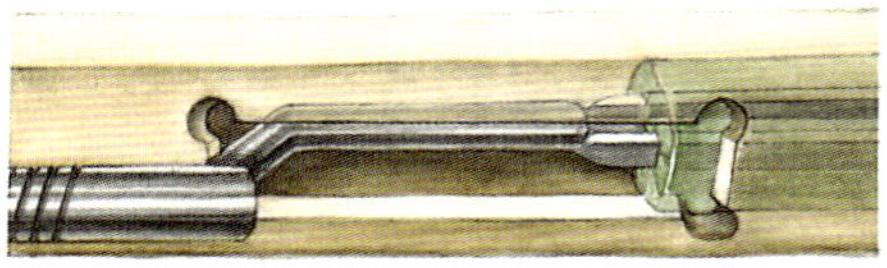
c

Fig. 4.**68a–c** Removing fractured stems through a femoral window.
a Stem fracture between the proximal and middle thirds of the implant. Removing the proximal fragment.
b Small window over the fracture. Cement in the window is removed, and a hole is drilled in the distal fragment with a carbide-tipped bit.
c If a distal window is cut over the distal tip of the stem, a longer revision stem must be implanted to bridge the defect.

After drilling the hole in the stem, the surgeon drives the distal fragment proximally by impacting a center punch until the hole disappears beneath the bone. The transverse force must be compensated for by hand or with a bone hook. If necessary, the surgeon drills a second hole and continues to drive the implant out with the center punch (Fig. 4.**69a**) until it can be removed (Fig. 4.**69b**). The revision implant usually does not have to be longer than the original implant, because except for the proximal window, the femur is generally stable.

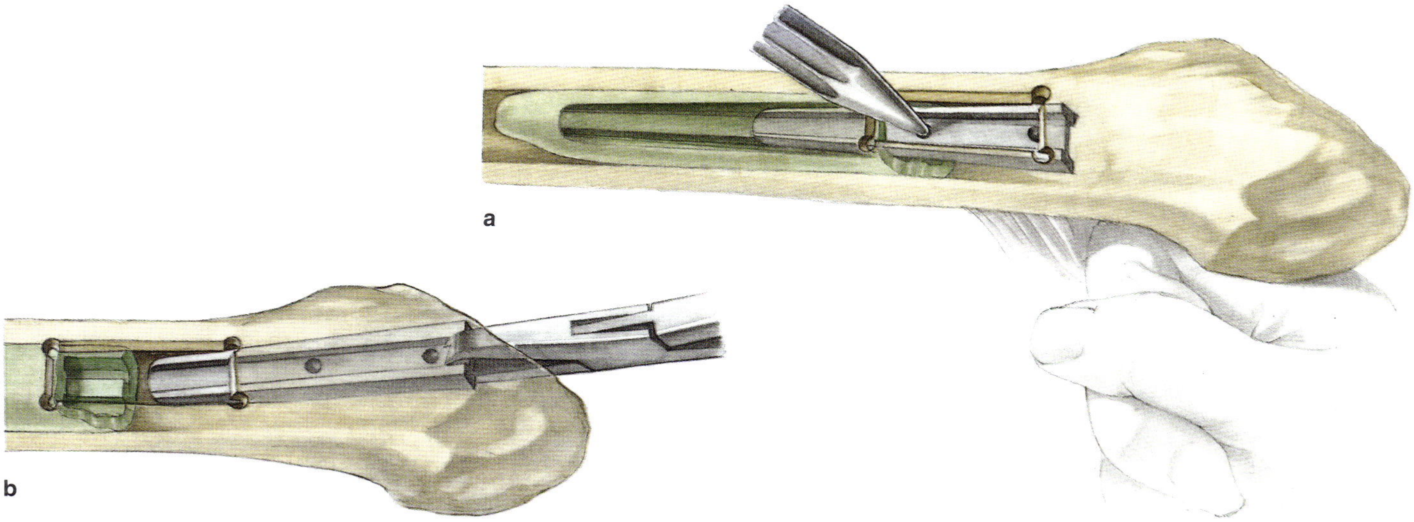

Fig. 4.**69a** and **b** Extracting the distal fragment.

a The distal fragment is driven proximally with a center punch. If necessary, additional holes are drilled. The transverse force must be compensated for by hand or with a bone hook.
b Removing the distal fragment.

Drilling a Hole through the Implant and Attaching a Bifurcate Extractor

A less invasive procedure is to drill through the proximal end of the distal fragment through a hole drilled in the femur, attach a bifurcate extractor to the fragment, and extract the fragment by applying extraction force axially (Zabel's method). This method is feasible only if there is sufficient space anteriorly and posteriorly to the fragment to insert the forks of the extractor.

First the surgeon removes the cement anteriorly and posteriorly to the fragment and inserts the forks above and below the stem. A jig mounted on the shaft of the extractor guides the bit as the surgeon drills a hole through the femoral cortex (Fig. 4.**70**).

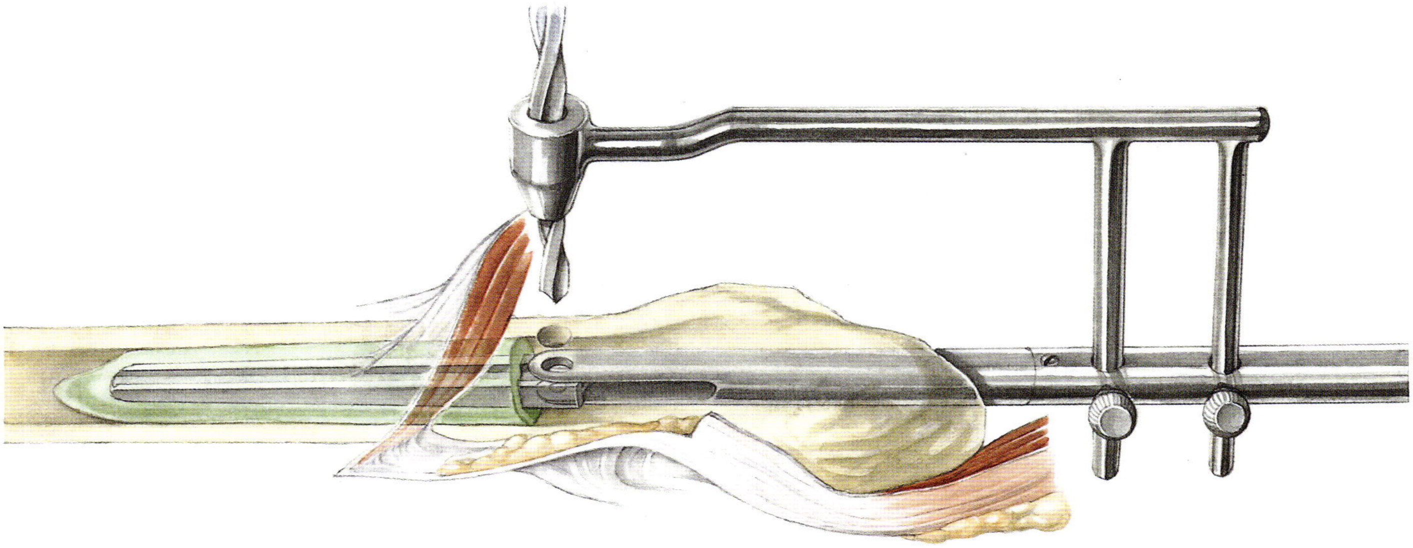

Fig. 4.**70** Removing a distal fragment by attaching a bifurcate extractor to the fragment (Zabel's method). A hole is drilled in the proximal femur over the proximal end of the distal fragment using a jig mounted on the shaft of the extractor.

Then a drill sleeve is inserted into the jig and the hole in the bone, and the surgeon drills into the implant through the hole in the anterior fork (Fig. 4.**71 a**). Then the extractor is withdrawn to avoid damaging the threading on its posterior fork, and the surgeon drills all the way through the implant (Fig. 4.**71 b**). A narrow Lambotte osteotome can be inserted under the proximal fragment to protect the posterior cortex. The cutting edge of the bit has been known to separate shortly before the implant is completely penetrated. If the separated edge cannot be removed through the hole in the bone and the implant or pushed through it posteriorly, then the procedure has failed. Once the hole has been drilled all the way through the stem, the forks of the extractor are reinserted. The surgeon securely attaches the extractor to the stem with a metal screw. The metal screw has a tapered point; it can thus better engage the threads in the posterior fork (Fig. 4.**71 c**). Once the extractor is attached, the fragment is easily removed (Fig. 4.**72**). If a posterior approach is used, the drilling can be done from posterior, since a hole in the linea aspera does not weaken the bone nearly as much as a posterior window.

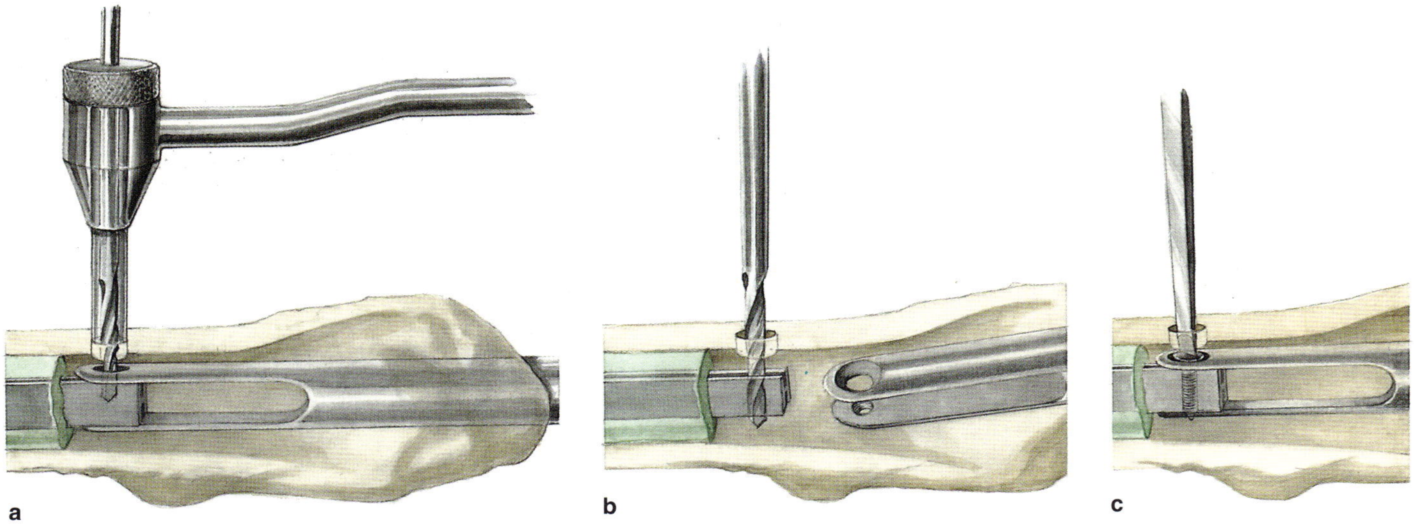

Fig. 4.**71 a**–**c** Drilling through the stem and attaching the extractor.

a A hole is drilled into the implant through a drill sleeve inserted into the jig and the hole in the bone and through the hole in the anterior fork.

b Drilling through the stem after removing the extractor.

c Attaching the distal fragment to the extractor.

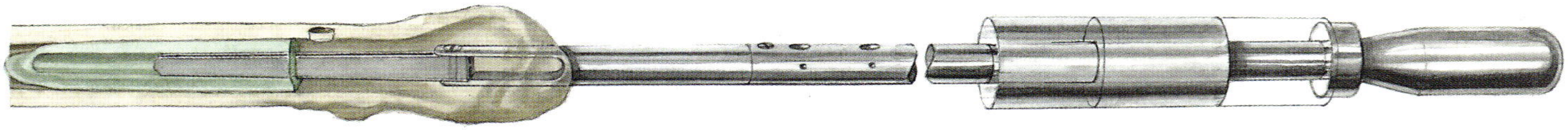

Fig. 4.**72** Extracting the distal fragment. Force is applied axially.

Drilling an Axial Hole with an Undercut and Attaching an Extractor with a Distal Toe

First the surgeon removes the cement around the implant proximally. A high-speed end-cutting tool is used to drill an axial hole in the fractured face of the fragment. The tool is centered with a drill guide. The drill guide's distal, tapered recess fits over the proximal end of the distal fragment (Fig. 4.**73**). Then a side-cutting tool is used to ream an undercut at the bottom of the hole (Fig. 4.**74**).

This undercut engages the toe of an extractor. The toe is fixed in the undercut by pushing a lateral blade opposite the toe distally through a longitudinal groove. Because the groove is shallower distally than proximally, it forces the blade out of the extractor laterally, pressing the toe into the undercut (Fig. 4.**75a**). The blade is advanced distally by threading a cannulated T-handle onto the extractor. The extractor is prevented from rotating while the cannulated T-handle is twisted because a long hex wrench passes through the cannulated T-handle into the butt end of the extractor (Fig. 4.**75b**).

When the foot of the extractor has been fixed in the undercut, a slap hammer is attached to the proximal end of the cannulated T-handle and the stem fragment is extracted (Fig. 4.**76**).

This procedure (Harris' method) is not invasive, but requires a sufficiently large fracture face and specialized instrumentation.

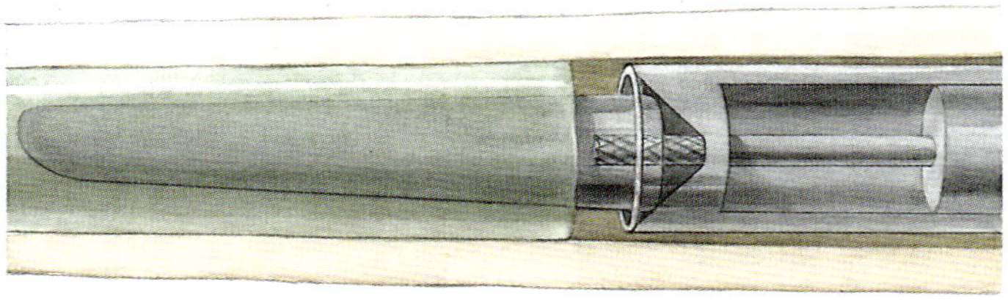

Fig. 4.**73** Drilling an axial hole with an undercut for attaching an extractor with a toe (Harris' method). Drilling the axial hole. An end-cutting tool is centered with a drill guide with a distal tapered recess.

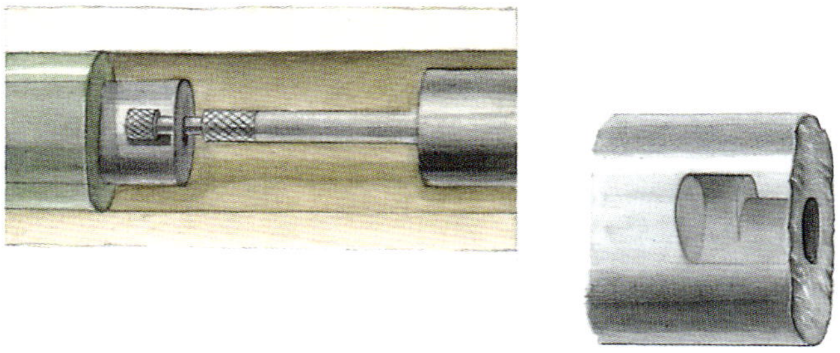

Fig. 4.**74** A side-cutting tool is used to ream an undercut at the bottom of the hole.

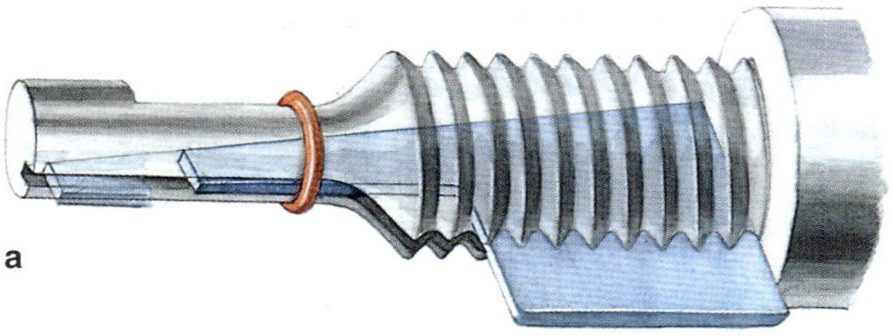

a

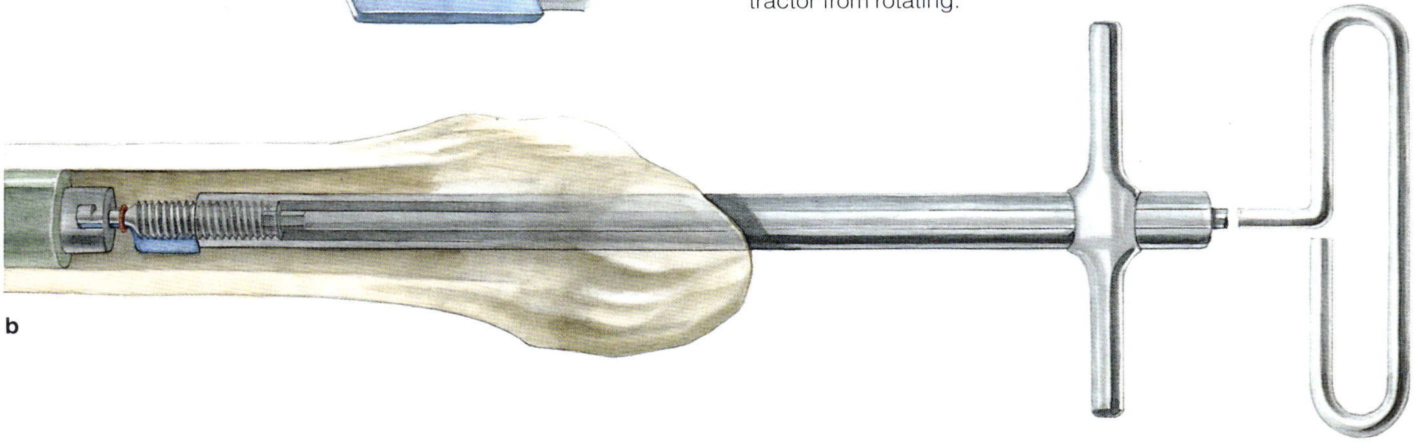

b

Fig. 4.**75a** and **b** Attaching the extractor.

a The extractor has a distal toe. A lateral blade (blue) is forced out of the extractor laterally as it is advanced distally through a longitudinal groove. This presses the foot into the undercut. A rubber ring holds the blade in the groove.

b The blade is advanced distally by threading a cannulated T-handle onto the extractor. A long hex wrench prevents the extractor from rotating.

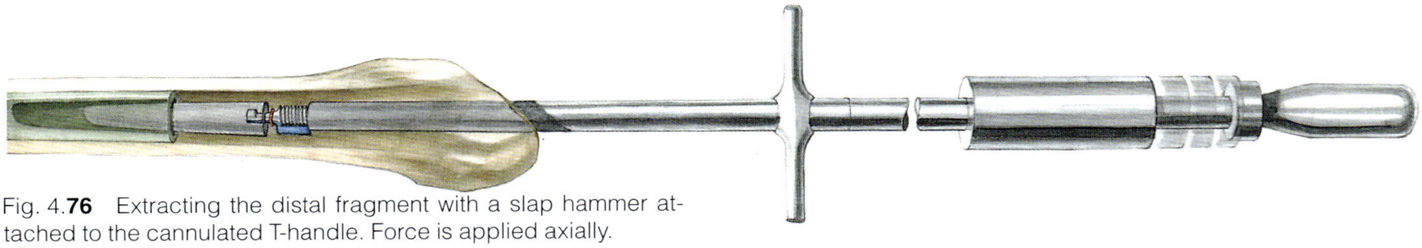

Fig. 4.**76** Extracting the distal fragment with a slap hammer attached to the cannulated T-handle. Force is applied axially.

Using a Hollow Reamer to Soften the Cement

Another procedure that is not invasive, but is not without risk to the femur, is advancing a hollow reamer around the distal fragment until the reamer jams in the cement remains between it and the fragment. The reamer and fragment together are then extracted using a slap hammer (Collins' method). This requires sufficient space between implant and bone and a femur strong enough to withstand the torque that occurs when the reamer jams.

First enough cement is removed around the stem to permit inserting a suitable hollow reamer over the fragment. Then the surgeon reams until the cement, softened by the heat of friction that collects within the reamer, rehardens. This slows and finally jams the reamer. The inner surface of the hollow reamer is designed to improve cement adhesion (Fig. 4.**77**). The fragment is then extracted using a slap hammer attached to the hollow reamer (Fig. 4.**78**).

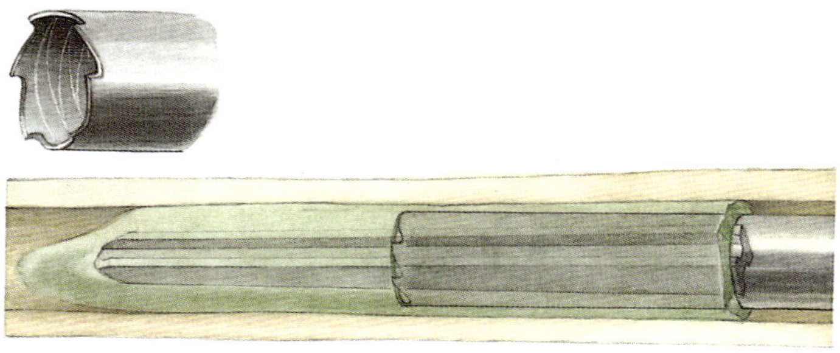

Fig. 4.**77** Using a hollow reamer to extract a distal fragment (Collis' method). Friction warms and softens the cement within the hollow reamer.

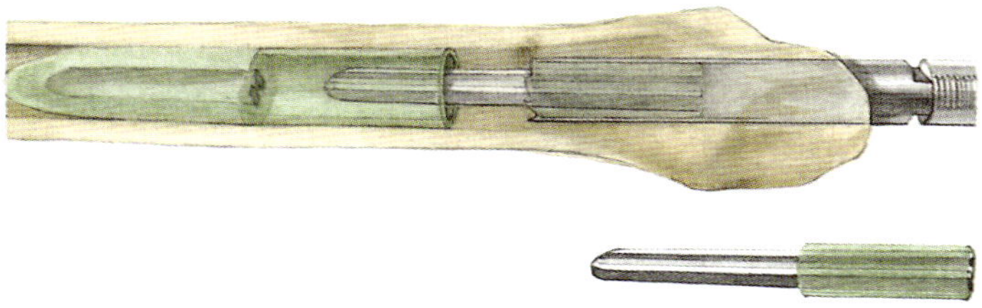

Fig. 4.**78** A slap hammer is attached after the rehardened cement jams the hollow reamer, and then the fragment is extracted.

Removing Cemented Acetabular Cups

After exposing the acetabulum (Fig. 4.**79**), the surgeon uses a spoon-shaped gouge with a curved shaft to disrupt the interface between the polyethylene and the cement at several sites as far as the surrounding bone permits. This should be done with caution, especially near the roof of the acetabulum because this area is often weakened and the remaining bone here is important to stability. If the blade is inserted precisely at the polyethylene–cement interface, it and the curved shaft will follow the interface without migrating into the polyethylene or the cement. The surgeon continues to cut until the polyethylene cup has been detached (Fig. 4.**80**).

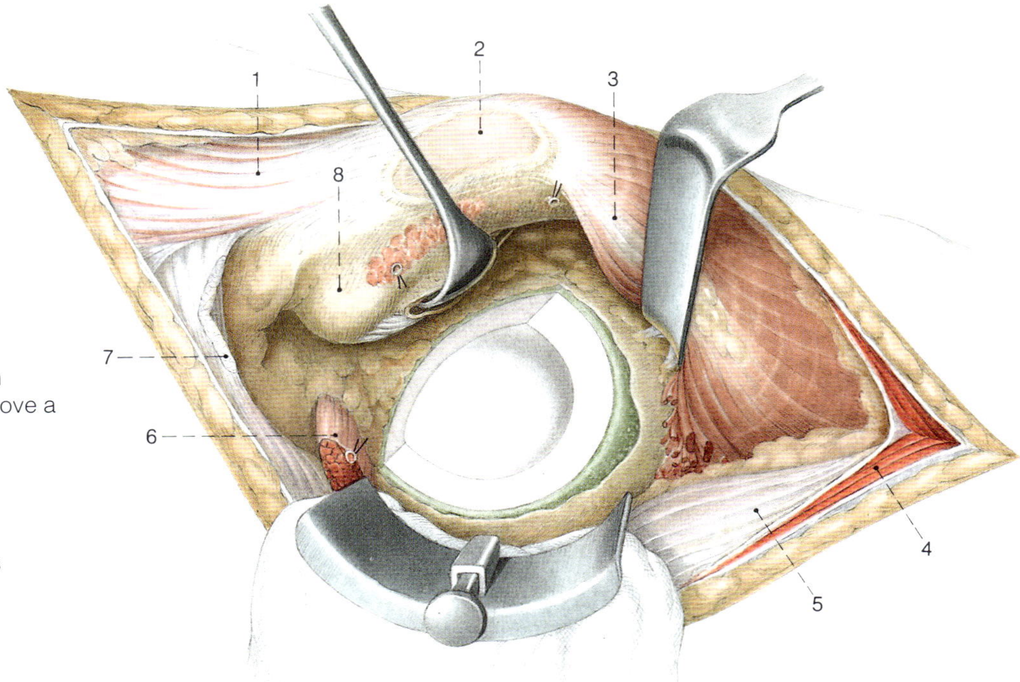

Fig. 4.**79** Exposing the acetabulum through a posterior approach to remove a cemented acetabular cup.

1 Vastus lateralis
2 Greater trochanter
3 Gluteus medius
4 Posterior fibers of the gluteus maximus
5 Inner surface of the gluteus maximus
6 Quadratus femoris
7 Incised gluteus maximus tendon
8 Lesser trochanter

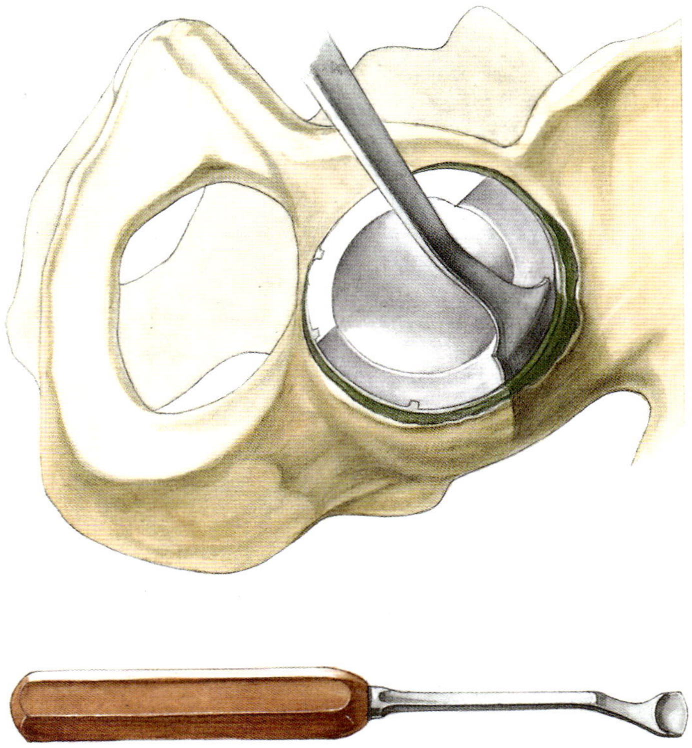

Fig. 4.**80** Disrupting the polyethylene–cement interface with a spoon-shaped gouge with a curved shaft. Avoid damaging the roof of the acetabulum.

The loosened acetabular cup is removed with a forceps. Using an osteotome as a lever over the rim of the acetabulum can damage the bone (Fig. 4.**81**). The spoon-shaped gouge is less effective in a metal-backed polyethylene cup because the blade is generally deflected off the structures on the convex side and into the cement.

If the polyethylene–cement interface cannot be disrupted in this manner without damaging the bone, the surgeon should drill a hole into the acetabular cup, use a tap and try to extract the acetabular component by pounding a mallet against the plate of the tap (Fig. 4.**82**).

If this does not loosen the acetabular component, it must be cut into segments that can be removed more easily. A narrow, extremely sharp Lambotte osteotome is best for this purpose. It should be narrow to minimize load to the floor of the acetabulum. The surgeon can ascertain when the chisel has penetrated into the cement through the polyethylene because the material feels harder and the sound is higher pitched (Fig. 4.**83**). A tap screwed into the cup can relieve the load on the bone while the surgeon cuts.

Once the acetabular component has been removed, the residual cement is divided into radial segments with an osteotome. Again, a narrow instrument is preferable. Cement pegs are then extracted from the cement retention holes in the acetabulum (Fig. 4.**84**).

Mushroom-shaped cement protrusions in the pelvis that are larger than the defect through which they passed should be removed in the presence of infection because they may be associated with a pelvic abscess. Removal is not necessary in aseptic cases unless the cement interferes with reconstruction of the acetabulum. To remove the cement without enlarging the defect, the cement protrusion is held at its acetabular flange of cement and carefully drilled (Fig. 4.**85**). Then a thin tap is advanced into the hole. It relieves load on the bone while the surgeon attempts to break up the protrusion with an osteotome. Often, the tap will split the cement so that chiseling is not necessary (Fig. 4.**86**). The segments of the cement can then be removed individually through the defect.

The surgeon should exercise extreme care when removing cement protrusions because it is possible to damage major vessels when doing so. This hazard is significantly increased where the surgeon attempts to remove a wire mesh intended to prevent protrusion that has failed, migrated into the pelvis, and become fused with pelvic soft tissue.

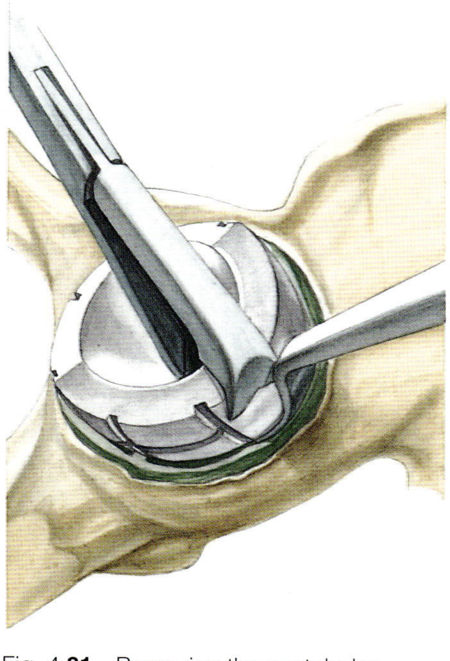

Fig. 4.**81** Removing the acetabular component.

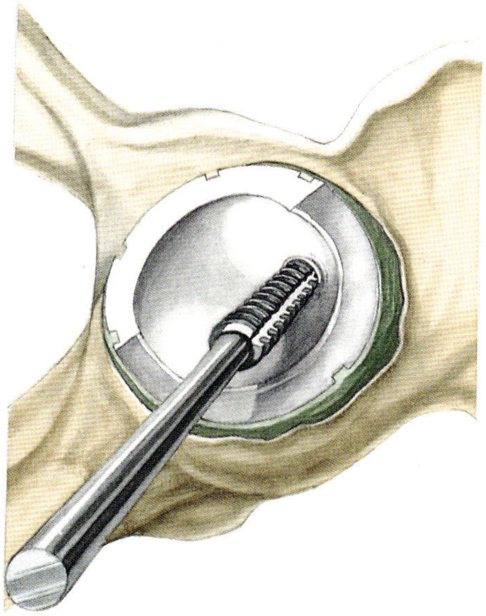

Fig. 4.**82** Drilling a hole in the acetabular component and extracting it with a tap.

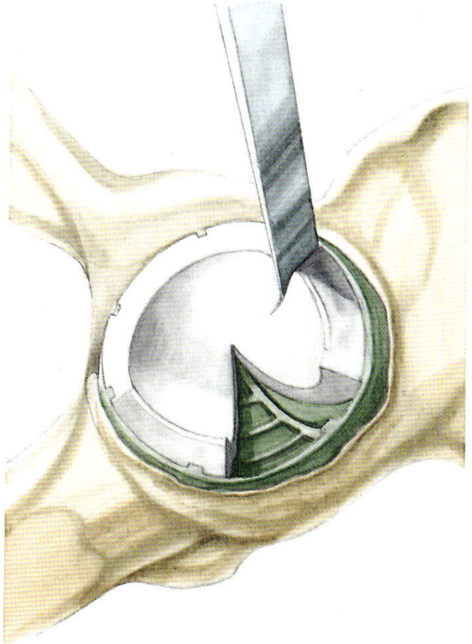

Fig. 4.**83** Dividing the acetabular component into radial segments with a narrow Lambotte osteotome.

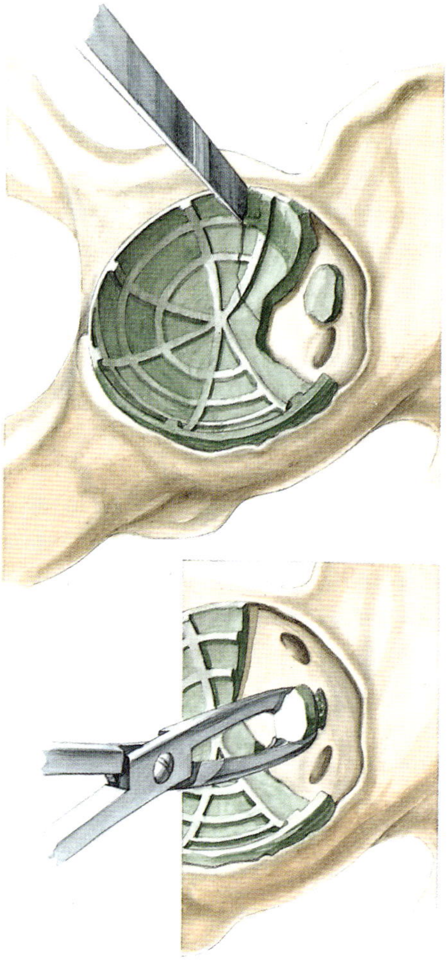

Fig. 4.**84** Dividing the residual cement into radial segments and extracting cement pegs from the cement retention holes in the acetabulum.

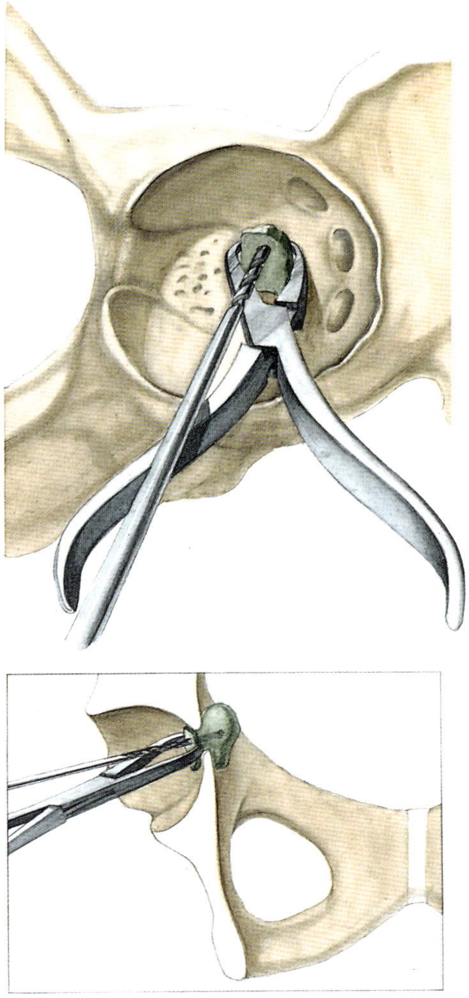

Fig. 4.**85** Drilling into a mushroom-shaped cement protrusion within the true pelvis. The cement is held in place at a cement flange in the acetabulum while it is drilled.

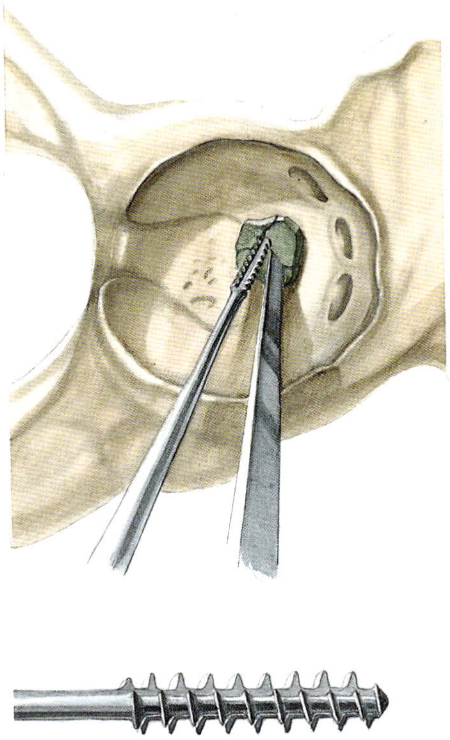

Fig. 4.**86** A tap relieves the load on the bone when cutting up the cement with the chisel.

Removing Cement with Ultrasound

A generator is used to produce a high-frequency alternating current. A cable conducts the current into the converter in the grip of the instrument. There, a reciprocal piezoelectric effect of the ceramic in the converter transforms the electricity into sound waves of the same frequency, which are conducted to the attached tool (Fig. 4.**87**).

A standing wave is created in the tool, with its peak energy at the tip of the tool. If the tool comes in contact with a thermoplastic material, such as polymethyl methacrylate or polyethylene, the material will be plasticized by the local warming that the vibration induces, only to solidify as soon as the tool is removed.

The cement in the femoral canal can be divided into flakes, stripped off the wall, and broken up transversely in the distal femoral canal. The tool is pressed with slight lateral motion into the cement. The site is irrigated with water (Fig. 4.**88**).

The surgeon can cut a ledge on the tip of a sliver of cement (Fig. 4.**89**) or cut a centered hole in the oblique face of a residual plug of cement (Fig. 4.**90**) to permit removing it with conventional instruments.

A polyethylene cup can be removed by disrupting the polyethylene–cement interface or by cutting it into segments (Fig. 4.**91**). The instrument can be used to divide the residual cement in the acetabulum into segments.

Mushroom-shaped cement protrusions into the pelvis can be retrieved even if there is no remaining flange of cement in the acetabulum to permit holding and breaking up the protrusion as described previously (Fig. 4.**92**, see also Fig. 4.**86**).

With continued bone contact, the tools can cause localized thermal necrosis, but no more than occurs when drilling or sawing. These areas should be removed with a reamer. If the tool is used around a metal implant, its tip will wear rapidly upon contact with the metal and further, ultrasonic energy eventually causes the tools to fracture.

This method is recommended as an aid in situations where conventional methods do not work. It complements instruments, such as the hammer, chisel, drill, etc.; it does not replace them.

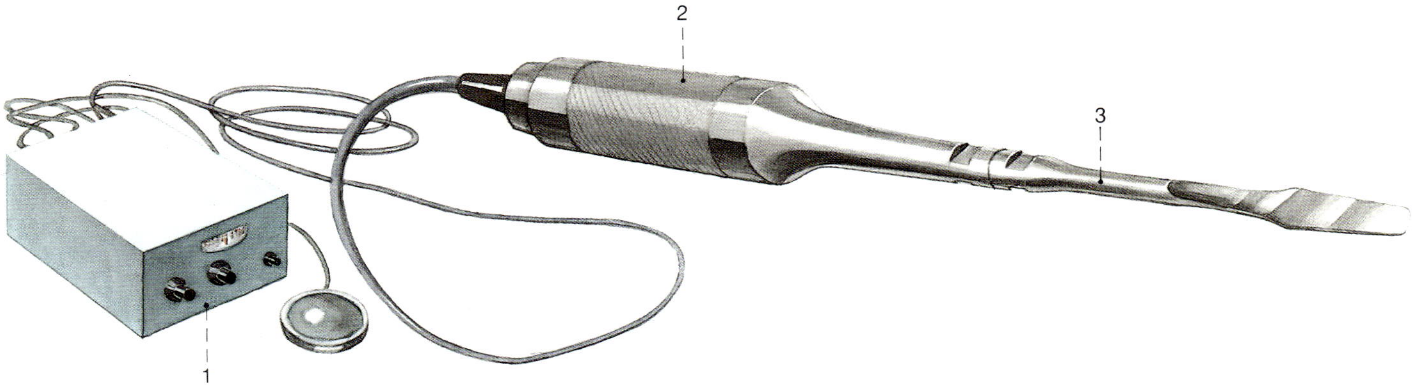

Fig. 4.**87** Ultrasonic equipment for removing cement. Generator, converter, and tool. Maximum ultrasonic vibrations occur at the tip of the tool.

1 Generator
2 Converter (grip)
3 Tool

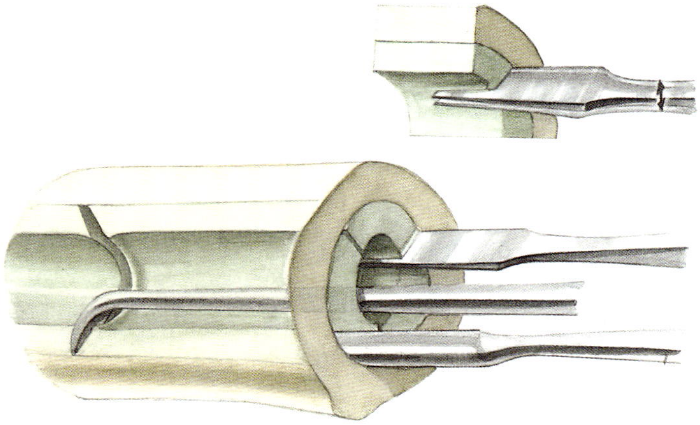

Fig. 4.**88** Dividing a cement mantle longitudinally and transversely. The tool is pressed with slight lateral motion.

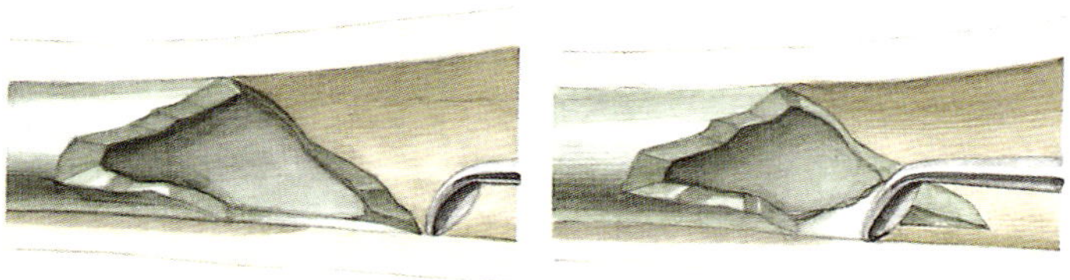

Fig. 4.**89** Cutting a ledge on a sliver of cement.

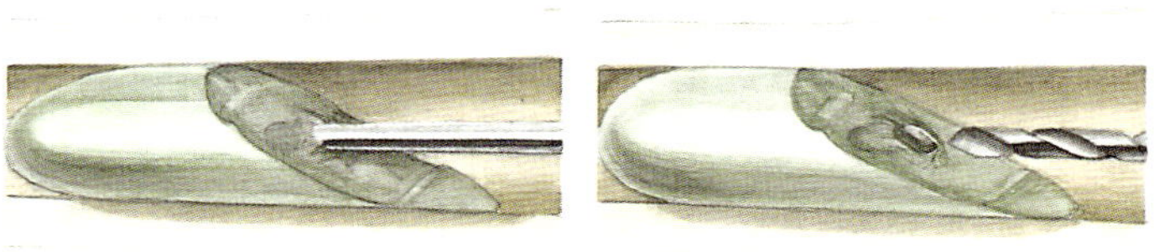

Fig. 4.**90** Cutting a hole in a residual plug of cement with an oblique face.

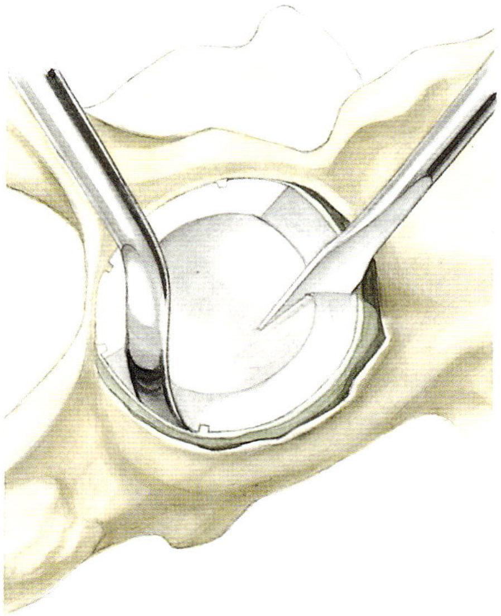

Fig. 4.**91** Removing an acetabular component. Disrupting the polyethylene–cement interface and segmenting the cup.

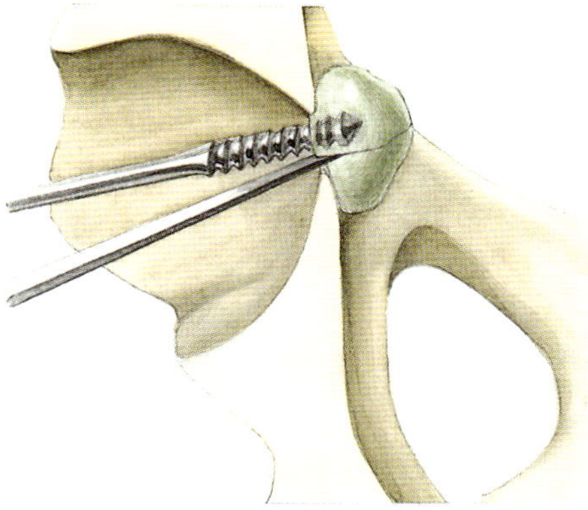

Fig. 4.**92** Holding a mushroom-shaped protrusion without a cement flange and breaking it up with an osteotome.

Removing Cementless Stems

Unless the stem is so loose that it can be extracted effortlessly, removing cementless stems is often difficult. The design of many cementless stems is not conducive to implant removal. Small areas of biological fixation or even connective tissue alone may adhere so firmly to the implant that removal of the shaft without invasive measures is impossible.

If the stem is collarless or has a removable collar and the surface of the stem is smooth, finely or longitudinally textured, then a narrow thin osteotome may be sufficient to disrupt the implant–bone interface (Fig. 4.**93**).

Collars that block access to the implant–bone interface and stems with a coarse complex surface structure designed to promote biologic fixation cause the most problems. This is particularly true in patients in whom good fixation has been achieved, but the stem must be replaced for other reasons. In such patients, it is best to split the lateral femur longitudinally past the tip of the implant rather than risk an uncontrolled femoral fracture by attempting to forcefully extract the implant. Although a strip of the vastus lateralis must be dissected off the linea aspera, the rest of the femur should still retain its soft-tissue attachments.

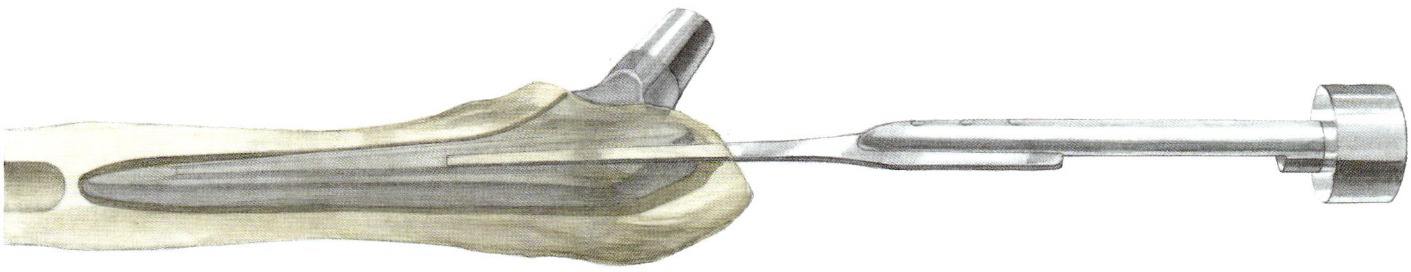

Fig. 4.**93** Removing a collarless cementless stem without coarse complex surface texturing. A narrow thin osteotome is used to disrupt the implant–bone interface.

In the transgluteal (Fig. 4.**94**) and transtrochanteric approaches (Fig. 4.**95**), the longitudinal osteotomy extends through the greater trochanter to a distal hole on the lateral femur. The osteotomy is performed through the greater trochanter because in typical cases the cancellous bone is healthy in this region and the osteotomy will heal well.

If a thin, flexible osteotome is used, only one distal hole is required to prevent cortical fracture distal to the osteotomy site while performing or subsequently spreading the osteotomy (see Fig. 4.**94**). If a standard osteotome is used, holes should be drilled at intervals corresponding to the width of the osteotome because a standard osteotome is more likely to cause cracking of the femoral bone (see Fig. 4.**95**).

In a posterior approach, the proximal osteotomy near the greater trochanter curves anteriorly to the anterior margin of the abductors. The surgeon dissects the anterior fibers of the abductors from the greater trochanter to avoid having to perform the proximal osteotomy right up to the anterior femur in thin cortical bone only (Fig. 4.**96**).

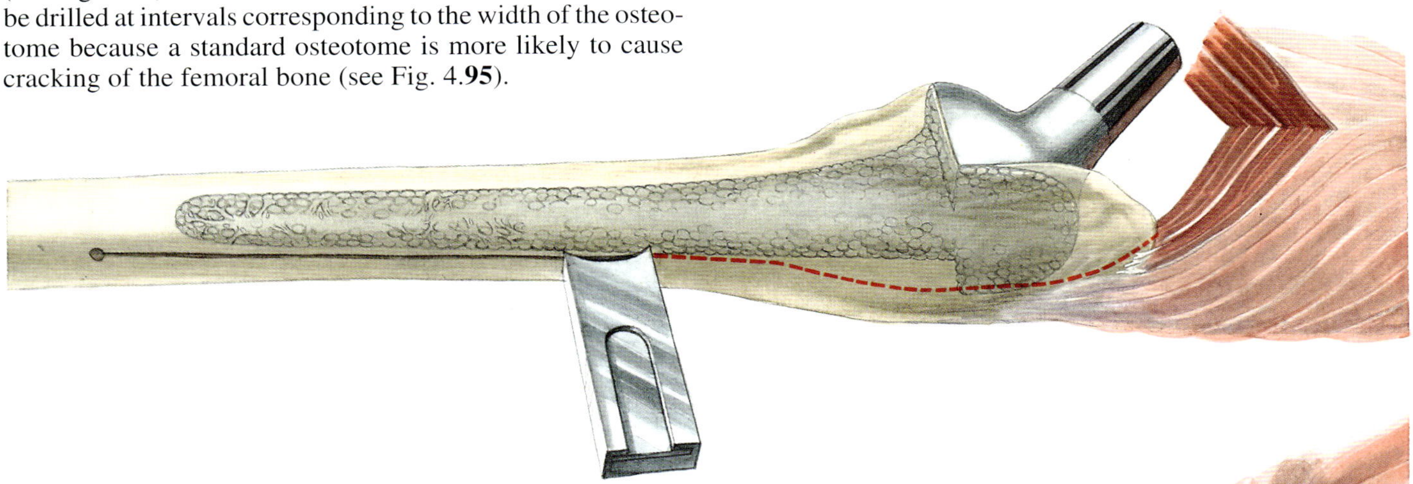

Fig. 4.**94** Removing a stem that is not conducive to removal. A lateral longitudinal osteotomy through the greater trochanter and femur is performed with a thin flexible osteotome in a blade guide. Drilling holes are not necessary (except for a distal hole). Transgluteal approach to the hip.

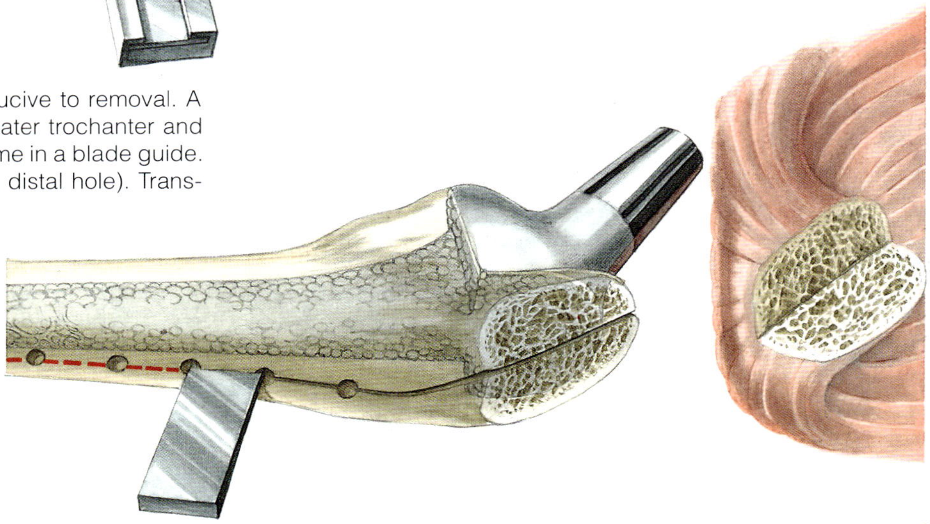

Fig. 4.**95** A lateral longitudinal osteotomy through the greater trochanter and femur is performed with a conventional osteotome. Holes are drilled at intervals corresponding to the width of the osteotome. Transtrochanteric approach to the hip.

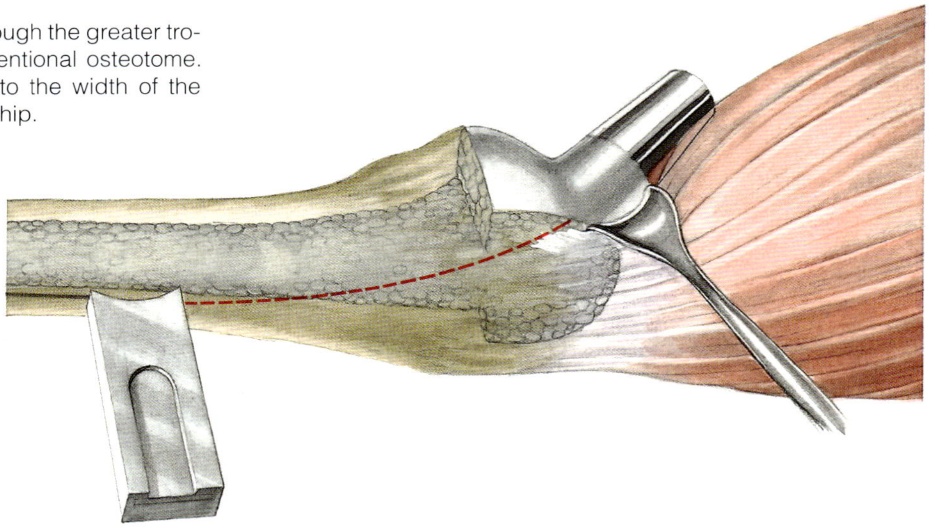

Fig. 4.**96** A lateral longitudinal osteotomy is performed with a wide flexible osteotome. The proximal osteotomy curves anteriorly. Posterior approach to the hip.

Next the surgeon spreads the osteotomy with two wide conventional osteotomes and attempts to extract the stem. Attempting to extract the stem by applying force diagonally—such as pounding on an impactor placed beneath the implant collar (Fig. 4.**97**, see also Fig. 4.**42**) or a center punch placed in a proximal hole (see Fig. 4.**45**)—is less effective and is more likely to cause a fracture than axial extraction using an extraction instrument attached directly to the taper (see Fig. 4.**46**).

If the stem cannot be removed in this manner, the surgeon dissects the vastus lateralis completely off the femur and performs a transverse osteotomy from the lateral distal hole to a hole drilled in the anteromedial femur. From this anteromedial hole, the surgeon performs a second longitudinal osteotomy (Fig. 4.**98 a**) and opens the anterior window created by these osteotomies (Fig. 4.**98 b**). A narrow Lambotte osteotome with a curved tip or a narrow curved saw blade (Fig. 4.**98 c**) is used to disrupt the implant–bone interface.

We do not recommend performing an osteotomy through the muscle on the anteromedial side, as in transfemoral removal of a loosened cemented stem in an extremely weakened femur (see Fig. 4.**66** and 4.**67**). Replacing a cementless stem is often an early revision procedure performed in a patient with good bone stock, where the femoral window can be expected to heal into a closed bony cylinder capable of full weight bearing. For this reason, the anterolateral osteotomy must be performed carefully after the vastus lateralis has been completely dissected from the femur to avoid uncontrolled fractures while attempting to open the window.

The surgeon can open a lateral window instead of an anterior window (see Figs. 4.**66** and 4.**67**). Again, this should be done carefully after the vastus lateralis has been dissected so that the femur will heal properly. The longitudinal osteotomies are performed close to the linea aspera and anteriorly or anterolaterally, respectively.

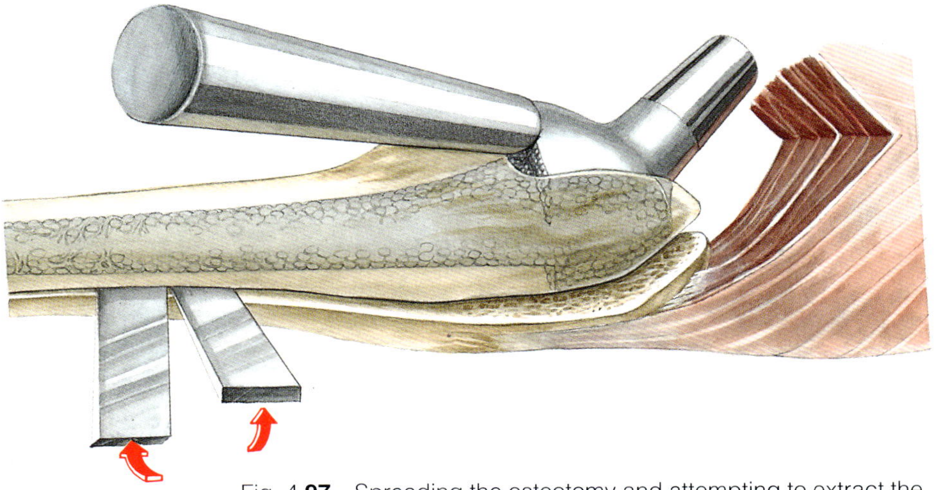

Fig. 4.**97** Spreading the osteotomy and attempting to extract the implant. An impactor placed beneath the implant collar places a transverse strain on the femur. Applying force axially with an extraction instrument attached directly to the taper is preferred (see Fig. 4.**46**).

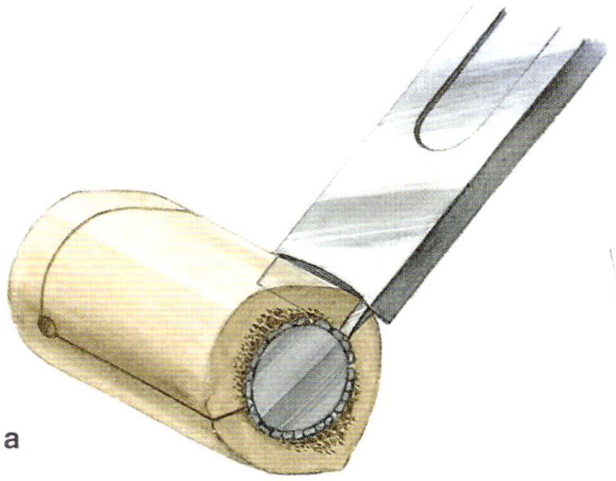

a

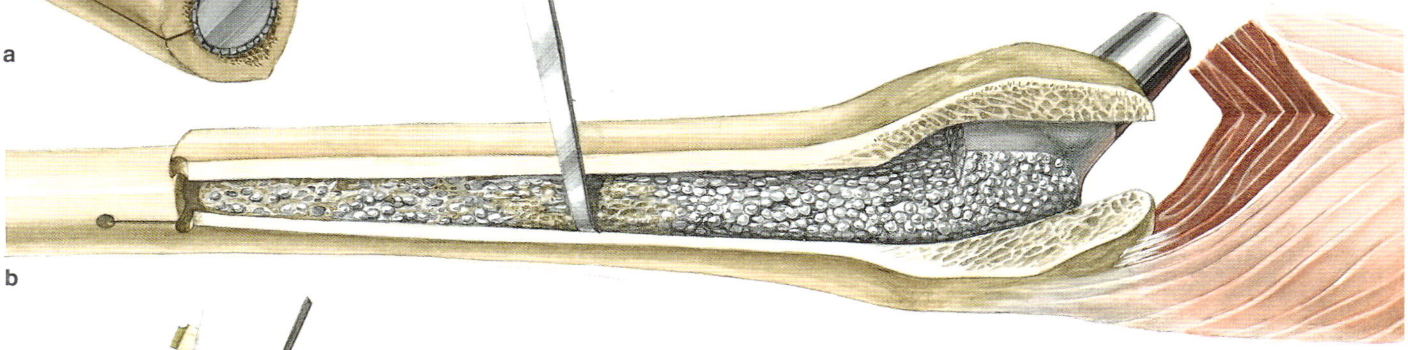

b

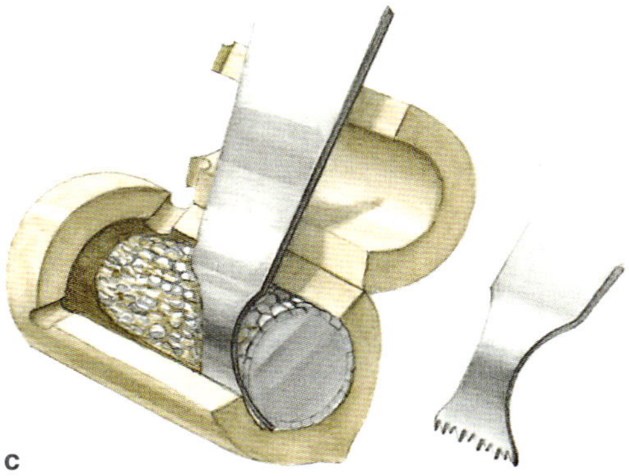

c

Fig. 4.**98 a–c** Large window covering the entire length of the implant–bone interface.
a A semicircular transverse osteotomy is performed between holes drilled over the distal tip of the implant. An anteromedial longitudinal osteotomy is performed with a flexible osteotome after the vastus lateralis has been dissected off the femur.
b Opening the window and disrupting the implant–bone interface with a narrow Lambotte osteotome with a curved tip.
c Disrupting the implant–bone interface with a narrow saw blade with a curved tip.

Removing Cementless Acetabular Components

As in cemented systems, removing a cementless acetabular component poses less of a problem than removing a cementless stem.

Before extracting the acetabular component, the surgeon removes bony ingrowth or connective tissue from the transverse undercuts in a threaded acetabular cup (Fig. 4.**99**). System-specific instruments that can produce high torque should be used with caution when unscrewing the cup to avoid pelvic fractures (Fig. 4.**100**). If a system-specific instrument is not available, the acetabular component can generally be unscrewed by turning it with a long, narrow impactor that engages the thread gaps. If the metal portion of the cup is designed as a ring, the surgeon can attempt to extract it with a hook after removing the polyethylene inlay (Fig. 4.**101**).

Ceramic acetabular components can be broken up with a sharp center punch (Fig. 4.**102**). The surgeon can introduce extracting force into the rear side of an acetabular component by driving a long, narrow impactor through the acetabular rim anterosuperiorly or posterosuperiorly depending on the approach used. This assumes that the acetabular bone is strong enough to permit this procedure (Fig. 4.**103**).

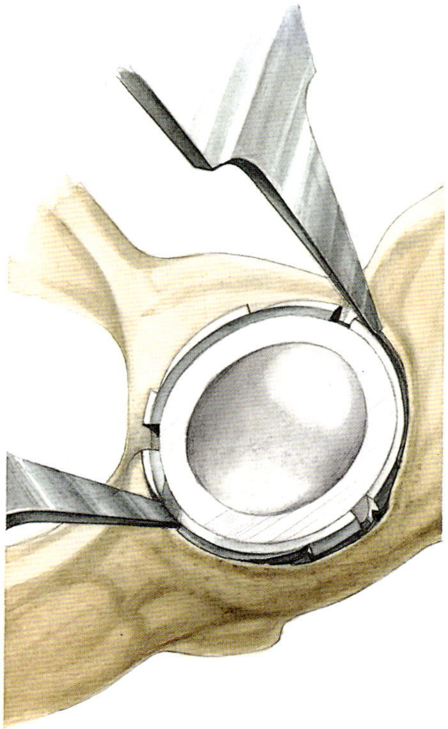

Fig. 4.**99** Removing cementless acetabular components. Using a narrow osteotome to remove bony ingrowth or connective tissue from the transverse undercuts in a threaded acetabular cup.

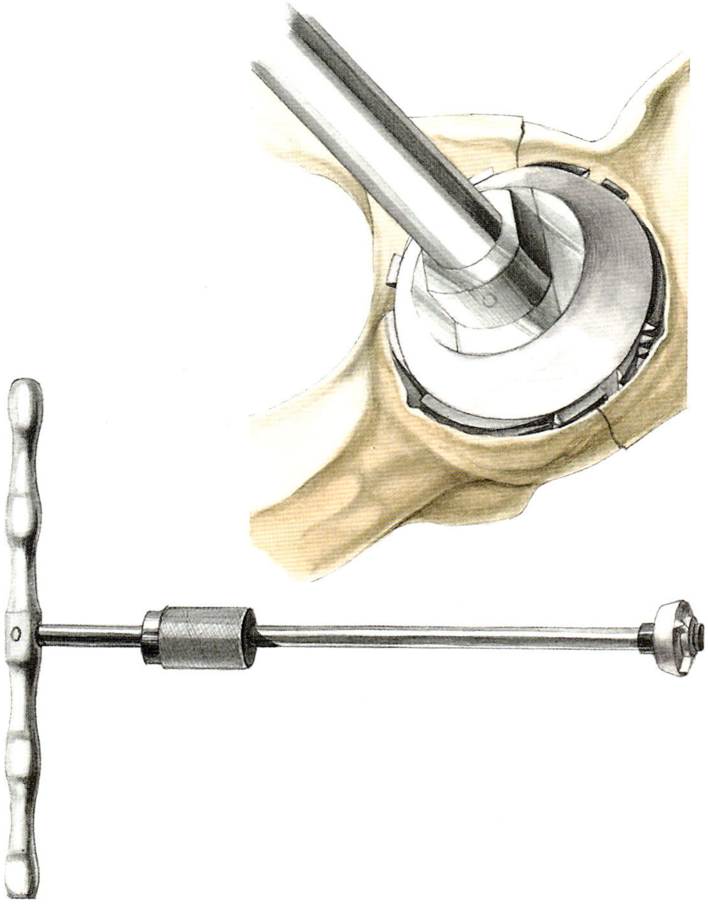

Fig. 4.**100** System-specific extraction instrument for threaded acetabular component that can produce high torque. Pelvic fracture may result.

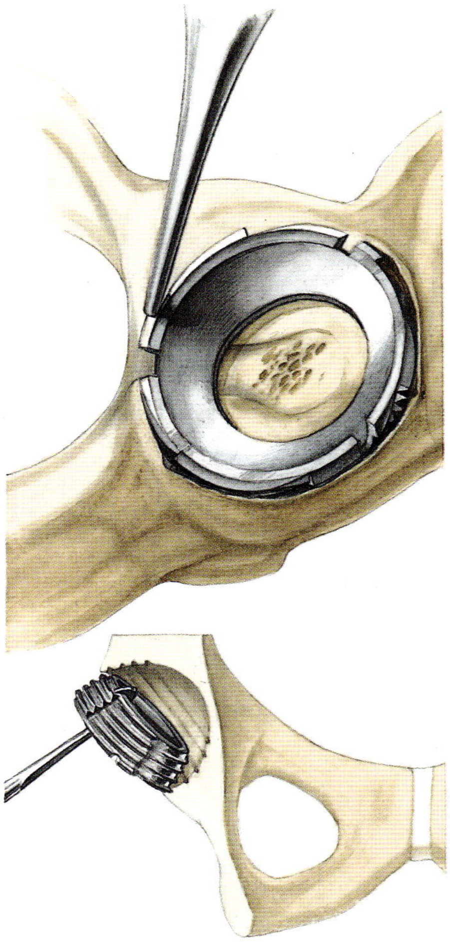

Fig. 4.**101** Extracting the acetabular component by turning it with an impactor that engages the thread gaps. Extracting a threaded ring with a hook.

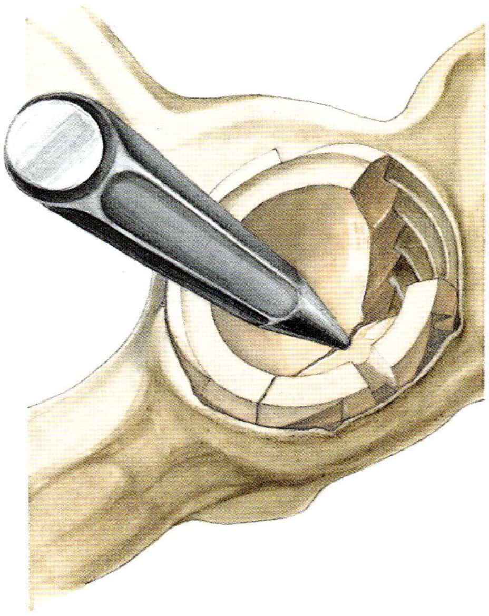

Fig. 4.**102** Destroying a ceramic acetabular component with a sharp center punch.

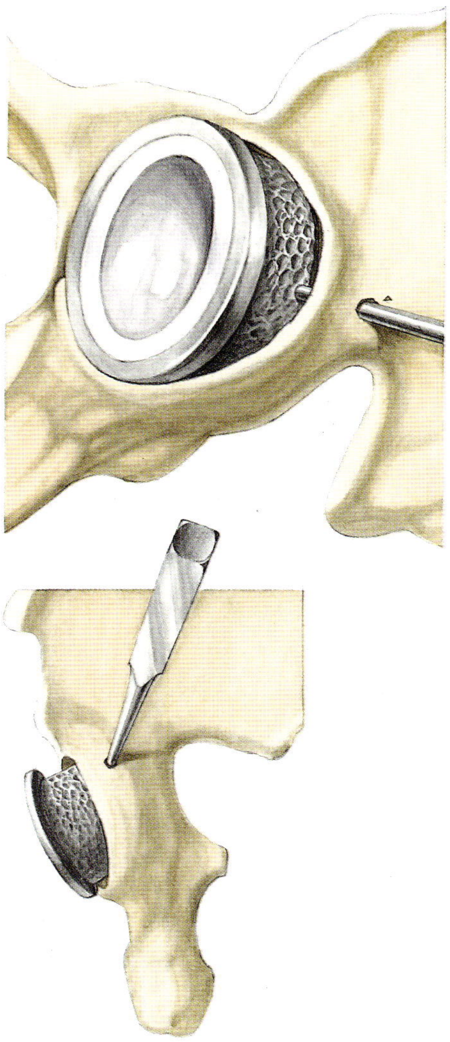

Fig. 4.**103** Introducing an extracting force into the rear side of an acetabular component by driving a long narrow impactor through the acetabular rim anterosuperiorly or posterosuperiorly.

Reimplanting Acetabular Components

Loosening of cementless and cemented components first widens the acetabulum concentrically. Furthermore, the cup can migrate superolaterally, superiorly, or superomedially (Fig. 4.**104 a**). In the sagittal plane, it will have a tendency to migrate anteriorly or posteriorly. Posterior migration is more problematic because the posterior rim of the acetabulum supports the cup more than the anterior rim.

When the acetabular component migrates superolaterally, it is no longer supported by the lateral part of the acetabular roof; depending on its position in the sagittal plane, it may also lack the support of the anterior or posterior acetabular rim. The floor of the acetabulum is generally intact (Fig. 4.**104 b**). The defect resembles hip dysplasia. Dysplasia is the most frequent condition preceding laterosuperior migration. This is particularly applicable in cases where the initial acetabular component was not implanted in the true acetabulum using an acetabular graft, but was implanted farther superiorly, sacrificing the roof of the dysplastic acetabulum.

When the acetabular component migrates superiorly, the roof of the acetabulum is shifted superiorly. The acetabular roof and the floor of the acetabulum are generally intact, but the roof is smaller and the floor protrudes into the pelvis because the dimensions of the bone superior to the acetabulum decrease superiorly (Fig. 4.**104 c**). Depending on the direction of migration in the sagittal plane, the anterior or posterior rim of the acetabulum is missing.

When the acetabular component migrates superomedially, the lateral part of the acetabular roof generally has the form of a bony ridge extending distally at an acute angle. The widened floor of the acetabulum is either thin but still present in the form of a thin periosteal layer of bone, or the bone separating the joint from the true pelvis is missing (or nearly so). We can therefore differentiate between closed protrusion (Fig. 4.**104 d**) or open protrusion (Fig. 4.**104 e**). If the acetabular component migrates farther anteriorly or posteriorly, the anterior or posterior rim of the acetabulum will be lost. In an open protrusion, these rims are the remaining connections between the ilium and the superior pubic ramus or the ischium. When one rim has been lost (e.g., the stronger posterior rim), a fatigue fracture can occur in the other (e.g. the weaker anterior rim). This interrupts the pelvic ring in the same manner as an acetabular resection (see Figs. 4.**136** and 4.**137**). The most frequent conditions that precede this severe defect are protrusion of the acetabulum, trauma, and excessive reaming of the acetabular floor and/or the anterior, posterior, or both rims (e.g. to implant an oversized acetabular component).

All diseases resulting in skeletal weakening contribute to the development of these defects.

In aseptic cases and young patients, the surgeon should always make an effort to fill defects with graft to permit secure reimplantation of the acetabular component. This is most successful in the presence of superior or superolateral and migration, or in the presence of closed protrusion following superomedial migration. Loss of the posterior rim complicates the correction. Open protrusion poses major problems. The limit of possible reconstruction can be reached when the anterior, posterior, or both acetabular rims are missing, and the pelvis is unstable.

Reconstructing the acetabulum with graft is not possible where transplant material is not available or fixation is not feasible. The patient's condition is a serious limiting factor; the patient may not tolerate complicated surgery and a postoperative period of partial weight bearing, thus necessitating a short procedure with immediate full weight bearing. A saddle prosthesis (see Fig. 4.**126**) is the alternative to a resection arthroplasty in these patients.

The resection arthroplasty requires no implants, which may be an advantage, and can provide satisfactory function. However, such hips are often unable to permit full weight bearing, and can telescope and cause pain if the pelvis does not provide a sufficient buttress for the femur and/or the proximal femur is shortened.

Arthrodesis is rarely an option in the presence of defects of this magnitude.

Please refer to the chapter on primary total hip arthroplasty for the surgical technique involved in implanting standard and enlarged revision acetabular components without grafting.

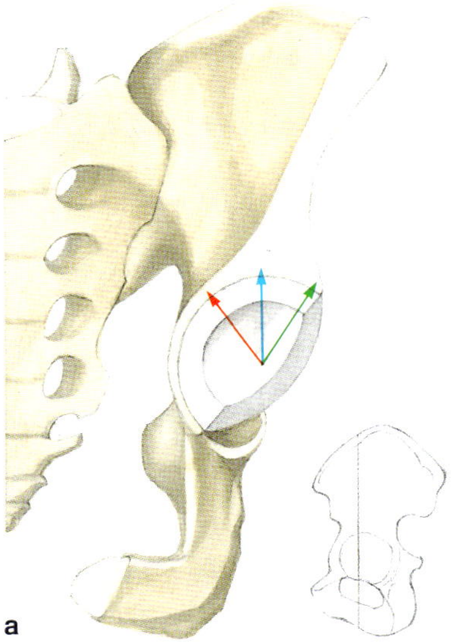

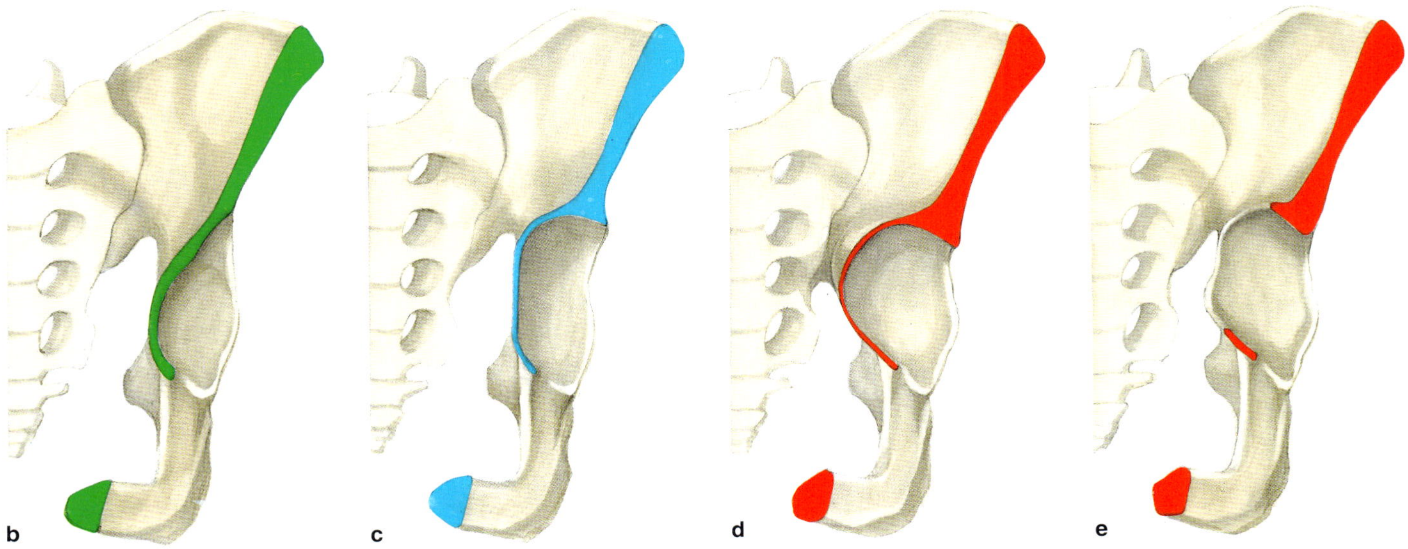

Fig. 4.**104a–e** Acetabular migration and the resulting defects.
a Directions of migration in the coronal plane.
b Defect caused by superolateral migration. Loss of the lateral part of the acetabular roof.
c Defect caused by superior migration. Diminished acetabular roof at a level higher up the pelvic bone and closed protrusion.
d Defect caused by superomedial migration. Closed protrusion.
e Defect caused by superomedial migration. Open protrusion.

Reconstructing the Acetabulum with Graft

Allograft taken from femoral heads is used, and occasionally autologous bone may provide graft material when the contralateral side also requires total hip arthroplasty and the contralateral femoral head may be used. Donors should be carefully screened and the allograft subjected to appropriate physical and chemical treatment to minimize transmission of tissue-borne diseases. The femoral heads can be used as structural or morsellized grafts (chips).

There are different and often conflicting opinions regarding the best size of a graft, the proportion of cortical to cancellous bone, and the extent of the graft integration; supporting data are often lacking. However, the following conditions are generally regarded as advantageous:

- Both recipient bone stock and allograft are of good quality
- The graft is surrounded by recipient bone stock on as many sides as possible
- High compressive forces act on the interface, and shear forces acting on fixation screws are minimized
- The construct has high primary stability (which is increased when cementing the acetabular component).

Structural Grafts

The bone is shaped to maximize the cancellous surface in contact with the recipient bone. If the area receiving the graft has a complex geometry, it can be shaped with a saw, reamer, or Luer forceps. This should be done conservatively because even the smallest portion of remaining pelvic bone is valuable. To accelerate graft integration, the surgeon uses a small drill bit to penetrate the cortex of the recipient bone at various sites.

The graft is fixed with cancellous screws with long or short threads depending on the fixation site. If indicated, a washer (which should rest on cortical bone of the graft) is used to prevent subsidence of the screw into the graft. The screws must act as lag screws, i.e., their threads should only lie in the recipient bone and should engage the cortex of the other side of the bone wherever possible. The surgeon drills a hole with a 3.2 mm bit through the graft and the recipient bone and then widens the hole within the graft to 4.5 mm (Fig. 4.**105a**). It is only necessary to cut threads in the presence of osteosclerosis. In this case, this is done only within the sclerotic layer of the recipient bone. Then the graft is fixed with the cancellous screw (Fig. 4.**105b**).

Screws inserted in a direction similar to that of the resultant force in the hip are best because shear forces acting on the screw are minimized. They produce a construct with high primary stability when there is a significant angle between the bone–graft interface and the resultant force in the hip. This means that the primary forces acting on the interface are compressive forces (Fig. 4.**105c**). Screws whose axis deviates significantly from the resultant force in the hip are less suitable because shear forces acting on the screw are maximized. These screws achieve only minimal primary stability when the bone–graft interface is nearly parallel to the resultant force in the hip because the primary forces acting on the interface are shear forces (Fig. 4.**105d**).

Morsellized Grafts

Bone chips are used to fill remaining gaps between the recipient bone and a structural graft, to seal sutures, and to fill defects surrounded on all sides by recipient bone (such as in a closed protrusion). Chips of increasing size are collected by reaming a resected femoral head, or with a bone mill or by cutting a femoral head into slices and breaking it up with Luer forceps. Fine chips are suitable for sealing sutures. Medium-grade chips are used for filling narrow gaps. The best compression and adhesion between the chips can be achieved with coarse chips.

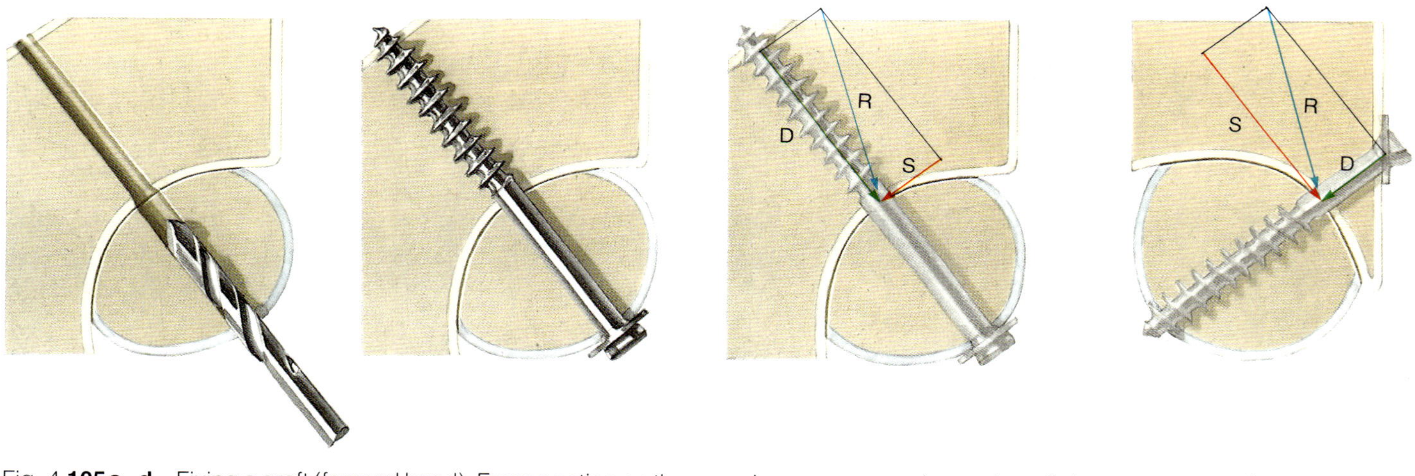

Fig. 4.**105a–d** Fixing a graft (femoral head). Forces acting on the fixation screw and bone–graft interface.
a Drilling through the graft and recipient bone with a 3.2-mm bit and widening the hole within the graft to 4.5 mm.
b Fixing the graft with a cancellous screw (lag screw). A washer is used if necessary.
c Large compression and small shear component forces acting on the screw and interface ensure good primary stability.
d Small compression and large shear component forces acting on the screw and interface result in poor primary stability.

R = Resultant force in the hip
D = Compressive component force
S = Shear component force

Reconstruction following Superolateral Migration of the Acetabular Component

Reconstruction following superolateral migration of the acetabular component (Fig. 4.**106**) is identical to primary reconstruction of a dysplastic hip. The surgeon resects the neck of the femoral head and contours the exposed cancellous bone to achieve intimate fit in the acetabulum (Fig. 4.**107**). Using a small drill bit, the surgeon penetrates the acetabular cortex at several sites and inserts the graft (Fig. 4.**108**). Any remaining gaps are filled with cancellous bone chips.

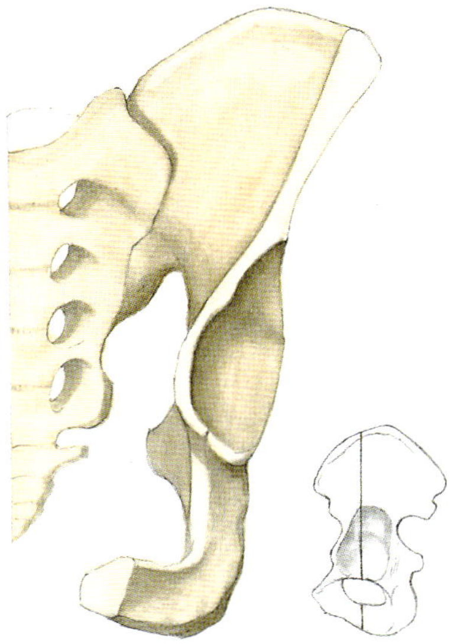

Fig. 4.**106** Damage caused by superolateral component migration.

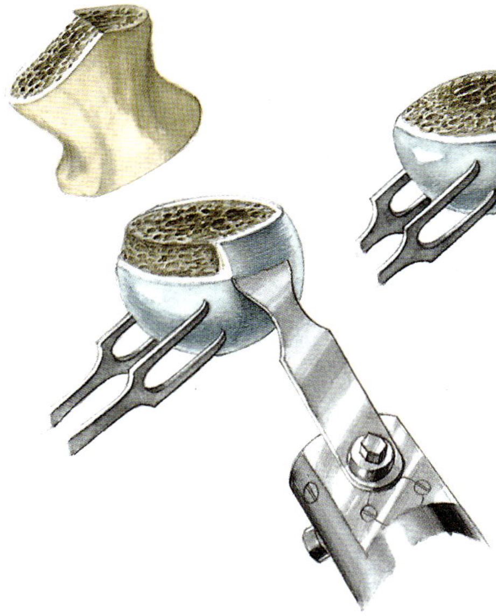

Fig. 4.**107** Contouring a cancellous surface to match the recipient bone.

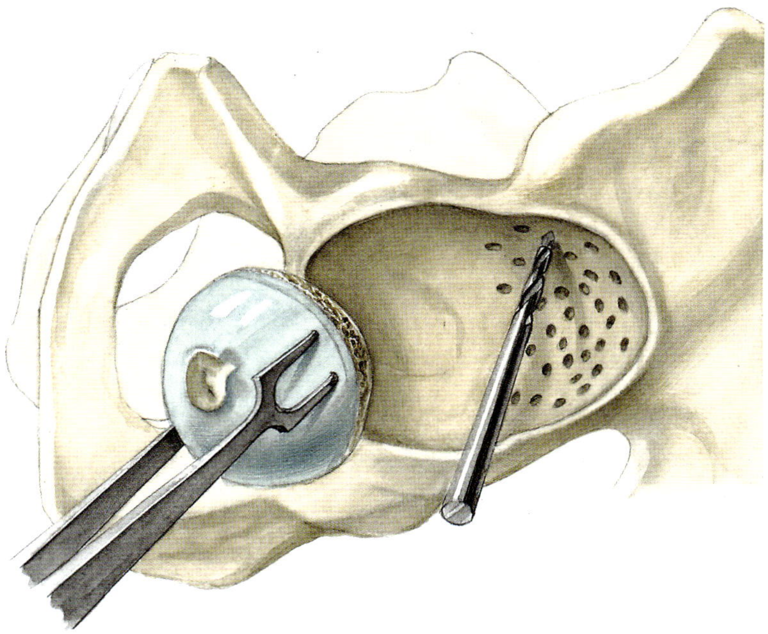

Fig. 4.**108** Perforating the cortex of the recipient bone and inserting the graft.

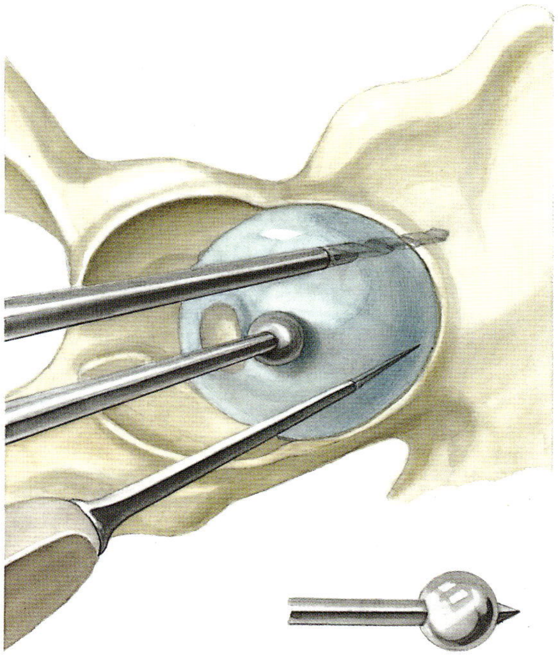

Fig. 4.**109** Holding the graft with a ball-tipped awl and a standard awl. A hole is drilled through the graft and the recipient bone with a 3.2-mm bit.

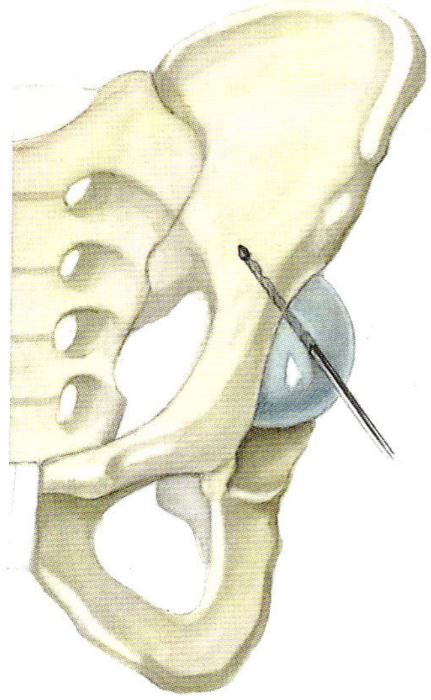

Fig. 4.**110** Hole drilled at a steep angle through the cortex of the inner table of the pelvis.

The graft is then pressed into the acetabulum with two ball-tipped awls or a ball-tipped awl and a standard awl. The awl inserted into the graft along a defined axis makes it easier for the surgeon to locate the cancellous surface of the graft after repeated corrections. With the graft in place, the surgeon drills a hole through the graft into the inner table of the pelvis using a 3.2 mm bit (Fig. 4.**109**). The hole within the graft is then widened with a 4.5 mm bit (see Fig. 4.**105 a**). Next, the surgeon selects a cancellous screw of the required length (long-thread screws are preferable) and fixes the graft (see Fig. 4.**105 b**). Without releasing the pressure on the awls, the surgeon inserts the second screw in the same manner.

Each hole should be as steep as possible to minimize shear forces acting on the screw (Figs. 4.**110** and see 4.**105 c**). The screws and washers should be inserted as close as possible to, but not within the inferior part of the graft which still has to be hollowed. Note, too, that most of the graft lies inferior to the screws. This means that optimum alignment, i.e., the axis of the screw is parallel to the resultant force in the hip, is seldom achieved in clinical practice.

When the graft appears to be sufficiently fixed, the surgeon hollows it with successively larger reamers (Fig. 4.**111**) until the acetabulum is large enough to accommodate the acetabular component. The graft is held with two ball-tipped awls to relieve the strain on the screws during reaming. An initial cavity should be formed before reaming. This prevents the initial reamer from migrating off the convex cortical and cartilaginous surface of the graft, and reduces the amount of graft that the reamer must remove. The cavity is best formed by incising the graft with a narrow, curved saw blade (Fig. 4.**111**, insert) or hollowing out the cavity with a spoon-shaped gouge (see Fig. 4.**80**). An alternative to reaming the graft in situ is to roughly prepare the graft before fixation. This procedure is prone to error, however. Before final reaming, the surgeon tightens the screws. If the posterior rim of the acetabulum is missing, the graft is fixed and reamed to form a posterior crescent, or a separate graft is fixed at that site.

Before fixing the graft, the remaining gaps between the pelvis and the graft are filled with medium-grade bone chips, remaining sutures are sealed with fine chips, and the graft and the recipient bone are keyed by drilling holes into their surfaces (Fig. 4.**112**). While the cement is being mixed, the acetabulum is packed with compresses to keep it dry and keep bone chips in place. Then the cement is applied. The illustration shows an anatomically shaped acetabular component (an anteroinferior segment has been removed) with a thin rim that traps the cement (Fig. 4.**113**). This form permits easy removal of excess cement anteriorly and inferiorly and eliminates the portion of the cup that could otherwise impinge the psoas tendon.

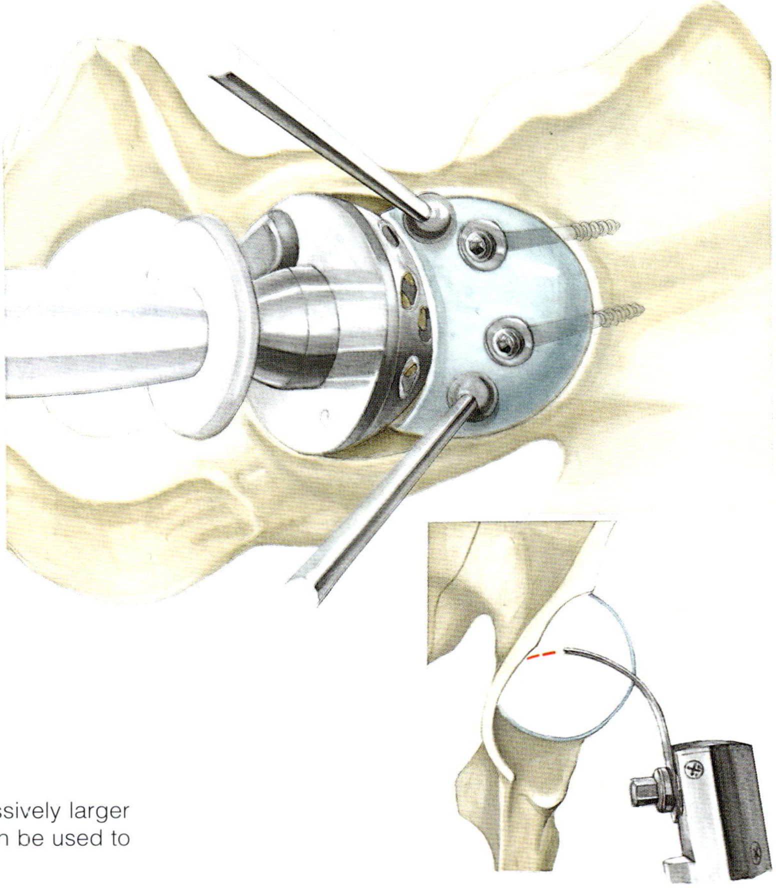

Fig. 4.**111** Hollowing out the fixed graft with successively larger acetabular reamers. A narrow, curved saw blade can be used to excavate the initial cavity.

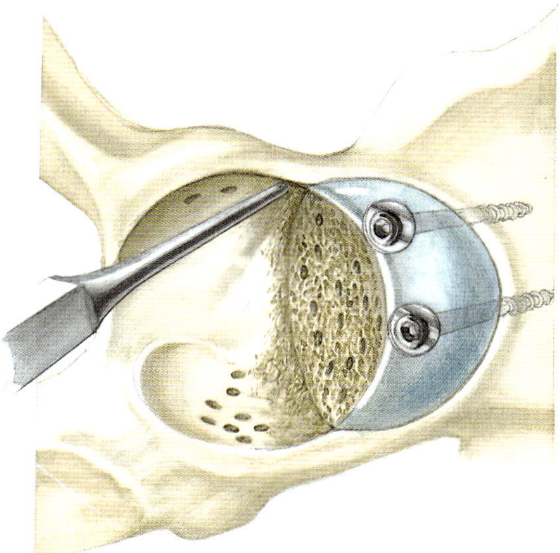

Fig. 4.**112** Filling remaining gaps and sealing sutures with cancellous chips. The recipient bone and the graft are keyed by drilling holes into their surfaces.

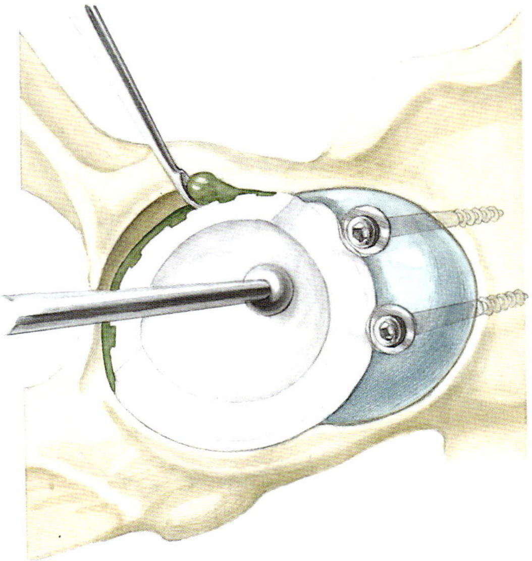

Fig. 4.**113** Cementing an anatomically shaped acetabular component.

Reconstruction following Superior Migration of the Acetabular Component

When the hip is reconstructed after superior migration of the acetabular component (Fig. 4.**114**), the femoral head is contoured so that part of it fits into the roof of the acetabulum (which is reduced in size and displaced superiorly) and part rests on the lateral cortex. The graft is fixed with one or two screws inserted superior to the new acetabular rim (Fig. 4.**115**), which is to be shifted inferiorly and laterally. After implanting and fixing the graft, the surgeon reams the new acetabulum.

The surgeon can significantly increase the stability of the graft during reaming by inserting an awl into it through the posterior acetabular rim (Fig. 4.**116**). The graft can be held with this awl alone when the surgeon is uncertain where to insert the screws. The awl is also used to hold a graft that is to be fixed with an "inside-out" technique. Where this type of fixation is desired, the screw is sunk into an initially reamed cavity in the graft, well into the cancellous bone. Then the surgeon alternately reams the cavity and sinks the screw further until the proper depth has been reached (Fig. 4.**116**, insert).

If the posterior acetabular rim is missing, the surgeon attempts to ream the graft to form a posterior crescent or fixes additional graft at that site. Next, the remaining gaps and sutures are filled with bone chips of suitable size. Finally, the surgeon keys the graft by drilling cement retention holes and cements the acetabular component.

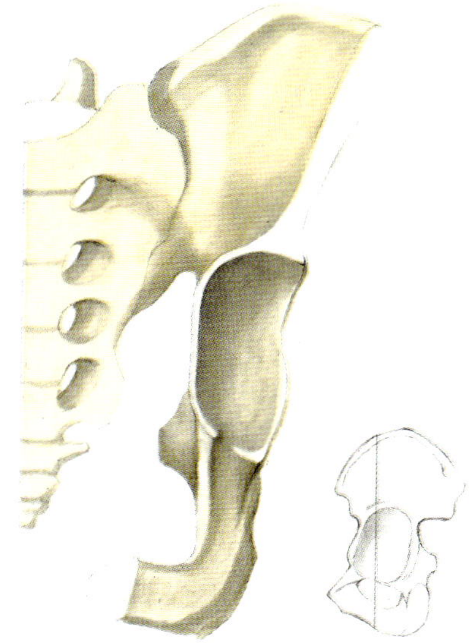

Fig. 4.**114** Damage caused by superior component migration.

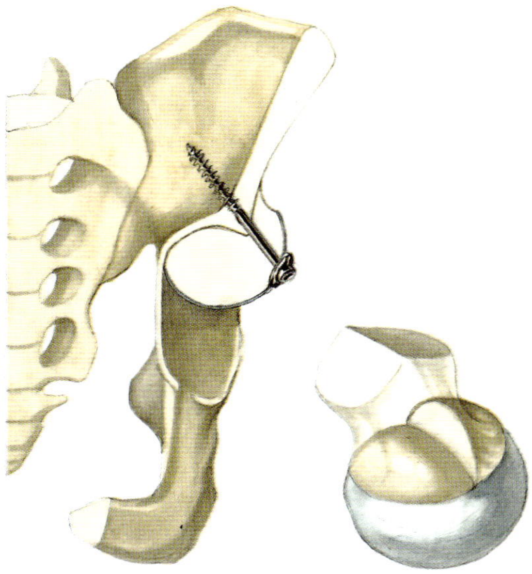

Fig. 4.**115** Contouring a graft to extend the acetabular roof and to displace it inferiorly. The graft is fixed with screws inserted superior to the new acetabular rim.

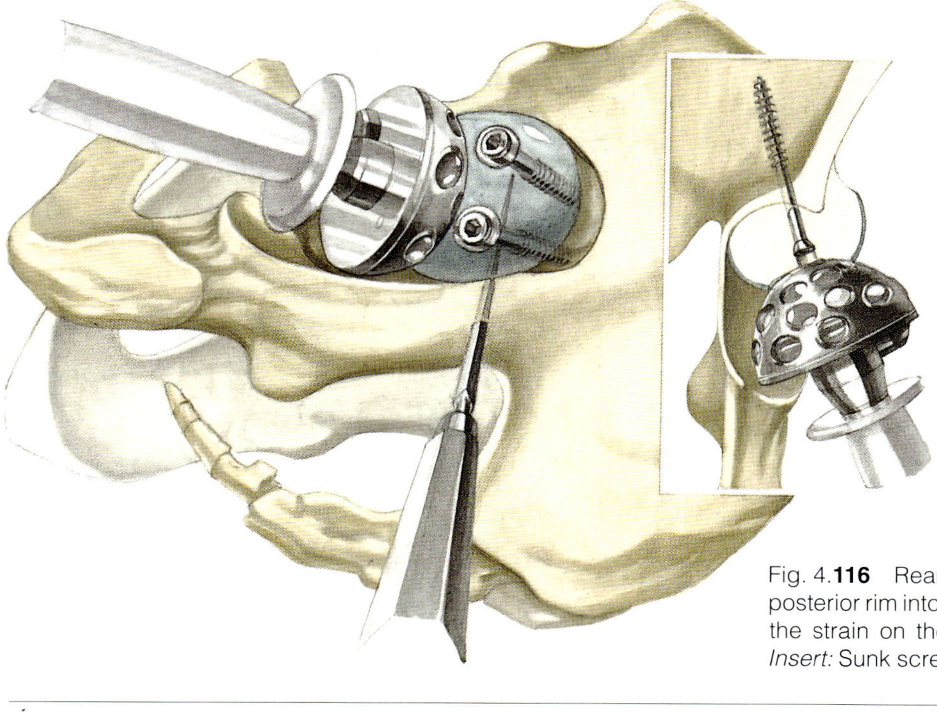

Fig. 4.**116** Reaming the graft. An awl inserted through the posterior rim into the graft and through the posterior rim relieves the strain on the screws while the surgeon reams the graft. *Insert:* Sunk screws in the graft.

Reconstruction following Superomedial Migration of the Acetabular Component

In areas where a thin periosteal layer of bone still separates the joint from the true pelvis after superomedial component migration (Fig. 4.**117a**), this layer can be used as a bed for a graft. The closed protrusion is filled with bone chips (Sloof's method). The best adhesion between the chips is achieved with chips obtained with a Luer forceps. The surgeon compresses the chips with a trial cup and then cements a collared acetabular cup in position (Fig. 4.**117b**). The collar relieves stress on the weakened acetabular floor. A polyethylene collar is advantageous because it can be trimmed to fit with a Luer forceps (Fig. 4.**117c**).

Where a central defect is present following superomedial component migration, the surgeon mobilizes the membrane of pelvic connective tissue with a small-hooked periosteal elevator if the defect is to be bridged with a structural graft (Fig. 4.**118**). This graft is taken from the superior portion of a resected femoral head, which is contoured to resemble a hat (Fig. 4.**119**). The top of the hat should have the same form as the defect (generally asymmetric) to prevent it from rotating when the inserted graft is reamed. If the defect is round, then the surgeon expands it slightly on one side to make it asymmetric. The brim of the hat should be thick and curved so that it covers a large area of the acetabular floor. After implanting the hat (Fig. 4.**120**), the surgeon carefully reams the acetabulum (Fig. 4.**121**), fills sutures with morsellized bone

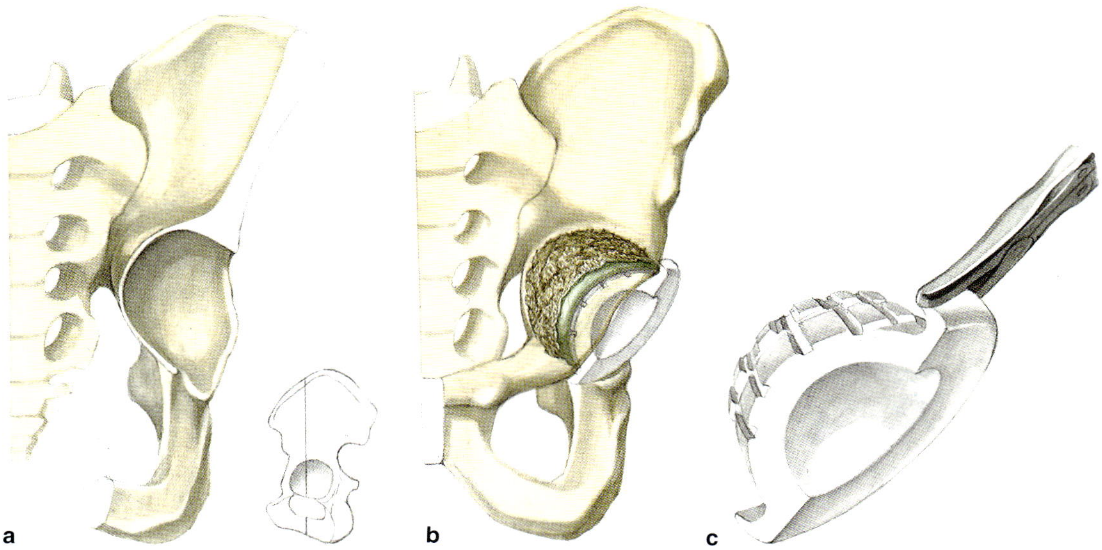

Fig. 4.**117** Damage caused by superomedial component migration. Closed protrusion. Morsellized graft (Sloof's method) and collared acetabular component.

a Closed protrusion.
b Filling the protruded acetabulum with chips (Sloof's method). Cementing a collared acetabular component.
c Trimming the collar.

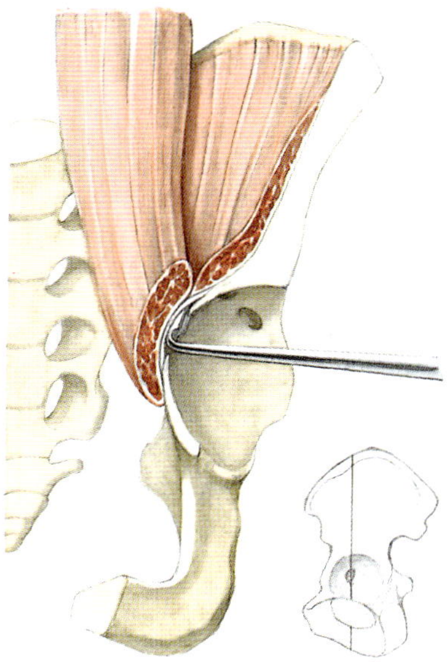

Fig. 4.**118** Damage caused by superomedial component migration: Central perforation. Mobilizing the connective tissue within the true pelvis to accommodate a structural graft.

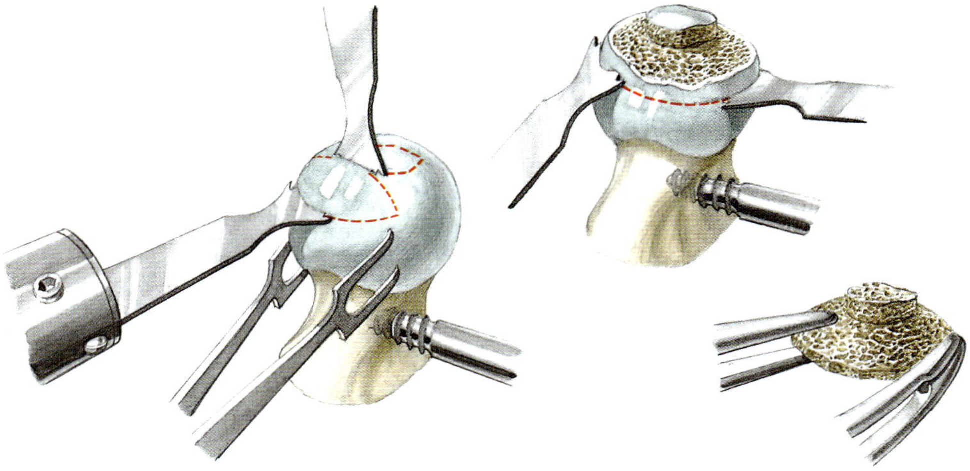

Fig. 4.**119** The graft resembles a hat.

(Fig. 4.**122**), and cements the acetabular component. Where the floor of the reconstructed acetabulum is thin, a collared acetabular cup is used.

Reconstruction is difficult when the floor of the acetabulum is missing completely after superomedial component migration and if the acetabulum opens into an expanding funnel that extends superiorly and medially (see Fig. 4.**104 e**). The surgeon must attempt to implant the femoral head into the inside of the bony ridge which represents the remains of the acetabular roof (Fig. 4.**123 a**), and insert the screws transversely above it from outside. Additional structural grafts are then impacted into the gap between the grafted femoral head and the inferior acetabular bone. The grafts are then hollowed out with a narrow, curved saw blade (see Fig. 4.**111**, insert), and the new acetabulum is carefully reamed to accommodate the acetabular component (Fig. 4.**123 b**). The cup must have a collar (see Fig. 4.**117 c**) because this type of construct does not have high stability. The primary forces acting on the transverse screws and the interface (which lies nearly parallel to the resultant force in the hip) are shear forces (see Fig. 4.**105 d**).

Reconstruction with screw fixation alone becomes very difficult where an open protrusion is accompanied by an absent anterior or (worse) posterior acetabular rim, or nearly impossible in cases where both are missing (see Fig. 4.**136**). These hips should be reconstructed using implants, such as metal acetabular cups with screw flanges and hooks, or alternatively, a saddle prosthesis (see Fig. 4.**126**) may be inserted.

When an acetabular cup with flanges is to be used, first a femoral head is implanted into the inside of the remaining acetabular roof and fixed with one or two cancellous screws (Fig. 4.**124**), as described previously (see Fig. 4.**123**). An initial cavity is excavated in the graft, which is then reamed. Generally, there is not enough anterior and/or posterior acetabular rim remaining to permit fastening additional structural grafts between the grafted head and the other parts of the acetabulum. Stability is achieved by screwing the flanges into the ilium and inserting the hook to engage the obturator foramen (Fig. 4.**125**).

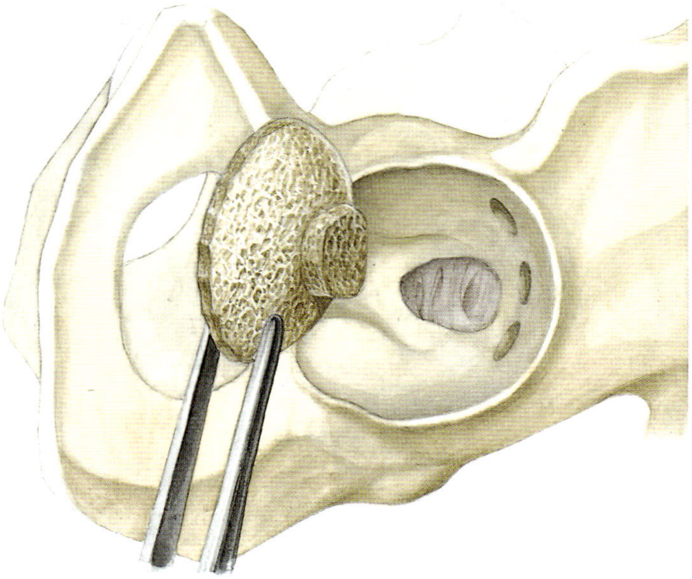

Fig. 4.**120** Inserting the hat-shaped acetabular graft.

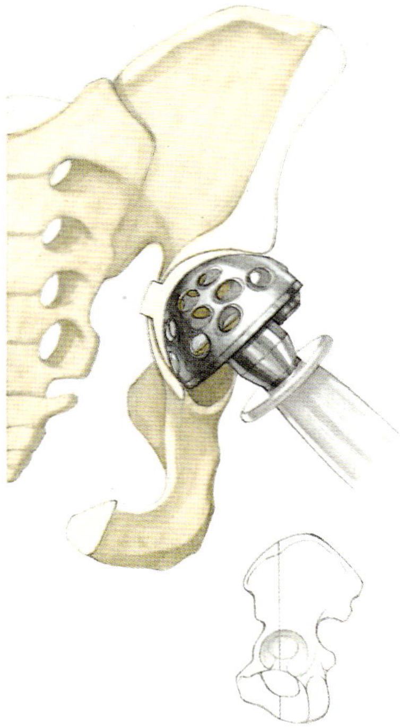

Fig. 4.**121** Reaming the graft. The top of the graft is shaped to match an asymmetrical perforation to prevent it from turning with a reamer.

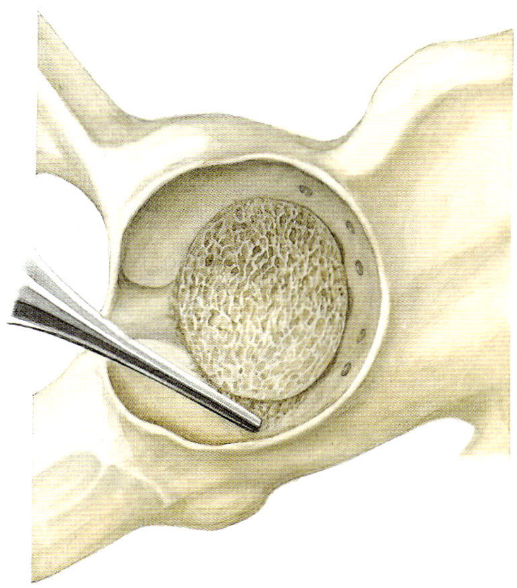

Fig. 4.**122** Filling remaining gaps and sealing sutures with cancellous chips. Cement retention holes are drilled in the recipient bone and the graft.

Long screw flanges require dissecting the anterior origins of the abductors off the ilium far enough to permit fastening screws in the flanges (see Fig. 4.**26**). Shorter flanges can be accommodated underneath the abductors after exposing the roof of the acetabulum through a posterior approach (see Fig. 4.**12**). The screws can be fastened to the ilium, if necessary, through the muscle.

After the flanges have been fixed, the surgeon inserts the hook to engage the obturator foramen (Fig. 4.**125**) or fastens a screw flange to the superior pubic ramus. If a hook is used, the bone superior to the obturator foramen is exposed by subperiosteal dissection to avoid damaging the obturator nerve. The hook can be attached through several inferior holes in the cup. Next, one or two screws are inserted superiorly into the graft through holes in the cup, and a polyethylene cup is cemented into it.

The screw flanges can be contoured to a certain degree if the implant does not fit, but the best method of dealing with extensive defects is to construct a model of the hip and manufacture an appropriate inplant. The accuracy of such a model depends on how successfully metallic artefacts caused by the old implant can be suppressed in the CT scans.

The graft and the hook in the obturator foramen or the screw flange on the superior pubic ramus provide a buttress to prevent the metal cup from tilting medially. However, it would be overly optimistic to assume that such a construct can close an open pelvic ring while restoring physiological stress transfer.

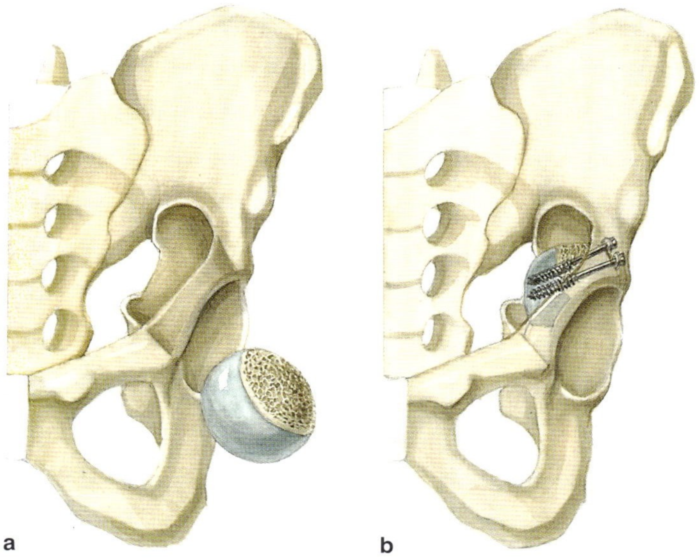

Fig. 4.**123a** and **b** Damage caused by superomedial component migration. Open protrusion where the anterior and posterior rims of the acetabulum are intact.

a Implanting a graft into the inside of the remains of the acetabular roof.

b The graft is fixed with screws inserted transversely above the acetabular roof. Additional structural grafts are impacted between the grafted femoral head and the inferior acetabular bone. Then the new acetabulum is reamed.

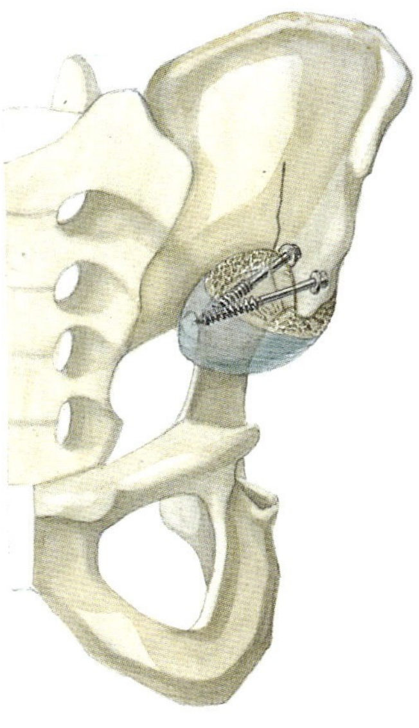

Fig. 4.**124** Damage caused by superomedial component migration. Open protrusion with loss of the anterior rim of the acetabulum accompanied by a fracture of the iliac wing. A graft is implanted into the inside of the remaining acetabular roof and then reamed.

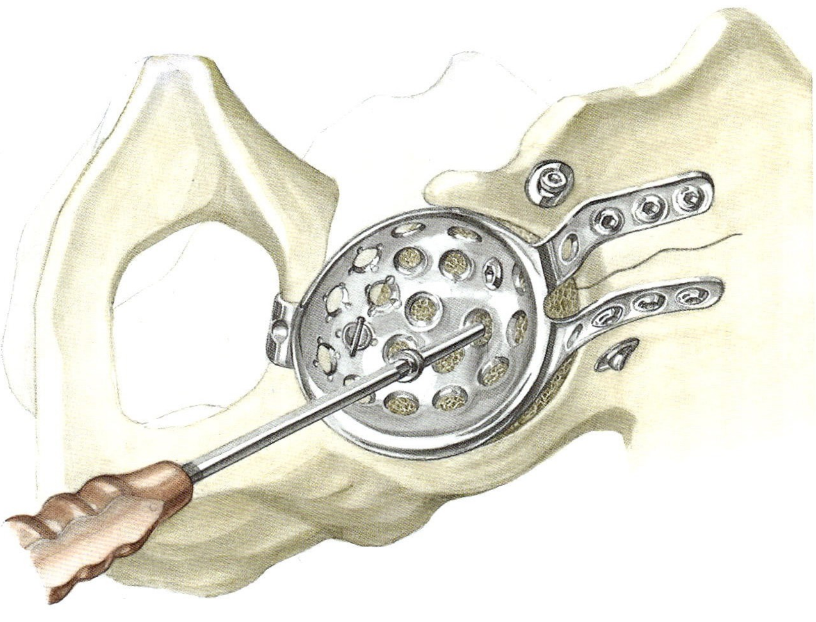

Fig. 4.**125** Implanting a metal acetabular cup with screw flanges on the iliac bone and a hook that engages the obturator foramen. The component is fixed to the graft with screws, and a polyethylene cup is cemented into it.

Saddle Prosthesis

Description of Implant

A metal saddle resting on a polyethylene-bearing sleeve rotates on a peg on a base. The base is available in several lengths (depending on the amount of bone loss) and is attached to the stem taper in place of a femoral head.

A set screw with a blunt tip engages a circumferential groove in the peg without placing any load on the metal. The set screw prevents the saddle and base from dislocating.

A locking pin within the conical recess of the base engages an eccentric slot in the face of the taper and prevents rotational instability within the conical mounting. This is necessary because unlike an implant with a spherical femoral head, axial torques (depending on the length of the base) can occur in a saddle prosthesis (Fig. 4.**126**).

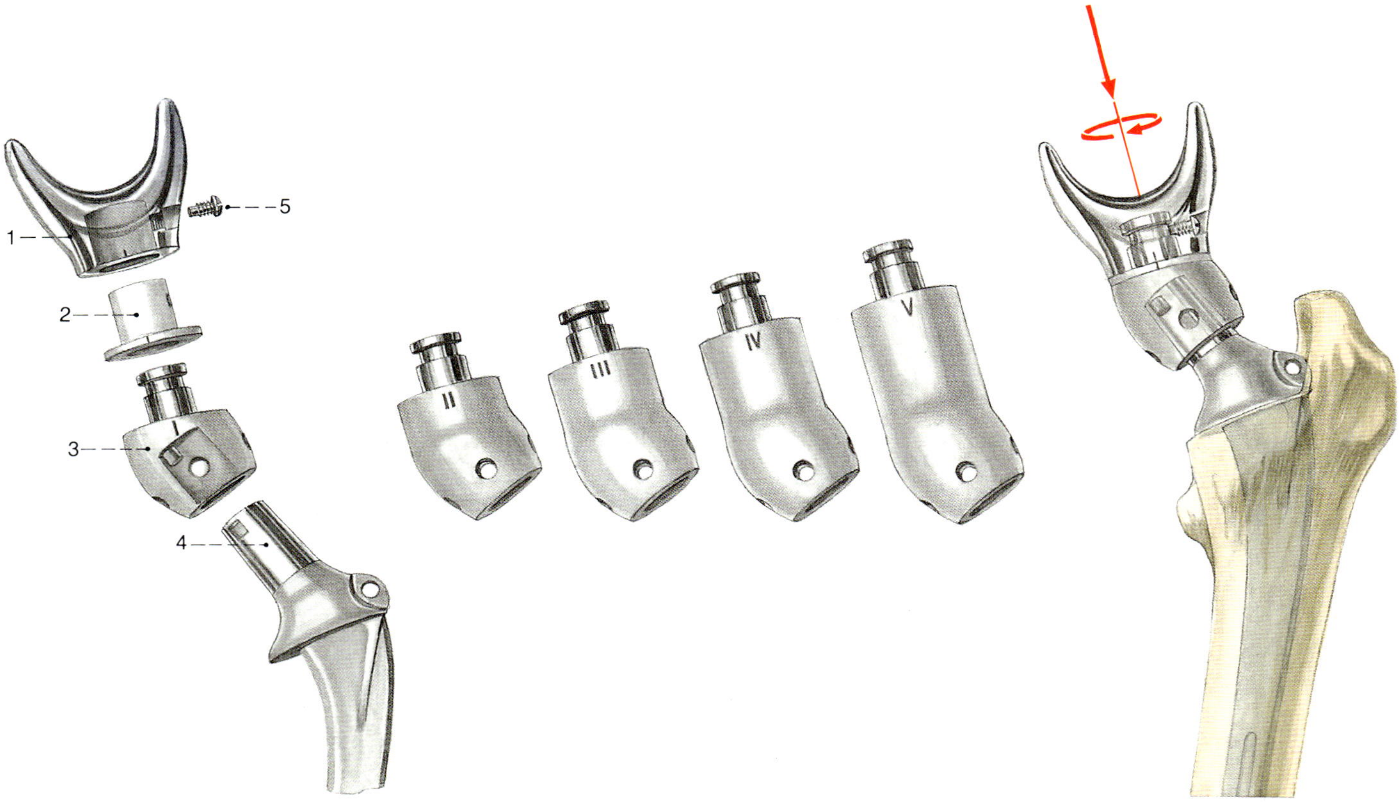

Fig. 4.**126** Saddle Prosthesis

1 Saddle
2 Bearing sleeve
3 Base with locking pin that engages taper
4 Taper with eccentric slot engaged by locking pin
5 Set screw for locking saddle to base

Anatomy

The saddle prosthesis articulates against a notch that the surgeon makes within the iliac remnants, as far medial as possible in stronger bone. One horn of the saddle lies within the true pelvis and is covered by the psoas major or the iliacus (Fig. 4.**127a**); the other is outside the pelvis and is coverd by the gluteus minimus (Fig. 4.**127b**).

The notch between the two horns of the saddle is perpendicular to the notch in the bone. Thus, when the site of articulation is inferior to the linea terminalis, the saddle horns generally lie within the coronal plane (depending on the sagittal direction of the inner wall of the lateral part of the small pelvis, see Fig. 4.**132**). If the site is superior to the linea terminalis within the bone of the large pelvis, the medial horn is more or less in anteversion (depending on the oblique curvature of the iliac wing, see Fig. 4.**137b**).

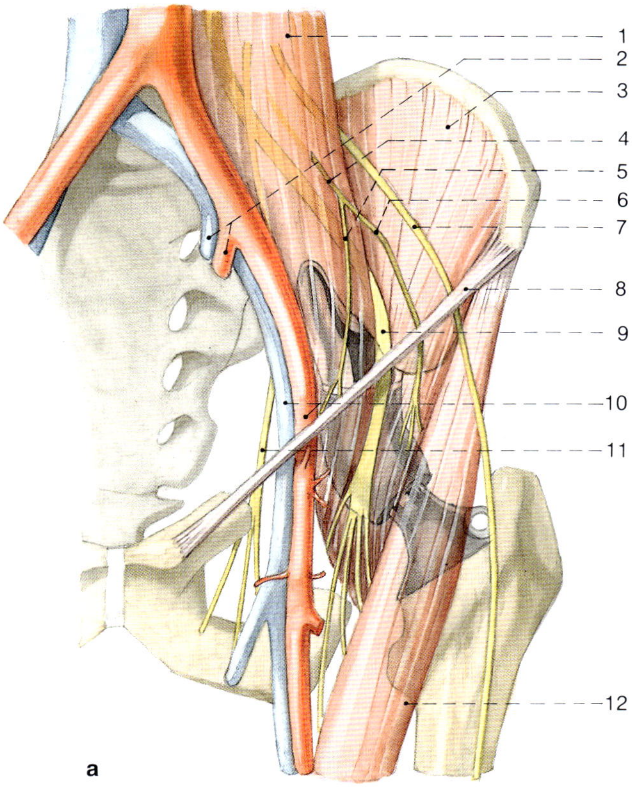

a

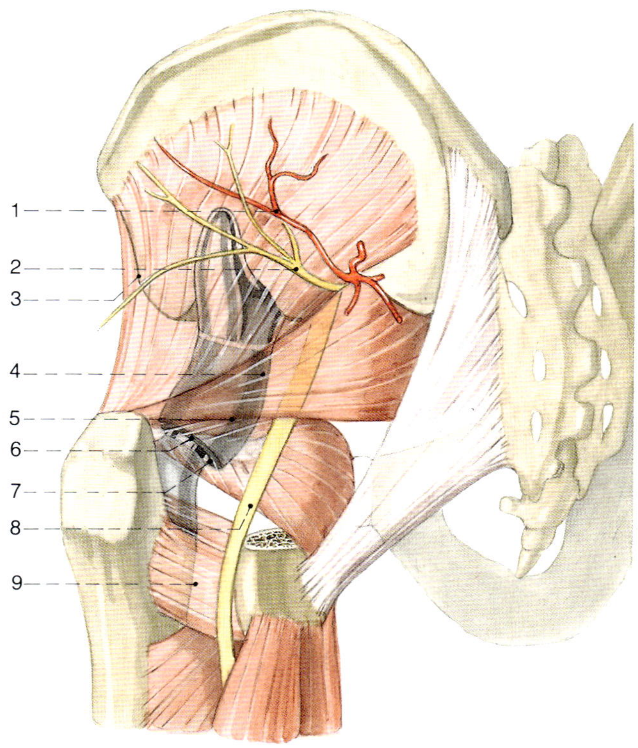

b

Fig. 4.**127a** and **b** Anatomy of the saddle articulation.

a Anterior view

1 Psoas major
2 Internal iliac artery and vein
3 Iliacus
4 Genitofemoral nerve
5 Genital branch
6 Femoral branch
7 Lateral femoral cutaneous nerve
8 Inguinal ligament
9 Femoral nerve
10 External iliac artery and vein
11 Obturator nerve
12 Sartorius

b Posterior view

1 Superficial branch of the superior gluteal artery
2 Superior gluteal nerve
3 Gluteus minimus
4 Piriformis
5 Superior gemellus
6 Obturator internus
7 Inferior gemellus
8 Sciatic nerve
9 Quadratus femoris

Motion

The articulation between the bone and the saddle permits the leg to be turned in any direction. Rotation, which a saddle articulation cannot provide, is made possible within the articulation between saddle and base. Thus, the prosthetic hip allows flexion, extension, adduction, abduction, and rotation like a ball and socket joint (Fig. 4.**128**).

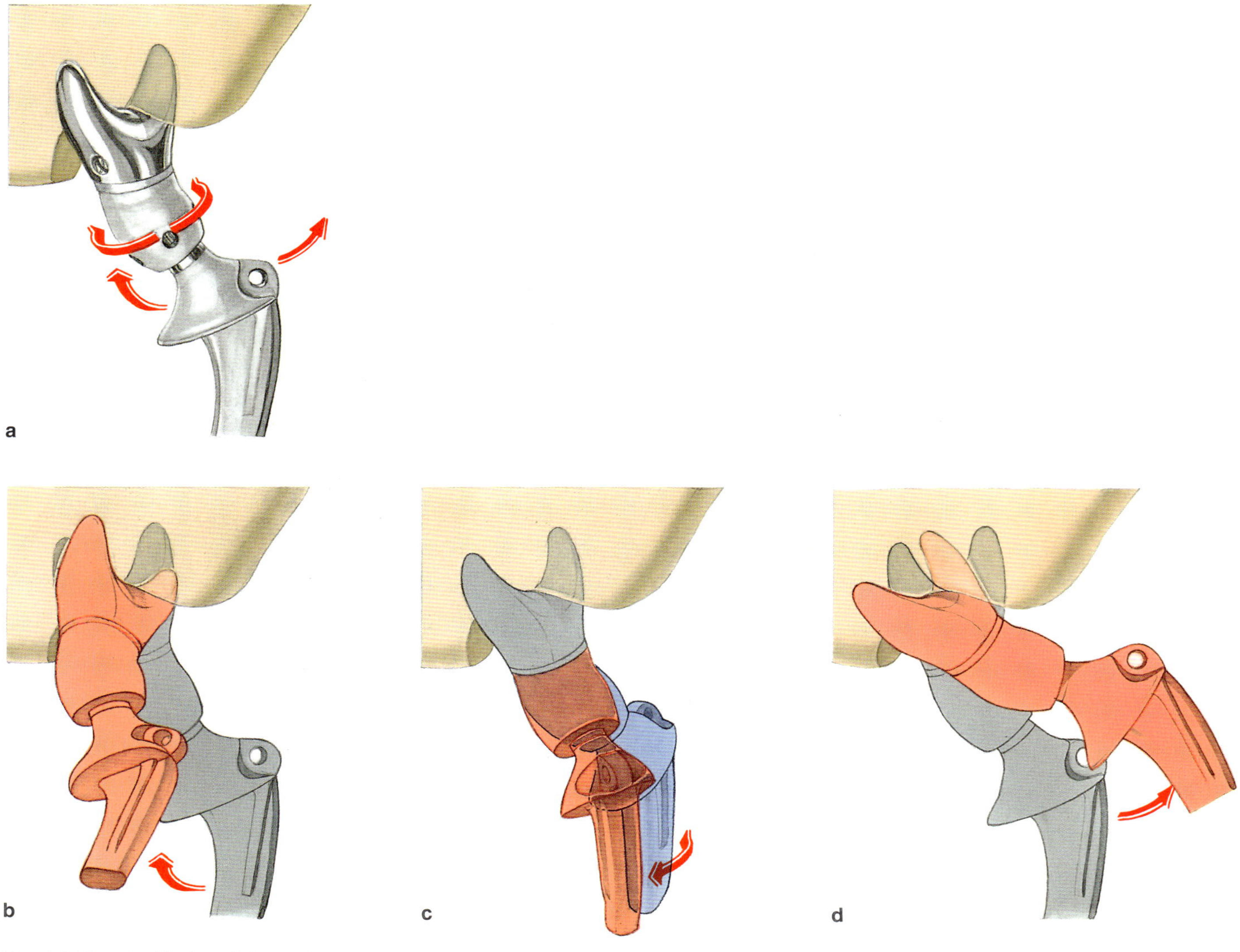

Fig. 4.**128a–d** Motion of the saddle articulation.
a The bone-saddle articulation permits turning the limb in any direction; the articulation between saddle and base allows rotation.
b Flexion
c Rotation
d Abduction

Statics

If the abductors are intact (which is unfortunately seldom the case when the saddle prosthesis is indicated) the patient will be able to stand on one leg because the prosthetic design preserves the physiological offset and thus the balance of moments (Fig. 4.**129a**). This also applies if the saddle articulates higher up the pelvic bone, provided all articulation sites and the implant's rotational axis and that of the bases lie within the resultant force (the higher up the pelvic bone, the farther medial and thus within the stronger iliac bone; Fig. 4.**129** and see Fig 4.**126**).

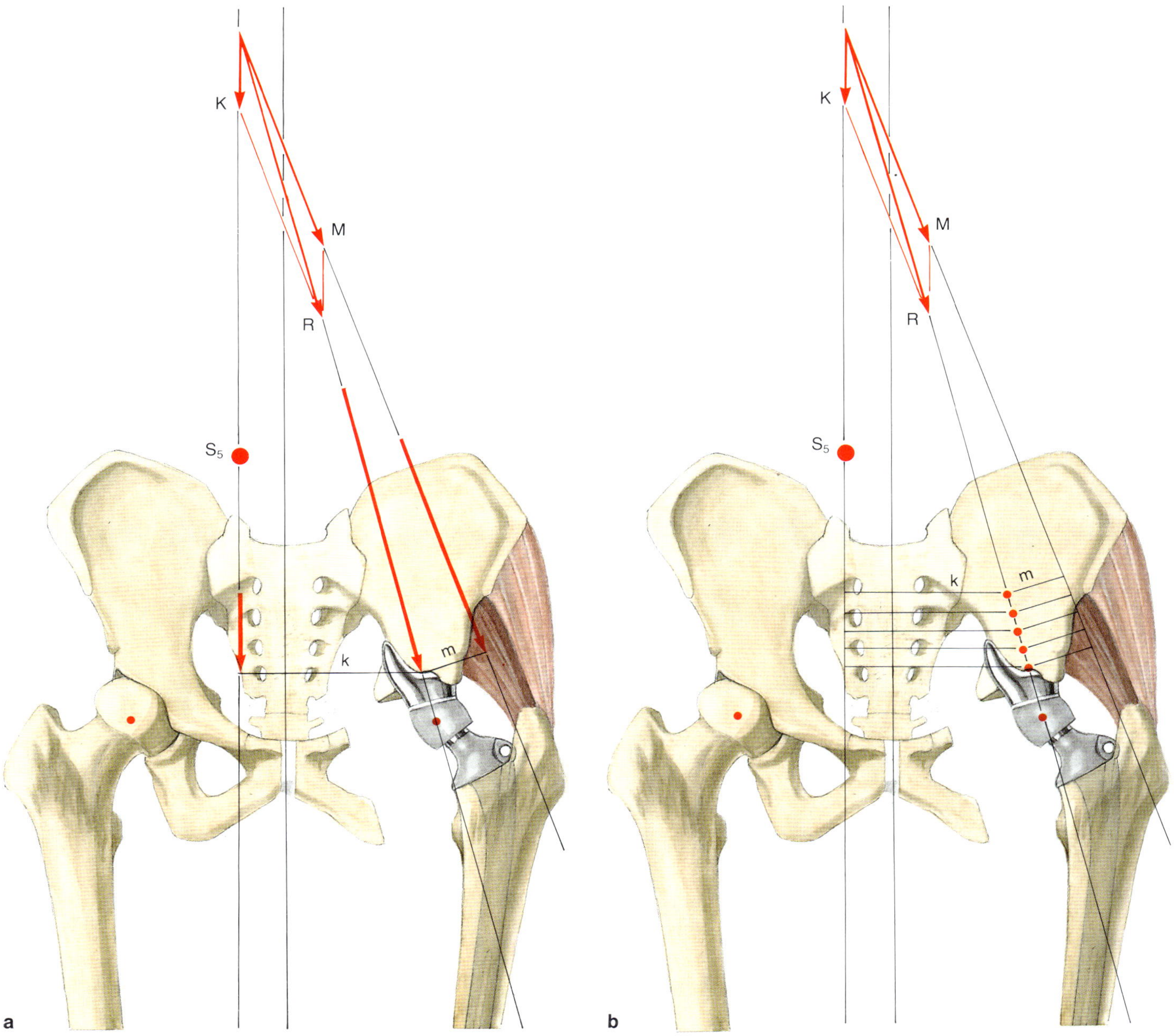

Fig. 4.**129a** and **b** Statics of the saddle articulation. Theoretical conditions for balance of moments (acc. to Pauwels; M · m = K · k)
a Articulation at the site of a ball and socket joint
b Articulation higher up the iliac bone

S_s = Body's center of gravity
K = Force of body weight
M = Force of abductors
R = Resultant force in the hip
k = Lever arm of K
m = Lever arm of M

These are the theoretical and idealized conditions. The conditions actually encountered at revision arthroplasty (and after resection of a tumor) are worse in the majority of cases.

After superolateral migration of the acetabular component the site of the saddle articulation is shifted into a medial position because the saddle articulates against a notch within the medial wall of the iliac bone (see Fig. 4.**132 b**). After superomedial migration of the cup the situation is vice versa, because the saddle articulates against the lateral wall of the iliac bone (see Fig. 4.**135 b**). Furthermore, if the saddle articulates higher up the pelvic bone there is an increased parallel superior displacement of the femur in the sagittal or coronal plane in flexion and abduction (Fig. 4.**130**). These circumstances alter the lever arms of all muscles and impair their function.

Ultimately, as with a ball and socket joint, function of the saddle arthroplasty depends on the quality of the remaining hip muscles. But exactly those muscles which are so important for function are often no longer present.

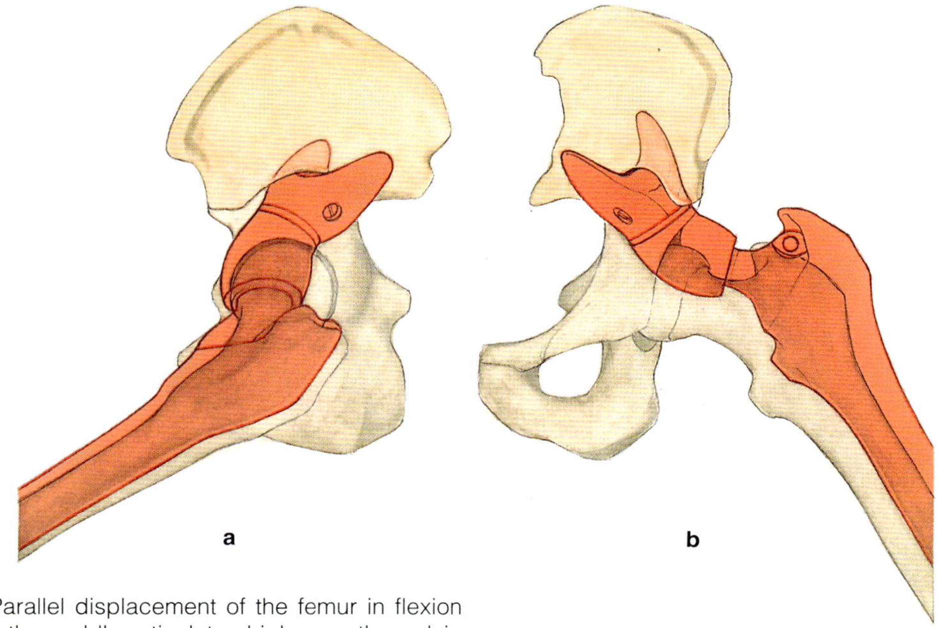

Fig. 4.**130 a** and **b** Parallel displacement of the femur in flexion and abduction when the saddle articulates higher up the pelvic bone.
a Flexion
b Abduction

Indication

The saddle prosthesis is indicated in revision total hip arthroplasty or tumor surgery when reconstruction of the acetabulum is no longer possible. Indications include lack of suitable graft material or a patient who is unable to tolerate more extensive surgery and/or is unable to comply with postoperative partial weight bearing, which is dictated by the insufficient stability of a reconstructed acetabulum.

Clinical considerations

Although a saddle prosthesis is appealing because of its straightforward surgical technique and because it allows immediate full weight bearing, the surgeon should first exhaust all options permitting implantation of a ball-and-socket joint. The surgeon should bear in mind that the saddle prosthesis has specific complications and should only use this implant when the acetabulum cannot be reconstructed by any other means. A resection arthroplasty, however, which the is main alternative at revision total hip arthroplasty, may result in a flail limb and in immobilization, expecially if loss of acetabular bone stock is associated with loss of the proximal femur.

Saddle Prosthesis following Superolateral Migration of the Acetabular Component

The floor of the acetabulum is generally intact after superolateral migration of the acetabular component (see Fig. 4.**104b**). It must be perforated. Using a narrow Lambotte osteotome, the surgeon carefully osteotomizes the thinnest part of the acetabular floor in a convex superior arc (Fig. 4.**131a**). Then he gradually removes bone with the Luer forceps until the opening is just large enough to accommodate the medial horn of the saddle (Fig. 4.**131b**). Thin bone of the acetabular floor inferior to this site does not have to be resected, but can be folded medially like a door.

A small hooked periosteal elevator is used to mobilize the pelvic soft tissue superiorly, anteriorly and posteriorly, creating a recess for the medial horn under the iliopsoas. The surgeon should be aware of the presence of the iliac vessls, which might be displaced and obscured by scars. Where the posteriorinferior acetabular rim interferes with extension, the surgeon removes parts of it (Fig. 4.**132a**). Any other bony structures obstructing movement of the leg are also resected.

After superolateral component migration, the articulation between the bone and the saddle is shifted medially, as is the femur. This is because the saddle articulates against a notch within the medial wall of the iliac bone (Fig. 4.**132b**).

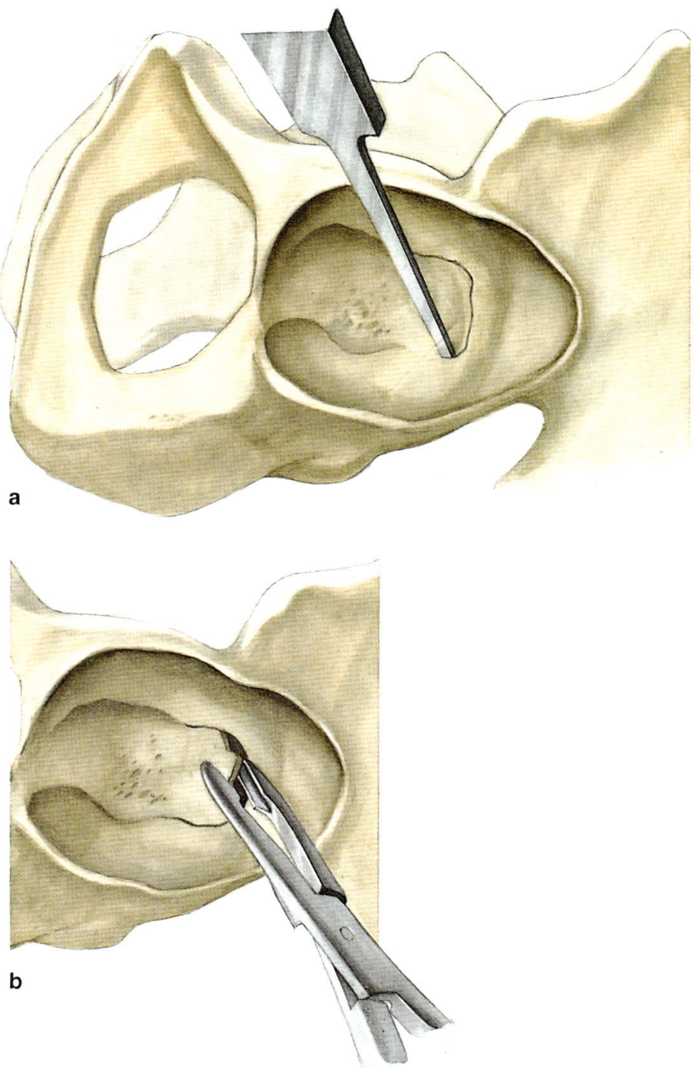
a

b

Fig. 4.**131a** and **b** Damage caused by superolateral component migration.
a Osteotomy of the acetabular floor
b Gradually opening the floor

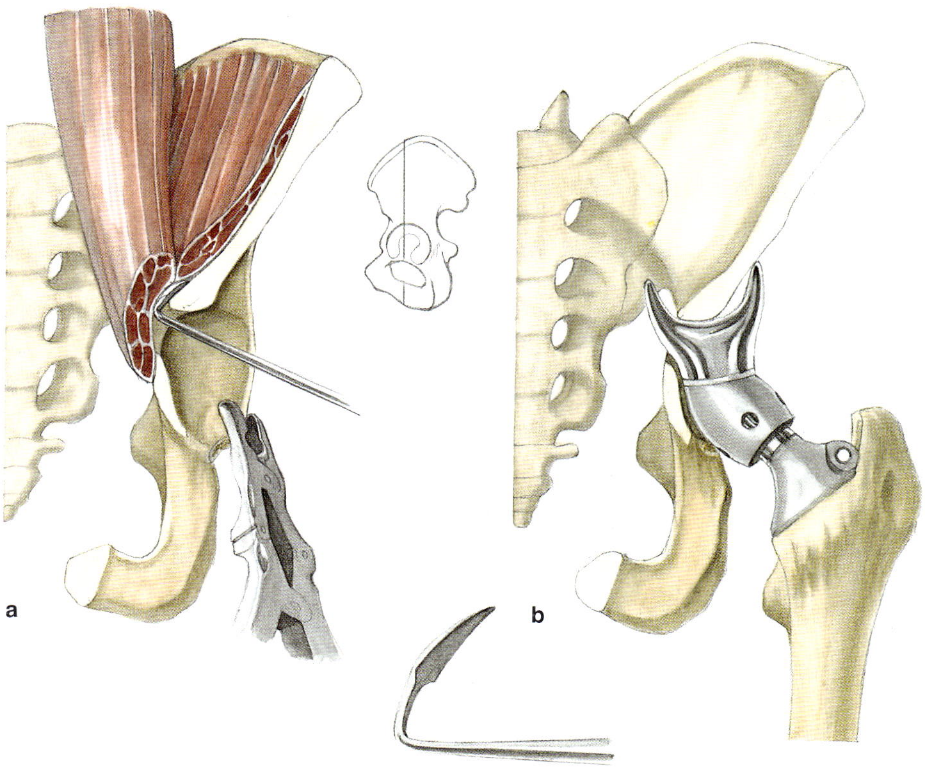
a

b

Fig. 4.**132a** and **b** Shaping a recess for the medial horn of the saddle prosthesis.
a Mobilizing the pelvic soft tissue. Removing parts of the inferior rim.
b After superolateral component migration, the articulation site is shifted medially.

Next the surgeon performs a trial reduction. The length of the base should be selected so that reduction is just barely possible with minimum play in the reduced joint. This may be difficult in the presence of extensive scar tissue. The limb is forced distally with an instrument attached to the lateral horn and/or traction is applied with a compress wrapped around the saddle (Fig. 4.**133**).

Before the saddle is finally attached onto the desired base, the base has to be securely impacted onto the taper (Fig. 4.**134**). Then the saddle is attached, the set screw inserted and the saddle prosthesis is finally reduced.

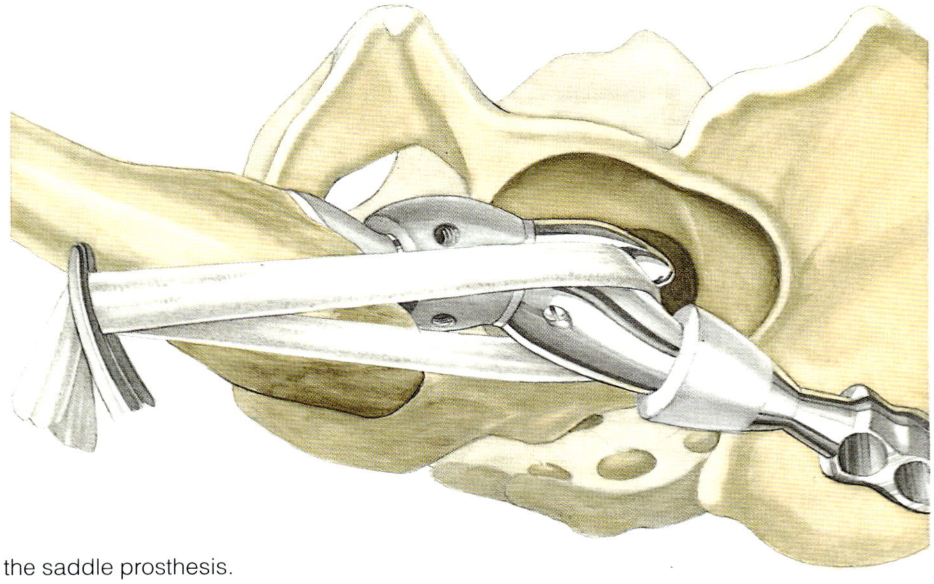

Fig. 4.**133** Reducing the saddle prosthesis.

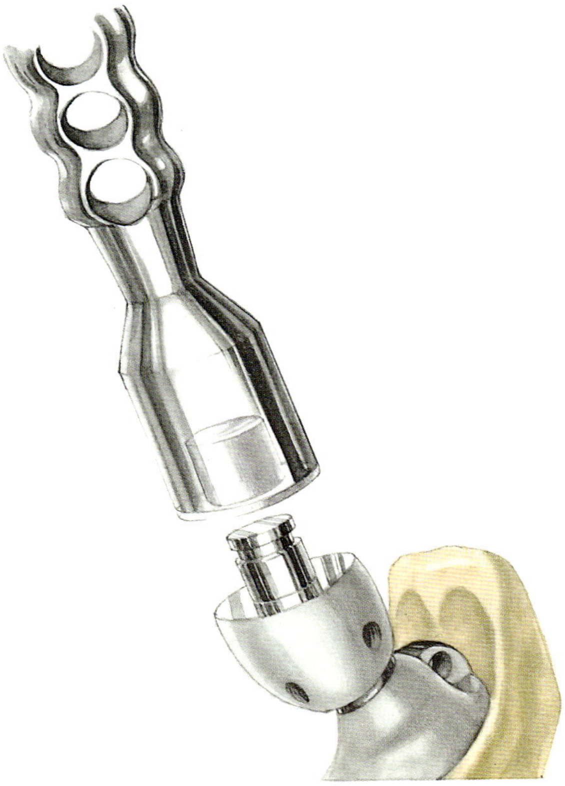

Fig. 4.**134** Impacting the base onto the taper.

Saddle Prosthesis following Superior and Superomedial Migration of the Acetabular Component

After superior and superomedial migration of the acetabular component (see Figs. 4.**104c,** 4.**104d,** and 4.**104e**), the notch for the saddle is made within the lateral part of the acetabular roof (Fig. 4.**135a**). Where the inner pelvis is separated from the joint by thin bone or a peristal layer in a closed protrusion, the floor of the acetabulum is opened so that the medial horn of the saddle prosthesis lies within the pelvis (Fig. 4.**135b**). The surgeon must ensure that the horn does not rest between the inner and outer tables of the pelvis. Again, bone that interferes with joint function may be resected. In an open protrusion (Fig. 4.**104e**), the procedure is easier. If the posterior and anterior acetabular rims are still present, it is sometimes not even necessary to shape a notch. Depending on how far the bony ridge, which represents the remains of the acetabular roof, projects, the site of the saddle articulation is shifted laterally (less so after superior migration).

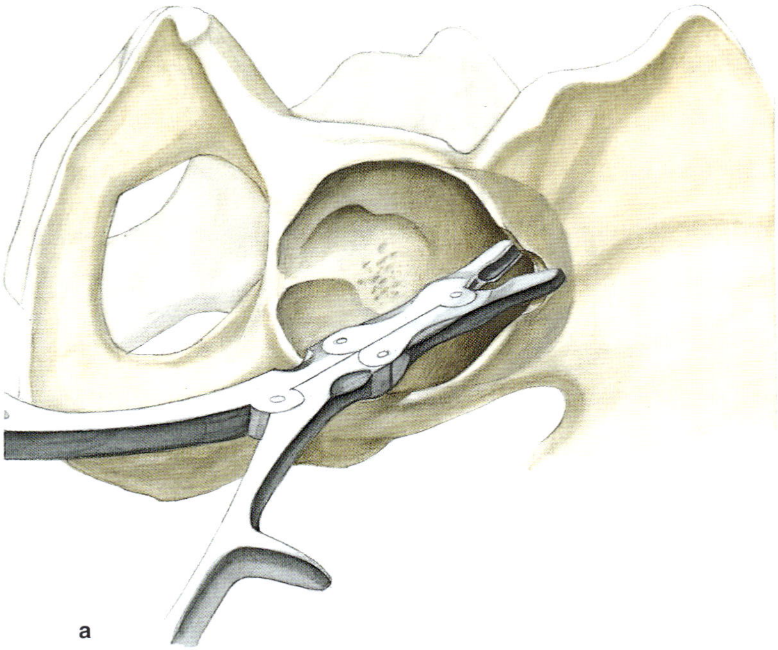

a

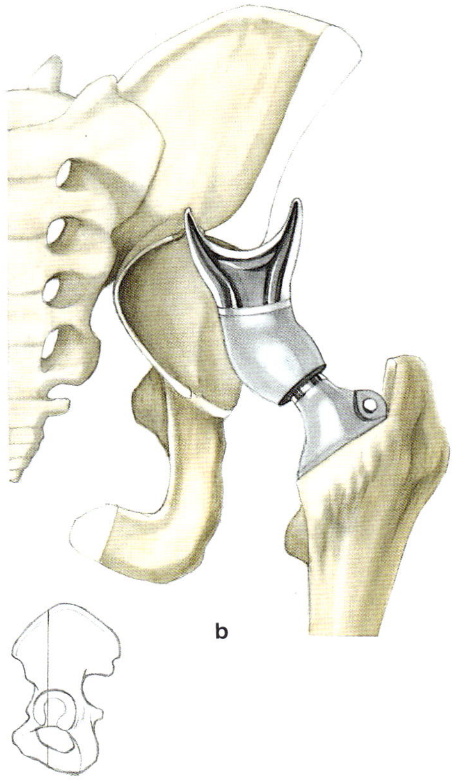

b

Fig. 4.**135a** and **b** Damage caused by superior and superomedial component migration with closed protrusion.
a Shaping the notch within the lateral remant of the acetabular roof.
b Opening the bone separating the acetabulum from the true pelvis to accommodate the medial horn of the saddle. After superomedial component migration, the articulation is shifted laterally.

Saddle Prosthesis in an Interrupted Pelvic Ring

Where the pelvic ring is partially or completely interrupted—as is generally the case in an open protrusion and interruption or loss of the anterior and/or posterior acetabular rim (Fig. 4.**136**)—the surgeon is faced with a situation that is similar to what occurs after resecting an acetabular tumor (see Fig. 4.**137**).

After resecting a tumor, the surgeon makes the notch within the distal margin of the ilium so that its depth matches that of the saddle (Fig. 4.**137**). In revision arthroplasty, osteotomizing the bone is often unnecessary if remains of the anterior or posterior acetabular rim or strong scar tissue with areas of pseudarthrosis are present.

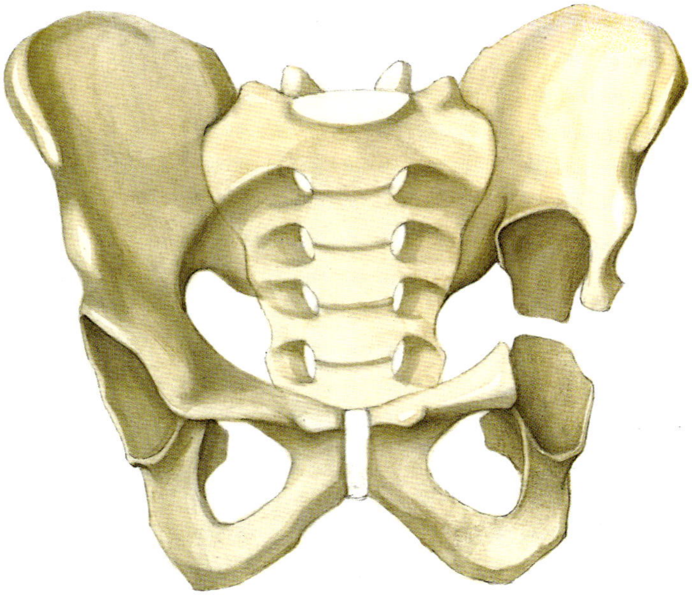

Fig. 4.**136** Interrupted pelvic ring at revision arthroplasty.

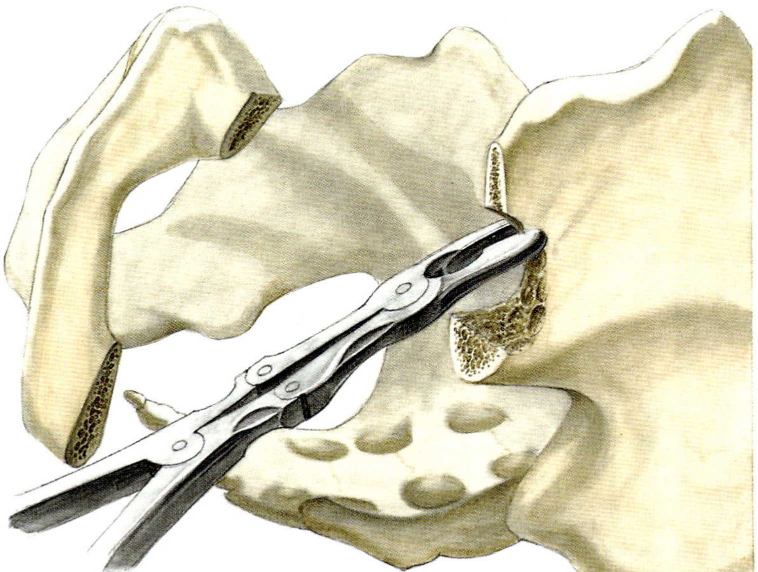

a

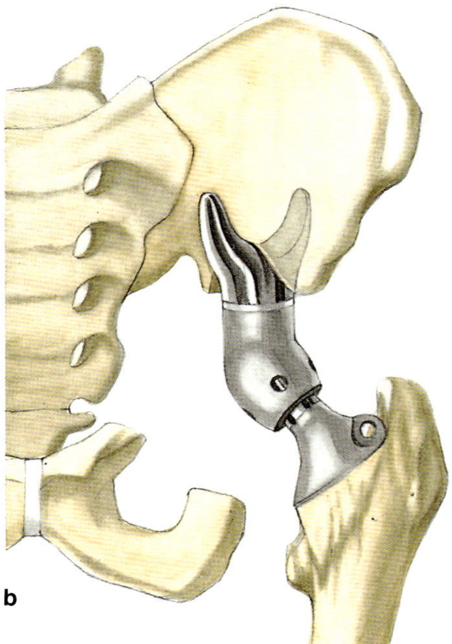

b

Fig. 4.**137 a** and **b** Interrupted pelvic ring after resection of an acetabulum and saddle arthroplasty.

a Making a notch within the iliac bone.
b Saddle prosthesis after reduction.

Dislocation between the Saddle and Bone

Most dislocations of the saddle articulation occur in the first few weeks postoperatively. The mechanism of dislocation is either "unhooking" or "drifting."

Where there is bone or strong scar tissue anterior and posterior to the articulation between saddle and bone, the saddle can dislocate only by "unhooking" due to insufficient tension in the soft tissue bridging the joint (Fig. 4.**138**). To dislocate in this manner, the prosthesis must travel a distance equal to the depth of the saddle—(far more than the distance required to dislocate a ball-and-socket joint). This mechanism of dislocation can be largely eliminated by selecting the length of the base so that reduction is just barely possible with minimum play in the reduced joint. In revision total hip arthroplasty, where there is often excessive soft-tissue tension due to scarring, this dislocation mechanism is rare. After resection of the acetabulum, however, the tension in the remaining soft tissue is generally reduced so that "unhooking" can occur more frequently. An increase in leg length must often be accepted in these patients.

Where the anterior and/or posterior acetabular rim is missing, the saddle can "drift" anteriorly and/or posteriorly while turning the leg depending on the respective defect (Fig. 4.**139 a**). This risk can be reduced by fixing a graft at the critical site, or by tying the saddle to the ilium with a loop of strong absorbable suture material. The loop is attached in such a manner that it prevents dislocation without restricting the joint's motion (Fig. 4.**139 b**). "Drift" dislocations generally occur following tumor surgery because the pelvic ring is interrupted after resection of an acetabular tumor. In contrast, the pelvic ring encountered in revision total hip arthroplasty is either intact or held together with areas of pseudarthrosis and scarring.

When dislocation occurs, the surgeon should first attempt closed reduction. This is often unsuccessful because the saddle twists as soon as one of the horns comes into contact with the bone. Where open reduction is indicated, a small incision (through which a finger can be inserted) may be sufficient. If this is not successful, the joint must be exposed. Surgical options include implanting a longer base, deepening the notch in the ilium, removing the structure that acts as a fulcrum, fixing a graft, or fastening the saddle with suture material.

The surgeon should assess the full range of motion intraoperatively to prevent undesired motion in the postoperative phase. If there is a significant risk of dislocation, the patient should be immobilized with an abduction pillow and short leg cast, an abduction cast (see Fig. 4.**175**), or light traction while the wound heals and should be fitted with an abduction orthosis then thereafter.

After a few weeks, a capsule will form around the saddle joint at a sufficient distance to permit joint movement. Ideally, the capsule will ossify, and the load-bearing area of the joint will sclerose (Fig. 4.**140**). Dislocations of the saddle are rare after these changes have taken place.

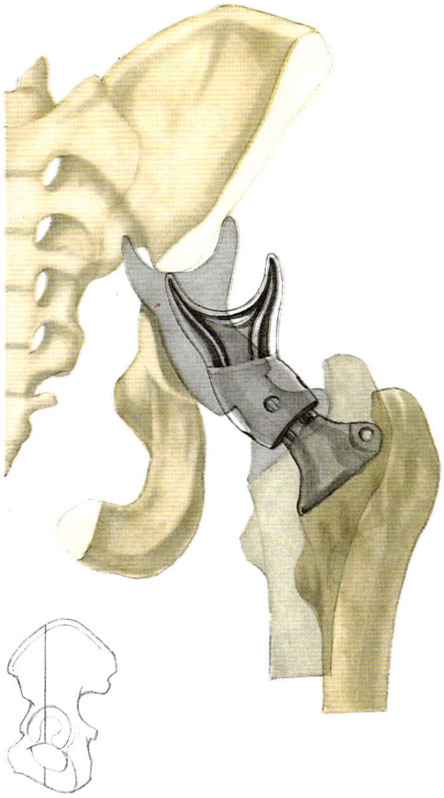

Fig. 4.**138** Dislocation where the saddle "unhooks" due to insufficient soft-tissue tension.

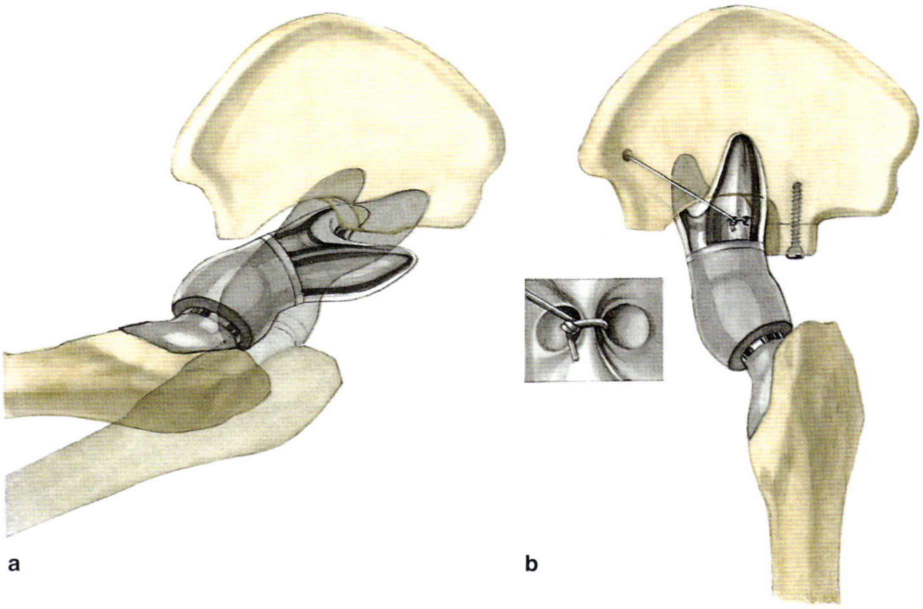

Fig. 4.**139 a** and **b** Dislocation where the saddle "drifts" along an interrupted pelvic ring.
a Saddle "drifts" posteriorly with the hip in flexion and/or abduction.
b Fixing a structural graft and tying the saddle.

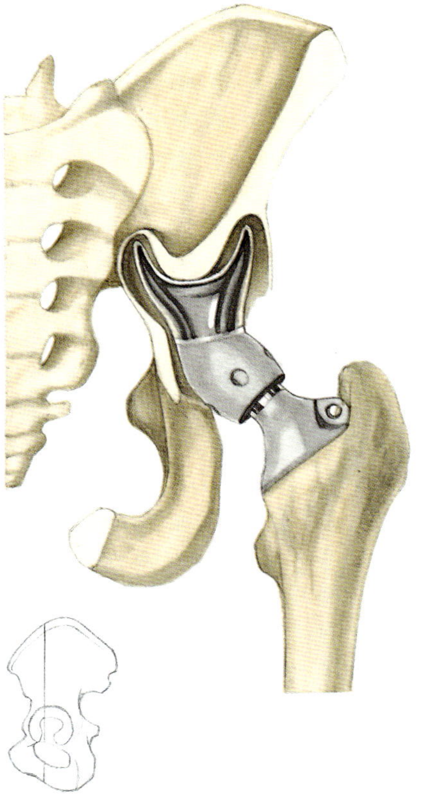

Fig. 4.**140** Formation of new bone around the horns of the saddle and sclerosis in the load-bearing area of the bone indicate successful stabilization and significantly reduced probability of dislocation between saddle and bone.

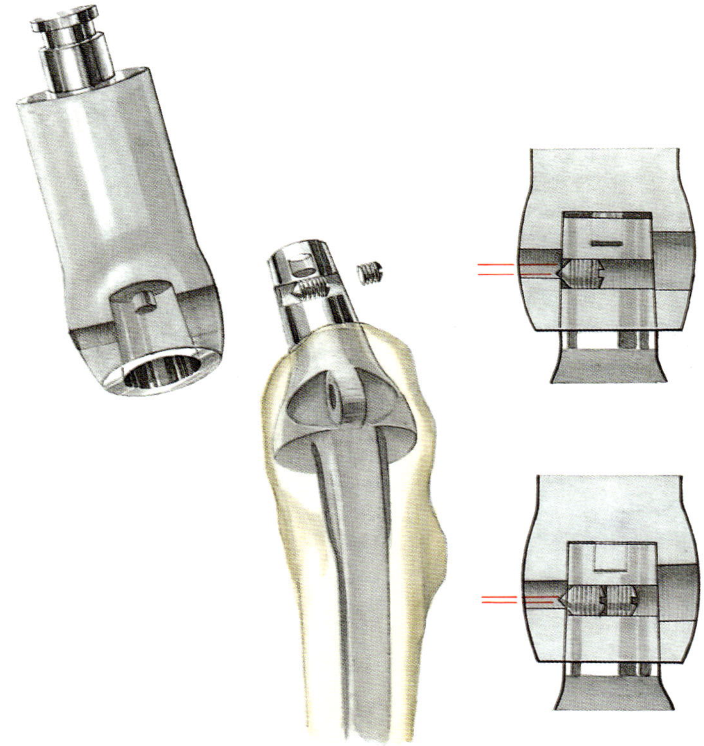

Fig. 4.**141** Saddle prosthesis with a "lost" set screw in the taper for extra long bases. The set screw is advanced through a posterior hole into an anterior hole in the base. The tip of the set screw engages the anterior hole eccentrically, drawing the base onto the taper. The set screw is blocked with a second blunt screw. The connection allows the taper to settle further.

Dislocation between the Base and Taper

Dislocations between the base and taper rarely occur in revision total hip arthroplasty because there is generally a great deal of tension in the soft tissue, and a short base is usually implanted. Using a long or an extra-long base in tumor surgery can induce varus forces that can damage the connection to the taper and cause loosening. This can result in dislocation between the base and taper, particularly in the presence of reduced tension in the soft-tissue and when surrounding bone or scar tissue prevent dislocation of the joint between saddle and bone.

This risk can be reduced by using a custom implant with an enlarged taper connection and/or by providing greater primary stability of the taper connection. This is achieved by using a stem with a "lost" screw in a threaded sagittal hole in the taper (Fig. 4.**141**).

The base is securely impacted onto the taper (see Fig. 4.**134**). Through a larger posterior hole in the base, the surgeon advances the "lost" set screw toward a narrower anterior hole in the base. The tapered tip of the set screw engages the anterior hole, achieving a tighter taper connection than is possible by impaction alone. The set screw is locked in place with a second blunt screw. Because the tip of the set screw engages the anterior hole eccentrically it does not prevent the taper connection from settling further (Fig. 4.**141**).

Superior Migration of the Saddle and Pelvic Fracture

Almost every saddle migrates a few millimeters during the first few months postoperatively as it forms its articular surface in the bone. New bone formation around the saddle horns and sclerosing of the surface of the bone articulating with the saddle are indications that the implant is stable and will not migrate further (see Fig. 4.**140**). However, some saddle arthroplasties show little or no bone reaction and varying rates of continued migration. In addition, a few traumatic and spontaneous fractures of the iliac wing have been known to occur.

If the saddle migrates rapidly or the iliac wing is fractured, the surgeon can attempt implantation of a metal acetabulum cup with screw flanges (see Fig. 4.**125**). If implantation is unsuccessful, the only remaining option is a resection arthroplasty, although this creates an unstable hip joint and a flail limb in the majority of cases.

Supplement: Mounting a Saddle Prosthesis on a Taper from a Different System

Where a saddle prosthesis is indicated and an existing stem from a different system without a slotted taper is to be utilized, the surgeon must achieve rotational stability at the taper by other means.

This is done by using a base without a locking pin but with four threaded holes on its lower circumference. The surgeon impacts the base onto the taper in neutral rotation, i.e., with the base inclined medially, as tightly as possible (see Fig. 4.**134**). Next, a drill guide is successively screwed into two or three of the threaded holes, and the surgeon drills holes through the guide into the taper using a carbide-tipped bit (Fig. 4.**142a**). After removing the base, the surgeon enlarges and deepens the holes with a larger bit (Fig. 4.**142b**). The base is then impacted onto the taper again, and the surgeon inserts set screws through the threaded holes of the base into the holes in the taper (Fig. 4.**142c**). Cement is pressed in the threaded holes over the set screws to secure them against loosening (Fig. 4.**142d**).

This an improvised solution. Transverse screws inserted into the taper may prevent the taper connection from settling further. This should only be done when the patient's condition contraindicates stem replacement and a saddle prosthesis is the only option available for mobilizing the hip.

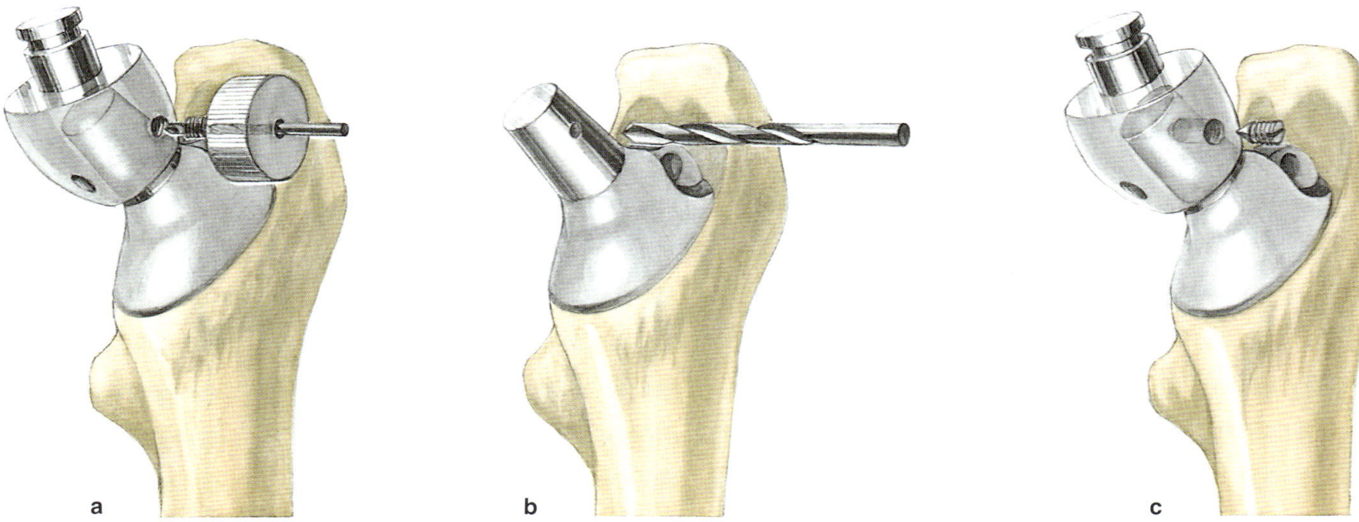

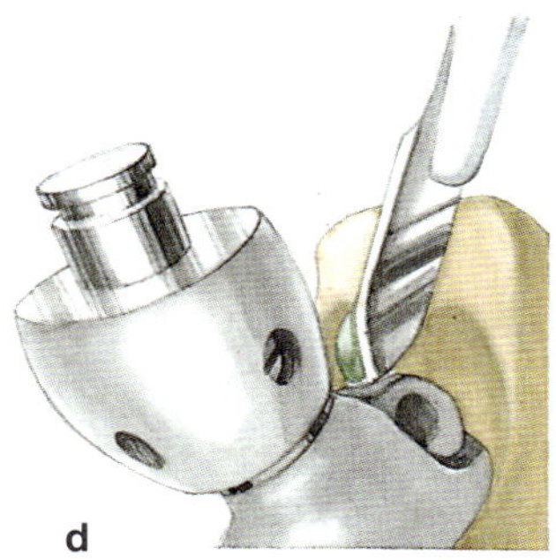

Fig. 4.**142a–d** Mounting a saddle prosthesis on a stem from a different system without a slotted taper. This is only indicated when other options are not available, since the set screw may prevent the taper connection from settling further.
a Using a guide to drill two or three holes in the taper.
b Enlarging and deepening the holes.
c Fixing the base with set screws.
d Securing the set screws with cement.

Reimplanting Femoral Components

Implanting long-stem femoral components is indicated in revision total hip arthroplasty when:

- Loosening has weakened the proximal femur, and the new stem must be fixed further distally
- Defects resulting from complications, such as a perforation or stem migration, or left by surgical procedures, such as a localized or full-length window or an osteotomy must be bridged
- A preoperative or intraoperative fracture occurs, and extramedullary internal fixation cannot provide sufficient stability

After femoral loosening reconstruction, graft should always be considered as an alternative to implantation of a long-stem femoral component. Where such attempts fail, subsequent revision surgery generally requires increasingly longer stems.

A long-stem implant is no longer indicated when even the femoral diaphysis is unable to provide sufficient support and only the distal femur remains intact. A total femoral prosthesis (see Fig. 4.**153**) is indicated in these patients. Given the uncertain fixation it offers, the distal femur alone is used to support implants only in palliative cases and in one-stage exchange operation (Buchholz' and Lodenkämper's method) to avoid introducing bacteria into the knee joint if the infection cannot be controlled by this measure.

Resection arthroplasty after loss of the proximal femur always leads to a shortened limb with poor functional results.

Please refer to the chapter on primary total hip arthroplasty for the surgical technique involved in implanting standard-length stems in patients with good bone stock.

Long-Stem Implants

Long-Stem Implants after Stem Loosening

Where loosening has damaged the proximal femur and the cortex is thin and widened, a longer stem must be implanted to permit anchoring the implant distally in intact bone.

Where the proximal femur is still intact and able to provide at least partial support for the stem, an anatomically shaped cemented stem may be implanted (Fig. 4.**143**). This stem may extend as far as the femoral diaphysis. Femoral heads with varying depths of the taper recess to provide different neck lengths should be available because proper soft-tissue tension is crucial to prevent dislocation and hip instability. Since revision arthroplasty is less durable than primary arthroplasty, good cement technique becomes particularly important (Please refer to the chapter on primary total hip arthroplasty). A cement restrictor is inserted prior to cementing the stem. Bone is used in aseptic cases; other materials include cellulose gauze or plastic. Tightly rolled cellulose gauze should be used, because it will be absorbed, it expands distal to the isthmus and usually does not slip further. This is not so with plastic cement restrictors, which can then become difficult to remove in subsequent revision surgery. A cement restrictor should rest immediately distal to the end of the stem to minimize the residual plug of cement that will have to be removed in any future revision.

If the proximal femur is completely incapable of supporting the implant, the stem should extend at least as far as the distal diaphysis and should have a larger cross section to minimize the risk of implant fatigue fracture. The implant may also require an anterior bow. In aseptic cases in which the proximal femur is absent or deficient, a polyethylene sleeve is used to minimize stem subsidence (Fig. 4.**144**). Radiographs at defined distances in two planes are required to determine the length, diameter, and anteversion of the stem and to calculate the dimensions of the polyethylene sleeve (see Figs. 4.**2** and 4.**3**). The sleeve dimensions are calculated generously because the sleeve can easily be shortened intraoperatively. The abductors, vastus and gluteal soft tissue, and even the fascia lata may be sutured to holes in the prosthetic greater trochanter. This minimizes the danger of early postoperative dislocation and improves formation of scar tissue joining the individual soft-tissue structures. However, the surgeon should not expect to achieve a permanent bond between soft tissue and implant.

An alternative to a polyethylene sleeve in aseptic patients is to cement a proximal femoral allograft to a long-stem implant. Remaining periosteal bone and muscles are attached to the graft in an attempt to achieve a permanent bond between the soft tissue and the graft.

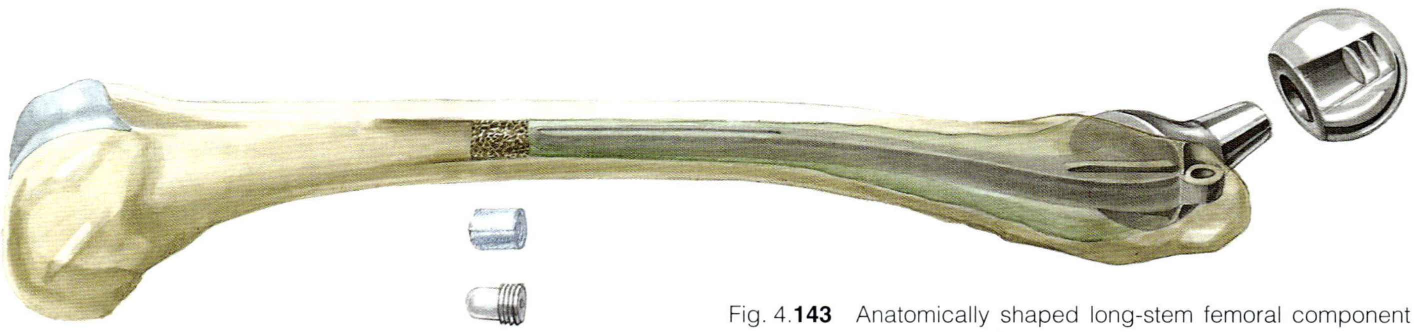

Fig. 4.**143** Anatomically shaped long-stem femoral component implanted in a proximal femur weakened by implant loosening. Femoral heads with taper recesses of varying depths. Cement restrictor of cancellous bone, rolled cellulose gauze, or plastic.

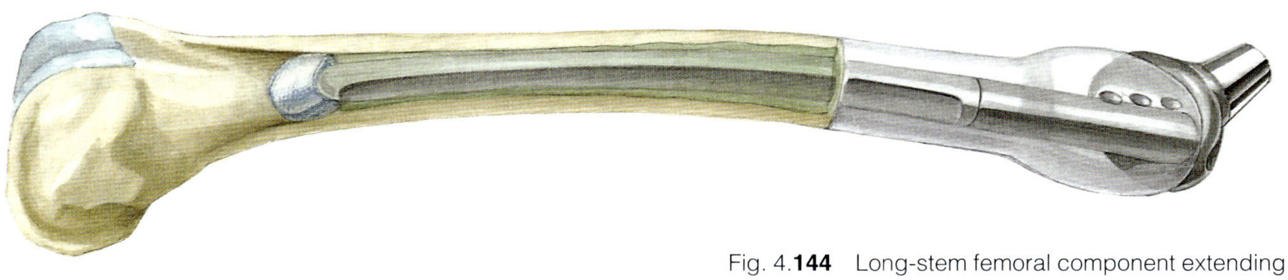

Fig. 4.**144** Long-stem femoral component extending to the distal end of the femoral diaphysis with an enlarged cross section and an anterior bow. A proximal polyethylene sleeve replaces the missing proximal femur. Cement restrictor of absorbable cellulose gauze.

Using Long-Stem Implants to Bridge Defects

If a shaft perforation occurs or a window is opened proximal to the distal end of the stem (see Figs. 4.**65a**, 4.**68a**, and 4.**68b**), the revision implant may be as short as the primary implant provided that be bone is stable (Fig. 4.**145a**).

A perforation or a window at the tip of the stem or distal to it requires implantation of a long-stem prosthesis to bridge the defect (Fig. 4.**145b**) because a defect at or distal to the top of the stem is a stress raiser with an increased risk of subsequent fracture. This applies especially when the defect interrupts the lateral cortex. There is no hard-and-fast rule for determining the length of the implant distal to the defect, but it should be proportional to the extent of the defect and the weakness of the bone.

While injecting the cement into the femoral canal, the surgeon holds a finger over any perforation or a smaller defect. A window is covered with a compress (Fig. 4.**146a**). The "lid" of the window is replaced while the cement is still soft, causing the cement to ooze out of the holes and the osteotomy gaps (Fig. 4.**146b**). The surgeon reopens the window, removes the cement from the holes and the osteotomy surfaces (Fig. 4.**146c**), and replaces the "lid" before the cement hardens. Where the bone is strong, the osteotomy gaps are small and beveled outward (see Fig. 4.**64c**), the lid sinks into the bone and fits tightly against the osteotomy surfaces (Fig. 4.**146d**; see Fig. 4.**145a**). The holes drilled at the corners of the window are filled with cancellous graft, if available. The chances for bony union are good in these cases.

Where the cortex is thin, the window does not fit tightly against the osteotomy surfaces. The window is reduced with a cerclage of suture material, and cancellous graft is inserted where possible. Even with cerclage and grafting, the chances for bony union are uncertain in these cases (see Fig. 4.**145b**).

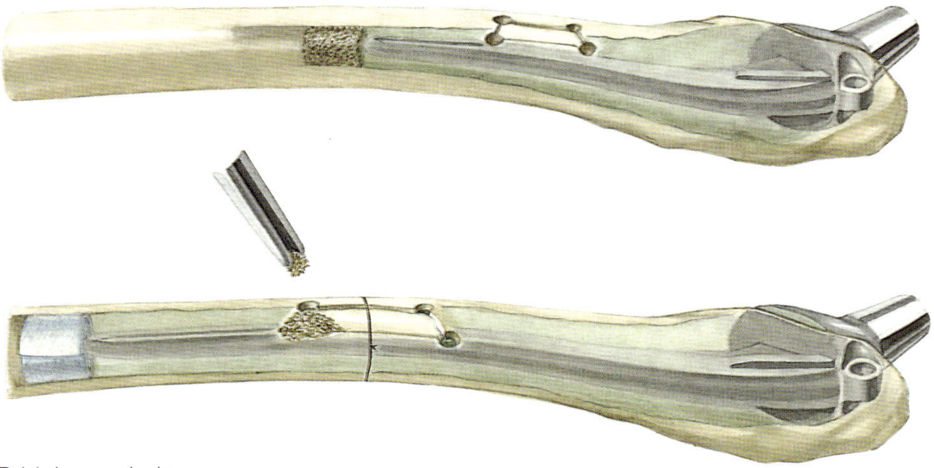

Fig. 4.**145a** and **b** Bridging a window.
a Anatomically shaped standard-length stem bridging a proximal cortical window in strong cortical bone. The window sinks into the bone and fits tightly against the osteotomy surfaces, which are beveled outward (see Fig. 5.**64c**). Cement restrictor of cancellous bone.
b Anatomically shaped long-stem implant bridging a distal window in thin cortical bone. The window does not fit tightly against the osteotomy surfaces and is held in place with a cerclage of suture material. Cancellous graft. Cement restrictor of absorbable cellulose gauze distal to the femoral isthmus.

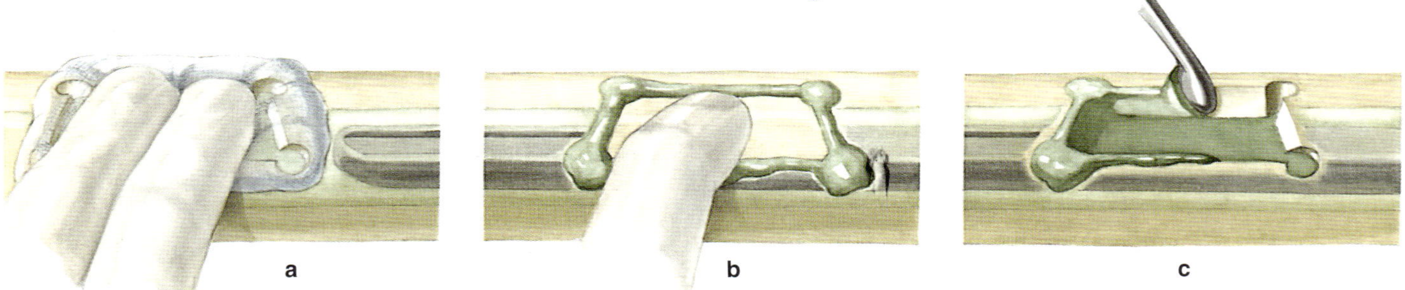

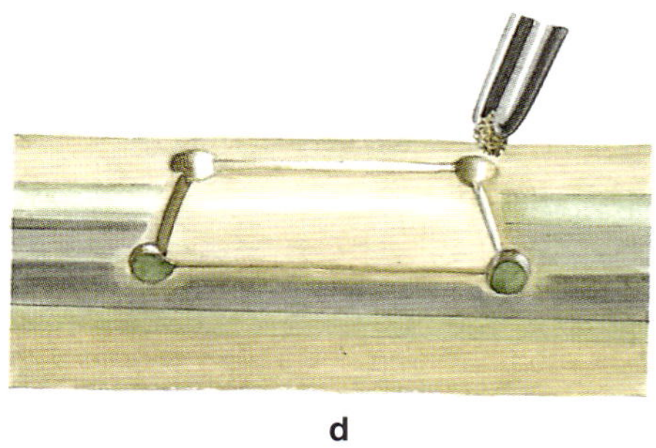

Fig. 4.**146a–d** Closing a window over a cemented stem.
a Holding a compress over the window while injecting the cement and inserting the stem.
b The "lid" is replaced before the cement hardens. Cement oozes out of the holes and the osteotomy gaps.
c The window is reopened and cement is removed from the holes and the osteotomy surfaces.
d The "lid" is reinserted so that it nests tightly against the beveled osteotomy surfaces. Holes are filled with cancellous graft.

When a long window has been cut in a femur with a strong cortex or such a femur is split longitudinally to remove a well-integrated cementless implant or one in the early stages of loosening (see Figs. 4.**94**–4.**98**), the osteotomy can generally be easily reduced (Fig. 4.**147**). This is true particularly when the surgeon carefully performs the osteotomy with a flexible osteotome under direct inspection after dissecting the vastus lateralis. The fragments are fixed with cerclage wire. Although the quality of the bone stock is generally good in these cases, the revision stem should be much longer than the original implant because the longitudinal osteotomy or long window significantly weakens the femur. We recommend reaming the inside of the femur slightly after fixing the reduced osteotomy with cerclage wire and before injecting the cement. This measure seals the sutures.

Often, an anatomic reduction is not possible. This is especially true when a transfemoral stem removal has been performed in a femur with an extremely weakened cortex without dissecting the vastus lateralis completely (see Figs. 4.**66** and 4.**67**). Generally, the fragments themselves are fractured.

The surgeon can then attempt to implant a cementless revision stem with a star-shaped cross section in the intact femoral diaphysis (Wagner's method). The surgeon opposes the osteotomized proximal femur or the fragments (without using cerclage) only by reattaching the partially dissected vastus lateralis (Fig. 4.**148a**).

Primary stability can also be achieved by implanting a cemented revision stem in the diaphysis (recommended when the damage extends to the diaphyseal bone itself). The distal section of the implant is cemented in the diaphysis, and the proximal fragments are opposed with the implant and fixed with cerclage. Additional cancellous bone chips may be inserted under the fragments (Fig. 4.**148b**). In both methods, fastening the fragments with cement is not recommended because the chances for osseous integration are uncertain. The fragments can migrate and lead to particulate wear problems. In both methods, callus may form on the fragments opposed to the proximal stem. The surgeon should not expect this bone to develop into a closed cylinder strong enough to provide support for a shorter implant. It does, however, at least preserve muscular origins and insertions.

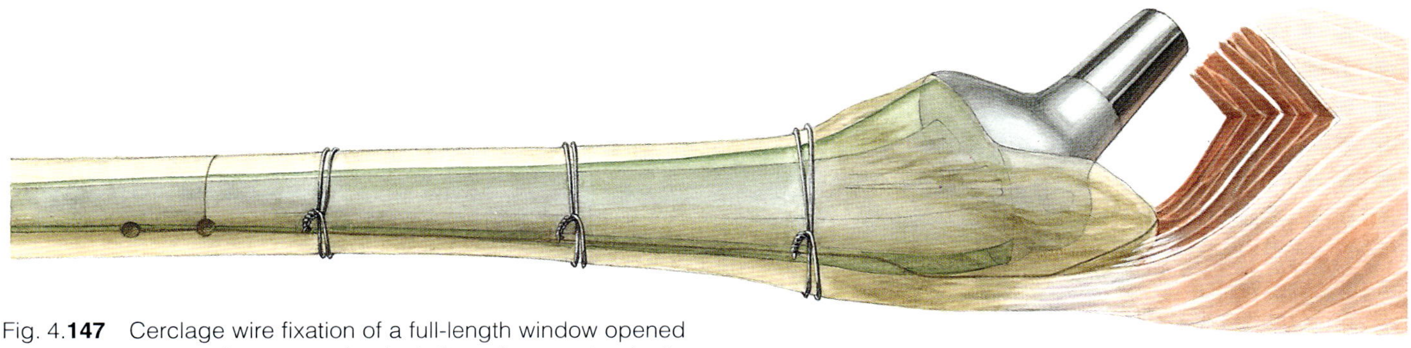

Fig. 4.**147** Cerclage wire fixation of a full-length window opened to remove a cementless stem. Implantation of an anatomically shaped long-stem revision implant.

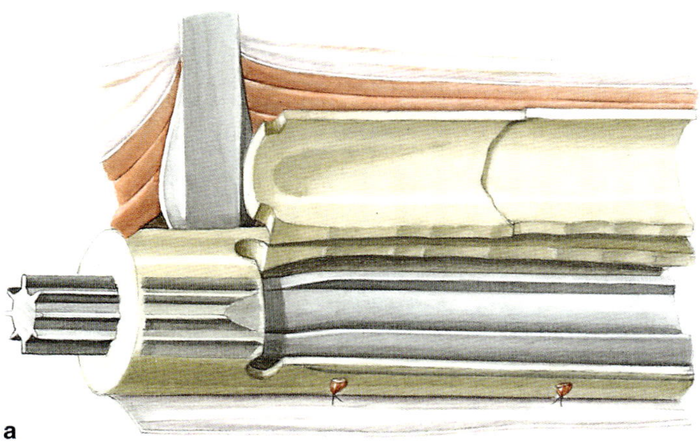

a

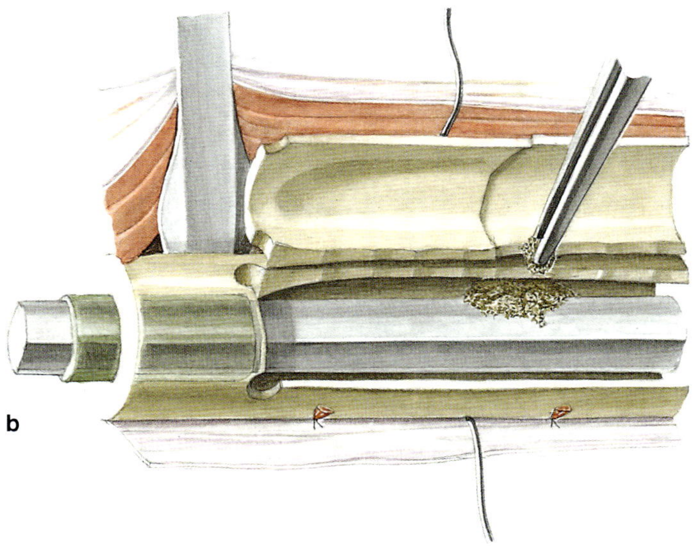

b

Fig. 4.**148a** and **b** Long-stem implant after transfemoral implant removal due to an extremely weakened proximal femur.

a Cementless revision implant. The stem has a star-shaped cross section for diaphyseal fixation (Wagner's method). The osteotomized proximal femur or the fragments are opposed with the proximal stem only by reattaching the vastus lateralis.

b The distal stem is cemented into the femoral diaphysis. After cancellous graft is inserted between the stem and the proximal bone, the proximal bone is opposed with the stem, and the construct is fixed with cerclage wire.

Long-Stem Implants after a Femoral Fracture and Internal Fixation

When loads are applied to the femur, peak stresses occur at the tip of the stem—in the transitional area between reinforced and unreinforced bone. Thus, when a stem is implanted, even forces below the normal fracture threshold can produce a fracture. The risk of fracture is increased if the integrity of the cortex has been compromised by a window, a perforation, or stem migration. This risk is also increased if there is only a short length of bone between two implants (i.e., a hip implant and a long-stem intracondylar knee implant). Intraoperative fractures occur when excessive force is applied when removing a stem that is not conducive to implant removal.

A fracture must be stabilized with a long-stem implant when:

- It compromises the fixation of a well-seated stem (Fig. 4.**149a**)
- A long-stem implant was indicated anyway to replace a loosened stem
- A stem fracture has occurred and the dislocated proximal fragment has caused a cortical fracture at the same site
- Internal fixation of a fracture which does not compromise the fixation of a well-seated implant is not possible because the plate would have to extend over the stem and the stem is too thick or the cortex too thin to permit fastening screws

Where a long-stem implant is indicated to stabilize a fracture, the surgeon combines a lateral approach to the femur with a transgluteal or transtrochanteric approach. These combinations permit repositioning the femur and trial reduction of the hip without producing significant torques around the femoral axis that might jeopardize the reduction of the fracture. The posterior approach to the hip should only be used when the surgeon expects that the reduced fracture can be well stabilized during the procedure.

Metal hose clamps are well suited for initially stabilizing a spiral fracture after the old stem is removed. Assuming the cortex is thick enough, they provide the required stability against stresses that occur when trial reduction is performed and the revision stem is implanted (Fig. 4.**149b**). The gaps for the hose clamps in the region of the linea aspera must be carefully dissected to prevent bleeding. Before the new implant is cemented, the surgeon should lightly ream the endosteal surface of the fracture to seal it if the condition of the femur permits it.

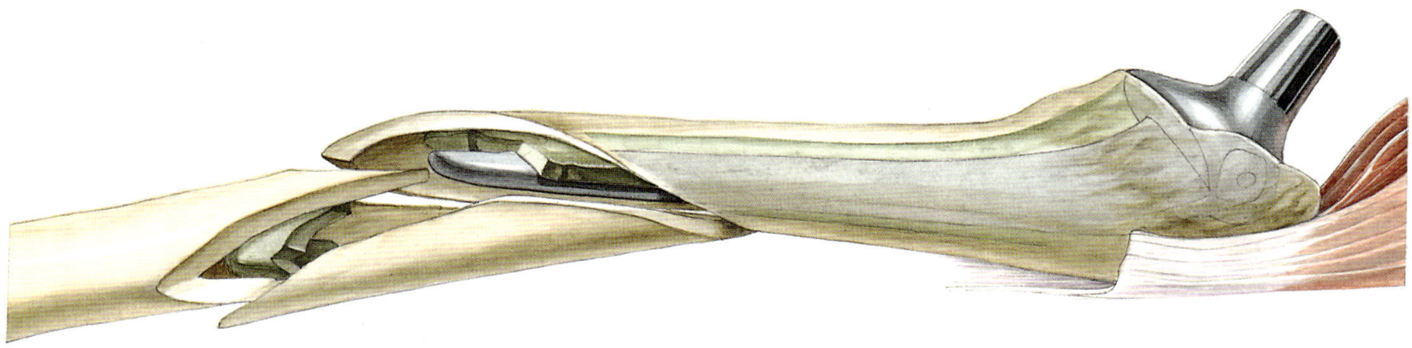

a

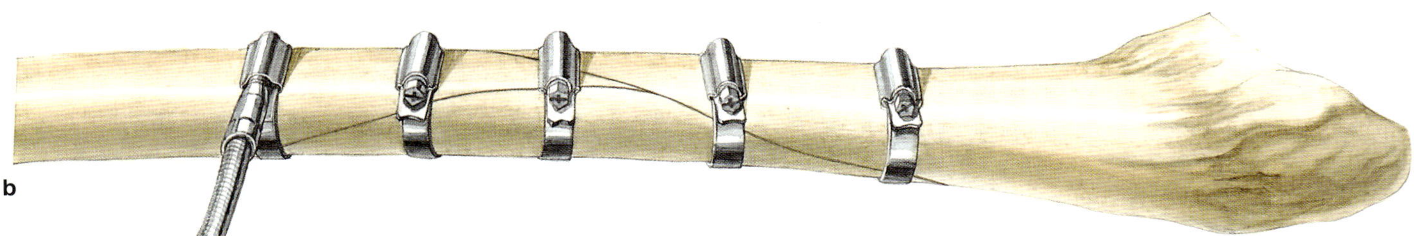

b

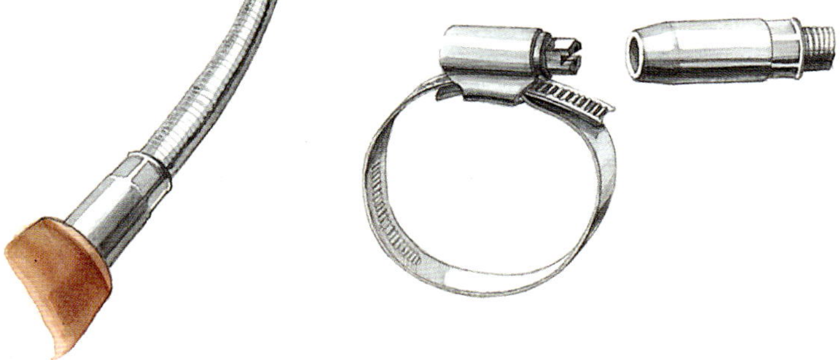

Fig. 4.**149a–d** Spiral fracture of the femur compromising the fixation of an implant. A long-stem implant is used to stabilize the fracture.
a The fracture compromises the stability of the old implant.
b The femoral shaft is stabilized with hose clamps.

If hose clamps of implant material were used, they may be left in place. If hose clamps of other material were used, they are replaced with cerclage wire (Fig. 4.**149c**). Double-wire cerclage provides better stability than single-wire cerclage. Regardless of whether pliers or a wire tightener are used, the surgeon should make sure that the ends of the wires are of equal length and that they are twisted applying uniform tension. Otherwise, one end of the wire will be twisted around the other, and one of the wires may break off without having created sufficient tension in the cerclage (Fig. 4.**149c**, insert). Cerclage wires applied to the tapered proximal femur tend to slip distally. This can be prevented by feeding them through a hole drilled in the lesser trochanter (Fig. 4.**149d**).

Where a fracture does not compromise the fixation of a well-seated implant, it can be stabilized with internal fixation. Transverse fractures are less likely to heal well than spiral fractures, particularly if the transverse fracture lies immediately distal to the tip of the stem as in the illustration (Fig. 4.**150**). Where the required plate or (in a distal fracture) condylar plate is so long that it extends over the stem, the screws are alternately inserted anterior and posterior to the stem to securely engage the bone. This is easier when a plate with widely staggered holes is used (Fig. 4.**150**, insert). If satisfactory screw fixation cannot be achieved, then a long-stem implant should be implanted to bridge the fracture.

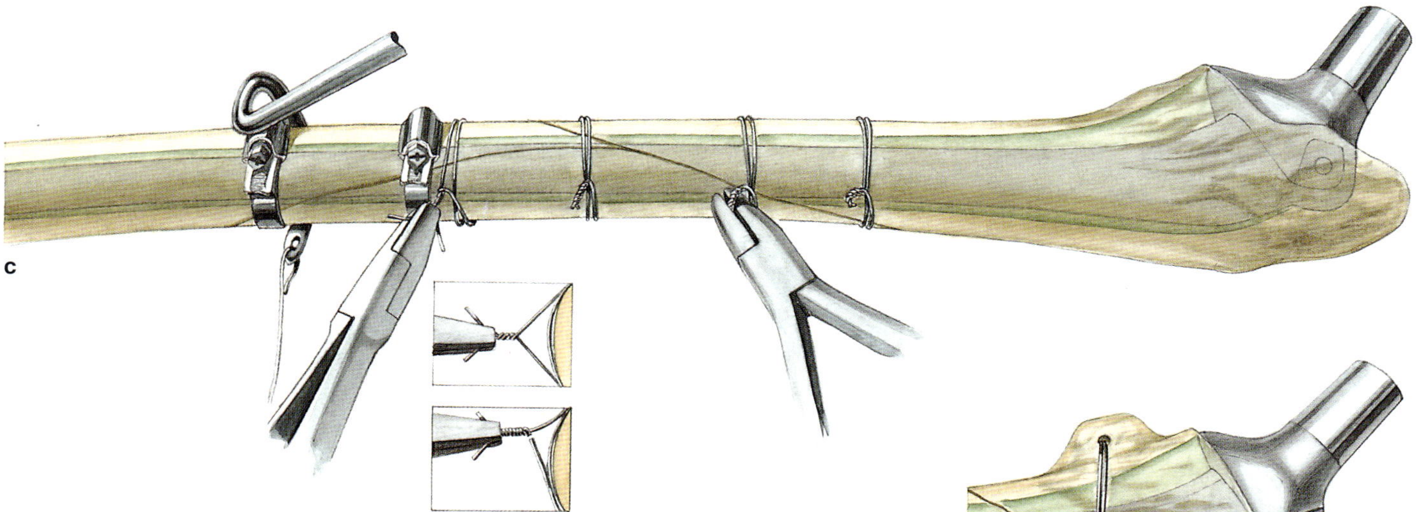

c

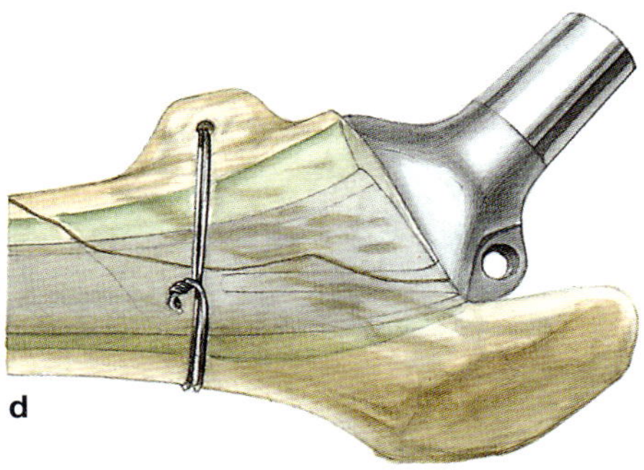

d

c Replacing the hose clamps by double-wire cerclages (left to right). Wire ends of equal length are twisted under constant tension. Twisting wire ends of unequal length together without applying tension causes one wire to twist around the other, and one will break off.

d Cerclage applied to the proximal femur is fed through a hole drilled in the lesser trochanter to prevent it from slipping distally.

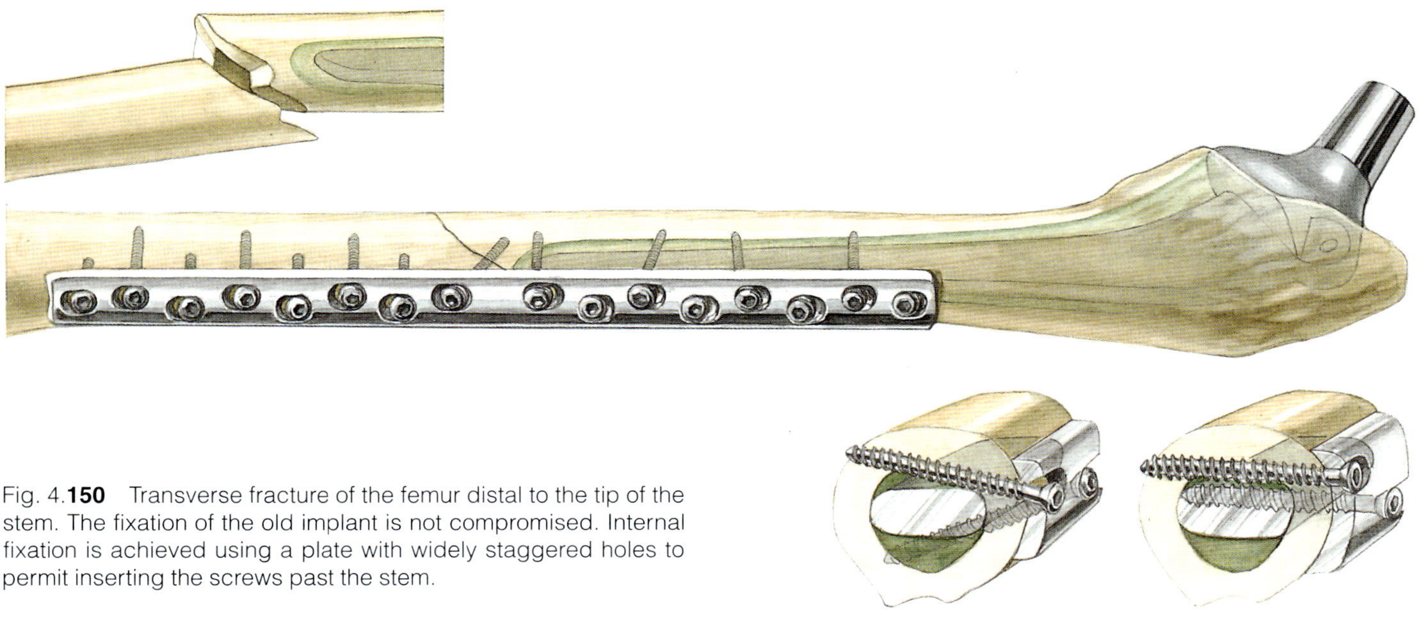

Fig. 4.**150** Transverse fracture of the femur distal to the tip of the stem. The fixation of the old implant is not compromised. Internal fixation is achieved using a plate with widely staggered holes to permit inserting the screws past the stem.

Reconstructing the Proximal Femur with Graft

To avoid long-stem implants, the surgeon can attempt to reinforce a proximal femur with a thin but intact cortex with allograft processed in a bone mill. The allograft is implanted in the femoral canal, the graft is compressed, and a cemented femoral component is implanted, either a stem with standard length or at least shorter than a long-stem femoral component, which would have been necessary without grafting.

The implant-specific instrumentation shown here for reconstructing the proximal femur (Ling and Gie's method) includes plastic bone plugs in different sizes, a guide wire with scale, which is screwed into the plugs with a guide wire extractor, and a slap hammer (Fig. 4.**151**).

Four tools are attached to the slap hammer in succession: a guide wire introducer, distal impactors of various sizes, stem-shaped proximal impactors (phantoms), and trial stems (Fig. 4.**152**). The slap hammer and the tools are cannulated so that they can be inserted on the guide wire. The proximal scale of the guide wire is visible through a window in the slap hammer and indicates the depth of the respective tool in the femoral canal.

First the guide wire is screwed on the plug using the guide wire extractor. Then, the surgeon removes the guide wire extractor and inserts the plug distally to the most distal resorption zone in the femoral canal using the guide wire introducer and the slap hammer. The surgeon selects the diameter of the plug so that it lodges firmly in the bone because it is the reference point for all further preparation of the femoral canal (Fig. 4.**152 a**).

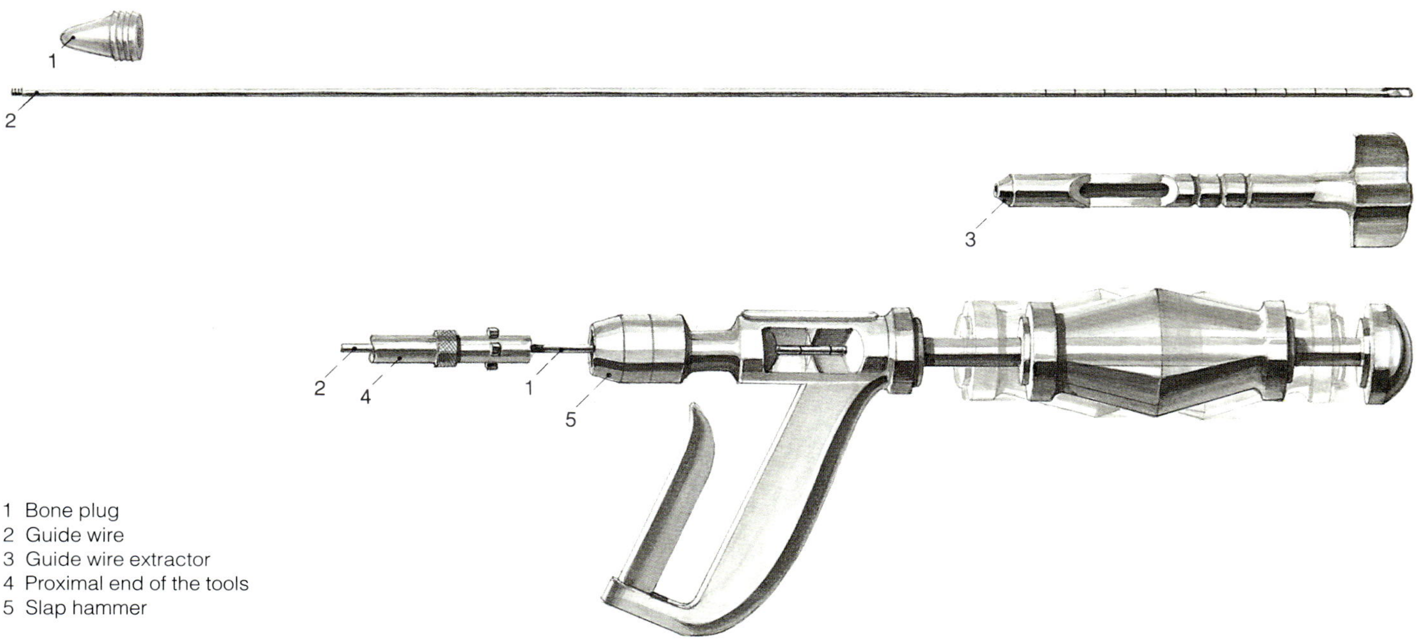

Fig. 4.**151** Implant-specific instrumentation to reconstruct the proximal femur with graft (Ling and Gie's method). Bone plug, guide wire with proximal scale, guide wire extractor for screwing the guide wire into and out of the bone plug, slap hammer for attaching four cannulated tools for preparing the femoral canal. The scale of the guide wire is visible through a window in the slap hammer and indicates the depth of the respective tool in the femoral canal.

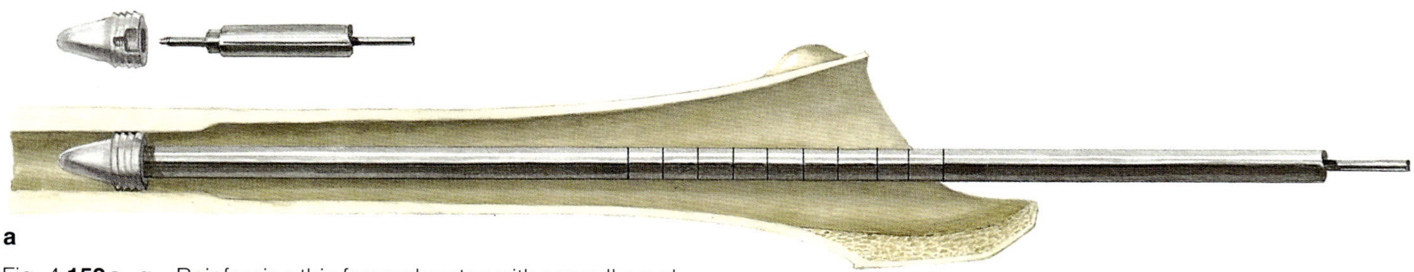

a

Fig. 4.**152 a–g** Reinforcing thin femoral cortex with cancellous allograft using the cannulated tools connected to the slap hammer.
a The plug and the guide wire are lodged in the femoral canal using the guide wire introducer. The scale on the guide wire introducer indicates the depth of the plug.

After removing the guide wire introducer, the surgeon attaches successively larger distal impactors to the slap hammer and checks how far distally they can be inserted before they come in contact with the cortex, recording the values displayed on the scale. The smallest distal impactor should be able to be inserted all the way down to the plug; the largest is the diameter of the femoral canal at half the planned depth of the stem. Next, the surgeon compacts the bone chips inserted into the femoral canal proximal to the plug, beginning with the smallest distal impactor and ending with the largest impactor that will fit at that depth. To minimize the risk of fracturing the cortex, the respective impactor may only be inserted as far distally as the respective recorded measurement (Fig. 4.**152b**).

Next, the final distal impactor is replaced with a proximal impactor (phantom) that has the same shape as the desired stem, but slightly larger. The tip of the phantom is impacted into the compacted graft to a depth corresponding to the final position of the stem. This pushes the bone chips toward the cortex and slightly proximally (Fig. 4.**152c**).

The surgeon partially extracts the phantom, inserts more bone chips into the gap between the phantom and the cortex, pushes them distally with straight and corner impactors, and reimpacts the phantom to its original depth. This is repeated until the gap has been filled and the graft compacted up to the proximal end of the femur. If at any time the phantom cannot be fully impacted, a phantom that is size smaller is introduced, and then the original phantom is used again. The graft should be compressed until the phanton can no longer be removed by hand and must be extracted with the slap hammer (Fig. 4.**152d**).

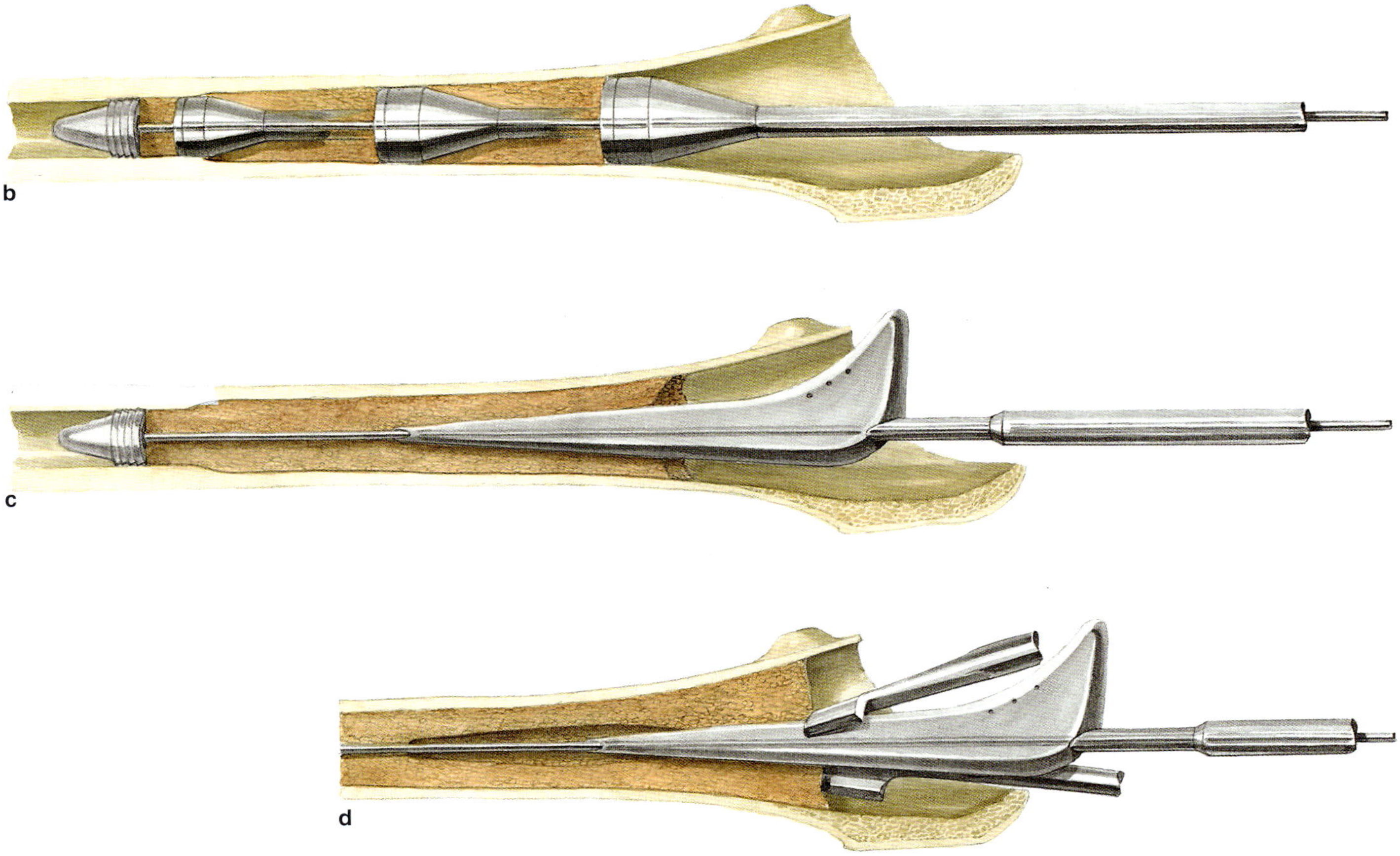

b Compacting the bone chips proximal to the bone plug with successively larger distal impactors up to half the planned depth of the stem.
c A phantom pushes the bone chips toward the cortex and slightly proximally.
d The phantom is partially extracted. More bone chips are inserted into the gap between the phantom and the cortex. The chips are pushed distally with straight and corner impactors, and compacted with the phantom.

Next, a reduction trial adapter is used to replace the phantom with a trial stem of the same size. The guide wire and adapter are then removed (Fig. 4.**152e**) and the hip joint is reduced using an appropriate trial head.

If the trial reduction is satisfactory, the guide wire is reinserted through the trial stem into the plug. The trial stem is then extracted again using its adapter. The surgeon next inserts a small distal impactor to the distal end of the impression left within the graft by the trial stem and hollows out a space for the tube of the cement gun and the stem centering plug (Fig. 4.**152f**).

After removing the small distal impactor and the guide wire, the surgeon injects the cement into the femoral canal and implants the final stem. The final stem is slighty smaller than the phantom to provide space for the cement mantle around the stem (Fig. 4.**152g**).

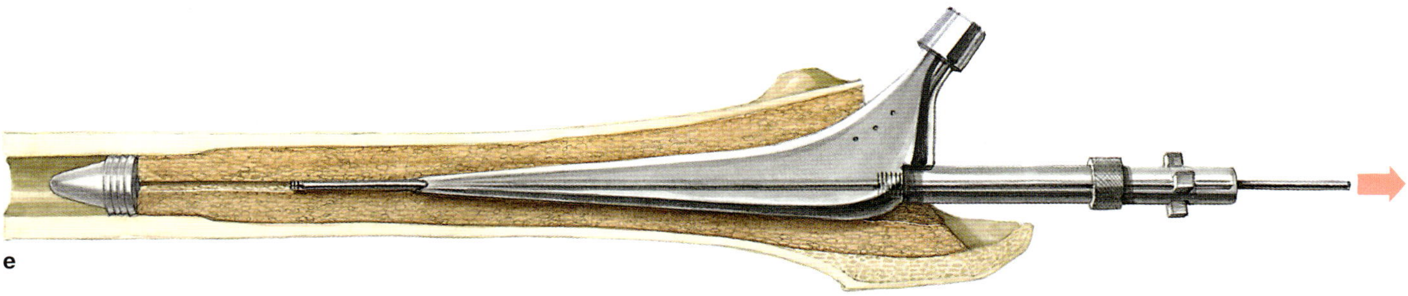

e

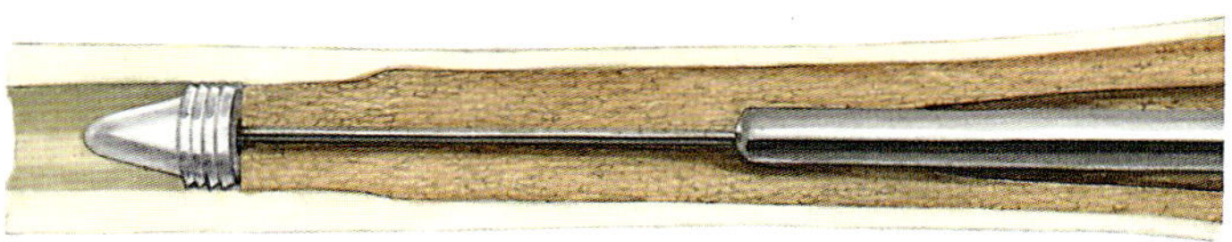

f

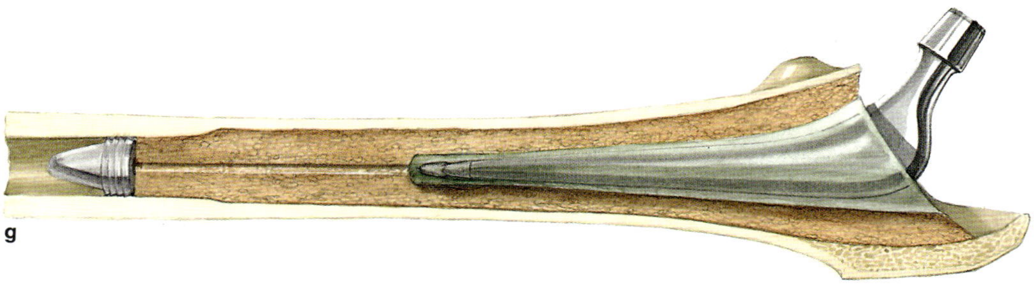

g

e The phantom is replaced with a trial stem of the same size (with taper), which is attached to the slap hammer with a reduction trial adapter. The guide wire and adapter are removed, and a trial reduction is performed.

f The guide wire is reinserted and the trial stem is replaced with a small distal impactor. This widens the distal end of the canal within to accommodate the tube of the cement gun and the stem centering plug.

g Cement injection and stem implantation. The final stem is slightly smaller than the phantom.

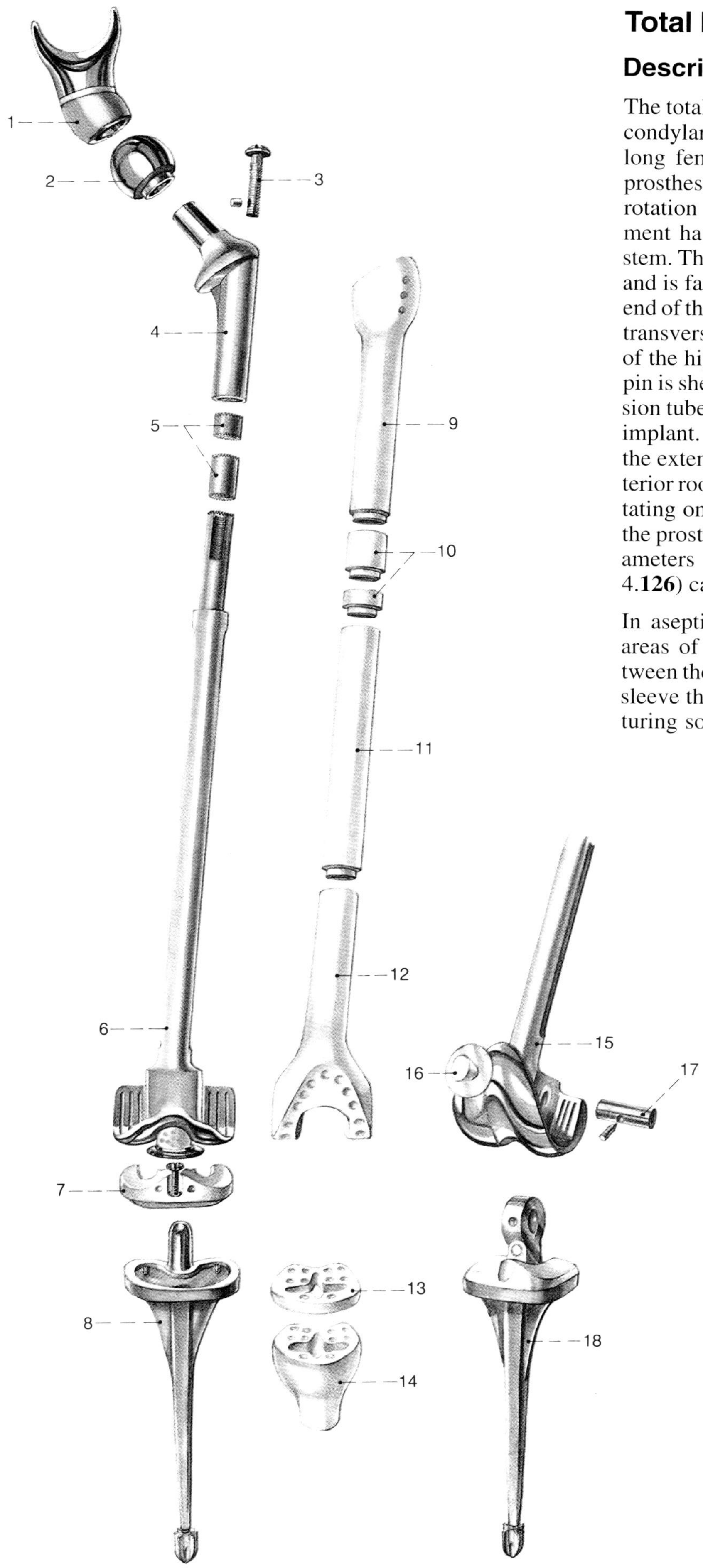

Total Femoral Prosthesis

Description of Implant

The total femoral prosthesis (Fig. 4.**153**) consists of an intracondylar knee prosthesis with a straight or anteriorly curved, long femoral stem and a modular hip segment. The knee prosthesis may be a hinge prosthesis, with or without tibial rotation and with or without a patellar shield. The hip segment has a tube under its collar instead of a conventional stem. The tube fits over the proximal end of the femoral stem and is fastened with a screw in an axial hole in the proximal end of the stem. A locking pin of polyethylene, inserted into a transverse hole in the centering screw before final assembly of the hip segment, prevents the screw from loosening. The pin is sheared off as the screw is tightened. One or two extension tubes of different lengths can be inserted to lengthen the implant. Teeth in the ends of the proximal end of the stem and the extension tubes mesh with corresponding teeth in the interior roof of the tube. They prevent the hip segment from rotating on the stem and permit varying of the anteversion of the prosthetic femoral neck. Femoral heads with different diameters and neck lengths or a saddle prosthesis (see Fig. 4.**126**) can be impacted onto the taper.

In aseptic cases, polyethylene sleeves are used to replace areas of lost bone stock and maintain proper distance between the remaining bone on the prosthetic stem. A proximal sleeve that simulates the greater trochanter has holes for suturing soft tissue. There is a diaphyseal sleeve, and a distal

Fig. 4.**153** Total femoral prosthesis.

1 Saddle prosthesis
2 Femoral head
3 Screw with locking pin
4 Hip segment
5 Extension tubes
6 Femoral component (rotating hinge without patellar shield)
7 Polyethylene tibial bearing with screw
8 Tibial component (rotating hinge)
9 Proximal femoral polyethylene sleeve
10 Femoral polythylene extension segments
11 Diaphyseal femoral polyethylene sleeve (femoral)
12 Distal femoral polyethylene sleeve (femoral)
13 Polyethylene tibial tray
14 Proximal tibiac polyethylene sleeve (tibial)
15 Femoral component (pure hinge with patellar shield)
16 Patellar button
17 Axis with set screw
18 Tibial component (pure hinge)

sleeve that replaces the femoral condyles. A polyethylene tibial tray compensates for slight shortening of the tibia, and a tibial polyethylene sleeve for the loss of the tibial condyles.

All components are dimensioned according to radiographs (see Fig. 4.**2** and 4.**3**). The base length of the total femoral prosthesis (without extension tubes) should be slightly shorter than necessary. Planning should include a short extension tube and a medium-length femoral head to match the length according to the radiograph to permit intraoperative adjustments so that the system can be lengthened or shortened as required, to compensate for measuring errors or unforeseen situations. The surgeon should also bear in mind that resecting scar tissue and bone reduces tension in the soft-tissue bridging the implant and that increasing the circumference of the construct by implanting sleeves can increase longitudinal tension.

Function

The total femoral prosthesis assumes the load-bearing functions of the femur. The slender stem is inserted through cylindrical bone or residual bone that can be reconstructed to form a cylinder. This means that regional muscular origins and insertions can be preserved, and the function of at least one of the two prosthetic joints will approximate that of the natural joint, i.e., knee function in total femur replacement after a total hip arthroplasty (see Fig. 4.**154**–4.**169**) and hip function in total femur replacement after a total knee arthroplasty, will be improved, because in these cases either the femoral condyles or the proximal femur can be preserved.

When soft tissue can be fixed to polyethylene sleeves (see Fig. 4.**169**), the surgeon should not expect to achieve a permanent bond between soft tissue and implant. In aseptic cases, allograft can be opposed with the stem instead of polyethylene sleeves. Here, there is at least a chance achieving a permanent bond between the muscles, graft, and implant.

Indications

A total femoral prosthesis is indicated when a long-stem implant has loosened and only the distal femur is still able to support an implant (Fig. 4.**154a**). The decision to implant a total femoral prosthesis is easier to make if implantation of an intracondylar prosthesis with an intramedullary stem is indicated anyway due to diseases of the knee with severe insufficiency of the knee ligaments, and the stem of the intracondylar prosthesis would overlap the stem of the hip implant (Fig. 4.**154b**), or if loosening of a long-stem hip implant is accompanied by a distal femoral fracture (Fig. 4.**154c**).

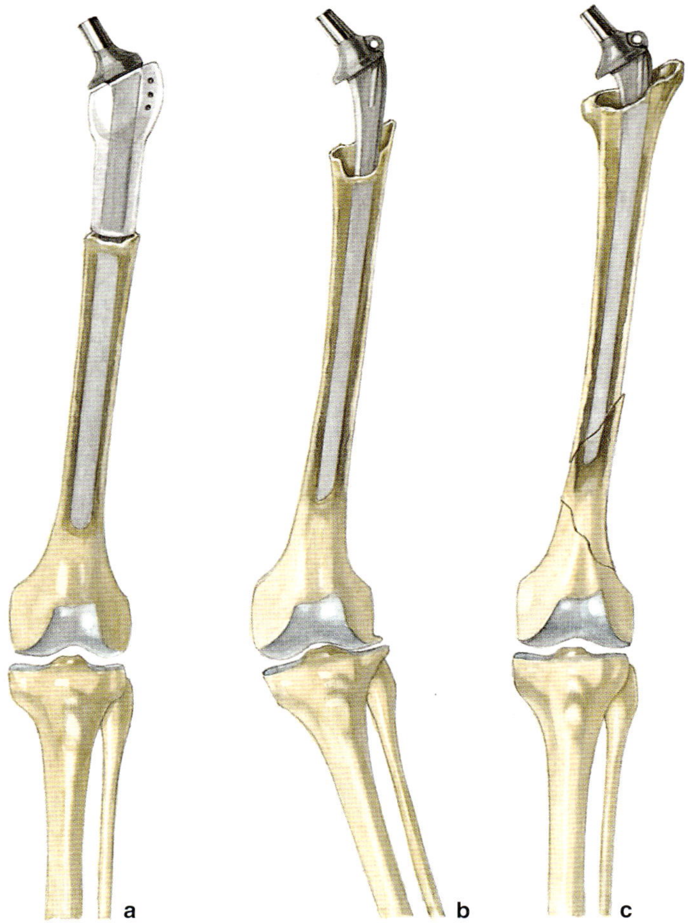

Fig. 4.**154a–c** Indications for a total femoral prosthesis after a total hip implant.

a Loosening of a long-stem implant. Diaphysis is no longer able to support an implant.
b Concomitant severe valgus osteoarthritis of the knee.
c Concomitant fracture of the distal femur.

Implanting a Total Femoral Prosthesis after Total Hip Arthroplasty

An approach to the hip with the patient supine (such as the transgluteal approach shown in the illustration) combined with a lateral approach to the femur and knee provides the best exposure of the femur (Fig. 4.**155** and see Fig. 4.**37**).

Where the proximal femur is absent or deficient, the surgeon can also make an incision posterior to the scarred proximal vastus and distal gluteal soft tissue even with the patient supine. Since the insertions of the short muscles of the hip are missing, dislocating the hip relaxes the soft tissue and provides good access to the periacetabular region even through this posterior approach to the hip in these cases. A transverse incision of scarred proximal vastus and distal gluteal soft tissue is only recommended if the surgeon intends to shorten it.

To minimize the risk of contaminating the large wound, the surgical site is exposed in three stages: first the hip is exposed, then the femur, and finally the knee. In keeping with standard practice in total joint arthroplasty, moistened cloths are sutured to the fascia lata to protect the subcutaneous tissue (see Fig. 4.**7** and Fig. 4.**169**).

The illustration (Fig. 4.**155**) shows a loosened and migrated long-stem implant that extends past the femoral diaphysis, an absent proximal femur, distal window, cortical fracture, and osteoarthritis of the knee. In this example (Fig. 4.**156**), a total femoral prosthesis with a rotating hinge prothesis without a patellar shield has been chosen as a revision implant. The femoral stem has an anterior bow corresponding to that of the residual anatomic femur. A polyethylene sleeve replaces the proximal femur.

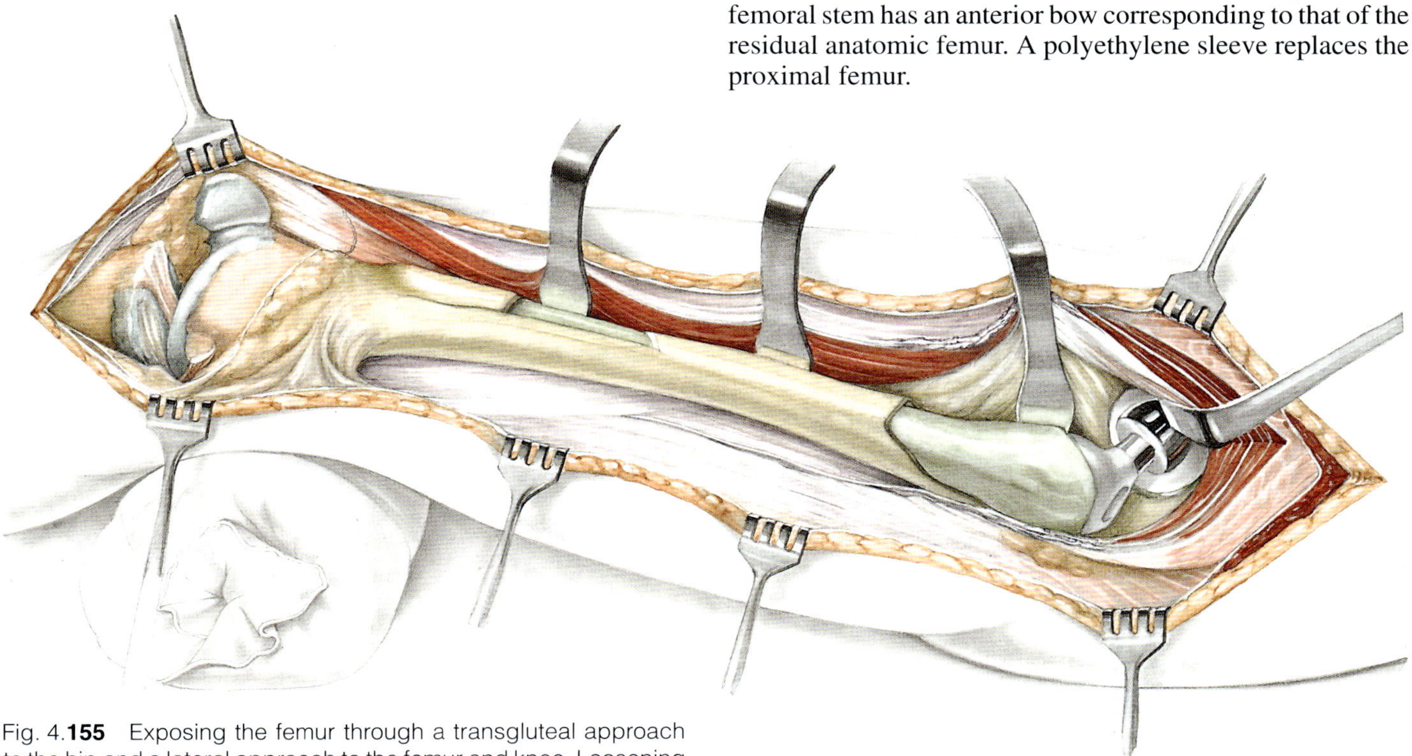

Fig. 4.**155** Exposing the femur through a transgluteal approach to the hip and a lateral approach to the femur and knee. Loosening of a long-stem implant, missing proximal femur, distal window, cortical fracture, migration of the distal tip of the stem, osteoarthritis of the knee.

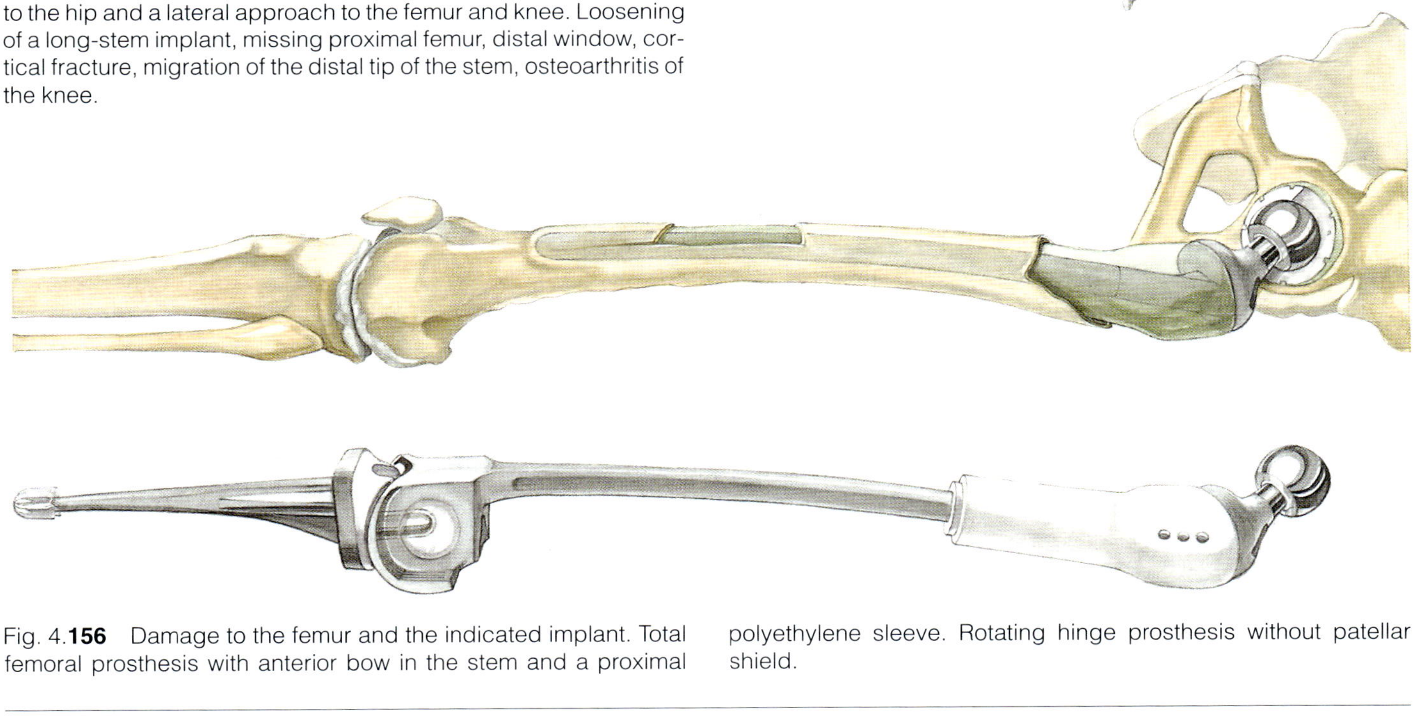

Fig. 4.**156** Damage to the femur and the indicated implant. Total femoral prosthesis with anterior bow in the stem and a proximal polyethylene sleeve. Rotating hinge prosthesis without patellar shield.

After removing the loosened stem and cement (Fig. 4.**157**), the surgeon exposes the knee (Fig. 4.**158a**), opens and reams the femur from distally, and performs a femoral intracondylar osteotomy using a femoral jig (Fig. 4.**158b**). After introducing the jig completely, the femoral condyles are contoured to match the jig, i.e., the runners of the implant.

Next a protective metal cap is screwed onto the proximal end of the femoral stem of the total femoral prosthesis, and the surgeon attempts to impact the femoral component into the femur from the knee. If this is not successful even with an anteverted femoral stem, a proximal femoral wedge osteotomy is performed (Fig. 4.**159**).

The surgeon then resects a section of the posterior condyles to match the runners of the femoral component and removes the proximal end of the femur to achieve an even transverse surface (Fig. 4.**160**).

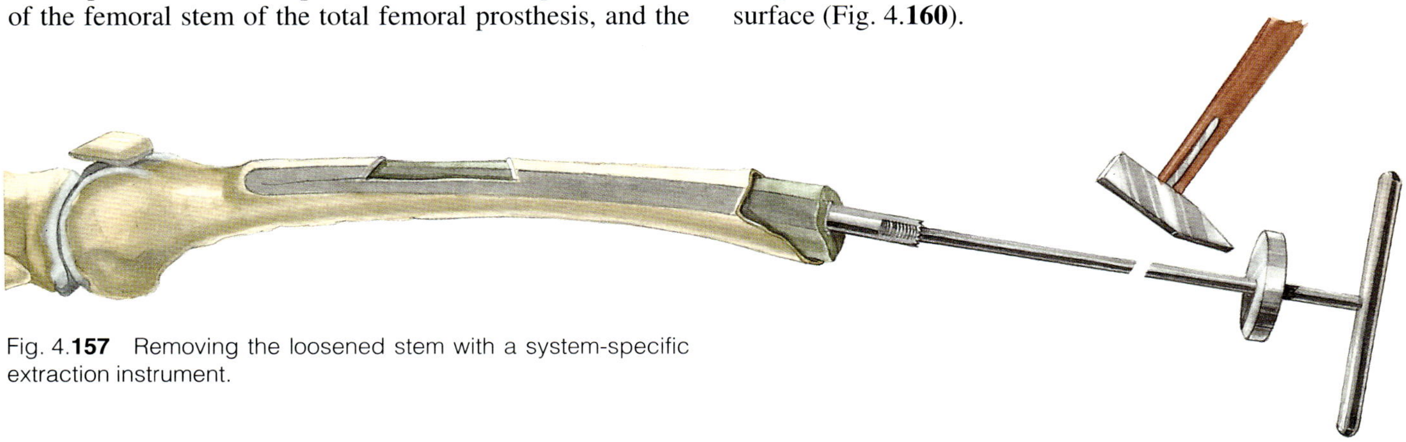

Fig. 4.**157** Removing the loosened stem with a system-specific extraction instrument.

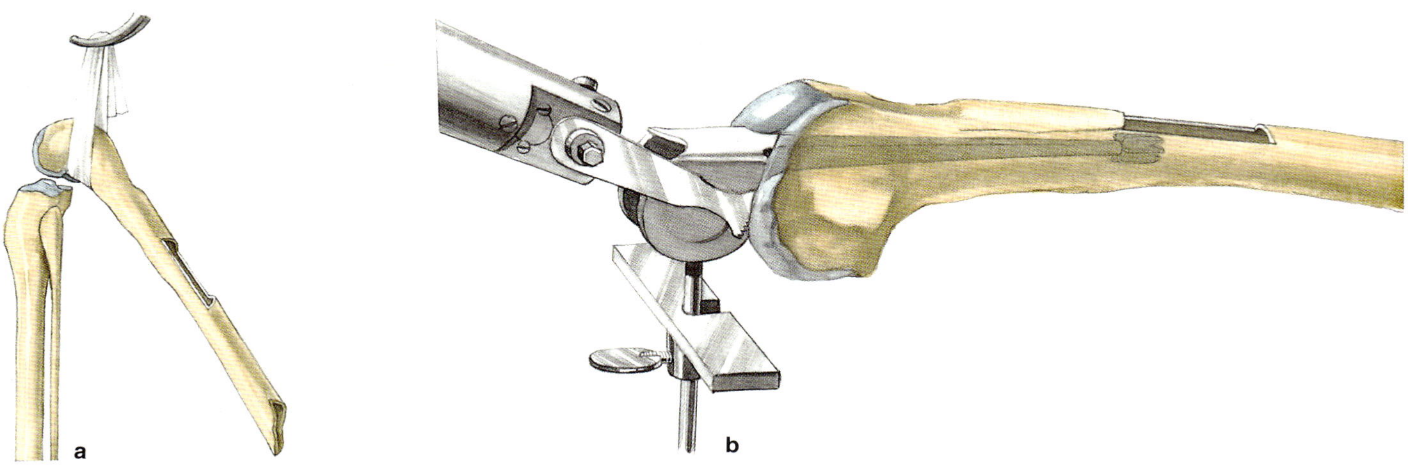

Fig. 4.**158a** and **b** Preparing the knee.
a Exposing the knee.
b Removing intracondylar bone with a femoral jig.

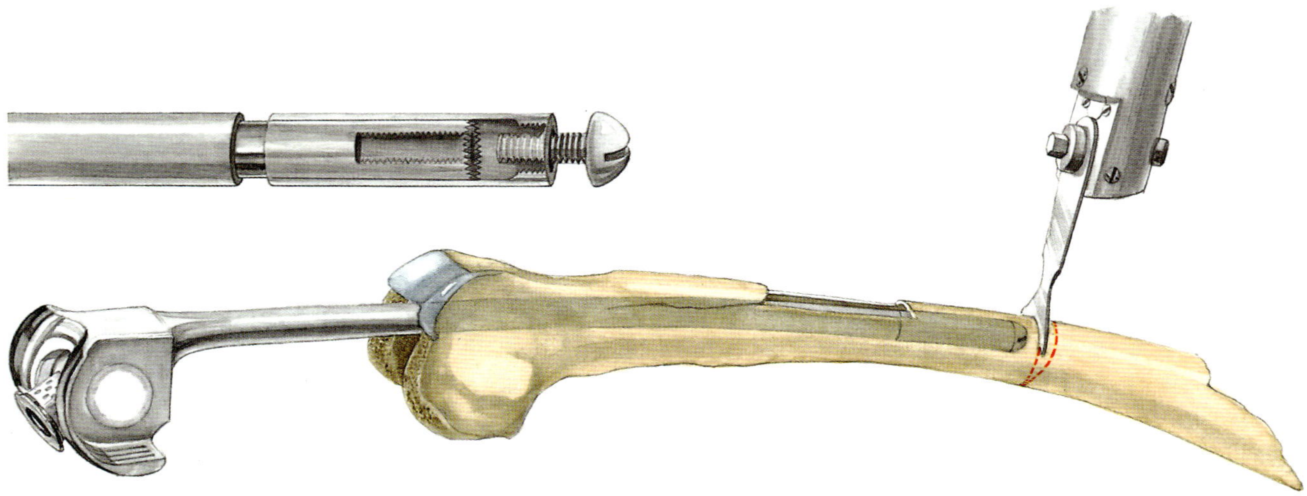

Fig. 4.**159** After the femoral condyles have been contoured, a protective cap is attached to the femoral component of the total femoral prosthesis, which is then impacted into the femur. A wedge osteotomy is performed to permit impacting the implant.

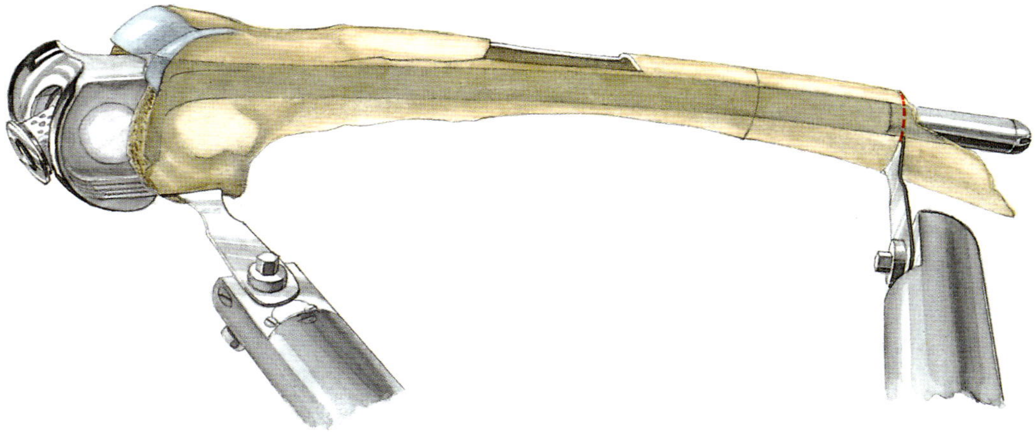

Fig. 4.**160** Resecting a section of the posterior femoral condyles and the proximal end of the femur.

Pushing the stem through a long narrow femoral canal can produce an offset in the distal end of the femoral component so that the femoral box of the prosthetic knee does not fit between the condyles despite a correct intracondylar osteotomy (Fig. 4.**161 a**). If the lateral offset is only slight, the surgeon resects some more intracondylar bone (Fig. 4.**161 b**). This procedure should not be attempted in the presence of a larger offset, because it might produce a joint in which one of the femoral runners projects laterally or where the patella no longer articulates properly with the patellar gliding path. To avoid this, the surgeon performs a supracondylar transverse osteotomy to correct the offset (Fig. 4.**161 c**). Next, the required tibial osteotomy is performed using a tibial jig (Fig. 4.**162**).

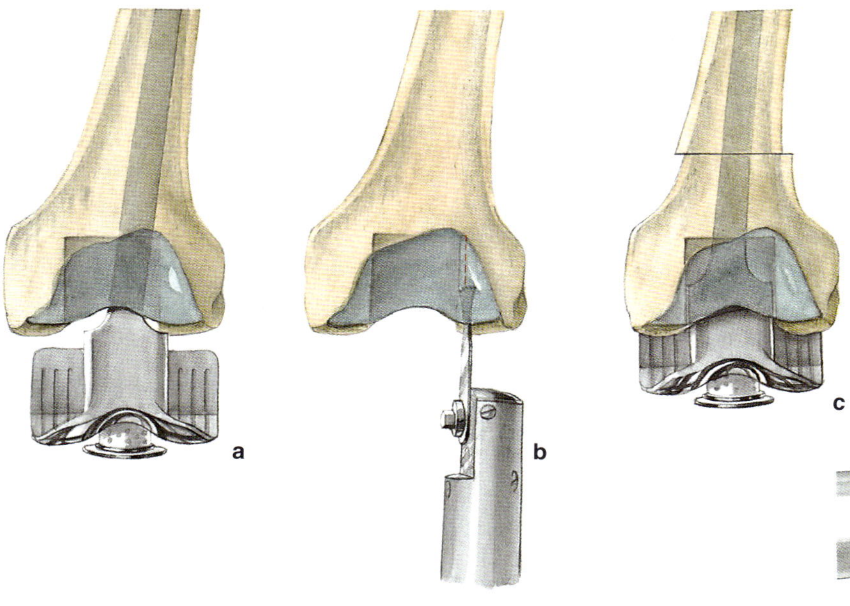

Fig. 4.**161 a–c** Compensating for an offset between the implant and the intracondylar osteotomy.
a The femoral box does not fit into the osteotomy.
b Widening the osteotomy to correct a slight offset.
c Supracondylar transverse osteotomy to correct a larger offset.

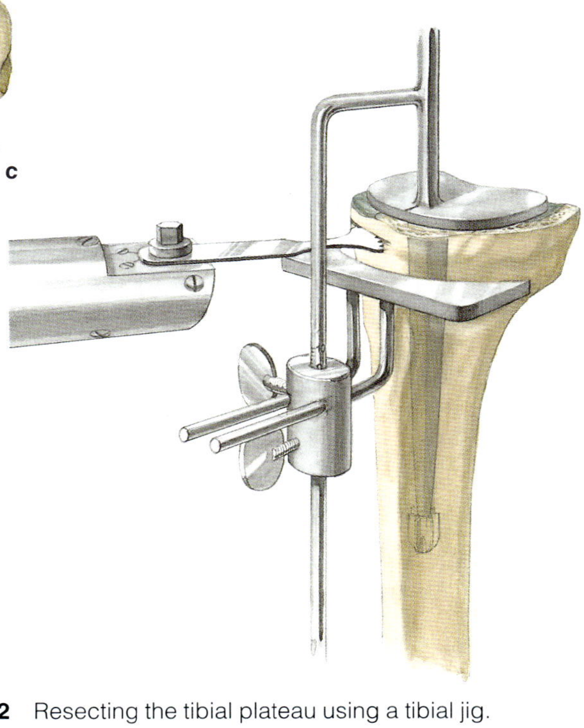

Fig. 4.**162** Resecting the tibial plateau using a tibial jig.

Then the surgeon assesses the tension in the soft-tissue bridging the hip (Fig. 4.**163**).

For this purpose the tibial component is inserted, the femoral component (with a protective cap) is pushed through the femur, and the surgeon reduces the knee. Trial reduction of the knee is performed without first inserting the tibial bearing because this needlessly complicates the procedure.

Next, the protective cap is removed from the proximal end of the stem, and the hip segment is attached with the required anteversion. The surgeon now performs a trial reduction of the hip to assess the stem length and that of the neck of the head (length of the base if a saddle prosthesis is used). If the hip cannot be reduced, an extension tube may be removed or a head with a shorter neck (or saddle prosthesis base) impacted; if the hip dislocates easily, an additional extension tube or a head with a longer neck (or base) may be indicated.

The resulting leg length is of secondary importance. Where no extension cylinder or only a short one is required, a short screw is used to fasten the hip segment. Where a longer extension tube is required, a long screw is necessary (Fig. 4.**163**, insert). The locking pin should not be inserted during trial reduction.

If trial reduction of the hip is satisfactory, the polyethylene sleeve is shortened to the required length (Fig. 4.**164**). The remaining femoral bone should be pushed distally when measuring to ensure good apposition between the condyles and the runners of the femoral component.

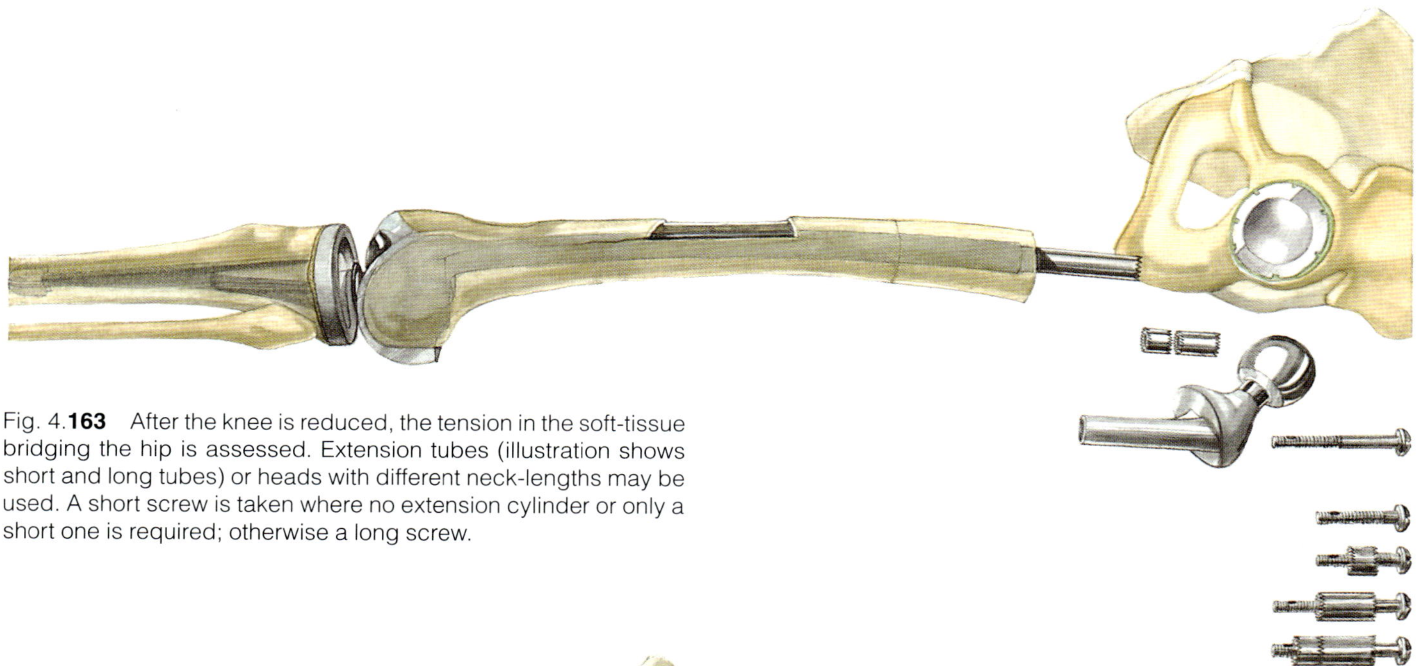

Fig. 4.**163** After the knee is reduced, the tension in the soft-tissue bridging the hip is assessed. Extension tubes (illustration shows short and long tubes) or heads with different neck-lengths may be used. A short screw is taken where no extension cylinder or only a short one is required; otherwise a long screw.

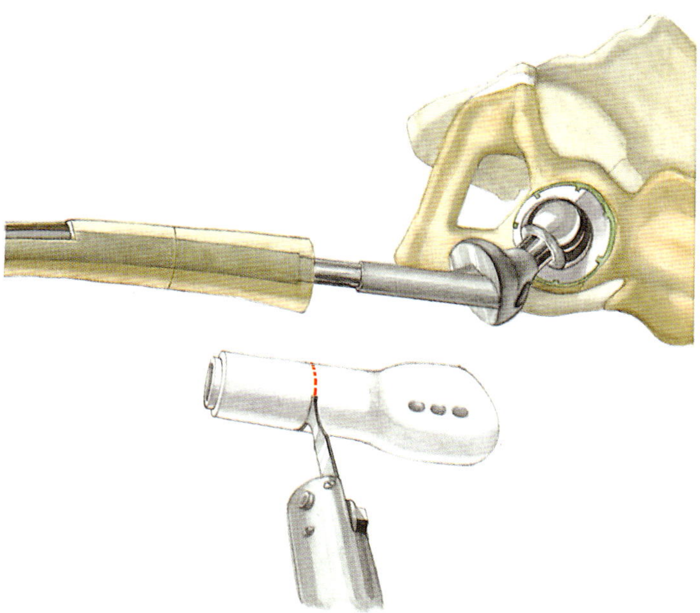

Fig. 4.**164** Measuring and shortening the polyethylene sleeve with the hip and knee reduced and the femur pushed distally.

Next, the hip segment (with extension tubes if indicated) and the polyethylene sleeve are assembled (Fig. 4.**165**), and the hip is reduced again to assess proper sleeve length.

If the sleeve is only slightly too long, the teeth of the proximal end of the stem (or extension tube) and in the tube of the hip segment will not mesh, and rotational instability in the proximal connection will result. If this is the case, the surgeon shortens the sleeve again. If the sleeve is too short, a new sleeve is used if available, or the old sleeve is shortened further and is combined with a femoral polyethylene extension segment. When the surgeon is certain that the proximal connection is stable and the sleeve cannot be moved, the hip is reduced again.

If the trial reduction of the hip with the polyethylene sleeve is satisfactory as well (Fig. 4.**166**), the prosthesis is implanted.

First, the tibial component is cemented. The femoral canal is then filled with cement, and the femoral component is reinserted into the remaining femur with its protective cap in place. The proximal end of the femur is held closed as long as possible to prevent cement from escaping. The bone is pressed distally while the cement hardens. Reducing the knee while the cement is still soft provides a good buttress to press the femur against. Residual cement that escapes through osteotomy gaps or defects is removed while still soft. After the cement hardens, the surgeon removes the screw from the protective cap from the femoral component and extracts it with an extraction instrument (Fig. 4.**167**).

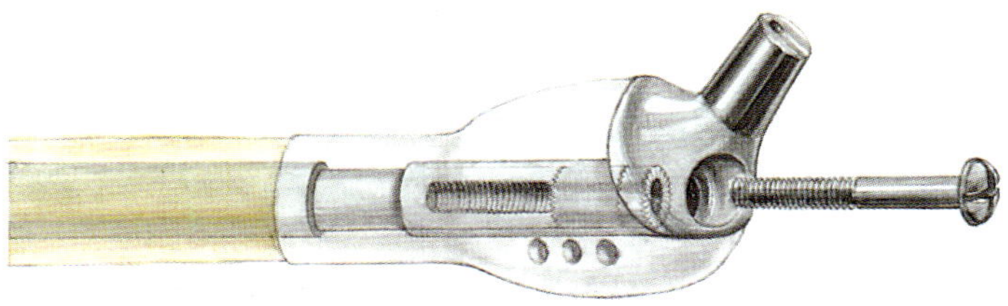

Fig. 4.**165** Assembling the hip segment with extension tubes and proximal polyethylene sleeve.

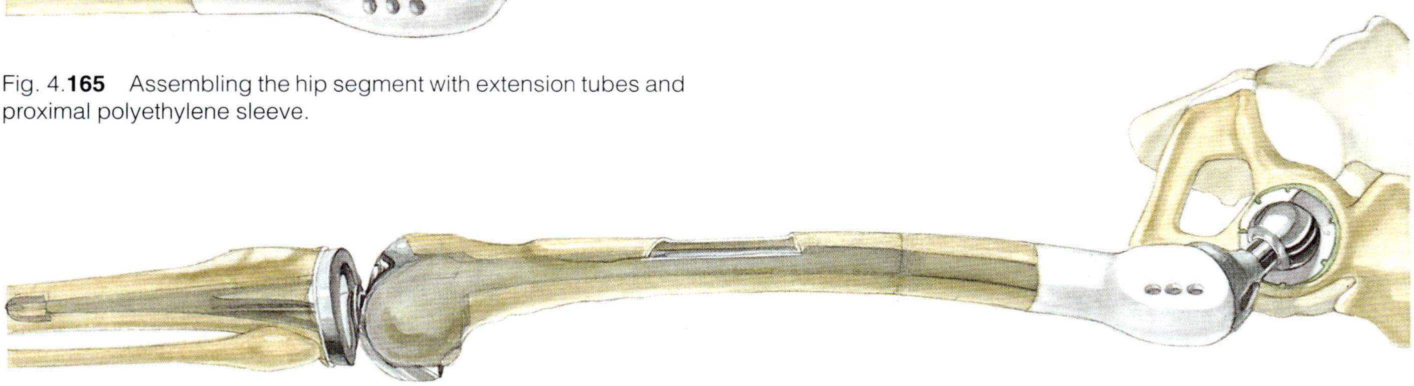

Fig. 4.**166** Trial reduction with proximal polyethylene sleeve.

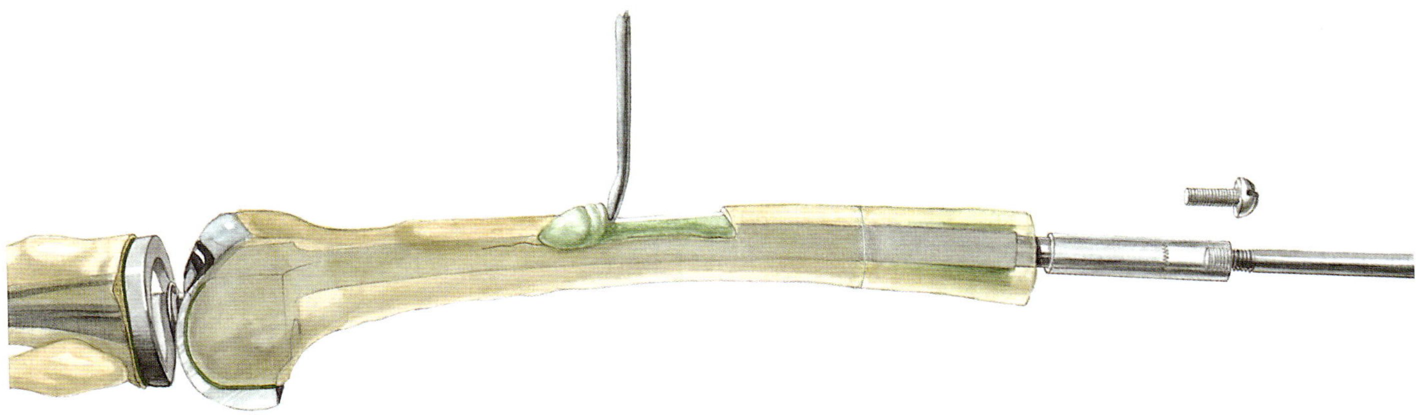

Fig. 4.**167** Cementing the tibial and then the femoral component. Removing excess cement and the protective cap.

Finally, the assembled hip segment (with polyethylene sleeve and extension tube if indicated) is attached to the proximal end of the femoral stem in the desired anteversion. The locking pin is inserted into the screw to prevent it from loosening and the screw is tightly fixed (Fig. 4.**168**). Then the hip is reduced in its final position. The surgeon dislocates the knee, inserts the tibial tray, and reduces the knee again.

The vastus and gluteal soft tissues are sutured to holes drilled in the prosthetic greater trochanter. This fixation minimizes the danger of early postoperative dislocation and permits the individual soft-tissue structures to heal together. However, the surgeon should not expect to achieve a permanent bond between soft tissue and implant (Fig. 4.**169**).

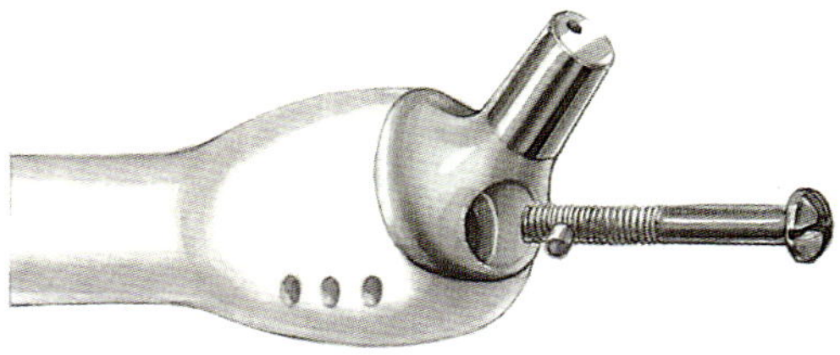

Fig. 4.**168** Final assembly of the hip segment. The locking pin is inserted to prevent the screw from loosening.

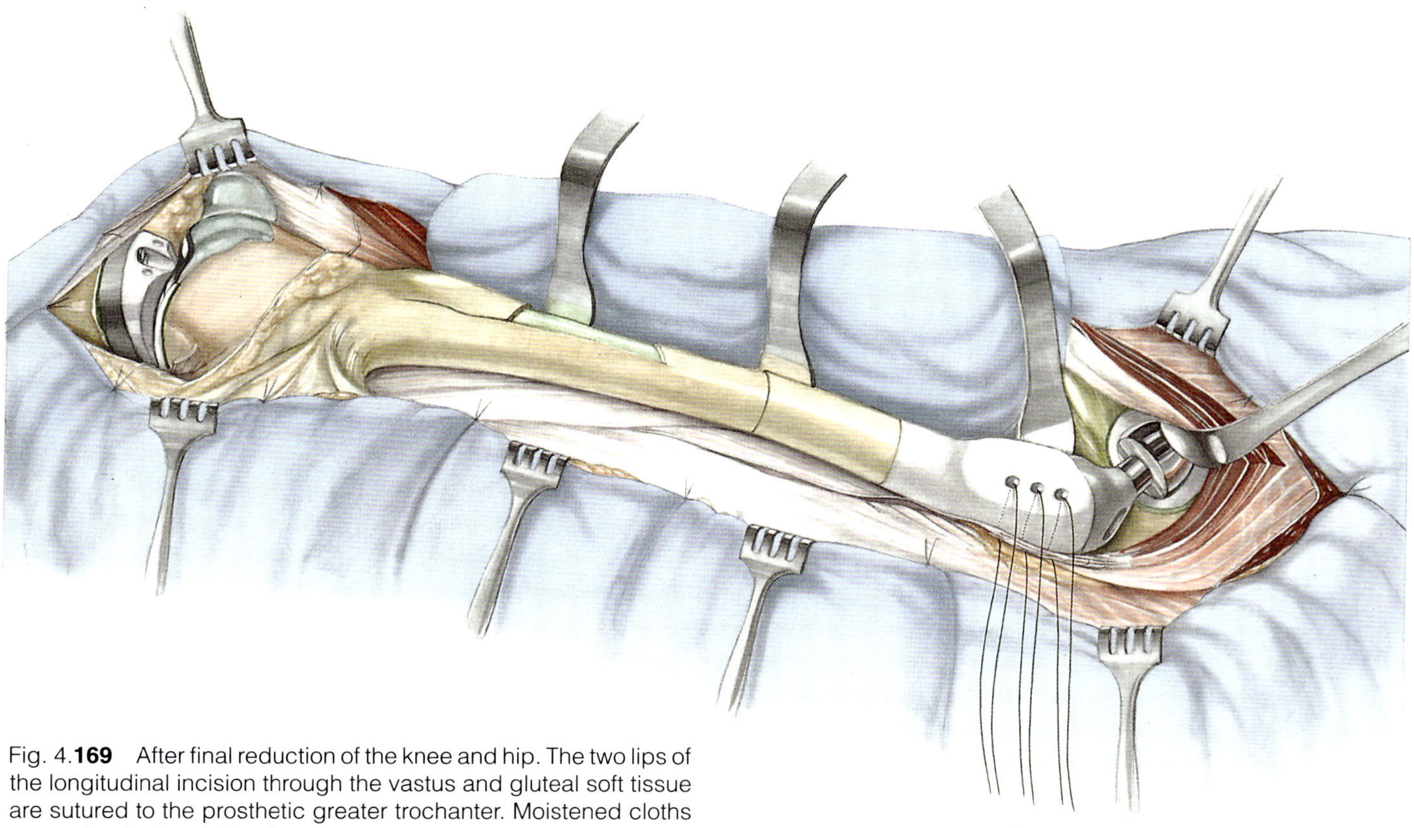

Fig. 4.**169** After final reduction of the knee and hip. The two lips of the longitudinal incision through the vastus and gluteal soft tissue are sutured to the prosthetic greater trochanter. Moistened cloths sutured to the fascia lata have prevented the subcutaneous tissue from drying during the entire procedure.

Soft-Tissue Reconstruction and Closure

Posterior Approach to the Hip

After a posterior approach (see Fig. 4.**9**–4.**17**), the surgeon reattaches the external rotators with tendinous insertions into the femur (Fig. 4.**170**). These include the piriformis, the obturator internus, and the tendon of the gluteus maximus (if it was incised to improve exposure). The piriformis and the obturator internus can only be reattached if the stumps of their tendons are long enough, i.e., if they were transected as close as possible to their femoral insertions on the trochanteric fossa (see Fig. 4.**10**). The gluteus maximus tendon can only be sutured if it was incised a few millimeters from the femoral insertion. The tendon of the obturator externus has generally disappeared into the deep layer of the wound. The muscle fibers of the gemellus muscles and the quadratus femoris insert directly into the femur, and thus cannot be reattached. Reinserting the piriformis, obturator internus and the maximus minimizes the risk of posterosuperior dislocation.

Since it is difficult to reattach the tendons to their original insertions on the trochanteric fossa and doing so would create too much soft-tissue tension (dissection during the approach almost always shortens them), the surgeon sutures their tendons to the medial side of the posterior fibers of the gluteus medius near the greater trochanter.

First the surgeon gathers the tendons of the piriformis and the obturator internus with sutures. A transverse stitch is made through the tendons and the anterior and posterior ends of the sutures are reinserted so they emerge through the transected face (Fig. 4.**170**, insert).

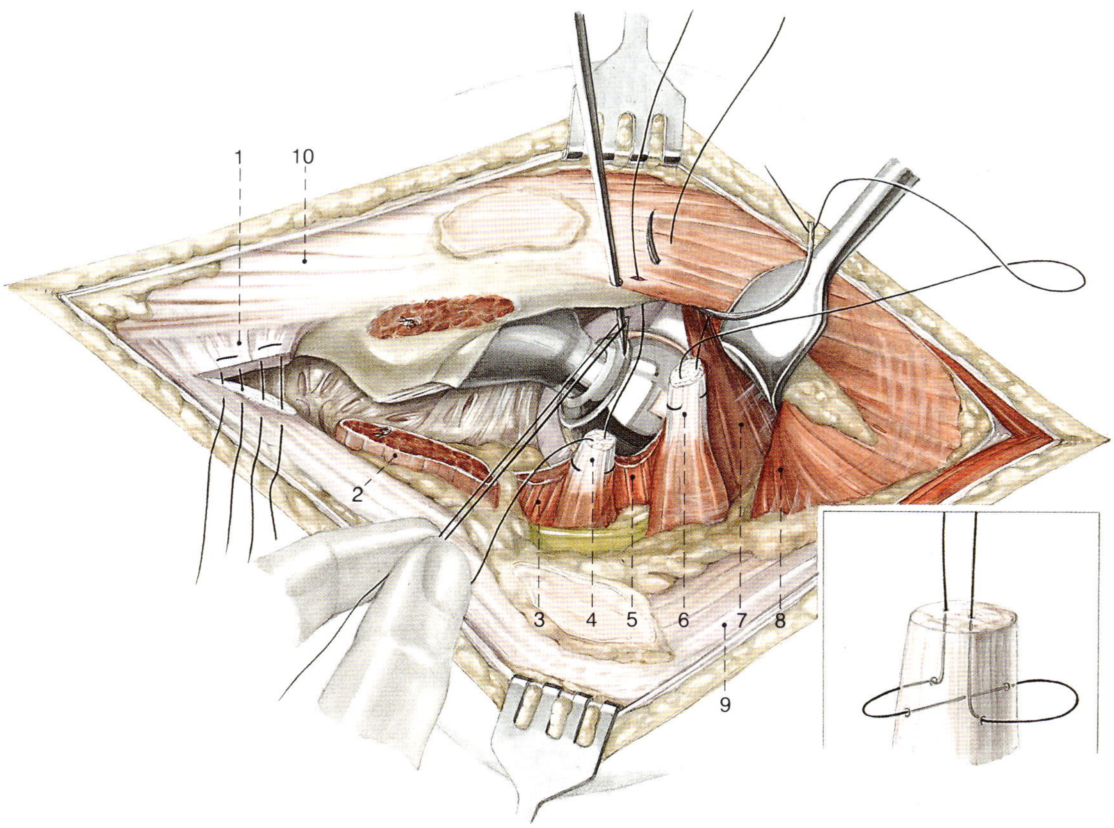

Fig. 4.**170** Soft-tissue reconstruction and closure after a posterior approach. The piriformis and obturator internus tendons are reattached to muscle or sutured to bone via drill holes. The tendon of the gluteus maximus is sutured. Insert shows technique.

1 Gluteus maximus tendon
2 Quadratus femoris
3 Inferior gemellus
4 Obturator internus tendon
5 Superior gemellus
6 Piriformis tendon
7 Gluteus minimus
8 Gluteus medius
9 Gluteus maximus
10 Vastus lateralis

To ensure that the sutures will strangle as few muscle fibers of the abductors as possible, the surgeon lifts the posterior margin of the gluteus medius with the hip in internal rotation and places a stitch from medial to distal and lateral parallel to the fibers with a large needle. The surgeon should remain as close as possible to the lateral aspect of the apex of the greater trochanter. The needle should require considerable effort to penetrate the dense tissue of the insertion so that the surgeon can be certain that the sutures will not pull out. When the tendons of both the piriformis and obturator internus are gathered, the respective pairs of sutures are tied. This is best done with the hip in neutral or external rotation. This generally pulls the gemellus muscles toward the femur because of their lateral connection to the tendons. An alternative technique is to suture the tendons to the proximal posterior greater trochanter via drill holes. The tension of the tendons must not be too great. Otherwise, an external rotation contracture might result, which could cause the tendons to ossify or tear. It is best not to reattach the tendons if proper tension cannot be achieved.

If the tendon of the gluteus maximus also requires suturing, the surgeon delays tying the sutures of the external rotators until the sutures of the gluteus maximus tendon have also been made. Depending on the length of the incision, two or three vertical mattress stitches are made in which the sutures emerge from the incised edges of the tendon so that the incised edges are not turned inward or outward. After all the sutures have been placed, the surgeon ties them with the hip in a neutral position or external rotation.

In revision total hip arthroplasty with extensive posterior scarring or ossification where parts of the external rotators were excised with the adhesions, these muscles cannot be reattached.

The surgical site is then closed in layers over subfascial and subcutaneous drains.

Transtrochanteric Approach to the Hip

After a transtrochanteric approach (see Fig. 4.**18**–4.**26**), the trochanter fragment must be refixed. This is best done with a wire suture (Müller's method; Fig. 4.**171**).

Before cementing the stem, the surgeon inserts a loop of wire (1.3–1.5 mm in diameter) though the lateral cortical bone distal to the greater trochanter. The loop of wire is bent superiorly. The ends of the wire are fed out of the femoral canal—one anteriorly, the other posteriorly. After the stem has been cemented, the wire ends are fed from medial to lateral through the insertion of the abductors immediately proximal to the trochanter fragment. Next, the surgeon pulls the trochanter fragment distally to the greater trochanter with a forceps. If the surgeon feels strong resistance after leg length has been increased or the femur laterally displaced, this will generally be due to adhesions on the inside of the abductors. While applying traction to the fragment, the surgeon palpates the tightened strands and incises them transversely until the fragment is sufficiently mobilized. The fragment is then pushed into its anatomic position on the osteotomy surface of the greater trochanter with ball-tipped awls. The wires are straightened, traction is applied, and they are bent distally around the proximal edge of the trochanter fragment. Then the surgeon feeds one of the wire ends through the loop, bends it proximally, and twists it together with the other end. A wire tightener or pliers can be used (see Fig. 4.**149 c**). The twisted ends are cut off, bent into hooks, and pressed into shallow holes drilled in the cortex. An alternative is to feed both wire ends through the loop, bend them proximally while applying strong traction, and press them into holes drilled in the cortex.

If the greater trochanter was osteotomized without a transverse incision in the vastus lateralis on the distal greater trochanter (see Fig. 4.**21**), the trochanter fragment is reattached

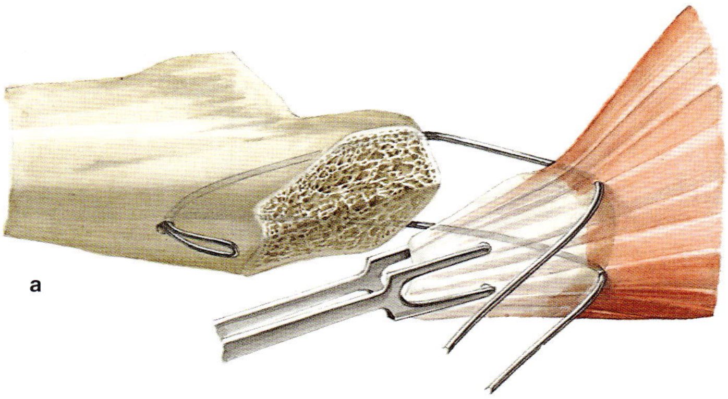

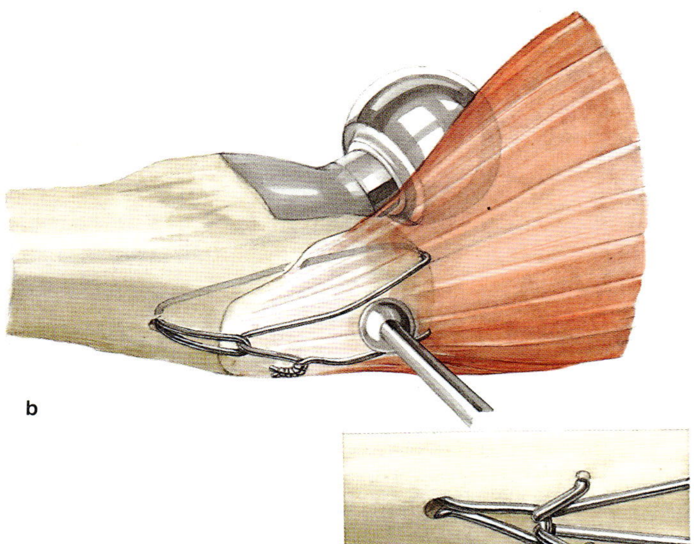

Fig. 4.**171 a** and **b** Reattaching a chevron osteotomy of the greater trochanter after a transtrochanteric approach (Müller's method).
a Wire suture.
b Reattaching the trochanter fragment. The wire ends are twisted together after one of the ends has been fed through the loop, or both are fed through the loop, bent into hooks, and pressed into shallow holes drilled in the cortex.

in the same manner. In this case, the wire loop must also be fed through the vastus lateralis.

If the external rotators were dissected, they can be reattached in the same manner as after a posterior approach. After a transtrochanteric approach it is best to reattach the tendons of the external rotators to the greater trochanter via drill holes instead of suturing them to the abductors (see Fig. 4.**170**).

Sometimes it is not possible to perform the osteotomy as steeply as planned during the approach (see Fig. 4.**20**), i.e., an osteotomy is performed at a wide angle to sagittal plane. In such a case, the locking wire suture will not function as tension band in a strict sense because the tension of the abductors does not create friction to compress the osteotomy and relieve stress on the wire. The only compression is produced by the wire itself. Additionally, a flat osteotomy of the greater trochanter often means that the only bone available for fixing the trochanter fragment is the distal, anterior, and/ or posterior cortex—without cancellous bone in the middle. The cancellous bone is often absent even after a steep osteotomy when the greater trochanter was hollowed out during previous surgery (either to implant a stem which necessitates this or for no apparent reason).

In such a case, the surgeon removes the cement from the shoulder of the revision implant before it hardens and fills the defect with cancellous graft (Fig. 4.**172**). A wedge or section of bone can be inserted to shift the insertion of the abductors laterally and increase their lever arm. Compression of the osteotomy can be increased by adding a cerclage around the proximal femur. To prevent the cerclage from slipping, it is placed proximal to the lesser trochanter, or under the collar while the implant is cemented.

Nonunion of the trochanter fragment can be treated in the same manner after preparing the surfaces of the osteotomy. Where the greater trochanter is absent or deficient after nonunion, the surgeon should not attempt to attach the trochanter fragment to the implant or cement. In this case, the abductors are mobilized as far distally as possible so that they can be sutured to the proximally mobilized tendinous tissue of the proximal vastus lateralis. If the surgeon can successfully join these muscles, then the fragment can be excised. If the results are not entirely satisfactory, the fragment should be left in place because excising it would open a posterior gap.

The surgical site is then closed in layers over drains.

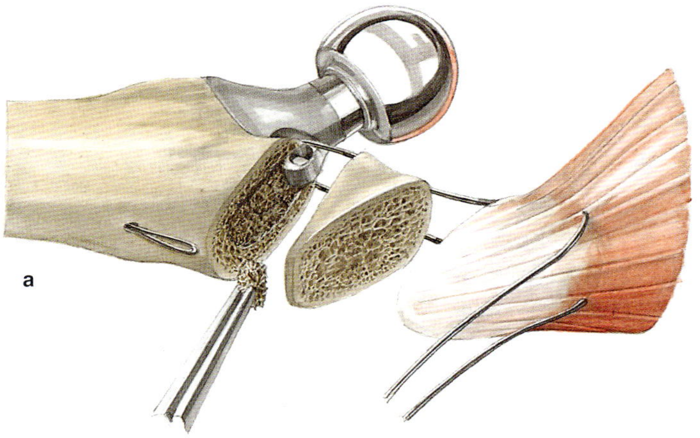

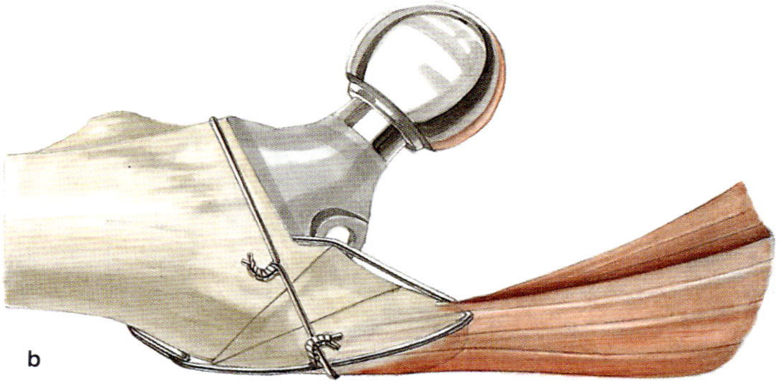

Fig. 4.**172a** and **b** Reattaching a trochanter fragment after a transtrochanteric approach in combination with grafting.

a Cancellous graft at the shoulder of the stem. Allograft from a femoral neck is implanted to shift the trochanter fragment laterally.

b Cerclage in addition to wire suture.

Transgluteal Approach to the Hip

After a transgluteal approach (see Fig. 4.**27**–4.**30**), the surgeon places two or three deep sutures proximal to the apex of the greater trochanter where tendinous septa penetrate the abductors. The anterior and posterior segments of the abductors are then joined with fascial sutures (Fig. 4.**173**). Depending on whether the vastus lateralis was split parallel to its fibers or dissected entirely from the femur (see Fig. 4.**27**), the surgeon either closes the fascia or sutures it to the intermuscular septum and the distal greater trochanter. The dissected tendons of the piriformis and the obturator internus are reattached in the same manner as in a posterior approach (see Fig. 4.**170**).

The surgical site is then closed in layers over drains.

After Distally Extended Approaches

If one of the approaches to the hip was extended distally (see Figs. 4.**31**–4.**37**), the surgeon sutures the vastus lateralis to the intermuscular septum after placing subfascial drains. The remaining fascial lip of the vastus lateralis is often too weak for this purpose. If the knee was exposed through a lateral approach, a drain is placed and the capsule and fascia are closed in a single layer. Subfascial drains are placed before the fascia lata is closed. Then the skin is sutured.

The drains should not be inserted directly through subcutaneous tissue, particularly in very slender patients. The tip is conducted diagonally out through the subcutaneous tissue for a few centimeters after crossing the fascia and then conducted out through the skin so that the channel to the joint can be closed by a valve mechanism postoperatively (Fig. 4.**173**, insert).

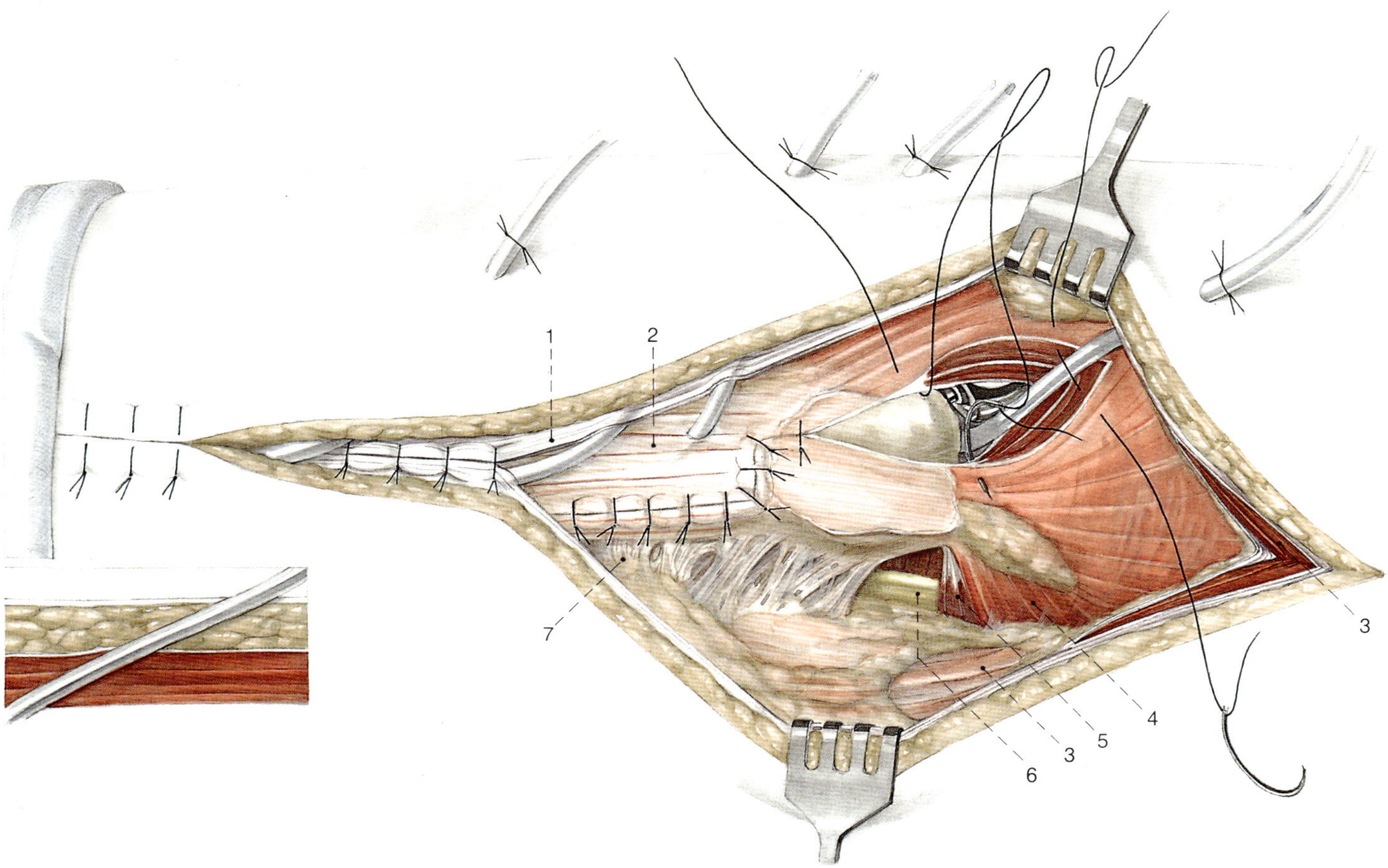

Fig. 4.**173** Soft-tissue reconstruction and closure after a transgluteal approach that has been extended distally. The fascia of the gluteus medius is sutured. Deep suture at the proximal aspect of the greater trochanter. Vastus and gluteal tendinous tissue is sutured over the greater trochanter. The fascia of the vastus lateralis is closed. Skin suture. The drains should penetrate the subcutaneous fat diagonally, not directly (insert).

1 Fascia lata
2 Vastus lateralis
3 Gluteus maximus
4 Gluteus medius
5 Piriformis
6 Sciatic nerve
7 Gluteus maximus tendon

Postoperative Management

Postoperative Surgical Management

The drains are removed on postoperative day two, and sutures between postoperative days 12 and 14. If a hematoma or diffuse swelling has increased skin tension and the sutures are free of irritation, then the surgeon removes first only some of the sutures or leaves all of them in place longer.

Subcutaneous administration of heparin as anticoagulant therapy is continued until the patient is out of bed for 2 to 3 hours every day. Conversion to coumarin anticoagulants is indicated in patients requiring longer immobilization or with increased risk of deep venous thrombosis. Treating all patients with anti-inflammatory agents for a few days is recommended as heterotopic ossification prophylaxis. Therapy should be continued for 4 weeks postoperatively in high-risk patients unless contraindicated.

Dislocation, hematoma, impairments to wound healing, or periprosthetic infection may be indications for surgery in the early postoperative period.

Dislocation

Hip dislocations generally occur early in the postoperative period, rarely late, and primarily in the direction of muscles weakened during the surgical approach. After a posterior approach, most dislocations are posterosuperior; after a transtrochanteric approach posterosuperior or anterosuperior; after a transgluteal approach, the direction is generally anterosuperior. The risk of dislocation increases where reattachment of the external rotators was not possible, the sutures did not hold, or the tendons of the external rotators were excised with adhesions and ossification; risk of dislocation is also increased if fixation of a trochanter fragment fails, and when the tendinous soft tissue becomes detached from the anterior greater trochanter after a transgluteal approach. Stability is further endangered when the function of other hip muscles is compromised because they have been destroyed or have lost their insertions on the proximal femur.

Aside from muscular insufficiency, the implant itself can cause dislocation. The acetabular component may have been implanted too steeply and with improper anteversion so that it does not engage the femoral head sufficiently. If the leg was shortened, tension in the entire soft-tissue may be insufficient. If the anteversion of the femoral head is too great, the greater trochanter can impinge the acetabular component in external rotation. This forces the head anteriorly. If the femoral neck is retroverted, the anterior soft-tissue and pelvic bone can force the head posteriorly out of the acetabular component in internal rotation. Medial displacement of the femur due to an implant with a large neck–shaft angle can cause the implant to impinge the pelvis in rotation so that it acts as an anterior or posterior fulcrum. In obese patients, the effect of this medial displacement is enhanced by increased compressive forces in the soft tissue. Medial displacement also changes the direction of the resultant force in the hip (similarly to a valgus osteotomy). The resultant force is now steeper due to the steeper angle of the force of the abductors and intersects the acetabulum farther lateral.

When dislocation occurs, it is reduced using fluoroscopy, either immediately after intervenous administration of a sedative or general anesthesia is performed. General anesthesia is preferable to regional anesthesia; greater relaxation is achieved, and its duration is temporary. This also avoids requiring the patient to sit or lie in a lateral position in pain while the local anesthesia is administered.

Open reduction is indicated if the joint repeatedly dislocates. The procedure depends on the reason for dislocation; often several are combined. These procedures include:

- Excising the membrane that forms in the dislocation cavity after repeated dislocation and prevents proper healing.
- Correcting malalignment of the acetabular component either by replacing the component or—in palliative cases—by attaching a polyethylene spacer to raise the rim of the acetabular component where coverage is insufficient (Fig. 4.**174**).
- Correcting reduced leg length either with a longer femoral head (with a custom model if necessary) or, if that fails, replacing the stem and implanting a revision stem further proximally in the femur.
- Correcting excessive anteversion or retroversion of the femoral neck.
- Correcting medial displacement by replacing the stem with one with a smaller neck–shaft angle.
- Reattaching the external rotators after a posterior approach, trochanter fragment after a transtrochanteric approach, or the anterior vastus and gluteal tendinous soft tissue after a transgluteal approach, if reattachment of the respective structures has failed.
- Distally displacing the insertions of the abductors by a trochanteric osteotomy.
- Moving the tendon of the gluteus maximus or the psoas to the greater trochanter, depending on whether internal rotation or external rotation is desired.
- Suturing the walls of a dislocation cavity.
- Doubling the fascia lata.

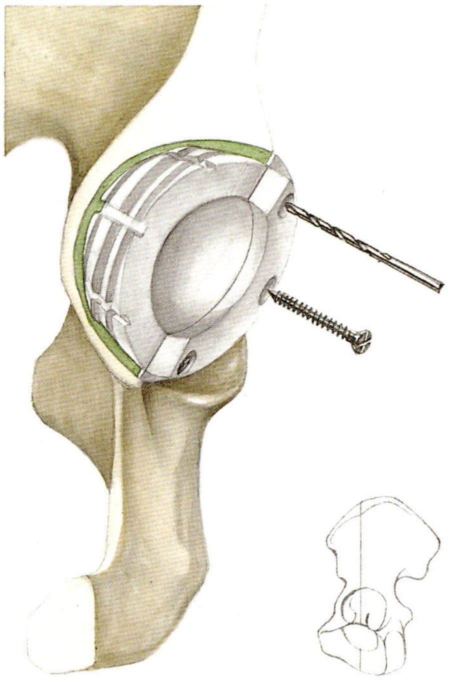

Fig. 4.**174** Attaching a polyethylene spacer to raise the rim of the acetabular component after repeated dislocation.

In rare cases of repeated dislocation where none of these procedures help, the surgeon may consider implanting a saddle prosthesis. To dislocate by "unhooking", the saddle must travel a distance equal to the depth of the saddle. This distance is greater than the distance required to dislocate a ball-and-socket joint (see Fig. 4.**138**). The saddle should be used only as a last resort however.

Following closed or open reduction, the patient should be immobilized according to the intraoperative assessment of the risk of recurrence.

Hematoma

A hematoma interferes with wound healing, bacterial contamination spreads more readily in a hematoma than in a joint without one, and an infected hematoma is an important vehicle for periprosthetic infection. For these reasons, hematomas are aspirated under sterile conditions in the operating room. Revision surgery is indicated when no fluid is obtained by aspirating the joint and there is a chance that the hematoma may discharge spontaneously.

A sterile hematoma that discharges before or after sutures are removed is an emergency—even if the opening is very small. In contrast to soft-tissue surgery, the surgeon must not wait and hope for the opening to close spontaneously because subcutaneous tissue will rapidly become contaminated. Bacterial migration to the subfascial region will soon occur. Immediate surgical intervention is indicated. General anesthesia is administered, all skin sutures are removed (if they are still in place), and a wedge-shaped skin incision is made the length of the entire wound down to the fascia. The incision should include the stitches. If a fascial gap is present and/or a subfascial source of bleeding is suspected, all fascial sutures are removed as well. The joint area is cleaned of all coagulants, aggressive lavage is performed, subcutaneous and subfascial hemostasis is obtained, and the joint area is drained. The fascia is then closed with absorbable sutures, the subcutaneous area is drained, and the wound is closed. Several days of immobilization and antibiotic therapy are recommended.

Microbiological examination of the subcutaneous and/or subfascial sample is always indicated. If initial microscopic examination reveals bacteria or there is macroscopic evidence of infection, an irrigation drainage must be placed.

Bleeding through the drains for a few days postoperatively is harmless. Danger of contamination is minimal via the canal of the drain in the subcutaneous tissue if the drain was conducted diagonally through the subcutaneous tissue for a few centimeters after crossing the fascia, and does not enter it directly through a thin layer of tissue (see Fig. 4.**173**, insert).

Disturbed Wound Healing and Periprosthetic Infection

Superficial disturbed wound healing generally occurs in the stitches or in areas where the lips of the skin incision are overlapped due to poor technique, particularly when the patient lies on the proximal end of a skin incision that has been extended too far posteriorly. Early surgical intervention is also indicated here. Where disturbed healing is localized, the surgeon may remove one or two sutures and wait a maximum of 24 hours. Intervention is indicated if the findings do not improve markedly because, like hematoma, disturbed wound healing is a major factor in periprosthetic infection.

As in removing a hematoma, the surgeon excises the skin and subcutaneous tissue the length of the entire wound down to the fascia. The incision should include the stitches. Often the skin can be closed primarily. Open treatment is recommended where local tissue swelling prevents healing. Here too, several days of immobilization and antibiotic therapy are recommended.

If a fascial gap is found during the procedure or preoperative aspiration reveals evidence of subfascial infection, an irrigation drainage must be considered. This can have a curing effect in the very early stages of a periprosthetic infection after primary replacement if treatment includes thorough cleaning of the joint and debridement. But removal of all implant material and radical excision of all infected soft tissue is necessary if periprosthetic infection becomes evident some weeks after primary replacement, and after revision arthroplasty in any case. Then, the author recommends immediate reimplantation of a new implant using specific antibiotic-loaded acrylic cement in a one-stage exchange operation (Buchholz' and Lodenkämper's method).

Physical Therapy

Dislocation Prophylaxis

Postoperatively, the patient is only allowed to lie supine. For the first week or two, the patient is fitted with an abduction pillow between the legs (Fig. 4.**175a**). As soon as the wound has healed sufficiently, the patient is permitted to lie and sleeps in a lateral position (initially only on the operated side). Lying or sleeping on the contralateral side should be allowed only later (after 4 weeks at the earliest), depending on the intraoperative assessment of dislocation risk, patient discipline, and muscle quality; a pillow should then be placed between the legs initially. If the patient lies on the contralateral side without a pillow between the legs, the operated leg may fall into adduction and internal rotation, which could dislocate the hip. The patient's night table should always be on the operated side so that bending over the night table will not place the hip in adduction.

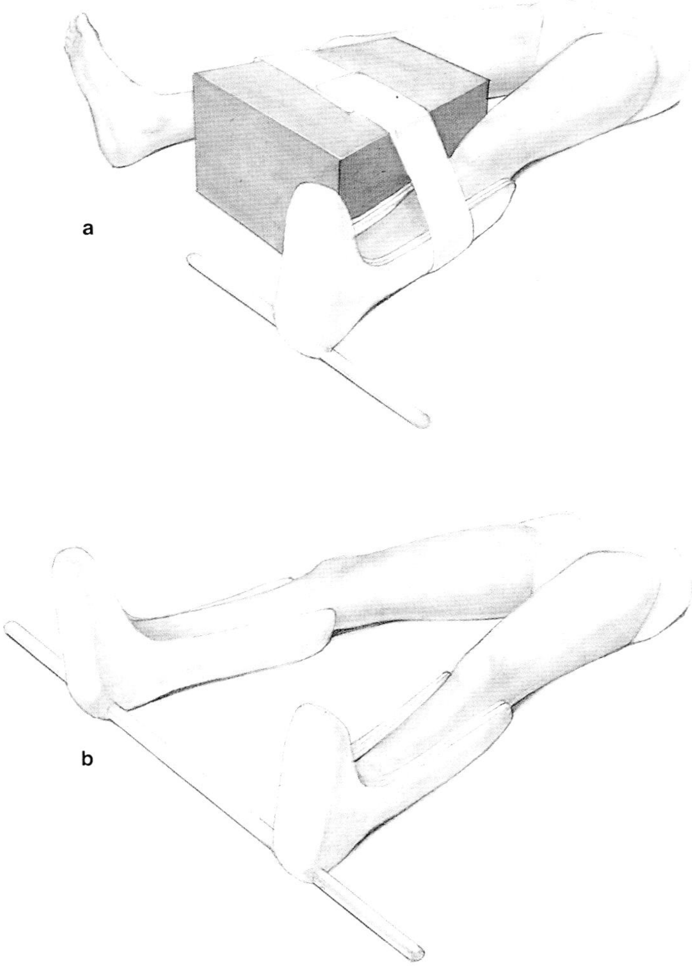

Fig. 4.**175a** and **b** Immobilization for dislocation prophylaxis.
a Abduction pillow. Short leg cast with transverse bar to prevent rotation (or place leg in a defined rotation).
b Abduction cast.

Additional measures are required where intraoperative assessment reveals significantly increased risk of dislocation, or where open or closed reduction of a dislocation has been performed. A long, well-padded, anteriorly open lower-leg cast with a transverse bar (Fig. 4.**175a**) is recommended for this purpose. The bar may be used to place the leg in the desired rotation. The "shoe" can be used to limit the patient's movements at night for a long time, even after initial mobilization. This promotes soft-tissue healing in the desired rotation. If greater immobilization is required, abduction cast in the form of two anteriorly open lower-leg casts connected with a transverse bar may be used (Fig. 4.**175b**). Where a high risk of dislocation exists, but the patient must be mobilized, the patient can be fitted with an abduction cast (or other appropriate orthopedic aid) extending to the knee of the operated leg.

Motion and Strength Exercises

In the absence of special considerations that indicate delayed mobilization, the patient begins exercises to improve motion and strengthen the hip on the second postoperative day. For 2 weeks, the patient only performs exercises supine; later, exercises in a prone and lateral position are added. After the sutures have been removed and the wound has healed, pool therapy is included (34 °C). All exercises avoid movements that entail a high risk of dislocation, i.e., adduction and external or internal rotation depending on the surgical approach used. The therapist should conduct the exercises patiently and should not tax the patient's tolerance. Strenuous exercise is counterproductive and leads to irritation and muscle tension. Particularly in patients where there is a probability of heterotopic ossification, exercises should not challenge the patient's tolerance.

Gait Training

Normally, the patient begins walking on postoperative day three. Initially, the patient uses a walker. Forearm crutches are added after sufficient confidence has been gained, and later, two canes are used for a period of several weeks. Three-point crutch walking permits partial weight bearing; four-point alternating crutch walking does not. A postoperative leg-length difference in is compensated for before gait training is begun.

When the patient should progress to the next respective walking aid depends on the individual, but the therapist should ensure that the patient always uses two walking aids. Walking with only one forearm crutch or cane causes the patient to assume an unbalanced posture.

Recommended activities for subsequent training include swimming, bicycle riding, or hiking with resilient shoes; sports involving sudden jarring stresses (tennis or jogging) or which involve risk of fracture (downhill skiing or horseback riding) are not advised. Like primary total hip arthroplasty, revision arthroplasty is not intended to restore the patient's ability to participate in sports.

Partial Weight Bearing

Cemented total hip implants permit immediate full weight bearing. Postoperative partial weight bearing is indicated after soft-tissue reconstruction or bone reconstruction with limited primary stability.

The surgeon must assess the extent and duration of weight bearing limitations. Detailed schedules (such as 8 weeks at 20 kg, followed by 4 weeks gradually increasing to full weight bearing) are standard procedure. Despite this, the surgeon should bear in mind that certain daily activities (bowel movement in bed, getting out of the bed, etc.) can place loads on the joint far in excess of body weight in spite of aid and conscious reliance on the unoperated leg. Unforeseen movements (such as stumbling) can result in stresses that are several times body weight. In the light of these considerations, partial weight bearing programs have serious limitations. Nevertheless, they are valuable in helping to discipline overactive patients, and they aid in teaching patients to walk consciously and carefully.

References

Bauer R, Kerschbaumer F, Poisel S, Oberthaler W. The transgluteal approach to the hip joint. Arch Orthop Traumat Surg. 1979; 95:47.

Bormann B, Schleinzer W. Autologe Bluttransfusion bzw. Eigenblutspende. Chir Gastroenterol. 1992; 8:2.

Buchholz HW. 1969. Das künstliche Hüftgelenk. Mat Med Nordmark. 1969; 21:613.

Buchholz HW, Engelbrecht E, Lodenkämper H, Röttger J, Siegel A, Elson RA. Management of deep infection of total hip replacement. Bone Jt Surg. 1981; 63B:342.

Caillouette JT, Gorab RS, Klapper RC, Anzel SH. Revision arthroplasty facilitated by ultrasonic tool cement removal. Orthop Review. 1991; 20:353,435.

Collis D, Dubrul W. The removal of fractured prosthetic components from medullary cavities: a new technique. Contemp Orthop. 1984; 8:61.

Endo-Klinik, eds. 1987. Primär- und Revisionsalloarthroplastik Hüft- und Kniegelenk. 10 Jahre Endo-Klinik Hamburg. Springer, Berlin 1987

Engelbrecht E, Engelbrecht H. Totalersatz des Femurs unter Verwendung der Hüft- und Kniegelenkstotalendoprothesen Modell "St. Georg." Chirurg. 1974; 45:231.

Foerster G. v. Wechsel von zementfreien Prothesen zu zementierten Endoprothesen. In: Stuhler T, ed. Hüftkopfnekrose Symposium, Nürnberg. Berlin: Springer 1990: 639.

Gie GA, Linder L, Ling RSM, Simon J-P, Slooff TJJH, Timperley AJ. Impacted cancellous allografts and cement for revision total hip arthroplasty. J Bone Jt Surg. 1993; 75-B:14.

Harris WH, White RE, Mitchel S, Barber F. A new technique for removal of broken femoral stems in total hip replacement. J Bone Jt Surg. 1981; 63:843.

Keller A. Spezialanfertigungen für den prothetischen Knochen- und Gelenkersatz. In: Endo-Klinik, ed. Primär- und Revisionsalloarthroplastik Hüft- und Kniegelenk. 10 Jahre Endo-Klinik. Springer: Hamburg, 1987: 293.

Ling RSM, Linder L, Timperley AJ. Histological findings in a case of cemented femoral revision treated by endosteal impaction grafting. Acta orthop scand. 1992; 63, Suppl. 248:29.

Mehrkens HH, Geiger P, Schleinzer W, Weindler M, Wollinsky KH, Pohland H. Vier Jahre Erfahrung mit dem autologen Transfusionskonzept Ulm (ATU). Infusionsther. 1990; 17, Suppl. 2:28.

Müller ME. Lessons of 30 years of total hip arthroplasty. Clin Orthop. 1992; 274:12.

Nieder E, Engelbrecht E. Die Sattelprothese, eine Alternative in Grenzsituationen des alloplastischen Hüftgelenkersatzes. In: Wolter D, ed. Osteolysen—pathologische Frakturen. 1. Paul-Sudeck-Symposium in Hamburg. Stuttgart: Thieme; 1982: 324.

Nieder E, Friesecke C. Mid-term results of 73 saddle prostheses, Endo-Model, at total hip revision arthroplasty. In: Limb salvage—Current trends. Proceedings 7th International Symposium on Limb Salvage. Singapore, 23–27 August 1993: 313.

Nieder E, Engelbrecht E, Röder U, Strickle E. Möglichkeiten der Anwendung von Ultraschallwerkzeug bei Endoprothesenwechsel. Chirurg. 1979; 50:257.

Nieder E, Engelbrecht E, Steinbrink K, Elson RA, Kasselt MR, Keller A. The saddle prosthesis for salvage of destroyed acetabulum. J Bone Jt Surg. 1990; 72-B:1014.

Nieder E, Engelbrecht E, Steinbrink K, Keller A. Modulares System für den Femurtotalersatz—Endo-Modell. Chirurg. 1983; 54:391.

Nieder E, Steinbrink K, Engelbrecht E, Siegel A. Verletzung von Beckengefäßen bei totalem Hüftgelenkersatz. Chirurg. 1979; 50:780.

Otto KB, Baars GW, Nieder E. Beckenknochendefekte in der Alloarthroplastik. Orthopäde. 1987; 16:261.

Otto KB, Baars GW, Nieder E. Alloarthroplastische Therapie der kongenitalen Hüftgelenkdysplasie. Orthopäde. 1989; 18:470.

Schleinzer W, Mehrkens H-H, Weindler M, Wollinsky K, Pohland H. Klinisches Konzept der autologen Transfusion: Hämodilution, maschinelle Autotransfusion, Plasmapherese, Eigenblutspende. Anästh Intensivmed. 1987; 28:235.

Schleinzer W, Singbartl G. 1991. Fremdblutsparende Maßnahmen in der operativen Medizin. CAT Symposium. Hamburg, 18.–19. Jan. 1991. Basel. Karger, 1993 (Beiträge zw Infusionstherapie, Vol. 29).

Sloof TJJH, Huiskes R, van Hom J, Lemmens AJ. Bone grafting in total hip replacement for acetabular protrusion. Acta orthop scand. 1984; 55:593.

Steinbrink K. 1987. Vorgehen bei ausgedehntem und völligem Knochensubstanzverlust des Femurs nach Schaftlockerung. Orthopäde. 1987; 16:277.

Steinbrink K. Total femoral prosthesis: 18 years experience in 147 cases. In: Limb salvage—Current trends. Proceedings 7th International Symposium on Limb Salvage. Singapore, 23–27 August 1993: 411.

Steinbrink K, Engelbrecht E, Fenelon GCC. The total femoral prosthesis: a preliminary report. J Bone Jt Surg. 1982; 64B:305.

Stühmer G, Weber BG, Mathys R. New set of instruments for the removal of implant and bone cement in the replacement of hip prostheses. In: Gschwend N, Debrunner HU, eds. Total Hip Prosthesis. Bern: Huber; 1976.

Wagner H. Revisionsprothese für das Hüftgelenk. Orthopäde. 1989; 18:438.

Wroblewski BM. A method of management of the fractured stem in total hip replacement. Clin Orthop. 1979; 141:71.

Zabel A, Nieder E. Auschlaginstrumentarium für gebrochene Hüftendoprothesen 53. Jahrestagung Deutsche Gesellschaft für Unfallheilkunde. 22–25 11 1989. Berlin (presentation).

Index